FENICHEL'S
Clinical Pediatric
Neurology

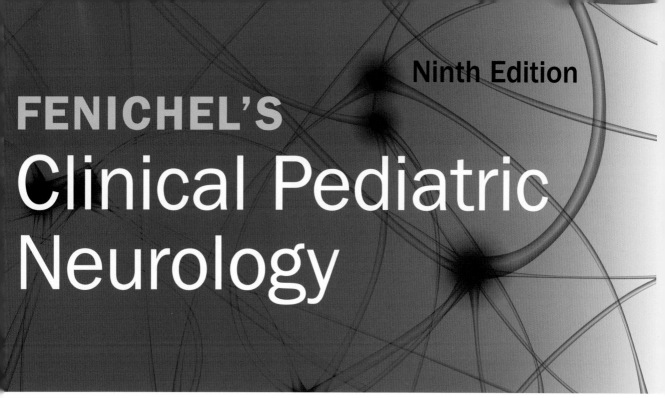

Ninth Edition

FENICHEL'S
Clinical Pediatric
Neurology

KAITLIN C. JAMES, MD

Assistant Professor of Pediatrics, Pediatric
Neurology
Vanderbilt Children's Hospital
Nashville, Tennessee

JESUS ERIC PIÑA-GARZA, MD

Professor of Neurology
Director, Pediatric Epilepsy
TriStar Children's Hospital at Centennial
Medical Center
Department of Neurology
TriStar Medical Group Children's Specialists
Nashville, Tennessee

ELSEVIER

Elsevier
1600 John F. Kennedy Blvd.
Ste 1800
Philadelphia, PA 19103-2899

FENICHEL'S CLINICAL PEDIATRIC NEUROLOGY, NINTH EDITION   ISBN: 978-0-323-93201-1

Notice

Practitioners and researchers must always rely on their own experience and knowledge in evaluating and using any information, methods, compounds or experiments described herein. Because of rapid advances in the medical sciences, in particular, independent verification of diagnoses and drug dosages should be made. To the fullest extent of the law, no responsibility is assumed by Elsevier, authors, editors or contributors for any injury and/or damage to persons or property as a matter of products liability, negligence or otherwise, or from any use or operation of any methods, products, instructions, or ideas contained in the material herein.

Previous editions copyrighted 2019, 2013, 2009, 2005, 2001, 1997 and 1993.

Content Strategists: Mary Hegeler, Melanie Tucker
Senior Content Development Specialists: Priyadarshini Pandey, Vasowati Shome
Content Development Manager: Somodatta Roy Choudhury
Publishing Services Manager: Shereen Jameel
Project Manager: Haritha Dharmarajan
Design Direction: Brian Salisbury

Printed in India

Last digit is the print number: 9   8   7   6   5   4   3   2   1

For our children

Kaitlin C. James
Jesus Eric Piña-Garza

PREFACE

The ninth edition of *Fenichel's Clinical Pediatric Neurology* presented us with unique challenges. We realized that the book needed significant updates; medical literature moves at lightning speed, and thousands of pertinent articles have been published since the eighth edition was released. The reader will find we covered some topics in more depth than others. Such decisions were made based on what we considered most helpful not just for the resident physician or non-neurologist but also for practicing pediatric neurologists who seek a quick update on their clinical knowledge. Our goal was to create a textbook that is practical, thorough, and not drowning in minutiae. In other words, we want the book to be *useful*. It needs to be complete enough to provide the reader with a well-rounded understanding of the subject while also not being *so* complete that your legs go numb when you hold it on your lap. We hope we have succeeded.

Kaitlin C. James, MD
Jesus Eric Piña-Garza, MD

ACKNOWLEDGMENTS

We wish first to acknowledge our mentor, Dr. Gerald Fenichel, who is quite rightly considered one of the pillars in the field of pediatric neurology. We offer our sincerest thanks to all the medical students and residents whom we have had the pleasure to teach over the years. And last but certainly not least, we wish to express our enormous gratitude to our patients and their families, whose strength, courage, and kindness cannot be overstated.

CONTENTS

1   Paroxysmal Disorders, 1

2   Altered States of Consciousness, 61

3   Headache, 95

4   Increased Intracranial Pressure, 113

5   Psychomotor Delay and Regression, 141

6   The Hypotonic Infant, 183

7   Flaccid Limb Weakness in Childhood, 208

8   Cramps, Muscle Stiffness, and Exercise Intolerance, 236

9   Sensory and Autonomic Disturbances, 249

10 Ataxia, 258

11 Hemiplegia, 281

12 Paraplegia and Quadriplegia, 299

13 Monoplegia, 317

14 Movement Disorders, 325

15 Disorders of Ocular Motility, 348

16 Disorders of the Visual System, 367

17 Lower Brainstem and Cranial Nerve Dysfunction, 381

18 Disorders of Cranial Volume and Shape, 403

19 Behavioral Neurology, 423

Index, 437

Paroxysmal Disorders

OUTLINE

Approach To Paroxysmal Disorders, 1
Paroxysmal Neurological Disorders of
    Newborns, 2
    Seizure Patterns, 2
    Seizure-Like Events, 4
Seizures in the Newborn, 5
    Differential Diagnosis of Seizures, 5
    Seizures due to Metabolic Derangements, 8
    Hypoxic-Ischemic Encephalopathy, 9
    Organic Acid Disorders and Aminoacidopathies, 10
    Treatment of Neonatal Seizures, 16
Paroxysmal Disorders in Children Less Than 2 Years
    Old, 18
    Apnea and Syncope, 18
    Normal Self-Stimulatory Behavior, 19
    Hereditary Hyperekplexia, 20
    Febrile Seizures, 20
Epilepsies Exacerbated By Fever, 21
    SCN1A-Related Disorders, 21
    Dravet Syndrome, 22
    Genetic Epilepsy With Febrile Seizures
        Plus, 22

    Nonfebrile Seizures in Children Under the Age
        of 2 Years, 22
    Migraine, 26
Paroxysmal Neurological Disorders of
Childhood, 26
    Paroxysmal Dyskinesias, 26
    Sleep Disorders, 27
    Hyperventilation Syndrome, 29
    Syncope, 29
    Staring Spells, 30
    Eyelid Myoclonia With or Without Absences
        (Jeavons Syndrome), 31
    Myoclonic Seizures, 33
    Focal Seizures, 36
    Generalized Seizures, 41
Managing Seizures, 43
    Antiepileptic Drug Therapy, 43
    Management of Status Epilepticus, 51
    The Ketogenic Diet, 54
    Vagal Nerve Stimulation, 55
    Surgical Approaches to Childhood Epilepsy, 55
References, 56

Paroxysmal neurological disorders (PNDs) are characterized by the sudden onset of neurological symptoms and stereotyped recurrence. In children, such events often clear completely. Examples of paroxysmal disorders include epilepsy, migraine, periodic paralysis, and paroxysmal movement disorders.

APPROACH TO PAROXYSMAL DISORDERS

The diagnosing physician rarely witnesses the paroxysmal event. It is important to obtain the description of the event from the observer or a video recording and not secondhand, as information easily becomes distorted if transferred from the observer to the parent and then to you. Most "spells" are not seizures, and epilepsy is not a diagnosis of exclusion. Physicians often misdiagnose syncope as a seizure, as many people stiffen and tremble at the end of a faint. The critical distinction is that syncope is associated with pallor and preceded by dimming of vision, and a feeling of lightheadedness or clamminess, whereas seizures are rarely preceded by these things. Also, the patient with syncope has a fast recovery of consciousness and coherence if allowed to remain supine postictal.

Spells seldom remain unexplained when viewed. Because observation of the spell is critical to diagnosis, ask the family to record the spell. Most families either own or can borrow a camera or a cell phone with video capability. Always ask the following two questions: Has this happened before? Does anyone else in the family have similar episodes? Often, no one offers this important information until requested. Episodic symptoms that last only seconds and cause no abnormal signs usually remain unexplained and often do not warrant diagnostic testing. The differential diagnosis of paroxysmal disorders is somewhat different in the neonate, infant, child, and adolescent, and is therefore presented best by age groups.

PAROXYSMAL NEUROLOGICAL DISORDERS OF NEWBORNS

Seizures are the main paroxysmal disorder of the newborn, occurring in 1.8%–3.5% of live births in the United States, and an important feature of neurological disease.[1] Uncontrolled seizures may contribute to further brain damage. Brain glucose decreases during prolonged seizures and excitatory amino acid release interferes with DNA synthesis. Therefore seizures identified by electroencephalography (EEG) that occur without movement in newborns are important to identify and treat. The challenge for the clinician is to differentiate seizure activity from normal neonatal movements and pathological movements caused by other mechanisms (Box 1.1).

The long-term prognosis in children with neonatal seizures is better in term newborns than in premature newborns.[2] However, the etiology of the seizures is the primary determinant of prognosis.

Seizure Patterns

Seizures in newborns, especially in the premature, are poorly organized and difficult to distinguish from normal activity. The absence of myelinated pathways for seizure propagation may confine seizures originating in one hemisphere and make them less likely to spread beyond the contiguous cortex or to produce secondary bilateral synchrony.

Box 1.2 lists clinical patterns that have been associated with epileptiform discharges in newborns. This classification is useful but does not do justice to the rich variety of patterns actually observed, nor does the classification account for the 50% of prolonged epileptiform discharges on the EEG without visible clinical changes. Generalized tonic-clonic seizures rarely occur. Many newborns suspected of having generalized tonic-clonic seizures are actually *jittery* (see Jitteriness section). Newborns paralyzed to assist mechanical ventilation pose an additional problem in seizure identification. In this circumstance, the presence of rhythmic increases in systolic arterial blood pressure, heart rate, and oxygenation desaturation should alert physicians to the possibility of seizures.

The term *subtle seizures* encompasses several different patterns in which tonic or clonic movements of the limbs are lacking, for example, tonic deviation of the eyes. One of the most common manifestations of seizures in young infants is behavioral arrest and unresponsiveness. The behavioral arrest is only obvious when the child is very active, which is not common in a sick neonate and therefore often goes unnoticed.

The definitive diagnosis of neonatal seizures often requires EEG monitoring. A split-screen 16-channel video EEG is the ideal means for monitoring. An amplitude-integrated EEG is also a useful monitoring

---

BOX 1.1   Movements That Resemble Neonatal Seizures
• Benign nocturnal myoclonus[a]
• Jitteriness[a]
• Nonconvulsive apnea
• Normal movement
• Opisthotonos
• Pathological myoclonus

[a]The most common conditions and the ones with disease-modifying treatments.

BOX 1.2   Seizure Patterns in Newborns
• Apnea with tonic stiffening of the body
• Focal clonic movements of one limb or both limbs on one side[a]
• Multifocal clonic limb movements[a]
• Myoclonic jerking
• Paroxysmal laughing
• Tonic deviation of the eyes upward or to one side[a]
• Tonic stiffening of the body

[a]The most common conditions and the ones with disease-modifying treatments.

technique. Seizures in the newborn may be widespread and electrographically detectable even when the newborn is not convulsing clinically.

Focal Clonic Seizures

Clinical features. Repeated, irregular slow clonic movements (1–3 jerks/second) affecting one limb or both limbs on one side are characteristic of focal clonic seizures. Rarely do such movements sustain for long periods, and they do not "march" as though spreading along the motor cortex. In an otherwise alert and responsive full-term newborn, unifocal clonic seizures always indicate a cerebral infarction or hemorrhage, or focal brain dysgenesis. In newborns with states of decreased consciousness, focal clonic seizures may indicate a focal infarction superimposed on a generalized encephalopathy.

Diagnosis. During the seizure, the EEG may show a unilateral focus of high-amplitude sharp waves adjacent to the central fissure. The discharge can spread to involve contiguous areas in the same hemisphere and can be associated with unilateral seizures of the limbs and adverse movements of the head and eyes. The interictal EEG may show focal slowing, sharp waves, or amplitude attenuation.

Newborns with focal clonic seizures should be immediately evaluated using head ultrasound and/or magnetic resonance imaging (MRI) with diffusion-weighted images. Head ultrasound is easily and quickly performed at the bedside of sick neonates, which in practice makes it the preferred initial imaging choice. MRI is necessary to fully evaluate abnormal findings on the head ultrasound. Bedside computed tomography (CT) or ultrasound is acceptable for less stable neonates unable to make the trip to the MRI suite or tolerate the time needed for this procedure.

Multifocal Clonic Seizures

Clinical features. In multifocal clonic seizures, migratory jerking movements are noted in first one limb and then another. Facial muscles may be involved as well. The migration appears random and does not follow expected patterns of epileptic spread. Sometimes prolonged movements occur in one limb suggesting a focal rather than a multifocal seizure. Detection of the multifocal nature comes later, when nursing notes appear contradictory concerning the side or the limb affected or the video demonstrates independent abnormal movements of the extremities. Multifocal clonic seizures are ordinarily associated with severe, generalized cerebral disturbances such as hypoxic-ischemic encephalopathy (HIE), but may also represent benign neonatal convulsions when noted in an otherwise healthy neonate.

Diagnosis. Standard EEG usually detects multifocal epileptiform activity. Twenty-four-hour video-EEG monitoring is the best diagnostic test to confirm diagnosis.

Myoclonic Seizures

Clinical features. Brief, nonrhythmic extension and flexion movements of the arms, the legs, or all limbs characterize myoclonic seizures. They constitute an uncommon seizure pattern in the newborn, but their presence suggests severe, diffuse brain damage.

Diagnosis. No specific EEG pattern is associated with myoclonic seizures in the newborn. Myoclonic jerks often occur in babies born to drug-addicted mothers. Whether these movements are seizures, jitteriness, or myoclonus (discussed later) is uncertain. Myoclonus noticed in an otherwise normal newborn may be a normal involuntary motion, such as benign myoclonus of drowsiness or sleep.

Tonic Seizures

Clinical features. The characteristic features of tonic seizures are extension and stiffening of the body, usually associated with apnea and upward deviation of the eyes. Tonic posturing without the other features is rarely a seizure manifestation.

Diagnosis. Tonic seizures in premature newborns are often a symptom of intraventricular hemorrhage and an indication for ultrasound study. Tonic posturing also occurs in newborns with forebrain damage, not as a seizure manifestation, but as a disinhibition of brainstem reflexes. Prolonged disinhibition results in *decerebrate posturing*, an extension of the body and limbs associated with internal rotation of the arms, dilation of the pupils, and downward deviation of the eyes. Decerebrate posturing is often a terminal sign in premature infants with intraventricular hemorrhage caused by pressure on the upper brainstem (see Chapter 4).

Tonic seizures and decerebrate posturing look similar to *opisthotonos*, a prolonged arching of the back not necessarily associated with eye movements. The cause of opisthotonos is probably meningeal irritation. It occurs in kernicterus, infantile Gaucher disease, and some aminoacidurias.

Seizure-Like Events

Apnea

Clinical features. An irregular respiratory pattern with intermittent pauses of 3–6 seconds, often followed by 10–15 seconds of hyperpnea, is a common occurrence in premature infants. The pauses are not associated with significant alterations in heart rate, blood pressure, body temperature, or skin color. Immaturity of the brainstem respiratory centers causes this respiratory pattern, termed *periodic breathing*. The incidence of periodic breathing correlates directly with the degree of prematurity. Apneic spells are more common during active than quiet sleep.

Apneic spells of 10–15 seconds are detectable at some time in almost all premature and some full-term newborns. Apneic spells of 10–20 seconds are usually associated with a 20% reduction in heart rate. Longer episodes of apnea are almost invariably associated with a 40% or greater reduction in heart rate. The frequency of these apneic spells correlates with brainstem myelination. Even at 40 weeks conceptional age, premature newborns continue to have a higher incidence of apnea than do full-term newborns. The incidence of apnea sharply decreases in all infants at 52 weeks conceptional age. Apnea with bradycardia is unlikely to be a seizure. Apnea with tachycardia raises the possibility of seizure and should be evaluated with simultaneous video EEG recording.

Diagnosis. Apneic spells in an otherwise normal-appearing newborn are typically a sign of brainstem immaturity and not a pathological condition. The sudden onset of apnea and states of decreased consciousness, especially in premature newborns, suggests an intracranial hemorrhage with brainstem compression necessitating immediate ultrasound examination.

Apneic spells are almost never a seizure manifestation unless associated with tonic deviation of the eyes, tonic stiffening of the body, or characteristic limb movements. However, prolonged apnea without bradycardia, and especially with tachycardia, is a seizure until proven otherwise.

Management. Short episodes of apnea do not require intervention. The rare epileptic apnea requires the use of anticonvulsant agents.

Benign Infantile Myoclonus of Sleep

Clinical features. Sudden jerking movements of the limbs during sleep occur in normal people of all ages (see Chapter 14). They appear primarily during the early stages of sleep as repeated flexion movements of the fingers, wrists, and elbows. The jerks do not localize consistently, stop with gentle restraint, and end abruptly with arousal. When prolonged, the usual misdiagnosis is focal clonic or myoclonic seizures.

Diagnosis. The distinction between benign nocturnal myoclonus and seizures or jitteriness is that benign nocturnal myoclonus occurs solely during sleep, is not activated by a stimulus, and the EEG is normal.

Management. Treatment is unnecessary, and education and reassurance are usually sufficient. Rarely, a child with violent myoclonus experiences frequent arousals disruptive to sleep, and a small dose of clonazepam may be considered. Videos of children with this benign condition are very reassuring for the family to see and are available on the internet.

Jitteriness

Clinical features. Jitteriness or tremulousness is an excessive response to stimulation. Touch, noise, or motion provokes a low-amplitude, high-frequency shaking of the limbs and jaw. Jitteriness is commonly associated with a low threshold for the Moro reflex, but it can occur in the absence of any apparent stimulation and be confused with myoclonic seizures.

Diagnosis. Jitteriness usually occurs in newborns with perinatal asphyxia, along with the occurrence of seizures. EEG monitoring, the absence of eye movements or alteration in respiratory pattern, and the presence of stimulus activation distinguish jitteriness from seizures. Newborns of addicted mothers and newborns with metabolic disorders are often jittery (see the following sections on Neonatal Abstinence Syndrome and Seizures due to Metabolic Derangements).

Management. Reduced stimulation decreases jitteriness. However, newborns of addicted mothers require sedation to facilitate feeding and to decrease energy expenditure.

Neonatal Abstinence Syndrome

Marijuana, cocaine, alcohol, narcotic analgesics (hydrocodone and oxycodone), hypnotic sedatives (lorazepam and alprazolam), and central nervous system (CNS) stimulants (amphetamine or methylphenidate) are the nonprescribed drugs most commonly used during pregnancy. Marijuana and alcohol do not cause drug dependence in the fetus and are not associated with withdrawal symptoms, although ethanol can cause fetal alcohol syndrome. Hypnotic sedatives, such as barbiturates, do not ordinarily produce withdrawal symptoms unless the ingested doses are very large. Phenobarbital has a sufficiently long half-life in newborns that sudden withdrawal does not occur. The prototype of narcotic withdrawal in the newborn is with heroin or methadone, but a similar syndrome occurs with codeine and propoxyphene. Cocaine and methamphetamine also cause significant withdrawal syndromes.

Similar but milder symptoms are common with the use of prescribed drugs in pregnancy such as selective serotonin reuptake inhibitors (SSRIs), including fluoxetine, sertraline, citalopram, escitalopram, and paroxetine.

Clinical features. Symptoms of opiate withdrawal are more severe and tend to occur earlier in full-term (first 24 hours) than in premature (24–48 hours) newborns. The initial feature is jitteriness, present only during the waking state, which can shake an entire limb. Irritability, a shrill, high-pitched cry, and hyperactivity follow. The newborn seems hungry, but has difficulty feeding and vomits afterward. Diarrhea and other symptoms of autonomic instability are common.

Myoclonic jerking is present in 10%–25% of newborns undergoing withdrawal. Whether these movements are seizures or jitteriness is not clear. Definite seizures occur in fewer than 5%. Maternal use of cocaine during pregnancy is associated with premature delivery, growth restriction, and microcephaly. Newborns exposed to cocaine, in utero or after delivery through breast milk, often show features of cocaine intoxication, including tachycardia, tachypnea, hypertension, irritability, and tremulousness.

Diagnosis. Suspect and anticipate drug withdrawal in every newborn whose mother has a history of substance abuse. Even when such a history is not available, the combination of jitteriness, irritability, hyperactivity, and autonomic instability should provide a clue to the diagnosis. Careful questioning of the mother concerning her use of prescription and nonprescription drugs is imperative. Blood, urine, and meconium analyses identify specific drugs.

Management. Symptoms remit spontaneously in 3–5 days, but appreciable mortality occurs among untreated newborns. Benzodiazepines or chlorpromazine 3 mg/kg/day may relieve symptoms and reduce mortality. Secretion of morphine, meperidine, opium, and methadone in breast milk is insufficient to cause or relieve addiction in the newborn. The following medications and doses may be used for narcotic withdrawal: oral morphine 0.04 mg/kg every 3–4 hours, oral methadone 0.05–0.1 mg/kg every 6 hours, or oral clonidine 0.5–1 µg/kg every 3–6 hours.[3] Levetiracetam 40 mg/kg/day is a good option for seizures.

The occurrence of seizures in itself does not indicate a poor prognosis. The long-term outcome relates more closely to the other risk factors associated with substance abuse in the mother.

SEIZURES IN THE NEWBORN

Differential Diagnosis of Seizures

Seizures are a feature of almost all brain disorders in the newborn. The time of onset of the first seizure indicates the probable cause (Box 1.3). Seizures occurring during the first 24 hours, and especially in the first 12 hours, are usually due to HIE. Sepsis, meningitis, and subarachnoid hemorrhage (SAH) are next in frequency, followed by intrauterine infection, and trauma. Direct drug effects, intraventricular hemorrhage at term, and pyridoxine and folinic acid dependency are relatively rare causes of seizures but are important to consider as they are treatable conditions.

The more common causes of seizures during the period from 24 to 72 hours after birth are intraventricular hemorrhage in premature newborns, SAH, cerebral contusion in large full-term newborns, and sepsis and meningitis at all gestational ages. The cause of unifocal clonic seizures in full-term newborns is often cerebral infarction or intracerebral hemorrhage. MRI with diffusion-weighted images is diagnostic. Cerebral dysgenesis may cause seizures in neonates and remains an important cause of seizures throughout infancy and childhood. All other conditions are relatively rare. Newborns with metabolic disorders are usually lethargic and feed poorly before the onset of seizures. Seizures are rarely the first clinical feature. After 72 hours, the initiation of protein and glucose feedings makes inborn errors of metabolism, especially aminoaciduria, a more important consideration. Box 1.4 outlines a battery of screening tests for metabolic disorders. Transmission of herpes simplex infection occurs during delivery and symptoms begin during the second half of the first week. Conditions that cause early and late seizures include cerebral dysgenesis, cerebral infarction, intracerebral hemorrhage, and familial/genetic neonatal seizures.

BOX 1.3 Differential Diagnosis of Neonatal Seizures by Peak Time of Onset

24 Hours
- Bacterial meningitis and sepsis[a] (see Chapter 4)
- Direct drug effect
- Hypoxic-ischemic encephalopathy[a]
- Intrauterine infection (see Chapter 5)
- Intraventricular hemorrhage at term[a] (see Chapter 4)
- Laceration of tentorium or falx
- Pyridoxine dependency[a]
- Subarachnoid hemorrhage[a]

24–72 Hours
- Bacterial meningitis and sepsis[a] (see Chapter 4)
- Cerebral contusion with subdural hemorrhage
- Cerebral dysgenesis[a] (see Chapter 18)
- Cerebral infarction[a] (see Chapter 11)
- Neonatal abstinence syndrome
- Glycine encephalopathy
- Glycogen synthase deficiency
- Hypoparathyroidism-hypocalcemia
- Idiopathic cerebral venous thrombosis
- Incontinentia pigmenti
- Intracerebral hemorrhage (see Chapter 11)
- Intraventricular hemorrhage in premature newborns[a] (see Chapter 4)
- Pyridoxine dependency[a]
- Subarachnoid hemorrhage
- Tuberous sclerosis
- Urea cycle disturbances

72 Hours–1 Week
- Cerebral dysgenesis (see Chapter 18)
- Cerebral infarction[a] (see Chapter 11)
- Familial neonatal seizures
- Hypoparathyroidism
- Idiopathic cerebral venous thrombosis[a]
- Intracerebral hemorrhage (see Chapter 11)
- Kernicterus
- Methylmalonic acidemia
- Nutritional hypocalcemia[a]
- Propionic acidemia
- Tuberous sclerosis
- Urea cycle disturbances

1–4 Weeks
- Adrenoleukodystrophy, neonatal (see Chapter 6)
- Cerebral dysgenesis (see Chapter 18)
- Fructose dysmetabolism
- Gaucher disease type 2 (see Chapter 5)
- GM_1 gangliosidosis type 1 (see Chapter 5)
- Herpes simplex encephalitis[a]
- Idiopathic cerebral venous thrombosis[a]
- Ketotic hyperglycinemias
- Maple syrup urine disease, neonatal[a]
- Tuberous sclerosis
- Urea cycle disturbances

[a]The most common conditions and the ones with disease-modifying treatments.

BOX 1.4 Screening for Inborn Errors of Metabolism That Cause Neonatal Seizures

Blood Glucose Low
- Fructose 1,6-diphosphatase deficiency
- Glycogen storage disease type 1
- Maple syrup urine disease

Blood Calcium Low
- Hypoparathyroidism
- Maternal hyperparathyroidism

Blood Ammonia High
- Argininosuccinic acidemia
- Carbamyl phosphate synthetase deficiency
- Citrullinemia
- Methylmalonic acidemia (may be normal)
- Multiple carboxylase deficiency
- Ornithine transcarbamylase deficiency
- Propionic acidemia (may be normal)

Blood Lactate High
- Fructose 1,6-diphosphatase deficiency
- Glycogen storage disease type 1
- Mitochondrial disorders
- Multiple carboxylase deficiency

Metabolic Acidosis
- Fructose 1,6-diphosphatase deficiency
- Glycogen storage disease type 1
- Maple syrup urine disease
- Methylmalonic acidemia
- Multiple carboxylase deficiency
- Propionic acidemia

Benign Familial Neonatal Seizures

This condition, now referred to as one of the self-limited familial epilepsy syndromes, should be suspected in neonates or infants with multifocal brief motor seizures and otherwise normal function, especially when a family history of similar events is present. This is usually associated with mutations that affect the potassium or the sodium channels. Most cases result from autosomal dominant pathogenic variants of the *KCNQ2*, *KCNQ3*, or *PRRT2* genes, although the disorder is genetically heterogeneous and other mutations have been described.[4]

Clinical features. Brief multifocal clonic seizures develop during the first week, sometimes associated with apnea. The delay of onset may be as long as 4 weeks. With or without treatment, the seizures usually stop spontaneously within the first months of life. Febrile seizures occur in up to one-third of affected children; some have febrile seizures without first having neonatal seizures. Epilepsy develops later in life in as many as one-third of affected newborns. The seizure types include nocturnal generalized tonic-clonic seizures and simple focal orofacial seizures.

Diagnosis. Suspect the syndrome when seizures develop without apparent cause in a healthy newborn. Laboratory tests are normal. The EEG often demonstrates multifocal epileptiform discharges and may be normal interictally. A family history of neonatal seizures supports the diagnosis but is not always present. The detection of causative mutations may abbreviate further diagnostic testing and be of some reassurance as most cases are benign; however, poor outcomes have been described.

Management. Oxcarbazepine is typically the most effective anticonvulsant. The duration of treatment needed is unclear. We often treat infants for about 6 months, after which we discontinue treatment if the child remains seizure free and the EEG has normalized. In our experience levetiracetam is ineffective in this condition.

Bilirubin Encephalopathy

Unconjugated bilirubin is bound to albumin in the blood. *Kernicterus*, a yellow discoloration of the brain that is especially severe in the basal ganglia and hippocampus, occurs when the serum unbound or free fraction becomes excessive. An excessive level of the free fraction in an otherwise healthy newborn is approximately 20 mg/dL (340 µmol/L). Kernicterus was an important complication of hemolytic disease from maternal-fetal blood group incompatibility, but this condition is now almost unheard of in most countries. The management of other causes of hyperbilirubinemia in full-term newborns is not difficult. Critically ill premature infants with respiratory distress syndrome, acidosis, and sepsis are the group at greatest risk. In such newborns, lower concentrations of bilirubin may be sufficient to cause bilirubin encephalopathy, and even the albumin-bound fraction may pass the blood-brain barrier.

Clinical features. Three distinct clinical phases of bilirubin encephalopathy occur in full-term newborns with untreated hemolytic disease. Hypotonia, lethargy, and a poor sucking reflex occur within 24 hours of delivery. Bilirubin staining of the brain is already evident in newborns during this first clinical phase. On the second or third day, the newborn becomes febrile and shows increasing tone and opisthotonic posturing. Seizures are not a constant feature but may occur at this time. Characteristic of the third phase is apparent improvement with normalization of tone. This may cause second thoughts about the accuracy of the diagnosis, but the improvement is short-lived. Evidence of neurological dysfunction begins to appear toward the end of the second month, and the symptoms become progressively worse throughout infancy.

In premature newborns, the clinical features are subtle and may lack the phases of increased tone and opisthotonos.

The typical clinical syndrome after the first year includes extrapyramidal dysfunction, usually athetosis, which occurs in virtually every case; disturbances of vertical gaze, upward more often than downward in 90%; high-frequency hearing loss in 60%; and intellectual disability in 25%. Survivors often develop a choreoathetoid form of cerebral palsy.

Diagnosis. In newborns with hemolytic disease, the basis for a presumed clinical diagnosis is a significant hyperbilirubinemia and a compatible evolution of symptoms. However, the diagnosis is difficult to establish in critically ill premature newborns, in whom the cause of brain damage is more often asphyxia than kernicterus. The MRI may show the targeted areas in the basal ganglia.

Management. Maintaining serum bilirubin concentrations below the toxic range, either by phototherapy or exchange transfusion, prevents kernicterus. Once kernicterus has occurred, further damage can be limited, but not reversed, by lowering serum bilirubin concentrations. Diazepam and baclofen are often needed for the management of dystonic postures associated with the cerebral palsy.

Seizures due to Metabolic Derangements

Hypocalcemia

The definition of hypocalcemia is a blood calcium concentration less than 7 mg/dL (1.75 mmol/L). The onset of hypocalcemia in the first 72 hours after delivery is associated with low birth weight, asphyxia, maternal diabetes, transitory neonatal hypoparathyroidism, maternal hyperparathyroidism, and the DiGeorge syndrome (DGS). Later-onset hypocalcemia occurs in children fed improper formulas, in maternal hyperparathyroidism, and in DGS.

Hypoparathyroidism in the newborn may result from maternal hyperparathyroidism, or it may be a transitory phenomenon of unknown cause. Hypocalcemia occurs in less than 10% of stressed newborns and enhances their vulnerability to seizures, but it is rarely the primary cause.

DGS is associated with microdeletions of chromosome 22q11.2.[5] Disturbance of cervical neural crest migration into the derivatives of the pharyngeal arches and pouches explains the phenotype. Organs derived from the third and fourth pharyngeal pouches (thymus, parathyroid gland, and great vessels) are hypoplastic.

Clinical features. The 22q11.2 deletion syndrome is phenotypically variable and encompasses several similar phenotypes, including DGS and *velocardiofacial syndrome* (VCFS). The acronym CATCH is used to describe the phenotype of cardiac abnormality, T-cell deficit, clefting (multiple minor facial anomalies), and hypocalcemia.[6] The identification of most children with DGS is in the neonatal period with a major heart defect, hypocalcemia, and immunodeficiency. Diagnosis of children with VCFS comes later because of cleft palate or craniofacial deformities.

The initial symptoms of DGS may be due to congenital heart disease, hypocalcemia, or both. Jitteriness and tetany usually begin in the first 48 hours after delivery. The peak onset of seizures is on the third day, but a 2-week delay may occur. Many affected newborns die of cardiac causes during the first month; survivors fail to thrive and have frequent infections secondary to the failure of cell-mediated immunity.

Diagnosis. Newborns with DGS come to medical attention because of seizures and heart disease. Seizures or a prolonged QT interval brings attention to hypocalcemia. Molecular genetic testing confirms the diagnosis.

Management. Management requires a multispecialty team, including cardiology, immunology, medical genetics, and neurology. Plastic surgery, dentistry, and child development contribute later on. Hypocalcemia generally responds to parathyroid hormone or to oral calcium and vitamin D.

Hypoglycemia

A transitory, asymptomatic hypoglycemia is detectable in 10% of newborns during the first hours after delivery and before initiating feeding. Asymptomatic, transient hypoglycemia is not associated with neurological impairment later in life. Symptomatic hypoglycemia may result from stress or inborn errors of metabolism (Box 1.5).

BOX 1.5   Causes of Neonatal Hypoglycemia

- **Primary transitional hypoglycemia**[a]
  - Complicated labor and delivery
  - Intrauterine malnutrition
  - Maternal diabetes
  - Prematurity
- **Secondary transitional hypoglycemia**[a]
  - Asphyxia
  - Central nervous system disorders
  - Cold injuries
  - Sepsis
- **Persistent hypoglycemia**
  - Aminoacidurias
  - Maple syrup urine disease
  - Methylmalonic acidemia
  - Propionic acidemia
  - Tyrosinosis
- **Congenital hypopituitarism**
- **Defects in carbohydrate metabolism**
  - Fructose 1,6-diphosphatase deficiency
  - Fructose + intolerance
  - Galactosemia
  - Glycogen storage disease type 1
  - Glycogen synthase deficiency
- **Hyperinsulinism**
- **Organic acidurias**
  - Glutaric aciduria type 2
  - 3-Methylglutaryl-CoA lyase deficiency

[a]The most common conditions and the ones with disease-modifying treatments.

Clinical features. The time of onset of symptoms depends on the underlying disorder. Early onset is generally associated with perinatal asphyxia, maternal diabetes, intracranial hemorrhage, and late-onset with inborn errors of metabolism. Hypoglycemia is rare and mild among newborns with classic maple syrup urine disease (MSUD), ethylmalonic-adipic aciduria, and isovaleric acidemia, and is invariably severe in those with 3-methylglutaconic aciduria, glutaric aciduria type 2, and disorders of fructose metabolism.

The syndrome includes any of the following symptoms: apnea, cyanosis, tachypnea, jitteriness, high-pitched crying, poor feeding, vomiting, apathy, hypotonia, seizures, and coma. Symptomatic hypoglycemia is often associated with later neurological impairment.

Diagnosis. Neonatal hypoglycemia is defined as a whole blood glucose concentration of less than 20 mg/dL (1 mmol/L) in premature and low-birth-weight newborns, less than 30 mg/dL (1.5 mmol/L) in term newborns during the first 72 hours, and less than 40 mg/dL (2 mmol/L) in full-term newborns after 72 hours. Finding a low glucose concentration in a newborn with seizures prompts an investigation into the cause of the hypoglycemia.

Management. Intravenous (IV) administration of glucose normalizes blood glucose concentrations, but the underlying cause must be determined before providing definitive treatment.

Hypoxic-Ischemic Encephalopathy

Asphyxia at term is usually an intrauterine event, and hypoxia and ischemia occur together; the result is HIE. *Acute systemic* and *severe asphyxia* often leads to death from circulatory collapse. Survivors are born comatose. Lower cranial nerve dysfunction and severe neurological deficits are the rule.

Less severe and systemic, prolonged asphyxia is the usual mechanism of HIE in surviving full-term newborns.[7] The fetal circulation accommodates reductions in arterial oxygen by maximizing blood flow to the brain, and to a lesser extent the heart, at the expense of other organs.

HIE may present as mild, moderate, or severe. Most severe forms have a clear cause, such as cord prolapse, uterine rupture, placental abruption, maternal trauma, or cardiorespiratory collapse. Exact diagnostic criteria for severe HIE vary among institutions but commonly include a gestational age greater than 35 or 36 weeks, cord pH less than or equal to 7, base deficit of 12–15, and Apgar of 5 or less at 10 minutes with an ongoing need for resuscitation. The treating physician may use these diagnostic criteria to determine eligibility for therapeutic cooling.

Clinical experience indicates that fetuses may be subject to considerable hypoxia without the development of brain damage. Any episode of hypoxia sufficiently severe to cause brain damage also causes derangements in other organs. Newborns with mild HIE always have a history of irregular heart rate and usually pass meconium. Those with severe HIE may have lactic acidosis, elevated serum concentrations of hepatic enzymes, enterocolitis, renal failure, and fatal myocardial damage.

Clinical features. Mild HIE is relatively common. The newborn is lethargic but conscious immediately after birth. Other characteristic features are jitteriness and irritability. Muscle tone is normal or increased at rest, tendon reflexes are normoreactive or hyperactive, and ankle clonus is usually elicited. Sympathetic overactivity and autonomic instability do not occur in mild HIE. The Moro reflex is complete, and a single stimulus generates repetitive extension and flexion movements. Seizures are not an expected feature, and their occurrence suggests concurrent hypoglycemia, the presence of a second condition or a more significant HIE.

Symptoms diminish and disappear during the first few days, although some degree of over-responsiveness may persist. Newborns with mild HIE often recover normal brain function completely.

Newborns with *severe HIE* are stuporous or comatose immediately after birth, and respiratory effort is usually periodic and insufficient to sustain life. Seizures begin within the first 12 hours. Hypotonia is severe, and tendon reflexes, the Moro reflex, and the tonic neck reflex are absent as well. Sucking and swallowing are depressed or absent, but the pupillary and oculovestibular reflexes are present. Most of these newborns have frequent seizures, which may appear on EEG without clinical manifestations. They may progress to status epilepticus. The response to anticonvulsant drugs is usually incomplete. Generalized increased intracranial pressure characterized by coma, bulging of the fontanelles, loss of pupillary and oculovestibular reflexes, and respiratory arrest often develops between 24 and 72 hours of age.

The newborn may die at this time or may remain stuporous for several weeks. The encephalopathy begins to subside after the third day, and seizures decrease in frequency and eventually may stop. Jitteriness is common as the child becomes aroused. Tone increases in the limbs during the succeeding weeks. Counsel families to expect neurological sequelae in newborns with severe HIE; however, the degree of long-term neurological deficits may be difficult to accurately predict.

Diagnosis. Clinical and laboratory findings are used to determine the severity of HIE and eligibility for treatment protocols. EEG, head ultrasound, and MRI are useful adjunctive tests, and continuous EEG monitoring is necessary for every neonate with severe HIE particularly when undergoing therapeutic whole-body cooling. In mild HIE, the EEG background rhythms are normal or lacking in variability. In severe HIE, the background is always abnormal and shows suppression of background amplitude. The degree of suppression correlates well with the severity of HIE. The worst case is a flat EEG or one with a burst-suppression pattern. A bad outcome is invariable if the amplitude remains suppressed for 2 weeks or a burst-suppression pattern is present at any time. Epileptiform activity may be present but is less predictive of the outcome than background suppression.

MRI with diffusion-weighted images are helpful to determine the full extent of injury. The basal ganglia and thalamus are often affected.

Management. The management of HIE in newborns requires immediate attention to derangements in several organs and correction of acidosis. Clinical experience indicates that control of seizures and maintenance of adequate ventilation and perfusion increases the chance of a favorable outcome. Whole-body cooling with continuous EEG monitoring is the standard of care.[8] Continuous EEG monitoring is needed as seizures are often subclinical in newborns; if seizures are present at any time during cooling, the EEG should be continued until at least 24 hours after rewarming as seizures may recur once the brain's metabolic demands increase.

A separate section details the treatment of seizures in newborns. The use of IV levetiracetam is our first choice,[9] but often fails. Intravenous lacosamide shows promise in several early reports and may have the added benefit of not increasing apoptosis, although research is preliminary.[10] Seizures in neonates with HIE follow a temporal pattern and often have an explosive onset, followed by a longer period of increased control.[11] The incidence of later epilepsy among infants who had neonatal seizures caused by HIE is 30%–40%. Continuing

antiepileptic therapy after the initial seizures have stopped does not seem to influence, significantly if at all, whether the child goes on to develop epilepsy as a lifelong condition.

Organic Acid Disorders and Aminoacidopathies

Aminoacidopathy is a general term that may refer to any disorder of organic or amino acid metabolism. "Organic acidemia" typically refers to four specific organic acid disorders involving the branched-chain amino acids. We use the general term "aminoacidopathy" when discussing nonketotic hyperglycinemia, and "organic acidemia" when discussing maple syrup urine disease (MSUD), isovaleric acidemia, methylmalonic acidemia (MMA), and propionic acidemia. All of these disorders can cause catastrophic metabolic crises and seizures in the newborn. Hyperammonemia is a common feature (Box 1.6). Glycine may be elevated in multiple different disorders, but all except nonketotic hyperglycinemia will be associated with concurrent ketosis.

A characteristic of organic acid disorders is the accumulation of compounds, usually ketones, or lactic acid that causes acidosis in biological fluids.[12] Among the dozens of organic acid disorders are abnormalities in vitamin metabolism, lipid metabolism, glycolysis, citric acid cycle, oxidative metabolism, glutathione metabolism, and 4-aminobutyric acid metabolism. The clinical presentations vary considerably and several chapters contain descriptions. Here we will focus on those that cause neonatal seizures.

BOX 1.6 Causes of Neonatal Hyperammonemia

- Liver failure
- Primary enzyme defects in urea synthesis
  - Argininosuccinic acidemia
  - Carbamyl phosphate synthetase deficiency
  - Citrullinemia
  - Ornithine transcarbamylase deficiency
- Other disorders of amino acid metabolism
  - Glycine encephalopathy
  - Isovaleric acidemia
  - Methylmalonic acidemia
  - Multiple carboxylase deficiency
  - Propionic acidemia
- Transitory hyperammonemia of prematurity

Nonketotic Hyperglycinemia

A defect in the glycine cleaving system causes glycine encephalopathy (nonketotic hyperglycinemia). Inheritance is autosomal recessive.[13]

Clinical features. Both severe and attenuated forms exist. In the severe form, affected newborns are normal at birth but become irritable and refuse feeding anytime from 6 hours to 8 days after delivery. The onset of symptoms is usually within 48 hours, but delays by a few weeks occur in attenuated forms. *Hiccupping* is an early and continuous feature; some mothers relate that the child hiccupped in utero as a prominent symptom. Progressive lethargy, hypotonia, respiratory disturbances, and myoclonic seizures follow. Some newborns survive the acute illness, but cognitive impairment, epilepsy, and spasticity characterize the subsequent course.

In milder forms, the onset of seizures occurs after the neonatal period. The developmental outcome is better, but does not exceed moderate cognitive impairment.

Diagnosis. During acute encephalopathy, the EEG demonstrates a burst-suppression pattern, which evolves into hypsarrhythmia during infancy. The MRI may be normal or may show agenesis or thinning of the corpus callosum. Delayed myelination and atrophy are later findings. Hyperglycinemia and especially elevated concentrations of glycine in the cerebrospinal fluid (CSF) in the absence of hyperammonemia, organic acidemia, or valproic acid treatment establish the diagnosis. Confirmatory molecular genetic testing demonstrates biallelic pathogenic mutations in the *GLDC* or *AMT* genes.

Management. No therapy has proven to be effective. Hemodialysis provides only temporary relief of the encephalopathy, and diet therapy has not been successful in modifying the course. Diazepam, a competitor for glycine receptors, in combination with choline, folic acid, and sodium benzoate, may control seizures but has no significant effect on developmental outcome. Oral administration of sodium benzoate at doses of 250–750 mg/kg/day can reduce the plasma glycine concentration into the normal range. This substantially reduces but does not normalize CSF glycine concentration. L-Carnitine 100 mg/kg/day may increase the glycine conjugation with benzoate. It has been reported that dextromethorphan 5–35 mg/kg/day divided into four doses is helpful in lowering levels of glycine.[14]

Disorders of Branched-Chain Amino Acids

Branched-chain aminoacidopathies encompass four distinct disorders: MSUD, isovaleric acidemia, MMA, and propionic acidemia. All four can present in the neonatal period, often after the initiation of feeds.

Metabolic crises are clinically characterized by vomiting and lethargy with or without new neurologic deficits. *These crises are life-threatening and should be treated as such.* Many institutions have specific treatment guidelines in place.

Maple syrup urine disease. An almost complete absence (less than 2% of normal) of branched-chain ketoacid dehydrogenase (BCKD) causes the neonatal form of MSUD. BCKD is composed of six subunits, but the main abnormality in MSUD is a deficiency of the E1 subunit on chromosome 19q13.1–q13.2. Leucine, isoleucine, and valine cannot be decarboxylated, and accumulate in blood, urine, and tissues (Fig. 1.1). See

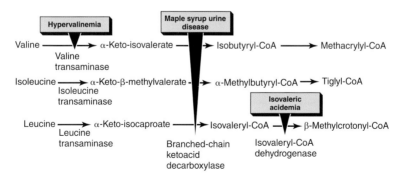

Fig. 1.1 Branched-Chain Amino Acid Metabolism. Transaminase system, branched-chain α-ketoacid dehydrogenase, isovaleryl-CoA dehydrogenase, α-methyl branched-chain acyl-CoA dehydrogenase, propionyl-CoA carboxylase (biotin cofactor), methylmalonyl-CoA racemase, and methylmalonyl-CoA mutase (adenosylcobalamin cofactor).

Chapters 5 and 10 for descriptions of later-onset forms. Transmission of the defect is by autosomal recessive inheritance.[15]

Clinical features. Affected newborns appear healthy at birth but lethargy, feeding difficulty, and hypotonia develop after ingestion of protein. A progressive encephalopathy develops by 2–3 days postpartum. The encephalopathy includes lethargy, intermittent apnea, opisthotonos, and stereotyped movements such as "fencing" and "bicycling." Coma and central respiratory failure may occur by 7–10 days of age. Seizures begin in the second week and are associated with the development of cerebral edema. Once seizures begin, they continue with increasing frequency and severity. Without therapy, cerebral edema becomes progressively worse and results in coma and death within 1 month.

Diagnosis. Plasma amino acid concentrations show increased plasma concentrations of the three branch-chained amino acids. MSUD is a standard part of newborn screening tests, but affected infants may become symptomatic before the result of the newborn screen returns. Urine classically smells like maple syrup. Ketonuria in any newborn should prompt further metabolic evaluation; infants with MSUD will not have associated hypoglycemia or hyperammonemia. Measures of enzyme in lymphocytes or cultured fibroblasts previously served as a confirmatory test; however, the availability of molecular genetic testing makes this unnecessary in most cases. A specific multigene panel can be used to confirm the results of abnormal newborn screens. Perform comprehensive genetic testing when the newborn screen is not available. Heterozygotes have diminished levels of enzyme activity.

Management. Hemodialysis may be necessary to correct the life-threatening metabolic acidosis. A trial of thiamine (10–20 mg/kg/day) improves the condition in a *thiamine-responsive MSUD variant*. Correct dehydration, electrolyte imbalance, and metabolic acidosis. Consult with a dietician to initiate a leucine-restricted diet while ensuring adequate isoleucine and valine supplementation. Special formulas are available that are free of branched-chain amino acids. Give natural proteins only in limited, quantified doses; infants may be fed breast milk but this must be expressed and carefully measured. Ongoing surveillance of amino acid concentrations is critical. Newborns diagnosed in the first 2 weeks and treated rigorously have the best prognosis.

Isovaleric Acidemia

Isovaleric acid is a fatty acid derived from leucine. The enzyme isovaleryl-CoA dehydrogenase converts isovaleric acid to 3-methylcrotonyl-CoA (see Fig. 1.1). Genetic transmission is autosomal recessive inheritance and results from biallelic mutations in the *IVD* gene.

Clinical features. Variable phenotypes are associated with the same enzyme defect ranging from an acute, overwhelming disorder of the newborn to a chronic infantile or even asymptomatic form. Newborns with the acute disorder are normal at birth but within a few days become lethargic, refuse to feed, and vomit. The clinical syndrome is similar to MSUD except that the urine smells like "sweaty feet" instead of maple syrup and laboratory evaluation reveals hyperammonemia, which is not seen in MSUD. Early detection and treatment have led to improved survival over the last couple of decades.

Diagnosis. The disorder is frequently discovered on routine newborn screening. Symptomatic newborns may have hyperammonemia and lactic acidosis. Molecular genetic testing is available. The clinical phenotype correlates not with the percentage of residual enzyme activity, but with the ability to detoxify isovaleryl-CoA with glycine.

Management. Dietary restriction of protein, especially leucine, decreases the occurrence of later neurological deficits. L-Carnitine, 50 mg/kg/day, is a beneficial supplement to the diet of some children with isovaleric acidemia. In acutely ill newborns, oral glycine, 250–500 mg/day, in addition to protein restriction and carnitine, lowers mortality. Arachidonic acid, docosahexaenoic acid, and vitamin B_{12} may become deficient and require supplementation in patients treated with dietary restriction of protein. Close monitoring and prompt treatment of attacks are vital.[16]

Methylmalonic Acidemia

D-Methylmalonyl-CoA is racemized to L-methylmalonyl-CoA by the enzyme D-methylmalonyl racemase and then isomerized to succinyl-CoA, which enters the tricarboxylic acid cycle. The enzyme D-methylmalonyl-CoA mutase catalyzes the isomerization. The cobalamin (vitamin B_{12}) coenzyme adenosylcobalamin is a required cofactor. The diagnosis of isolated MMA encompasses several possible defects in this pathway. The most common phenotype is the infantile or non-B12-responsive form, which is also the most severe. Partial deficiency or B12-responsive phenotypes, as well as methylmalonyl-CoA epimerase deficiency, can present in infancy but may not become symptomatic until later in life. Genetic transmission of the several defects in this pathway is by autosomal recessive inheritance with biallelic pathogenic mutations in the *MMAA, MMAB, MCEE, MMADHC,* or *MMUT* genes.[17] Propionyl-CoA, propionic acid, and methylmalonic acid accumulate and cause hyperglycinemia and hyperammonemia.

Clinical features. In the infantile/non-B12-responsive form, the symptoms appear during the first week after delivery and include lethargy, failure to thrive, recurrent vomiting, dehydration, respiratory distress, and hypotonia after the initiation of protein feeding. Leukopenia, thrombocytopenia, and anemia are present in more than one-half of patients. Intracranial hemorrhage may result from a bleeding diathesis. Treatment must be initiated promptly to avoid the development of hyperammonemic encephalopathy. The outcome for newborns with complete mutase deficiency has improved over the past several years; however, survivors typically have recurrent acidosis, basal ganglia infarcts during periods of metabolic crisis, movement disorders, and intellectual disability.

Diagnosis. Suspect the diagnosis in any newborn with metabolic acidosis, especially if associated with ketosis, hyperammonemia, and hyperglycinemia. Testing for MMA is included in the newborn screen, and confirmatory genetic testing is available.

Management. Initially, the treating physician will not know if the infant is cobalamin-responsive or not. Vitamin B$_{12}$ supplementation is useful in some defects of adenosylcobalamin synthesis, and hydroxocobalamin administration is reasonable while awaiting the definitive genetic diagnosis. Maintain treatment with protein restriction (0.5–1.5 g/kg/day) and hydroxocobalamin (1 mg) weekly. As in propionic acidemia, oral supplementation of L-carnitine reduces ketogenesis in response to fasting. Long-term management of secondary complications such as growth failure, pancreatitis, functional immune impairment, cardiac disease, and liver and renal cancer requires a multidisciplinary approach.

Propionic Acidemia

Propionyl-CoA forms as a catabolite of methionine, threonine, and the branched-chain amino acids. Its further carboxylation to D-methylmalonyl-CoA requires the enzyme propionyl-CoA carboxylase and the coenzyme biotin (see Fig. 1.1). Isolated deficiency of propionyl-CoA carboxylase causes propionic acidemia. Transmission of the defect is autosomal recessive.

Clinical features. As with MMA, there is a range of phenotypes with the infantile form being both the most common and most severe. In newborns, the symptoms are nonspecific: feeding difficulty, lethargy, hypotonia, and dehydration. Untreated newborns rapidly become dehydrated, have generalized or myoclonic seizures, and become comatose.

Hepatomegaly caused by a fatty infiltration occurs in approximately one-third of patients. Neutropenia, thrombocytopenia, and occasionally pancytopenia may be present. A bleeding diathesis accounts for massive intracranial hemorrhage in some newborns. Children who survive beyond infancy may develop infarctions in the basal ganglia during periods of metabolic crisis, also known as "metabolic stroke."

Diagnosis. Consider propionic acidemia in any newborn with ketoacidosis or with hyperammonemia without ketoacidosis. Propionic acidemia is the probable diagnosis when the plasma concentrations of glycine and propionate and the urinary concentrations of glycine, methylcitrate, and β-hydroxypropionate are increased. While the urinary concentration of propionate may be normal, the plasma concentration is always elevated, without a concurrent increase in the concentration of methylmalonate.

Testing for propionic academia is included on some expanded newborn screens. Molecular genetic testing reveals biallelic pathogenic variants in the *PCCA* or *PCCB* genes, although enzymatic assays may still be necessary in some cases to confirm the diagnosis.[18]

Management. The newborn in ketoacidosis requires dialysis to remove toxic metabolites, parenteral fluids to prevent dehydration, and restriction of propriogenic precursors. Restricting protein intake to 0.5–1.5 g/kg/day decreases the frequency and severity of subsequent attacks. Oral administration of L-carnitine reduces the ketogenic response to fasting and may be useful as a daily supplement. Intermittent administration of non-absorbed antibiotics reduces the production of propionate by gut bacteria. Consider liver transplantation in patients with frequent episodes of metabolic crisis or hyperammonemia. As with other organic acid disorders, avoid stressors that may trigger metabolic crises, such as fasting, vomiting, or high protein loads.

Vitamin-Dependent Seizures

Pyridoxine dependency and folinic acid dependency are both present in the neonatal or early infantile period.

Pyridoxine Dependency

Pyridoxine dependency is a rare disorder transmitted as an autosomal recessive trait. Biallelic pathogenic variants in the *ALDH7A1* gene cause the disorder, which has variable phenotypic presentation ranging from typical to atypical.[19]

Clinical features. Newborns experience seizures soon after birth. The seizures are usually multifocal clonic at onset and progress rapidly to status epilepticus. Although presentations consisting of prolonged seizures and recurrent episodes of status epilepticus are typical, recurrent self-limited events, including partial seizures, generalized seizures, atonic seizures, myoclonic events, and infantile spasms also occur. The seizures only respond to pyridoxine. A seizure-free interval of up to 3 weeks may occur after pyridoxine discontinuation. The outcome is improved and cognitive deficits decreased with early diagnosis and treatment; nevertheless, intellectual disability is common particularly in the typical form.

Atypical features include late-onset seizures (up to age 2 years); seizures that initially respond to antiepileptic drugs and then do not; seizures that do not initially respond to pyridoxine but then become controlled; and prolonged seizure-free intervals (up to 5 months) occurring after stopping pyridoxine.

Diagnosis. Suspect the diagnosis in newborns with an affected older sibling or in newborns with daily seizures unresponsive to anticonvulsants, with a progressive course, and worsening EEGs. Characteristics of the typical/infantile-onset variety are intermittent myoclonic seizures, focal clonic seizures, or generalized tonic-clonic seizures. In our experience ictal apnea is a prominent symptom. The EEG is continuously abnormal because of generalized or multifocal spike discharges and tends to evolve into hypsarrhythmia. An IV injection of pyridoxine 100 mg stops the clinical seizure activity and often converts the EEG to normal in less than 10 minutes. However, sometimes 500 mg is required. When giving pyridoxine IV, arousals may look like improvements in the EEG since hypsarrhythmia is a pattern seen initially during sleep. Comparing the sleep EEG before and after pyridoxine is needed to confirm an EEG response. Supportive but nonspecific laboratory findings include plasma and urine elevations of α-aminoadipic semialdehyde; elevations of pipecolic acid in plasma and CSF; and characteristic findings in monoamine metabolite analysis of CSF. Genetic testing confirms the diagnosis.

Management. A lifelong dietary supplement of pyridoxine prevents further seizures. The International Consortium of PDE has published practice guidelines recommending doses of 100 mg/day for newborns and 30 mg/kg/day for infants with a maximum daily dose of 300 mg. The dose can be doubled for several days during periods of acute illness or stress; the only risk is that of a reversible sensory neuropathy, which we have never seen in this patient population. Initiate dietary therapy with reduced lysine intake. Recommend prenatal testing for all subsequent siblings, as pyridoxine supplements can be given to the mother during pregnancy, and treatment started immediately on delivery.[20]

Folinic Acid Dependency

Folinic acid dependency seizures are similar to pyridoxine dependency seizures. A case report of Ohtahara syndrome responsive to folinic acid was negative for the known *ALDH7A1* mutation associated with folinic acid and pyridoxine-dependent seizures and positive for an *STXBP1* mutation.[21] Additional case reports identified novel mutations in the folate receptor *FOLR1* gene.[22]

Clinical features. Infants develop seizures during the first week of life that are not responsive to anticonvulsants or pyridoxine.

Diagnosis. A characteristic peak on CSF electrophoresis confirms the diagnosis, as does molecular genetic testing.[23]

Management. Treat the disorder with folinic acid (NOT FOLIC ACID) supplementation of 2.5–5 mg twice daily.

Seizures Resulting From Perinatal Infections

Virtually any severe infection can cause seizures in the newborn due to their impaired immune function. However, the infection of most concern is herpes simplex encephalitis.

Herpes Simplex Encephalitis

Herpes simplex virus (HSV) is a large DNA virus separated into two serotypes, HSV-1 and HSV-2. HSV-2 is associated with 80% of genital herpes and HSV-1 with 20%. Both subtypes are prevalent in the population. Transmission of HSV to the newborn can occur in utero, peripartum, or postnatally. However, 85% of neonatal cases are HSV-2 infections acquired during the time of delivery. The highest risk for perinatal transmission occurs when a mother with no prior HSV-1 or HSV-2 antibodies acquires either virus in the genital tract within 2 weeks before delivery (first-episode primary infection). Postnatal transmission can occur with HSV-1 through mouth or hand by the mother or other caregiver.

Clinical features. The clinical spectrum of perinatal HSV infection is considerable. Among symptomatic newborns, one-third have disseminated disease, one-third have localized involvement of the brain, and one-third have localized involvement of the eyes, skin, or mouth. Whether the infection is disseminated or localized, approximately half of infections involve the CNS. The overall mortality rate is over 60%, and 50% of survivors have permanent neurological impairment.

The onset of symptoms may be as early as the fifth day, but is usually in the second week. A vesicular rash is present in 30%, usually on the scalp after vertex presentation and on the buttocks after breech presentation. Conjunctivitis, jaundice, and a bleeding diathesis may be present. The first symptoms of encephalitis are irritability and seizures. Seizures may be focal or generalized and are frequently only partially responsive to therapy. Neurological deterioration is progressive and characterized by coma and quadriparesis.

Diagnosis. Culture specimens are collected from cutaneous vesicles, mouth, nasopharynx, rectum, or CSF. Polymerase chain reaction (PCR) is the standard for diagnosing herpes encephalitis. The EEG is always abnormal and shows multifocal spikes, initially more than the periodic triphasic pattern seen in older populations. The periodic pattern of slow waves usually suggests a destructive underlying lesion similar to stroke. The CSF examination shows a lymphocytic leukocytosis, red blood cells, and an elevated protein concentration.

Management. The best treatment is prevention. Cesarean section should be strongly considered in all women with active genital herpes infection at term, whose membranes are intact or ruptured for less than 4 hours.

IV acyclovir is the drug of choice for all forms of neonatal HSV disease. The dosage is 60 mg/kg/day divided into three doses, given IV for 14 days for skin/eye/mouth disease and 21 days for disseminated disease. All patients with CNS HSV involvement should undergo a repeat lumbar puncture at the end of IV acyclovir therapy to determine that the CSF is PCR negative and normalized. Therapy continues until documenting a negative PCR. Acute renal failure is the most significant adverse effect of parenteral acyclovir. Mortality remains 50% or greater in newborns with disseminated disease.

Trauma and Intracranial Hemorrhage

Neonatal head trauma occurs most often in large-term newborns of primiparous mothers. Prolonged labor and difficult extraction are usual because of fetal malpositioning or fetal-pelvic disproportion. A precipitous delivery may also lead to trauma or hemorrhage. Intracranial hemorrhage may be subarachnoid, subdural, or intraventricular. Intraventricular hemorrhage is discussed in Chapter 4.

Idiopathic cerebral venous thrombosis. The causes of cerebral venous thrombosis in newborns are coagulopathies, polycythemia, and sepsis. Cerebral venous thrombosis, especially involving the superior sagittal sinus, also occurs without known predisposing factors, probably due to the trauma even in relatively normal deliveries.

Clinical features. The initial symptom is focal seizures or lethargy beginning any time during the first month. Intracranial pressure remains normal, lethargy slowly resolves, and seizures tend to respond to anticonvulsants. The long-term outcome is uncertain and probably depends on the extent of hemorrhagic infarction of the hemisphere.

Diagnosis. CT venogram or MRI venogram is the standard test for diagnosis. CT venogram is a more sensitive and accurate imaging modality; however, MRI is preferred due to the absence of radiation.

Management. Anticoagulation may decrease the risk of thrombus progression, venous congestion leading to hemorrhage and stroke, and facilitate recanalization of the venous sinus. Response to therapy varies widely, and dosages of low molecular weight heparin frequently require readjustment to maintain therapeutic anti-Xa levels of 0.5–1 U/mL. A starting dose of 1.7 mg/kg every 12 hours for term infants, or 2.0 mg/kg every 12 hours for preterm infants, may be beneficial.[24] Ultimately, therapeutic decisions must incorporate treatment of the underlying cause of the thrombosis, if known.

Primary subarachnoid hemorrhage

Clinical features. Blood in the subarachnoid space probably originates from tearing of the superficial veins by shearing forces during a prolonged delivery with the head molding. Mild HIE is often associated with SAH, but the newborn is usually well when suddenly an unexpected seizure occurs on the first or second day of life. Lumbar puncture, performed because of suspected sepsis, reveals blood in the CSF. The physician may suspect a traumatic lumbar puncture; however, red blood cell counts in the first and last tube typically show similar counts in SAH and show clearing numbers in traumatic taps. Most newborns with SAHs will not suffer long-term sequelae.

Diagnosis. CT is useful to document the extent of hemorrhage. Blood is present in the interhemispheric fissure and the supratentorial and infratentorial recesses. EEG may reveal epileptiform activity without background suppression. This suggests that HIE is not the cause of the seizures and that the prognosis is more favorable. Clotting studies are needed to evaluate the possibility of a bleeding diathesis.

Management. Seizures usually respond to anticonvulsants. Specific therapy is not available for the hemorrhage, and posthemorrhagic hydrocephalus is uncommon.

Subdural hemorrhage

Clinical features. Subdural hemorrhage is usually the consequence of a tear in the tentorium near its junction with the falx. Causes of a tear include excessive vertical molding of the head in vertex presentation, anteroposterior elongation of the head in face and brow presentations, or prolonged delivery of the aftercoming head in breech presentation. Blood collects in the posterior fossa and may produce brainstem compression. The initial features are those of mild to moderate HIE. Clinical evidence of brainstem compression begins 12 hours or longer after delivery. Characteristic features include irregular respiration, an abnormal cry, declining consciousness, hypotonia, seizures, and a tense fontanelle. Intracerebellar hemorrhage is sometimes present. Mortality is high, and neurological impairment among survivors is common.

Diagnosis. MRI, CT, or ultrasound visualizes the subdural hemorrhages.

Management. Small hemorrhages do not require treatment, but surgical evacuation of large collections relieves brainstem compression.

Incontinentia Pigmenti (Bloch-Sulzberger Syndrome)

Incontinentia pigmenti is a rare neurocutaneous syndrome involving the skin, teeth, eyes, and CNS. Genetic transmission is X-linked, with pathogenic heterozygous mutations of *IKBKG* in affected females and pathogenic hemizygous mutations in males. The loss-of-function variant is lethal in male fetuses and results in miscarriage; virtually all affected males have 47-XXY or somatic mosaicism.[25]

Clinical features. The female-to-male ratio is 20:1. An erythematous and vesicular rash resembling epidermolysis bullosa is present on the flexor surfaces of the limbs and lateral aspect of the trunk at birth or soon thereafter. The rash persists for the first few months and a verrucous eruption that lasts for weeks or months replaces the original rash. Between 6 and 12 months of age, deposits of pigment appear in the previous area of rash in bizarre polymorphic arrangements. The pigmentation later regresses and leaves a linear hypopigmentation. Alopecia, hypodontia, abnormal tooth shape, and dystrophic nails may be associated. Some have retinal vascular abnormalities that predispose to retinal detachment in early childhood.

Neurological disturbances occur in fewer than half of the cases. In newborns, the prominent feature is the onset of seizures on the second or third day, often confined to one side of the body. Residual neurological handicaps may include cognitive impairment, epilepsy, hemiparesis, and hydrocephalus.

Diagnosis. The clinical findings and biopsy of the skin rash are diagnostic. The bases for diagnosis are the clinical findings and the molecular testing of the *IKBKG* gene.

Management. Neonatal seizures caused by incontinentia pigmenti usually respond to standard anticonvulsant drugs. The blistering rash requires topical medication and oatmeal baths. Regular ophthalmological examinations are needed to diagnose and treat retinal detachment.

Treatment of Neonatal Seizures

Animal studies suggest that continuous seizure activity, even in the normoxemic brain, may cause brain damage by inhibiting protein synthesis, breaking down polyribosomes, and via neurotransmitter toxicity. In premature newborns, an additional concern is that the increased cerebral blood flow associated with seizures will increase the risk of intraventricular hemorrhage. Protein binding of anticonvulsant drugs may be impaired in premature newborns and the free fraction concentration may be toxic, whereas the measured protein-bound fraction appears therapeutic.

The initial steps in managing newborns with seizures are to maintain vital function, identify and correct the underlying cause, that is, hypocalcemia or sepsis, when possible, and rapidly provide a therapeutic blood concentration of an anticonvulsant drug when needed.

In the past, treatment of neonatal seizures had little support based on evidence. Conventional treatments with phenobarbital and phenytoin seem to be equally effective or ineffective.[26] Levetiracetam, oxcarbazepine, and lamotrigine have been studied in infants as young as 1 month of age, demonstrating safety and efficacy.[27–31]

When treating neonatal seizures we must first answer two questions: (1) Is the treatment effective? Neonates have a different chloride transporter in the first weeks of life, and opening the chloride pore by gamma-aminobutyric acid (GABA) activation may result in a hyperexcitable state rather than an anticonvulsant effect. Furthermore, neuromotor dissociation has been documented when using phenobarbital in neonates, causing cessation of clinical convulsions while electrographic seizures continue. (2) Are the seizures worse than the possible unknown and known negative effects of medications in the developing brain, such as apoptosis? A few brief focal seizures may be acceptable in the setting of a resolving neonatal encephalopathy.

Antiepileptic Drugs

Levetiracetam. IV levetiracetam (100 mg/mL) provides a newer and safer option for the treatment of newborns. Because levetiracetam is not liver metabolized, but excreted unchanged in the urine, no drug-drug interactions exist. Use of the drug requires maintaining urinary output. We consider it an excellent treatment option and recommend it as initial therapy. The initial dose is 30–40 mg/kg; the maintenance dose is 40 mg/kg/day in the first 6 months of life, and up to 60 mg/kg/day between 6 months and 4 years. The maintenance dose is dependent on renal clearance. Reduce the dosage and dosing interval in neonates with hypoxic injury with associated lower renal function.

Oxcarbazepine. Oxcarbazepine suspension is a good option in neonates with functioning gastrointestinal tracts and a lower risk for necrotizing enterocolitis. Doses between 20 and 40 mg/kg/day for infants less than 6 months, and up to 60 mg/kg/day divided two or three times a day are adequate for older infants and young children. We find this drug helpful in all localization-related epilepsies, but particularly in benign neonatal and infantile epilepsies where levetiracetam is often less effective.

Phenobarbital. IV phenobarbital is a widely used drug for the treatment of newborns with seizures. However, its efficacy and safety remain controversial. The chloride transporters in newborns may convert phenobarbital into a proconvulsant or at least a less effective anticonvulsant. The possible antiseizure effect in this age group may be explained by extrasynaptic effects. A unitary relationship usually exists between the IV dose of phenobarbital in milligrams per kilogram of body weight and the blood concentration in micrograms per milliliter measured 24 hours after the load. A 20 μg/mL blood concentration is safely achievable with a single IV loading dose of 20 mg/kg injected at a rate of 5 mg/min. The usual maintenance dose is 4 mg/kg/day. Use additional boluses of 10 mg/kg, to a total of 40 mg/kg, for those who fail to respond to the initial load. In term newborns with intractable seizures from HIE, the use of this drug to achieve a burst-suppression pattern is an alternative (likely extrasynaptic effect). The half-life of phenobarbital in newborns varies from 50 to 200 hours.

Phenytoin. *Fosphenytoin sodium* is safer than phenytoin for IV administration. Oral doses of phenytoin are poorly absorbed in newborns. The efficacy of phenytoin in newborns is less than impressive and concerns exist regarding potential apoptosis. A single IV injection of 20 mg/kg at a rate of 0.5 mg/kg/min safely achieves a therapeutic blood concentration of 15–20 μg/mL (40–80 μmol/L). The half-life is long during the first week, and the basis for further administration is current knowledge of the blood concentration. Most newborns require a maintenance dosage of 5–10 mg/kg/day. We prefer fosphenytoin over phenobarbital when levetiracetam fails.

Lacosamide

Lacosamide is approved for use in children over the age of 4 years. Initial case series show good efficacy and tolerability in the neonatal population, but larger studies are needed.[32]

Duration of Therapy

Seizures caused by an acute, self-limited, and resolved encephalopathy, such as mild HIE, do not ordinarily require prolonged maintenance therapy. In most newborns, seizures stop when the acute encephalopathy is over. Therefore discontinuation of therapy after a period of complete seizure control is reasonable unless signs of permanent cortical injury are confirmed by EEG, imaging, or clinical examination. If seizures recur, reinitiate antiepileptic therapy.

In contrast to newborns with seizures caused by acute resolved encephalopathy, treat seizures caused by cerebral dysgenesis or symptomatic epilepsies continuously as most of them are lifetime epileptic conditions.

PAROXYSMAL DISORDERS IN CHILDREN LESS THAN 2 YEARS OLD

The pathophysiology of PNDs in infants is more variable than in newborns (Box 1.7). Seizures, especially febrile seizures, are the main cause of PNDs in infants and young toddlers, but apnea and syncope (breath-holding spells) are relatively common as well. Often the basis

---

BOX 1.7   Paroxysmal Disorders in Children Younger Than 2 Years

- Apnea and Breath-holding
  - Cyanotic[a]
  - Pallid
- Dystonia
  - Glutaric aciduria (see Chapter 14)
  - Transient paroxysmal dystonia of infancy
- Migraine
  - Benign paroxysmal vertigo[a] (see Chapter 10)
  - Cyclic vomiting[a]
  - Paroxysmal torticollis[a] (see Chapter 14)
- Seizures[a]
- Epilepsy triggered by fever
- Infection of the nervous system
- Simple febrile seizure
  - Febrile seizures
  - Nonfebrile seizures
- Benign familial infantile seizures
- Ictal laughter
- Generalized tonic-clonic seizures
- Focal seizures
  - Myoclonic seizures
  - Infantile spasms
  - Benign myoclonic epilepsy
  - Severe myoclonic epilepsy
  - Myoclonic status
  - Lennox-Gastaut syndrome
  - Stereotypies (see Chapter 14)

[a]The most common conditions and the ones with disease-modifying treatments.

---

for requested neurological consultation in infants with PNDs is the suspicion of seizures. The determination of which "spells" are seizures is difficult and relies more on obtaining a complete description of the spell than any diagnostic tests. Ask the parents to provide a sequential history. If more than one spell occurred, they should first describe the one that was best observed or most recent. After listening to the description of the event by a direct observer, the following questions should be included: What was the child doing before the spell? Did anything provoke the spell? Did the child's color change? If so, when and to what color? Did the eyes move in any direction? Did the spell affect one body part more than other parts?

In addition to obtaining a home video of the spell, ambulatory or prolonged video-EEG monitoring is the only way to identify the nature of unusual spells. Seizures characterized by decreased motor activity with indeterminate changes in the level of consciousness arise from the temporal, temporoparietal, or parieto-occipital regions, while seizures with motor activity usually arise from the frontal, central, or frontoparietal regions.

Apnea and Syncope

The definition of infant apnea is cessation of breathing for 15 seconds or longer, or for less than 15 seconds if accompanied by bradycardia. Premature newborns with respiratory distress syndrome may continue to have apneic spells as infants, especially if they are neurologically abnormal.

Apneic Seizures

Apnea alone is rarely a seizure manifestation. The frequency of apneic seizures relates inversely to age, more often in newborns than infants, and rare in children. Isolated apnea occurs as a seizure manifestation in infants and young children, but when reviewed on video, identification of other features becomes possible. Overall, reflux accounts for much more apnea than seizures in most infants and young children. Unfortunately, among infants with apneic seizures, diagnostic EEG abnormalities often only appear at the time of apnea. Therefore monitoring is required for diagnosis.

Breath-Holding Spells

Breath-holding spells with loss of consciousness occur in almost 5% of infants and young children. The cause is a disturbance in central autonomic regulation probably transmitted by autosomal dominant inheritance with incomplete penetrance. Approximately 20%–30% of parents of affected children have a history of the condition. The term *breath-holding* is a misnomer because breathing always stops at expiration. Both cyanotic and pallid breath-holding occur; cyanotic spells are three times more common than pallid spells. Most children experience only one or the other, but 20% have both.

The spells are involuntary responses to adverse stimuli. In approximately 80% of affected children, the spells begin before 18 months of age, and in all cases they start before 3 years of age. The last episode usually occurs by age 4 years and no later than age 8 years.

Cyanotic syncope

Clinical features. The usual provoking stimulus for cyanotic spells is anger, pain, frustration, or fear. The infant's sibling takes away a toy, the child cries, and then stops breathing in expiration. Cyanosis develops rapidly, followed quickly by limpness and loss of consciousness. Crying may not precede cyanotic episodes provoked by pain.

If the attack lasts for only seconds, the infant may resume crying on awakening. Most spells, especially the ones referred for neurological evaluation, are longer and are associated with tonic posturing of the body and trembling movements of the hands or arms. The eyes may roll upward. These movements are mistaken for seizures by even experienced observers, but they are probably a brainstem release phenomenon. Concurrent EEG shows flattening of the record, not seizure activity.

After a short spell, the child rapidly recovers and seems normal immediately; after a prolonged spell, the child first arouses and then goes to sleep. Once an infant begins having breath-holding spells, the frequency increases for several months and then declines, and finally ceases.

Diagnosis. The typical sequence of cyanosis, apnea, and loss of consciousness is critical for diagnosis. Cyanotic syncope and epilepsy are confused because of a lack of attention to the precipitating event. It is not sufficient to ask, "Did the child hold his breath?" The question conjures up the image of breath-holding during inspiration. Instead, questioning should be focused on precipitating events, absence of breathing, facial color, and family history. The family often has a history of breath-holding spells or syncope.

Between attacks, the EEG is normal. During an episode, the EEG first shows diffuse slowing and then rhythmic slowing followed by background attenuation during the tonic-clonic, tonic, myoclonic, or clonic activity.

Management. Education and reassurance. The family should be educated to leave the child in a supine position with airway protection until they recover consciousness. Picking up the child, which is the natural act of the mother or observer, prolongs the spell. If the spells occur in response to discipline or denial of the child's wishes, we recommend caretakers comfort the child but remain firm in their decision, as otherwise, children may learn that crying translates into getting their wish. This may in turn reinforce the spells.

Pallid syncope

Clinical features. The provocation of pallid syncope is usually a sudden, unexpected, painful event such as a bump on the head. The child rarely cries but instead becomes white and limp and loses consciousness. These episodes are truly terrifying to behold. Parents invariably believe the child is dead and begin mouth-to-mouth resuscitation. After the initial limpness, the body may stiffen, and clonic movements of the arms may occur. As in cyanotic syncope, these movements represent a brainstem release phenomenon, not seizure activity. The duration of the spell is difficult to determine because the observer is so frightened that seconds seem like hours. Afterward, the child often falls asleep and is normal on awakening.

Diagnosis. Pallid syncope is the result of reflex asystole. Pressure on the eyeballs to initiate a vagal reflex provokes an attack. We do not recommend provoking an attack as an office procedure. The history alone is diagnostic.

Management. Pallid syncope can, in rare cases, be associated with cardiac arrhythmias or structural anomalies, and we recommend that all children with pallid syncopal episodes be evaluated by a cardiologist. Approximately 6% of children with syncope have an underlying cardiac cause.[33] We have treated one child with pallid breath-holding who was subsequently diagnosed with long QT syndrome, and another who was discovered to have an arrhythmia requiring pacemaker placement. Provided the cardiac workup is normal, reassurance remains the standard treatment.

Normal Self-Stimulatory Behavior

This behavior (previously mislabeled as "infantile masturbation" and later as "gratification disorder") is a normal, nonsexual behavior in young children.

Self-stimulation of the genitalia is a common sexual behavior in normal adolescents and adults. This is more often displayed publicly, without intention, in patients with cognitive impairment. Self-stimulatory behavior in younger children is usually seen in children with normal or advanced development who become aware of the different sensations around their genitalia.

Clinical features. Normal children, girls more than boys, are referred for suspected seizures due to a stereotyped scissoring posturing or bicycling-like motion of legs for seconds or minutes while lying in bed or on the floor. This is common during drowsiness and often followed by normal sleep.

Diagnosis. A good history and obtaining a video of the event are all we need for diagnosis.

Management. Reassure parents about the benign nonsexual nature of this behavior.

Hereditary Hyperekplexia

Hereditary hyperekplexia (HPX), formerly called a stiff-infant syndrome, is caused by impaired inhibitory glycinergic transmission. An exaggerated startle that does not habituate is pathognomonic. Inheritance may be autosomal dominant or autosomal recessive and is caused by pathogenic changes in the *GLRA1*, *GLRB*, or *SLC6A5* genes. Importantly, hyperekplexia is a symptom of various other acquired or genetic/metabolic conditions, many of which are not as benign as HPX. Therefore the workup of an infant with an exaggerated startle may be extensive. Both autosomal dominant and autosomal recessive forms exist.[34]

Clinical features. The onset is at birth or early infancy. When the onset is at birth, the newborn may appear hypotonic during sleep and develop generalized stiffening on awakening. Tonic apneic episodes cause significant cyanosis in some infants and may be life-threatening. Infants and children experience an exaggerated startle response, sometimes followed by generalized stiffening. Congenital hernias, sleep disorders, epilepsy, and developmental delay occur in some patients.[35] Apnea and an exaggerated startle response are associated signs. Hypertonia in the newborn is unusual. Rigidity diminishes but does not disappear during sleep. Tendon reflexes are brisk, and the response spreads to other muscles.

The stiffness resolves spontaneously during infancy, and by 3 years of age most children are normal; however, episodes of stiffness may recur during adolescence or early adult life in response to startle, cold exposure, or pregnancy. Throughout life, affected individuals show a pathologically exaggerated startle response to visual, auditory, or tactile stimuli that would not startle normal individuals. In some, the startle is associated with a transitory, generalized stiffness of the body that causes falling without protective reflexes, often leading to injury. The stiffening response is often confused with the stiff person syndrome (see Chapter 8).

Other findings include periodic limb movements in sleep and hypnagogic (occurring when falling asleep) myoclonus. Intellect is usually normal.

Diagnosis. A family history of startle disease helps the diagnosis but often is lacking. In startle disease, unlike startle-provoked epilepsy, the EEG is always normal. Infants with recurrent episodes of exaggerated startle responses are often referred due to concern for infantile spasms, and prolonged EEG monitoring may be needed to confirm the episodes are not epileptic. MRI brain is obtained to rule out acquired causes of hyperekplexia. Genetic testing is available and confirms the diagnosis.

Management. Clonazepam is the most useful agent to reduce the attack frequency. Valproate, clobazam, phenytoin, and carbamazepine have been used with variable success. Tonic apneic episodes can be aborted by forcefully flexing the head and legs in toward the trunk. Affected infants get better with time.

Febrile Seizures

An infant's first seizure often occurs at the time of fever. Three explanations are possible: (1) an infection of the nervous system; (2) an underlying seizure disorder in which the stress of fever triggers the seizure, although subsequent seizures may be afebrile; or (3) a *febrile seizure*, a genetic age-limited condition in which seizures occur only with fever. Nervous system infection is discussed in Chapters 2, 4, and 5. Children who have seizures from encephalitis or meningitis do not wake up immediately afterward; they are usually obtunded or comatose. The distinction between epilepsy and simple febrile seizures is sometimes difficult and may require time rather than laboratory tests.

Epilepsy specialists who manage monitoring units have noted that a large proportion of adults with intractable seizures secondary to mesial temporal sclerosis have prior histories of febrile seizures as children. The reverse is not true. Among children with febrile seizures, mesial temporal sclerosis is a rare event.[36]

Clinical features. Febrile seizures not caused by infection or another definable cause occur in approximately 4% of children. Only 2% of children whose first seizure is associated with fever will have nonfebrile seizures (epilepsy) by age 7 years. The most important predictor of subsequent epilepsy is an abnormal neurological or developmental state. *Complex febrile seizures*, defined as prolonged, focal, or multiple seizures within a 24-hour period, and a family history of epilepsy slightly increase the probability of subsequent epilepsy.

A single, brief, generalized seizure occurring in association with fever is likely to be a simple febrile seizure. The seizure need not occur during the time when the fever is rising. "Brief" and "fever" are difficult to define. Parents do not time seizures. When a child has a seizure, seconds seem like minutes. A prolonged seizure is one that is still in progress after the family has contacted the doctor or has left the house for the emergency room. Postictal sleep is not part of seizure time.

Simple febrile seizures are familial; multiple genes and inheritance patterns have been identified, although our genetic understanding of this disorder remains incomplete. One-third of infants who have a first simple febrile seizure will have a second one at the time of a subsequent febrile illness, and half of these will have a third febrile seizure. The risk of recurrence increases if the first febrile seizure occurs before 18 months of age or at a body temperature less than 40°C. More than three episodes of simple febrile seizures are unusual and suggest that the child may later have nonfebrile seizures.

Diagnosis. Any child thought to have an infection of the nervous system should undergo a lumbar puncture for examination of the CSF. Approximately one-quarter of children with bacterial or viral meningitis have seizures. After the seizure from CNS infection, prolonged obtundation is expected.

In contrast, infants who have simple febrile seizures usually look normal after the seizure. Lumbar puncture is unnecessary following a brief, generalized seizure from which the child recovers rapidly and completely, especially if the fever subsides spontaneously or is otherwise explained.

Blood cell counts, measurements of glucose, calcium, electrolytes, urinalysis, EEG, and cranial CT or MRI on a routine basis are not cost-effective and we discourage their use in patients with simple febrile seizures. Individual decisions for laboratory testing depend on the clinical circumstance. Obtain an EEG on every infant who is not neurologically normal or who has a family history of epilepsy. Infants with complex febrile seizures may benefit from an EEG or MRI.

Management. Because only one-third of children with an initial febrile seizure have a second seizure, treating every affected child is unreasonable. Treatment is unnecessary in the low-risk group with a single, brief, generalized seizure. No evidence has shown that a second or third simple febrile seizure causes epilepsy or brain damage. Of note, many clinicians give parents strict instructions to monitor and treat fever immediately to avoid febrile seizures. While this is helpful, it is not always possible, and in many cases the parent only realizes the child has a fever because the child seizes. This leads to unnecessary guilt and stress for parents, and a feeling that they harmed their child by failing to recognize and treat the fever quickly enough. Parents should always be reassured that febrile seizures are not their fault. We always offer families the option to have diazepam gel or midazolam nasal spray available for prolonged or acute repetitive seizures.

At the time of presentation, it is not possible to know with certainty that seizures are simply febrile and not the initial manifestation of an underlying epilepsy. We consider the use of anticonvulsant medication in the following situations:

1. Complex febrile seizures in children with neurological deficits.
2. Recurrent simple or complex febrile seizures in children with a strong family history of epilepsy.
3. Febrile status epilepticus.
4. Febrile seizures with a frequency higher than once per quarter.

EPILEPSIES EXACERBATED BY FEVER

SCN1A-Related Disorders

The most common epilepsies exacerbated by fever are caused by pathogenic variants in the *SCN1A* gene, which lead to various syndromes, including Dravet syndrome (DS) and genetic epilepsy with febrile seizures plus (GEFS+). DS in particular is highly associated with loss-of-function *SCN1A* mutations; GEFS+ is more heterogeneous and is associated with multiple other genetic variants as well as some *SCN1A* gain-of-function mutations. Undoubtedly our classification of these disorders will continue to evolve as we gain further understanding of their complex genetics.

Dravet Syndrome

Clinical features. DS is suspected in children with complex febrile seizures evolving into difficult-to-control epilepsies, exacerbated by antiseizure medications with sodium blocking mechanism of action (carbamazepine, oxcarbazepine, phenytoin, or lamotrigine). The first seizures are frequently febrile and prolonged, and can be generalized or focal clonic in type. Febrile and nonfebrile seizures recur, sometimes as status epilepticus. Generalized myoclonic or atonic seizures appear after 1 year of age. Complex partial seizures with secondary generalization may also occur. Coincident with the onset of myoclonic/atonic seizures are the slowing of development and the gradual appearance of ataxia and hyperreflexia.

Diagnosis. The diagnosis is based on the phenotype, but genetic testing is increasingly important. Up to 80% of patients have a mutation on *SCN1A* with a negative effect on sodium channel function. Genetic testing (positive in 80% of cases) is helpful and may prevent further unnecessary EEGs or imaging studies.

Management. Avoid sodium channel drugs. Medications such as levetiracetam,[37] divalproex sodium, topiramate, zonisamide, rufinamide, and management with a ketogenic diet are good options. Epidiolex (cannabinoid) is a US Food and Drug Administration (FDA)–approved drug for the treatment of DS. Fintepla (fenfluramine) was recently approved for use, and clinical trials show such significant efficacy in DS that we recommend clinicians consider initiating it as soon as the diagnosis is confirmed.[38] Patients should have a soft helmet to prevent head injury during seizure-related falls. Encourage parents to take a class in cardiopulmonary resuscitation (CPR). A written emergency room protocol that families carry with them is often helpful. Prenatal counseling and genetic testing of the patient's siblings should be considered.

Genetic Epilepsy With Febrile Seizures Plus

Clinical features. GEFS+ was previously termed generalized epilepsy with febrile seizures plus until it was discovered that focal seizures occur in the disorder as well. Suspect GEFS+ in patients with family histories of generalized or focal epilepsies and recurrent febrile seizures. GEFS+ presents with a broad range of phenotypes, and clinical manifestations may vary among family members. As mentioned previously, it is most commonly associated with pathogenic mutations of the *SCN1A* gene, although multiple other genes have been identified, including *SCN1B* and *GABRG2*.[39]

Diagnosis. The diagnosis has traditionally been based on the phenotype, which is highly variable regarding manifestations, prognosis, and response to treatment. Genetic testing identifying clinically significant pathogenic variants may help clarify the diagnosis.

Management. Wide-spectrum antiseizure medications are recommended, including divalproex sodium, levetiracetam, zonisamide, topiramate, clobazam, and perampanel. Lacosamide and lamotrigine are helpful in some cases. GEFS+ may be caused by mutations not involving the voltage-gated sodium channel, and sodium channel drugs can be used with caution.

Nonfebrile Seizures in Children Under the Age of 2 Years

Disorders that produce nonfebrile seizures in infants and young toddlers are not substantially different from those that cause nonfebrile seizures in childhood (see the following section). Major risk factors for the development of epilepsy in infancy and childhood are congenital malformations (especially migrational errors), neonatal seizures and insults, and a family history of epilepsy. Epilepsies that tend to present specifically in this age group include benign familial neonatal and infantile epilepsy (discussed in the previous section on neonatal seizures) and various types of symptomatic epilepsy.

Multiple studies have been done to evaluate the recurrence risk and prognosis of unprovoked seizures in young children. Estimates vary widely depending on the population and the methods used, but in general the recurrence rate is higher in children with neurological or developmental abnormalities, focal seizures, younger age, and abnormal EEG results (particularly focal discharges).[40,41]

Intractable epilepsy in children less than 2 years of age is often associated with later cognitive impairment. The seizure types with the greatest probability of cognitive impairment in descending order are infantile spasms, myoclonic/atonic, tonic-clonic, complex partial, and simple partial.

Myoclonus, Spasms, and Myoclonic Seizures

Infantile spasms. Infantile spasms are age-dependent seizures that occur with an incidence of 25 per 100,000 live births in the United States and Western Europe. An underlying cause can be determined in approximately 75% of patients; congenital malformations and perinatal asphyxia are common causes, and tuberous sclerosis accounts for 20% of cases in some series (Box 1.8).

BOX 1.8 **Neurocutaneous Disorders Causing Seizures in Infancy**

- Incontinentia pigmenti
  - Seizure type
    - Neonatal seizures
    - Generalized tonic-clonic
  - Cutaneous manifestations
    - Erythematous bullae (newborn)
    - Pigmentary whorls (infancy)
    - Depigmented areas (childhood)
- Linear nevus sebaceous syndrome
  - Seizure type
    - Infantile spasms
    - Lennox-Gastaut syndrome
    - Generalized tonic-clonic
  - Cutaneous manifestation
    - Linear facial sebaceous nevus
- Neurofibromatosis
  - Seizure type
    - Generalized tonic-clonic
    - Partial complex
    - Partial simple motor
  - Cutaneous manifestations
    - Café au lait spots
    - Axillary freckles
    - Neural tumors
- Sturge-Weber syndrome
  - Seizure type
    - Epilepsia partialis continua
    - Partial simple motor
    - Status epilepticus
  - Cutaneous manifestation
    - Hemifacial hemangioma
- Tuberous sclerosis
  - Seizure type
    - Neonatal seizures
    - Infantile spasms
    - Lennox-Gastaut syndrome
    - Generalized tonic-clonic
    - Partial simple motor
    - Partial complex
  - Cutaneous manifestations
    - Abnormal hair pigmentation
    - Adenoma sebaceum
    - Café au lait spots
    - Depigmented areas
    - Shagreen patch

The combination of infantile spasms, agenesis of the corpus callosum (as well as other midline cerebral malformations), and retinal malformations is referred to as *Aicardi syndrome*.[42] Affected children are always females, and genetic transmission of the disorder is an X-linked dominant trait with hemizygous lethality in males.

Clinical features. The peak age at onset is between 4 and 7 months, and onset almost always occurs before 1 year of age. The spasm can be a flexor, extensor, or mixed movement. Spasms generally occur in clusters during drowsiness, feedings, and shortly after the infant awakens from sleep. A rapid flexor spasm involving the neck, trunk, and limbs followed by a tonic contraction sustained for 2–10 seconds is characteristic. Less severe flexor spasms consist of dropping of the head, abduction of the arms, or flexion at the waist. Extensor spasms resemble the second component of the Moro reflex: the head moves backward and the arms suddenly spread. Whether flexor or extensor, the movement is usually symmetrical and brief and tends to occur in clusters with similar intervals between spasms. Spasms often upset the infant, and she may fuss or cry during the cluster.

When the spasms are secondary to an identifiable cause (symptomatic), the infant is usually abnormal neurologically or developmentally at the onset of spasms. Microcephaly is common in this group. Prognosis depends on the cause, the interval between the onset of clinical spasm and hypsarrhythmia, and the rapidity of treatment and control.

Idiopathic spasms characteristically occur in children who had been developing normally at the onset of spasms and have no history of prenatal or perinatal disorders. Neurological findings, including head circumference, are normal. It was previously thought that 40% of children with idiopathic spasms would be neurologically normal or only mildly cognitively impaired subsequently. Some of these children may have had benign myoclonus. With improvement in diagnostic testing, idiopathic infantile spasms are less frequent.

Diagnosis. The delay from spasm onset to diagnosis is often considerable. Infantile spasms are so unlike the usual perception of seizures that even experienced pediatricians may be slow to realize the significance of the movements. Colic or gastroesophageal reflux is often the first diagnosis because of the sudden flexor movements and is treated several weeks before suspecting seizures.

EEG helps differentiate infantile spasms from benign myoclonus of early infancy (Table 1.1). The EEG is

TABLE 1.1 Electroencephalographic (EEG) Appearance in Myoclonic Seizures of Infancy

Seizure Type	EEG Appearance
Infantile spasms	Hypsarrhythmia
	Slow spike and wave
	Burst suppression
Benign myoclonus	Normal
Benign myoclonic epilepsy	Spike and wave (3 cps)
	Polyspike and wave (3 cps)
Severe myoclonic epilepsy	Polyspike and wave (>3 cps)
Lennox–Gastaut syndrome	Spike and wave (2–2.5 cps)
	Polyspike and wave (2–2.5 cps)

cps, Cycles per second.

the single most important test for diagnosis. However, EEG findings vary with the duration of recording, sleep state, duration of illness, and underlying disorder. *Hypsarrhythmia* is the usual pattern recorded during the early stages of infantile spasms. A chaotic and continuously abnormal background of very high voltage and random slow waves and spike discharges are characteristic. The spikes vary in location from moment to moment and are generalized but never repetitive. Typical hypsarrhythmia usually starts during active sleep, progresses to quiet sleep, and finally wakefulness as a progressive epileptic encephalopathy. During quiet sleep, greater interhemispheric synchrony occurs and the background may have a burst-suppression appearance.

The EEG may normalize briefly on arousal, but when spasms recur, an abrupt attenuation of the background or high-voltage slow waves appear. Within a few weeks, greater interhemispheric synchrony replaces the original chaotic pattern of hypsarrhythmia. The distribution of epileptiform discharges changes from multifocal to generalized, and background attenuation follows the generalized discharges.

Management. A practice parameter for the medical treatment of infantile spasms is available.[43] Adrenocorticotropic hormone (ACTH), the traditional treatment for infantile spasms, is effective for short-term treatment control of the spasms. ACTH has no effect on the underlying mechanism of the disease and is only a short-term symptomatic therapy. The ideal dosages and treatment duration are not established. ACTH gel is usually given as an intramuscular injection of 150 U/m²/day with a gradual tapering at weekly intervals over 6–8 weeks. Very high-dose oral prednisolone (8 mg/kg/day, maximum dose 60 mg/day) may be just as effective for short-term control as ACTH.[44] Even when the response is favorable, one-third of patients have relapses during or after the course of treatment with ACTH or prednisone.

Several alternative treatments avoid the adverse effects of corticosteroids and may have a longer-lasting effect. Clonazepam, levetiracetam,[45,46] and zonisamide[47] are probably the safest alternatives. Valproate monotherapy controls spasms in 70% of infants with doses of 20–60 mg/kg/day, but due to concern for fatal hepatotoxicity, it has limited use in this age group. This concern is higher in cases in which an underlying inborn error of metabolism is suspected. Mitochondrial disease may exist and increase the risk of liver failure even in the absence of valproate. Topiramate is an effective adjunctive treatment in doses up to 30 mg/kg/day.[48] At higher doses it may cause several side effects, including drowsiness and anorexia; the most significant is a possible metabolic acidosis at high doses due to its carbonic anhydrase activity. Such side effects would not be desirable in a less devastating epilepsy syndrome, but in this case we advise parents that we may need to tolerate some short-term side effects to protect the long-term function of their child's brain. Anorexia to the point of dehydration, profound sedation, failure to thrive, and significant metabolic acidosis indicate that modification of the treatment plan is necessary.

Vigabatrin is effective for treating spasms in children with tuberous sclerosis and perhaps cortical dysplasia.[49] This medication is also helpful in other etiologies. The main concern regarding vigabatrin is the loss of peripheral vision. Its use is justified in children with *West syndrome* (infantile spasms, developmental regression, and hypsarrhythmia) as most of them have cortical visual impairment as part of the epileptic encephalopathy and may actually gain functional vision if vigabatrin is effective.

Monotherapy for infantile spasms often fails, which suggests that early polypharmacy may provide better chances of controlling the progressive epileptic encephalopathy; clinical trials are ongoing at the time of publication. The authors often combine ACTH or prednisone with rapid titration of topiramate or vigabatrin. Ongoing trials with cannabidiol, allosteric modulation of GABA receptors, and dietary modifications may provide additional therapy options. Close follow-up with serial EEGs is essential for evaluation of treatment efficacy, and to determine the need for additional anticonvulsants. Always remember: time is brain!

Benign spasms of infancy

Clinical features. Benign spasms of infancy (previously referred to as benign myoclonus of infancy) is a rare disorder that is not well understood but appears to be harmless. Many series of patients with infantile spasms include a small number with normal EEG results. Such infants cannot be distinguished from others with infantile spasms by clinical features because the age at onset and the appearance of the movements are the same. The spasms occur in clusters, frequently at mealtime. Clusters increase in intensity and severity over a period of weeks or months and then abate spontaneously. After 3 months, the spasms usually stop altogether, and although they may recur occasionally, no spasms occur after 2 years of age. Affected infants are normal neurologically and developmentally and remain so afterward.

Diagnosis. Because the symptomatology is clinically indistinguishable from epileptic infantile spasms, a normal EEG *during a spasm* is required for diagnosis.

Management. Education and reassurance.

Benign myoclonic epilepsy.

Benign myoclonic epilepsy is a rare disorder comprising only a small percentage of childhood epilepsies. Its exact incidence is uncertain due to significant clinical overlap with myoclonic-astatic epilepsy (*Doose syndrome*, discussed later in this chapter).

Clinical features. Benign myoclonic epilepsy is a rare disorder of uncertain cause. Onset is between 4 months and 2 years of age. Affected infants are neurologically normal at the onset of seizures and typically remain so afterward. Brief myoclonic attacks characterize the seizures. These may be restricted to head nodding or may be so severe as to throw the child to the floor. The head drops to the chest, the eyes roll upward, the arms move upward and outward, and the legs flex. Myoclonic seizures may be single or repetitive, but consciousness is not lost. Seizures are often triggered by light (photosensitivity) and may occur more during drowsiness. No other seizure types occur in infancy, but generalized tonic-clonic seizures may occur in adolescence. Many patients have a family history of epilepsy, and pathogenic variants in *SLC2A1* and *HCN4* have been found in some cases.[50]

Diagnosis. EEG during a seizure shows generalized spike-wave or polyspike-wave discharges. The pattern is consistent with genetic generalized epilepsy.

Management. Valproate produces complete seizure control, but levetiracetam and zonisamide are safer options for initial treatment. Developmental outcome generally is good with early treatment, but cognitive impairment may develop in some children, particularly if seizures are not well controlled.

Early epileptic encephalopathy with burst suppression.

The term *epileptic encephalopathy* encompasses several syndromes in which an encephalopathy is associated with continuous epileptiform activity. Two distinct syndromes are recognized in this age group: early infantile epileptic encephalopathy (EIEE or *Ohtahara syndrome*) and early myoclonic epileptic encephalopathy (EMEE).[51]

Clinical features. EIEE presents with tonic spasms, and EMEE presents with myoclonic seizures. Seizures are explosive in onset and relentless in progression. Pathogenic variants of the *STXBP1*, *ARX*, *STK9*, and *CDKL5* genes cause more than 50% of EIEE cases. Many of these mutations are de novo but may require genetic counseling. Progression to infantile spasms and Lennox-Gastaut syndrome (LGS) is common, as with all epilepsies refractory to medical treatment.

Diagnosis. EEG demonstrates diffuse background suppression alternating with bursts of diffuse, high-amplitude, spike-wave complexes.

Management. Seizures are refractory or only partially responsive to most anticonvulsant drugs. The treating clinician typically cycles through several drugs alone and in combination to achieve some level of control. Topiramate, lacosamide, clobazam, vigabatrin, and levetiracetam are potential treatments. High-dose steroids, pyridoxine, and folinic acid are often trialed while awaiting definitive diagnosis.

Severe myoclonic epilepsy of infancy (Dravet syndrome).

Severe myoclonic epilepsy of infancy (DS) was described earlier in this chapter. Recurrent febrile seizures and febrile status epilepticus are typically the presenting symptoms.

Biotinidase deficiency.

Genetic transmission of this relatively rare disorder is an autosomal recessive trait.[52] The cause is defective biotin absorption or transport and was previously called *late-onset multiple (holo) carboxylase deficiency*.

Clinical features. The initial features in untreated infants with profound deficiency are seizures and hypotonia. Later features include hypotonia, ataxia, developmental delay, hearing loss, and cutaneous abnormalities.

In childhood, patients may also develop weakness, spastic paresis, and decreased visual acuity.

Diagnosis. Ketoacidosis, hyperammonemia, and organic aciduria are present. Newborn screen reveals biotinidase deficiency in serum and establishes the diagnosis. In profound biotinidase deficiency, mean serum biotinidase activity is less than 10% of normal. In partial biotinidase deficiency, serum biotinidase activity is 10%–30% of normal. Molecular genetic testing shows biallelic pathogenic variants of the *BTD* gene.

Management. Early, lifelong treatment with biotin 5–20 mg/day successfully reverses most of the symptoms and prevents neurologic deficits if started immediately. Provide vision aids, hearing aids, and developmental therapies as indicated. Avoid ingestion of raw eggs, as the egg-white protein avidin binds biotin and decreases the bioavailability of supplements.

Migraine

Clinical features. Migraine attacks are uncommon under the age of 2 years, but when they occur, the clinical features are often paroxysmal and suggest the possibility of seizures. Cyclic vomiting is probably the most common manifestation. Attacks of vertigo (see Chapter 10) or torticollis (see Chapter 14) may be especially perplexing, and some infants have attacks in which they rock back and forth and appear uncomfortable.

Diagnosis. The stereotypical presentation of *benign paroxysmal vertigo* is recognizable as a migraine variant. Other syndromes often remain undiagnosed until the episodes evolve into a typical migraine pattern. A history of migraine in one parent is essential for diagnosis.

Management. There is little if any evidence on migraine prophylaxis or abortive treatment in this age group. We have used small doses of amitriptyline (5 mg nightly) and cyproheptadine (2 mg once or twice daily) in cases requiring prophylaxis. A combination of ondansetron and ibuprofen given at the onset of symptoms is our preferred treatment for acute attacks; acetaminophen, prochlorperazine, or promethazine may also be used as abortive therapies.

PAROXYSMAL NEUROLOGICAL DISORDERS OF CHILDHOOD

Like infants, seizures are the usual first consideration for any paroxysmal episode of childhood. Seizures are the most common PND requiring medical consultation. Syncope, especially presyncope, is considerably more common, but diagnosis and management usually occur at home unless associated symptoms suggest a seizure.

Migraine is probably the most common etiology of PNDs in childhood; its incidence is 10 times greater than that of epilepsy. Chapters 2, 3, 10, 11, 14, and 15 describe migraine syndromes that may suggest epilepsy. Several links exist between migraine and epilepsy[53]: (1) ion channel disorders cause both, (2) both are genetic, paroxysmal, and associated with transitory neurological disturbances, (3) migraine sufferers have an increased incidence of epilepsy and epileptics have an increased incidence of migraine, and (4) they are both disorders associated with a hyperexcitable brain cortex. In children who have epilepsy and migraine, both disorders may have a common aura and one may provoke the other. Migraine with brainstem aura (see Chapter 10) and benign occipital epilepsy best exemplify the fine line between epilepsy and migraine. Characteristics of both are seizures, headache, and epileptiform activity. Children who have both epilepsy and migraine require treatment for each condition, but some drugs (valproate and topiramate) serve as prophylactic agents for both.

Paroxysmal Dyskinesias

Paroxysmal dyskinesia occurs in several different syndromes; the general term "dyskinesia" encompasses several different types of movements, including dystonia, chorea, athetosis, ballismus, and myoclonus. Paroxysmal kinesiogenic dyskinesia (PKD) is associated with pathogenic *PRRT2* mutations, as is paroxysmal kinesiogenic dyskinesia with infantile convulsions (PKD/IC) and benign familial infantile epilepsy. Paroxysmal nonkinesiogenic dyskinesia (PNKD) is caused by *PNKD* mutations. Both are inherited in an autosomal dominant pattern. Other rare causes of paroxysmal dyskinesia beginning in childhood or adolescence include *ADCY5*-related dyskinesia and paroxysmal exertion–induced dyskinesia (PED). The paroxysmal nature of dyskinesia differentiates these from other movement disorders, which will be discussed elsewhere (see Chapter 14).

Paroxysmal Kinesiogenic Dyskinesia

PKD was previously referred to as familial paroxysmal choreoathetosis. Pathogenic heterozygous *PRRT2* variants cause ~99% of cases. Genetic transmission is an autosomal dominant trait and the gene maps to chromosome 16p11.2; a small number of cases are caused by larger 16p11.2 deletions or biallelic pathogenic *PRRT2* variants.[54]

Clinical features. PKD usually begins in childhood. Sudden movement, startle, or changes in position precipitate an attack, which lasts less than a minute. Several attacks occur each day. Each attack may include dystonia, choreoathetosis, or ballismus (see Chapter 14) and may affect one or both sides of the body. Some patients have an "aura" described as tightness or tingling of the face, stomach, or limbs. Some *PRRT2* mutations can cause seizures; consider EEG if clinically warranted.

Diagnosis. The clinical features distinguish the diagnosis. Genetic testing is available.

Treatment management. Low dosages of carbamazepine or phenytoin are effective in stopping attacks. Other sodium channel drugs such as lamotrigine or oxcarbazepine may be beneficial. We have had less success with oxcarbazepine than carbamazepine.

Familial Paroxysmal Nonkinesiogenic Dyskinesia

Genetic transmission of PNKD is an autosomal dominant trait caused by mutations of the *PNKD* gene.[55]

Clinical features. PNKD usually begins in childhood or adolescence. Attacks of dystonia, chorea, and athetosis last from 5 minutes to several hours. Precipitants are alcohol, caffeine, hunger, fatigue, nicotine, and emotional stress. Preservation of consciousness is a constant during attacks and life expectancy is normal. The length of attacks and the fact that they are not precipitated by movement differentiates PNKD from PKD.

Diagnosis. Ictal and interictal EEGs are normal, and genetic testing is available.

Management. PNKD is difficult to treat, but clonazepam taken daily or at the first sign of an attack may reduce the frequency or severity of attacks. Gabapentin is effective in some children, and some case studies report efficacy with levetiracetam or acetazolamide. All affected families should receive genetic counseling.

ADCY5 Dyskinesia

This is a rare cause of paroxysmal dyskinesia presenting anywhere from infancy to late adolescence, with a wide range of phenotypes. Heterozygous pathogenic variants (or rarely, biallelic pathogenic variants) in the *ADCY5* gene cause the disorder. Inheritance is autosomal dominant with a small number of autosomal

recessive cases reported; most cases are secondary to de novo mutations.[56]

Clinical features. Hyperkinetic movements, including chorea, athetosis, dystonia, or myoclonus, are the presenting feature. Axial hypotonia and spasticity are common and can cause gross motor delays. Some affected individuals experience psychiatric symptoms, cardiomyopathy, intellectual disability, or epilepsy. Importantly, dyskinesias may persist during sleep, particularly in younger children, but EEG does not show any evidence of epilepsy. Patients may experience unexplained episodes of remission lasting days to weeks. Nonmyokymic facial twitches involving perioral or periocular muscles are common. Anxiety, stress, and drowsiness commonly exacerbate the movements.

Diagnosis. Genetic testing is available, and we recommend genetic counseling for affected families. EEG and brain MRI are normal.

Management. The disorder requires multidisciplinary care to address neurological, psychiatric, and developmental concerns. All patients should undergo cardiac evaluation. Tetrabenazine, trihexyphenidyl, clonazepam, or acetazolamide may be helpful in managing dyskinesias.

Paroxysmal Exertion–Induced Dyskinesia

Paroxysmal exertion–induced dyskinesia (PED) is caused by mutations in the *SLC2A1* gene. Other *SLC2A1* mutations cause the GLUT-1 deficiency syndrome, which is characterized by epileptic encephalopathy in addition to dyskinesia.[57]

Clinical features. In PED, attacks of chorea, athetosis, or dystonia are triggered by exercise or exertion and typically resolve in minutes to hours. Legs are the most frequently affected body parts.

Diagnosis. The clinical history suggests the appropriate genetic testing.

Management. The ketogenic diet or modified Atkins diet has been helpful in some patients. Levodopa or acetazolamide may be beneficial, but the disorder is so rare that no large-scale studies have been done.

Sleep Disorders

Certain sleep disorders can cause abnormal paroxysmal events in children.

Narcolepsy

Narcolepsy is a sleep disorder characterized by an abnormally short latency from sleep onset to rapid eye movement (REM) sleep. A person with narcolepsy attains REM sleep in less than 20 minutes instead of the usual 90 minutes. Characteristics of normal REM sleep are dreaming and severe hypotonia. In narcolepsy, these phenomena occur during wakefulness. Type 1 narcolepsy is associated with cataplexy, while type 2 occurs without cataplexy.

Human narcolepsy, unlike animal narcolepsy, is not a simple genetic trait.[58] Evidence suggests an immunologically mediated destruction of hypocretin-containing cells in human narcolepsy. An alternate name for hypocretin is *orexin*. Most cases of human narcolepsy with cataplexy have decreased hypocretin 1 in the CSF[59] and an 85%–95% reduction in the number of orexin/hypocretin-containing neurons.

Clinical features. Onset may occur at any time from early childhood to middle adulthood, usually in the second or third decade and rarely before age 5 years. The syndrome has five components:

1. *Narcolepsy* refers to short sleep attacks. Three or four attacks occur each day, most often during monotonous activity, and are difficult to resist. Half of the patients are easy to arouse from a sleep attack, and 60% feel refreshed afterward. Narcolepsy is usually a lifelong condition.
2. *Cataplexy* is a sudden loss of muscle tone induced by laughter, excitement, or startle. Cataplexy is the defining feature of type 1 narcolepsy but is absent in type 2. The patient may collapse to the floor and then arise immediately. Partial paralysis, affecting just the face or hands, is more common than total paralysis. Attacks may occur rarely or up to several times per day. They are embarrassing but usually do not cause physical harm.
3. *Sleep paralysis* occurs in the transition between sleep and wakefulness. The patient is mentally awake but unable to move because of generalized paralysis. Partial paralysis is less common. The attack may end spontaneously or when the patient is touched. Two-thirds of patients with narcolepsy-cataplexy also experience sleep paralysis once or twice each week. Occasional episodes of sleep paralysis may occur in people who do not have narcolepsy-cataplexy.
4. *Hypnagogic hallucinations* are vivid, sometimes frightening visual and auditory perceptions occurring at the transition between sleep and wakefulness, often described as a sensation of "dreaming while awake." Approximately half of the patients with narcolepsy experience hypnagogic hallucinations.
5. *Disturbed night sleep* occurs in 75% of cases and *automatic behavior* in 30%. Automatic behavior is characterized by the repeated performance of a function such as speaking or writing in a meaningless manner, or driving on the wrong side of the road or to a strange place without recalling the episode. These episodes of automatic behavior may result from partial sleep episodes.

Diagnosis. Syndrome recognition is determined by the clinical history. However, the symptoms are embarrassing or sound "crazy," and considerable prompting is required before patients divulge a full history. Narcolepsy can be difficult to distinguish from other causes of excessive daytime sleepiness. The multiple sleep latency test is the standard for diagnosis. Patients with narcolepsy enter REM sleep within a few minutes of falling asleep.

Management. Symptoms of narcolepsy tend to worsen during the first years and then stabilize, while cataplexy tends to improve with time. Two scheduled 15-minute naps each day and good sleep hygiene can reduce excessive sleepiness. Most patients also require pharmacological therapy.

Modafinil and armodafinil are first-line treatments for adults and often used "off-label" in children and adolescents due to their superior side effect profile as compared to traditional stimulants. Sodium oxybate (Xyrem) is an FDA-approved drug to treat cataplexy and excessive daytime sleepiness in children over 7 years old. SSRIs and tricyclic antidepressants help treat hallucinations, cataplexy, and sleep paralysis.[60]

Sleep (Night) Terrors and Sleepwalking

Sleep terrors and sleepwalking are partial arousals from nonrapid eye movement (NREM) sleep. A positive family history is common.

Clinical features. The onset usually occurs by 4 years of age and always by age 6 years. Two hours after falling asleep the child awakens in a terrified state, does not recognize people, and is inconsolable. An episode usually lasts for 5–15 minutes, but can last for an hour. During this time the child screams incoherently, may run if not restrained, and then goes back to sleep. Afterward, the child has no memory of the event.

Most children with sleep terrors experience an average of one or more episodes each week. Night terrors stop by 8 years of age in one-half of affected children but continue into adolescence in one-third.

Diagnosis. Half of the children with night terrors are also sleepwalkers, and many have a family history of either sleepwalking or sleep terrors. The history alone is the basis for diagnosis. A sleep laboratory evaluation often shows that children with sleep terrors suffer from sleep-disordered breathing.[61]

Management. Correction of the breathing disturbance often ends sleep terrors and sleepwalking.

Hyperventilation Syndrome

Hyperventilation induces alkalosis by altering the proportion of blood gases. This is easier to accomplish in children than in adults.

Clinical features. During times of emotional upset, the respiratory rate and depth may increase insidiously, first appearing like sighing and then as obvious hyperventilation. The occurrence of tingling in the fingers disturbs the patient further and may induce greater hyperventilation. Headache is an associated symptom. Allowing hyperventilation to continue may result in loss of consciousness.

Diagnosis. The observation of hyperventilation as a precipitating factor of syncope is essential to diagnosis. Often patients are unaware that they are hyperventilating, but probing questions elicit the history in the absence of a witness.

Management. Controlling respiration is the key to management. Age-appropriate mindfulness and meditation apps are abundantly available and often free, and most public libraries carry children's books regarding breathing exercises. Treat underlying comorbid anxiety with SSRIs when hyperventilation is frequent and disruptive.

Syncope

Syncope is a loss of consciousness because of a transitory decline in cerebral blood flow. The pathological causes include an irregular cardiac rate or rhythm, or alterations of blood volume or distribution. However, syncope is a common event in otherwise healthy children, especially in the second decade affecting girls more than boys. Diagnostic testing is rarely necessary.

Clinical features. The mechanism is a vasovagal reflex, which causes relaxation of arterial tone and produces peripheral pooling of blood. Stimuli that provoke the reflex include a sudden intense emotional experience, prolonged upright position in the setting of orthostasis, overextension or sudden decompression of viscera, the Valsalva maneuver, and stretching with the neck hyperextended. Fainting in a hot, crowded church is especially common. Usually, the faint occurs as the worshipper rises after prolonged kneeling.

Healthy children do not faint while lying down and rarely while seated. Fainting from anything but standing or arising suggests a cardiac arrhythmia and requires further investigation. The child may first feel presyncopal (described as "faint," "dizzy," or "light-headed") or may lose consciousness without warning. The face drains of color, and the skin is cold and clammy. The person often complains of nausea, feeling excessively hot or cold, and darkening of the vision (sometimes described as a dark mist rising in the visual field, other times described as "seeing spots"). With loss of consciousness, the child falls to the floor. The body may stiffen and the limbs may tremble or even have brief clonic movements resembling a seizure. The stiffening and trembling are especially common when keeping the child upright, which prolongs the reduced cerebral blood flow. A short period of confusion may follow, but recovery is complete within minutes.

Diagnosis. The criteria for differentiating syncope from seizures are a clear presyncopal prodrome, the precipitating factors, and the child's appearance. Seizures are unlikely to produce pallor and cold, clammy skin; similarly, it is unusual for seizures to produce an aura of dizziness. Diagnostic tests are not cost-effective when syncope occurs in expected circumstances, and the results of the clinical examination are normal. Recurrent orthostatic syncope requires the investigation of autonomic function, and any suspicion of cardiac abnormality deserves ECG monitoring. Always ask the child if irregular heart rate or beats occurred at the time of syncope or at other times.

Management. Infrequent syncopal episodes of obvious cause do not require treatment. Holding deep inspiration at the onset of symptoms may abort an attack.[62] Good hydration and avoiding sudden changes from prolonged supine into the standing position decrease orthostasis and orthostatic syncope.

Postural Orthostatic Tachycardia Syndrome

The postural orthostatic tachycardia syndrome (POTS) is increasingly diagnosed and has received quite a bit of attention in the lay press. For children and adolescents, diagnosis requires a heart rate increase of 40 beats per minute or more within the first 10 minutes of standing, in the absence of orthostatic hypotension.

Clinical features. Headaches, fatigue, palpitations, exercise intolerance, nausea, "brain fog," and color change or coldness in the extremities are common and can be debilitating. Approximately 50% of adult patients with POTS suffer from small fiber neuropathy; most patients have hypovolemia, and many have hypermobility or positive autoimmune markers. Elevated levels of norepinephrine on standing indicate increased sympathetic tone. There is a clear female preponderance, and the disorder is often misdiagnosed as anxiety. Anxiety is a common comorbidity but is not the cause of the condition.[63]

Diagnosis. Check the heart rate and blood pressure on lying, sitting, standing at 1 minute, and standing at 5 minutes. Tilt table testing can be done but is often difficult to obtain in the pediatric population. Consider QSART testing for patients with suspected autonomic neuropathy.

Management. Institutions vary as to whether neurologists or cardiologists manage patients with POTS. Encourage aggressive hydration with at least 2–3 L of water per day. Salt tablets or adding extra salt to the diet aids in increasing intravascular volume; compression stockings prevent blood pooling in the lower extremities. The patient must maintain some physical activity to avoid deconditioning, which worsens symptoms. Exercises that can be done in a reclining position are often tolerated the best; swimming is especially helpful for children and adolescents with joint hypermobility as there is minimal chance of impact injuries. Fludrocortisone, beta blockers, and midodrine can be helpful in cases in which conservative management is not effective. Treat associated disorders, including anxiety and depression.

Staring Spells

Daydreaming is a pleasant escape for people of all ages. Children feel the need for escape most acutely when in school and may stare vacantly out of the window to the place where they would rather be. Daydreams can be hard to break, and a child may not respond to verbal commands. Neurologists and pediatricians often recommend EEG studies for daydreamers. Sometimes the EEG shows sleep-activated central spikes or another abnormality not related to staring, which may lead the physician to prescribe inappropriate antiepileptic drug therapy. The best test for unresponsiveness during a staring spell is applying a mild noxious stimulus, such as pressure on the nail bed. Children with behavioral staring will have an immediate response and children with absence or focal seizures will have a decreased or no response.

Staring spells are characteristics of absence epilepsies and complex partial seizures. They are usually distinguishable because absence is brief (5–15 seconds) and the child feels normal immediately afterward, while focal seizures with impaired awareness usually last for more than 1 minute and are followed by fatigue and psychomotor slowing. The associated EEG patterns and the response to treatment are quite different, and the basis for appropriate treatment is precise diagnosis before initiating treatment.

Absence seizures occur in four epileptic syndromes: childhood absence epilepsy (CAE), juvenile absence epilepsy (JAE), juvenile myoclonic epilepsy (JME), and epilepsy with generalized tonic-clonic seizures alone (EGTCS). All four syndromes are genetic disorders with considerable phenotypic overlap. The most significant difference is the age at onset.

Childhood Absence Epilepsy

CAE usually begins between ages 5 and 8 years. As a rule, later onset is more likely to represent JAE, with a higher frequency of generalized tonic-clonic seizures, and persistence into adult life. CAE has been associated with multiple distinct genetic variants, many of which are not commonly tested on genetic epilepsy panels, and we recommend genetic testing only for unusual or refractory cases. Patients have an easily recognized phenotype, and the gene test provides limited if any additional benefit. At this point we only know susceptibility genes or alleles that predispose to this and other generalized genetic epilepsy syndrome such as juvenile absence, JMEs, and generalized epilepsies on awakening. It is not clear how many of these genetic factors need to coexist or what other environmental factors are required to produce clinical symptoms. This multifactorial complexity is the reason we often have patients with a negative family history with a clear phenotype.

Clinical features. The reported incidence of epilepsy in families of children with absence varies from 15% to 40%. Concurrence in monozygotic twins is 75% for seizures and 85% for the characteristic EEG abnormality.

Affected children are otherwise healthy, although attention-deficit hyperactivity disorder (ADHD) and specific learning disabilities are common comorbid conditions. Typical attacks last for 5–10 seconds and occur up to 100 times each day. The child stops ongoing activity, stares vacantly, sometimes with rhythmic movements of the eyelids or mouth, and then resumes activity. Aura and postictal confusion never occur. Longer seizures may last for up to 1 minute and are indistinguishable by observation alone from focal seizures. Associated features may include myoclonus, increased or decreased postural tone, picking at clothes, turning of the head, and conjugate movements of the eyes. Occasionally, prolonged absence status causes confusional states in children and adults. These often require emergency department visits.

A small percentage of children with absence seizures also have generalized tonic-clonic seizures. The occurrence of a generalized tonic-clonic seizure in an untreated child does not change the diagnosis or prognosis but changes medication selection for seizure control.

Diagnosis. The background rhythms in patients with typical absence seizures usually are normal. The interictal EEG pattern for typical absence seizures is a characteristic 3 Hz spike-and-wave pattern lasting less than 3 seconds that may cause no clinical changes (Fig. 1.2). Longer paroxysms of 3 cps spike-wave complexes are concurrent with the clinical seizure (ictal pattern). The amplitude of discharge is greatest in the frontocentral regions, but variants with occipital predominance may occur. Although the discharge begins with a frequency of 3 cps, it may slow to 2 cps as it ends.

Hyperventilation usually activates the discharge. The interictal EEG is usually normal, but brief generalized discharges are often seen.

Although the EEG pattern of discharge is stereotyped, variations on the theme in the form of multiple spike and wave discharges and bifrontal or bioccipital 3 Hz delta waves are also acceptable. During sleep, the discharges often lose their stereotypy and become polymorphic and change in frequency, but remain generalized. Once a correlation between clinical and EEG findings is made, looking for an underlying disease is unnecessary. The distinction between absence epilepsy and JME (see later discussion on myoclonic seizures) is the age at onset and absence of myoclonic seizures. JAE presents later, usually between the ages of 9 and 13 years, and absence seizures are less frequent than those seen in CAE.

Management. Ethosuximide and valproic acid are more effective than lamotrigine in controlling CAE without intolerable side effects. Ethosuximide has a smaller negative effect on attentional measures than valproic acid. There were no significant differences among the three groups with regard to discontinuation of treatment due to intolerable adverse events.[64]

Levetiracetam and zonisamide seem to work in a smaller percentage of patients, and topiramate is relatively ineffective for absence seizures.[65] If neither drug alone provides seizure control, use them in combination at reduced dosages or substitute another drug. The EEG becomes normal if treatment is successful, and repeating the EEG is useful to confirm the seizure-free state in some cases of continuing learning difficulties or accidents. We recommend confirming that children with concentration problems have adequately controlled seizures before beginning medication for suspected ADHD.

Refractory CAE presents unique challenges since drug choice is limited; avoid carbamazepine and oxcarbazepine as they can worsen seizures and cause absence status. Fycompa, clobazam, and the modified Atkins diet may be helpful in some patients. There is preliminary evidence to support the use of acetazolamide or amantadine in super-refractory cases.[66] In our experience surgical interventions such as the vagal nerve stimulation (VNS) are not effective; however, newer surgical therapies such as deep brain stimulation (DBS) show promise in initial clinical trials.[67]

Eyelid Myoclonia With or Without Absences (Jeavons Syndrome)

Jeavons syndrome is a distinct syndrome characterized by the triad of eyelid myoclonia with or without absence seizures, eye closure–induced generalized paroxysms, and EEG photosensitivity. It is classified as a generalized epilepsy but may represent an occipital epilepsy with rapid spreading.[68] However, frontal onset with rapid spreading is a known EEG pattern seen with clear generalized epilepsies such as absence epilepsy.

Clinical features. Children present between the ages of 2 and 14 years with eye closure–induced seizures (*eyelid myoclonia*), photosensitivity, and EEG paroxysms, which may be associated with clinical absence seizures. Eyelid myoclonia, a jerky upward deviation of the eyeballs and retropulsion of the head, is the key feature. The seizures are brief but occur multiple times per day. In

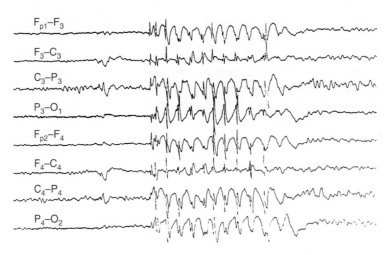

Fig. 1.2 Absence Epilepsy. A generalized burst of 3 cps spike-wave complexes appears during hyperventilation.

addition to eye closure, bright light, not just flickering light, may precipitate seizures. In many cases, Jeavons syndrome appears to be a lifelong condition. The eyelid myoclonia is resistant to treatment. The absences may respond to ethosuximide, divalproex sodium, and lamotrigine.

An apparently separate condition, *perioral myoclonia with absences*, also occurs in children. A rhythmic contraction of the orbicularis oris muscle causes protrusion of the lips and contractions of the corners of the mouth. Absence and generalized tonic-clonic seizures may occur. Such children are prone to develop absence status epilepticus.

Diagnosis. Reproduce the typical features with video/EEG.

Treatment. Treatment is similar to the other absence epilepsies: ethosuximide, lamotrigine, levetiracetam, divalproex sodium, or zonisamide.

Focal Seizures With Impaired Awareness

Consider focal seizures with impaired awareness if the staring child demonstrates decreased responsiveness for more than 30 seconds, followed by confusion or fatigue. Focal seizures arise in the cortex, most often the temporal lobe, but can originate from the frontal, occipital, or parietal lobes as well. Such seizures (discussed more fully in the section on Focal Seizures) may be symptomatic of an underlying focal disorder.

Clinical features. Impaired consciousness without generalized tonic-clonic activity characterizes focal

seizures with impaired awareness. Some level of altered mentation, lack of awareness, or amnesia for the event are essential features. They either occur spontaneously or are sleep-activated. Most last 1–2 minutes and rarely less than 30 seconds. Less than 30% of children report an aura. The aura is usually a nondescript unpleasant or "weird" feeling, but may also be a stereotyped auditory or visual hallucination or abdominal discomfort. The first feature of the seizure can be staring, automatic behavior, tonic extension of one or both arms, or loss of body tone. Staring is associated with a change in facial expression and followed by automatic behavior.

Automatisms are more or less coordinated, involuntary motor activity occurring during a state of impaired consciousness either in the course of or after an epileptic seizure and usually followed by amnesia. They vary from facial grimacing and fumbling movements of the fingers to walking, running, and resisting restraint. Automatic behavior in a given patient tends to be similar from seizure to seizure.

The seizure usually terminates with a period of postictal confusion, disorientation, or lethargy. Transitory aphasia is sometimes present with dominant hemisphere seizures. Secondary generalization is likely if the child is not treated or if treatment is abruptly withdrawn.

Focal status epilepticus is a rare event characterized by impaired consciousness, staring alternating with wandering eye movements, and automatisms of the face and hands. Such children may arrive at the emergency department in a confused or delirious state (see Chapter 2).

Diagnosis. The etiology of focal seizures with impaired awareness is heterogeneous, and a cause is often not determined. Contrast-enhanced MRI is an indicated study in all cases. It may reveal a low-grade glioma or dysplastic tissue, especially migrational defects.

Record an EEG in both the waking and sleeping states. Hyperventilation and photic stimulation typically are not useful as provocative measures. Results of a single EEG may be normal in the interictal period, but prolonged EEGs usually reveal either a spike or a slow-wave focus in the epileptogenic area. During the seizure a discharge of evolving amplitude, frequency, and morphology occurs in the involved area of cortex.

Management. All seizure medications with the exception of ethosuximide have similar efficacy in controlling partial seizures. We often select oxcarbazepine, levetiracetam, or lacosamide based on safety, tolerability, and potential side effects. Topiramate and divalproex sodium are good alternatives for migraine sufferers with debilitating headaches. Once daily medications (either extended-release formulation or those with long half-lives) provide the best chance of adherence to treatment. Families more easily remember to take once daily medicines, and they reduce toxicity by lowering peak levels while maintaining higher trough levels. Suggested medications are oxcarbazepine ER (Oxtellar XR), levetiracetam ER (Keppra XR), topiramate ER (Trokendi or Qudexy), lamotrigine ER (Lamictal XR), Divalproex (Depakote ER), perampanel (Fycompa), and zonisamide (Zonegran).

Surgery should be offered to good surgical candidates with pharmacoresistant epilepsy or unacceptable side effects. Consider a ketogenic diet and VNS for all other patients with partial response to treatments (discussed later in this chapter in the sections on Ketogenic Diet and Vagal Nerve Stimulation).

Myoclonic Seizures

Myoclonus is a brief, involuntary muscle contraction (jerk) that may represent: (1) a seizure manifestation, as in JME, (2) a physiological response to startle or to falling asleep, (3) an involuntary movement of sleep, or (4) an involuntary movement from disinhibition of the spinal cord (see Table 14.7). Myoclonic seizures are often difficult to distinguish from myoclonus (the movement disorder) on clinical grounds alone. Chapter 14 discusses *essential myoclonus* and other nonseizure causes of myoclonus.

Myoclonic-Astatic Epilepsy

Myoclonic-astatic epilepsy, also known as *Doose syndrome*, affects children aged 2–5 years. Potential genetic causes include pathogenic variants in *SYNGAP1*, *SLC6A1*, *KIAA2022*, and multiple others. It has been proposed that myoclonic-astatic epilepsy actually represents a manifestation of several distinct disorders rather than a single syndrome.[69]

Clinical features. Often the child does not come to medical attention until suffering a generalized tonic-clonic seizure; however, myoclonic and astatic seizures define the syndrome. Some children also experience absence seizures. Falls and injuries are common, as the child abruptly drops to the ground with no attempt to catch themselves. Although most children are developmentally normal before seizure onset, many develop behavior problems and speech delay.

Diagnosis. The clinical history suggests the diagnosis. EEG demonstrates generalized spike-wave and polyspike-wave discharges. Background rhythms are normal to mildly slow, and the brain MRI is normal. Genetic testing is often performed but usually not helpful.

Management. Valproic acid is the most effective treatment option. Levetiracetam, zonisamide, topiramate, and the ketogenic diet or modified Atkins diet are useful adjuncts. Many parents are taken aback by the relatively sudden appearance of developmental delays in their previously normal child; neuropsychological testing can assist in determining the child's educational and therapy needs. A soft helmet protects against head injuries. Be aware that families often struggle to find daycare centers or preschools willing to take on a child with frequent falls, whom they consider a liability. While many children outgrow the disorder, lifelong epilepsy and intellectual disability can occur.

Juvenile Myoclonic Epilepsy

JME is a hereditary disorder, probably inherited as an autosomal dominant trait.[70] It accounts for up to 10% of all cases of epilepsy. Many different genetic loci produce JME syndromes.

Clinical features. JME occurs in both genders with equal frequency. Seizures in children and their affected relatives may be tonic-clonic, myoclonic, or absence seizures. The usual age at onset of absence seizures is 7–13 years; of myoclonic jerks, 12–18 years; and of generalized tonic-clonic seizures, 13–20 years. JME may be difficult to differentiate from JAE in initial presentation.

The myoclonic seizures are brief and bilateral, but not always symmetric, flexor jerks of the arms, which may be repetitive. The jerk sometimes affects the legs, causing the patient to fall. The highest frequency of myoclonic jerks is in the morning. Consciousness is not impaired and the patient is aware of the jerking movement; some children feel distressed by their myoclonic jerks, which lead to a misdiagnosis of anxiety or nonepileptic spells. Seizures are precipitated by sleep deprivation, alcohol ingestion, and awakening from sleep.

Most patients also have generalized tonic-clonic seizures, and a third experience absence. All are otherwise normal neurologically, although attention problems and learning disabilities are potential comorbid conditions. The potential for seizures of one type or another continues throughout adult life.

Diagnosis. Delays in diagnosis are common, often until a generalized tonic-clonic seizure brings the child to medical attention. Ignoring the myoclonic jerks is commonplace. Suspect JME in any adolescent driver involved in a motor vehicle accident, when the driver has no memory of the event, but did not sustain a head injury. The interictal EEG in JME consists of bilateral, symmetrical spike, and polyspike-and-wave discharges of 3.5–6 Hz, usually maximal in the frontocentral regions (Fig. 1.3). Photic stimulation often provokes a discharge. Focal EEG abnormalities may occur.

Management. Levetiracetam is an excellent therapy, stopping seizures in almost all cases.[71] Other effective drugs include valproate, lamotrigine, zonisamide, and topiramate. We have found perampanel to provide control of generalized tonic-clonic seizures in patients' refractory to monotherapy when added to levetiracetam. Treatment is lifelong.

Lennox-Gastaut Syndrome

The triad of seizures (atypical absence, atonic, and myoclonic), 1.5–2 Hz spike-wave complexes on EEG, and cognitive impairment characterize the LGS. LGS is the description of *one stage* in the spectrum of a progressive epileptic encephalopathy. Nobody is born with LGS. LGS is the result of childhood-onset epilepsies refractory

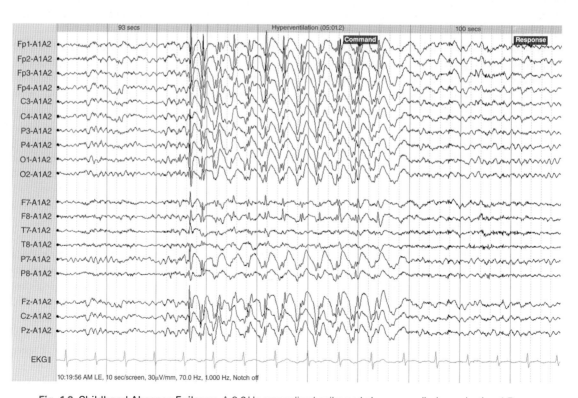

Fig. 1.3 Childhood Absence Epilepsy. A 3.2 Hz generalized spike and slow wave discharge lasting 4.5 seconds during hyperventilation.

to medical management, evolving into symptomatic generalized epilepsies with the characteristics described earlier. Adult-onset refractory epilepsy does not lead to LGS. The characteristics of the syndrome fade away in many survivors and the EEG may evolve into a multifocal pattern with variable seizure types. We often used the term Lennox-Gastaut spectrum (LG-little s) for the stages preceding and following the stage described by Lennox and Gastaut.

Clinical features. The peak age at onset is 3–5 years; less than half of the cases begin before age 2. Approximately 60% have an identifiable underlying cause, most frequently neurocutaneous disorders such as tuberous sclerosis, perinatal disturbances, and postnatal brain injuries. Twenty percent of children with LGS have a history of infantile spasms.

Most children are neurologically abnormal before seizure onset. Every seizure type exists in LGS, even a very small percentage of typical absences. Atypical absence seizures occur in almost every patient and drop attacks (atonic and tonic seizures) are essential for the diagnosis. A characteristic of atonic seizures is a sudden dropping of the head or body, at times throwing the child to the ground. Most children with the syndrome function suffer from cognitive impairment by 5 years of age.

Diagnosis. The diagnosis is based on the history of multiple seizure types, including drop attacks, developmental regression with high likelihood of cognitive impairment, childhood-onset epilepsy, and a large spectrum of EEG abnormalities. The spectrum of EEG abnormalities includes a slow posterior dominant rhythm, absence of normal physiological sleep structures (sleep spindles, K-complexes, and vertex waves), the generalized 1.5–2.5 Hz spike and slow wave discharges in early to middle stages, and generalized electrodecrements with fast activity and multifocal spike and slow waves.

In addition to EEG, diagnostic workup requires a thorough evaluation with special attention to skin manifestations that suggest a neurocutaneous syndrome (see Box 1.8). MRI is useful for the diagnosis of brain dysgenesis, postnatal disorders, and neurocutaneous syndromes. Genetic testing may or may not change management but is important for family genetic counseling, and is increasingly part of a comprehensive seizure evaluation, particularly in children with no apparent structural brain anomalies.

Management. Seizures are difficult to control even with a combination of drugs, diet, and surgery.

Cannabidiol, rufinamide, valproate, lamotrigine, topiramate, felbamate, clobazam, and clonazepam are usually the most effective drugs. Clinicians almost always try levetiracetam at some point, so it is frequently part of the treatment regimen although we find it unlikely to control seizures unless used at high doses in conjunction with other drugs. Fenfluramine (Fintepla) was recently approved for the treatment of LGS, although clinical data indicate that it is more effective for the treatment of DS.[72] Consider the ketogenic diet and surgery when drugs fail. VNS and corpus callosotomy are alternatives for drop attacks refractory to medications and diet.

Progressive Myoclonus Epilepsies

The term *progressive myoclonus epilepsies* is used to cover several progressive disorders of the nervous system characterized by: (1) myoclonus, (2) seizures that may be tonic-clonic, tonic, or myoclonic, (3) progressive mental deterioration, and (4) cerebellar ataxia, involuntary movements, or both. Some of these disorders are due to specific lysosomal enzyme deficiencies, whereas others are probably mitochondrial disorders (Box 1.9).

Lafora disease (progressive myoclonus epilepsy, Lafora type). Lafora disease is a rare hereditary disease transmitted by autosomal recessive inheritance.[73] A mutation in the *EPM2A* gene is responsible for ~50% of patients with Lafora disease; the remainder are caused by pathogenic variants in *NHLRC1*. Skin biopsy shows characteristic Lafora bodies composed of insoluble glycogen molecules.

Clinical features. Onset is between 11 and 18 years of age, with the mean at age 14 years. Tonic-clonic or myoclonic seizures are the initial feature in 80% of cases. Hallucinations from occipital seizures are common.

BOX 1.9 Progressive Myoclonus Epilepsies

- Ceroid lipofuscinosis, juvenile form (see Chapter 5)
- Glucosylceramide lipidosis (Gaucher type 3) (see Chapter 5)
- Lafora disease
- Myoclonus epilepsy and ragged-red fibers (see Chapter 5)
- Ramsay-Hunt syndrome (see Chapter 10)
- Sialidosis (see Chapter 5)
- Progressive myoclonus epilepsy type 1

Myoclonus becomes progressively worse, may be segmental or massive, and increases with movement. Confusion and psychiatric symptoms are common. Cognitive impairment begins early and is relentlessly progressive. Ataxia, spasticity, and involuntary movements occur late in the course. Death occurs within 10 years after the onset of symptoms.

Diagnosis. The EEG is normal at first and later develops nonspecific generalized polyspike discharges during the waking state. The background becomes progressively disorganized and epileptiform activity more constant. Photosensitive discharges are a regular feature late in the course. The basis for diagnosis is the detection of one of the two known associated mutations.

Management. The seizures become refractory to most anticonvulsant drugs. Valproic acid and clonazepam are the most effective drugs in myoclonic epilepsies. Divalproex is preferred when the diagnosis is known and mitochondrial disease is not suspected. Levetiracetam, zonisamide, perampanel, and topiramate can be used adjunctively. Treatment of the underlying disease is not available.

Progressive myoclonic epilepsy type 1. Progressive myoclonic epilepsy type 1 (EPM1, previously referred to as Unverricht-Lundborg syndrome) is clinically similar to Lafora disease, except that inclusion bodies are not present. Genetic transmission is by autosomal recessive inheritance caused by biallelic expansion repeats in *CSTB* or compound heterozygosity for a *CTSB* repeat expansion as well as a *CTSB* pathogenic variant. Most reports of the syndrome are from Finland and other Baltic countries, but distribution is worldwide. [74]

Clinical features. Onset is usually between 6 and 15 years of age. The main features are stimulus-sensitive myoclonus and tonic-clonic seizures. As the disease progresses, other neurological symptoms including cognitive impairment and ataxia appear.

Diagnosis. EEG shows marked photosensitivity. Genetic molecular diagnosis is available.

Management. Valproic acid is the preferred treatment; clonazepam is also approved for the treatment of myoclonic seizures and is often used as an adjunct. Levetiracetam, perampanel, topiramate, and zonisamide are additional options. Make sure the child has access to school accommodations, physical and occupational therapies, and adaptive devices. Treatment of the underlying disease is not available.

PRICKLE1-Related Disorders

The *PRICKLE1*-related disorders cause progressive neurodegeneration, ataxia, and myoclonic seizures, but are less common than Lafora disease or EPM1.

Clinical features. Onset is between 5 and 10 years of age. Myoclonic seizures, generalized tonic-clonic seizures, action myoclonus, spontaneous myoclonus, and dysarthria define the disorder in children with biallelic pathogenic variants, while children with heterozygous pathogenic variants present with myoclonic seizures, autism spectrum disorders, and developmental delays.[75]

Diagnosis. Molecular genetic testing reveals the diagnosis.

Management. As with other progressive myoclonus epilepsies, consider valproic acid as a first-line drug and use clonazepam, levetiracetam, perampanel, zonisamide, and topiramate for adjunctive treatment. Speech, physical, and occupational therapies comprise an essential part of treatment.

Focal Seizures

A note regarding terminology: The International League Against Epilepsy (ILAE) has modified seizure terminology multiple times over the last several years. The current preferred terminology is "focal seizures with impaired awareness" for complex partial seizures, and "focal seizures without impaired awareness" for simple partial seizures. We find these terms more precise but rather clunky for the reader. For this reason, we have elected to use a combination of old and new terminology in the following section.

This section discusses several different seizure types of focal cortical origin. Such seizures may be purely motor or purely sensory or may affect higher cortical function. The self-limited (previously called *benign*) focal childhood epilepsies are a common cause of partial seizures in children, encompassing self-limited epilepsy with centrotemporal spikes (SLECTS, previously called BECTS or benign Rolandic epilepsy) and occipital epilepsy of the Panayiotopoulos or Gastaut forms. The various partial epilepsy syndromes begin and cease at similar ages, have a similar course, and often occur in the members of the same family; however, precise genotype-phenotype correlations are not well understood.

Partial seizures are also secondary to underlying diseases, which can be focal, multifocal, or generalized. Neuronal migrational disorders and gliomas often cause intractable partial seizures.[76] MRI is a recommended study for all children with focal clinical seizures, seizures associated with an unexplained focal abnormality on EEG, or with a new or progressing neurological deficit.

Cerebral cysticercosis is an important cause of partial seizures in Mexico and Central America which is now common in the Southwestern United States,[77] and is becoming more common in contiguous regions. Ingestion of poorly cooked pork containing cystic larvae of the tapeworm *Taenia solium* causes the infection.

Any seizure that originates in the cortex may become a bilateral tonic-clonic seizure (secondary generalization). If the discharge remains localized for a few seconds, the patient experiences a focal seizure or an aura before losing consciousness. Often secondary generalization occurs so rapidly that a bilateral tonic-clonic seizure is the initial symptom. In such cases, cortical origin of the seizure may be detectable on EEG. However, normal EEG findings are common during a simple partial seizure and do not exclude the diagnosis.

Acquired Epileptiform Aphasia

Acquired aphasia in children associated with epileptiform activity on EEG is the Landau-Kleffner syndrome. The syndrome appears to be a disorder of auditory processing. The cause is unknown except for occasional cases associated with temporal lobe tumors.

Clinical features. Age at onset ranges from 2 to 11 years, with 75% beginning between 3 and 10 years. The first symptom may be aphasia or epilepsy. Auditory verbal agnosia is the initial characteristic of aphasia. The child has difficulty understanding speech and stops talking. "Deafness" or "autism" develops. Several seizure types occur, including generalized tonic-clonic, partial, and myoclonic seizures.[78] Atypical absence is sometimes the initial feature and may be associated with continuous spikes and slow waves during slow-wave sleep. Hyperactivity and personality change occur in half of affected children. The neurological examination is otherwise normal.

Recovery of language is more likely to occur if the syndrome begins before 7 years of age. Seizures cease generally by age 10 and always by age 15.

Diagnosis. Acquired epileptiform aphasia, as the name implies, is different from autism and hearing loss because the diagnosis requires that the child have normal language, hearing, and cognitive development before the onset of symptoms. The EEG shows multifocal spike discharges with a predilection for the temporal and parietal lobes. Involvement is bilateral in 88% of cases. An IV injection of diazepam may normalize the EEG and transiently improve speech, but this should not suggest that epileptiform activity causes the aphasia. Instead, both features reflect an underlying cerebral disorder. A portion of children respond to immune modulation, suggesting an inflammatory or autoimmune mechanism in some cases. Genetic causes are suspected and multiple candidate genes have been reported, including *GRIN2A, RELN, BSN, EPHB2,* and *NID2.*[79] Every child with the disorder requires cranial MRI to exclude the rare possibility of a temporal lobe tumor.

Management. Standard anticonvulsants usually control the seizures but do not improve speech. Corticosteroid therapy, especially early in the course, may normalize the EEG and provide long-lasting remission of aphasia and seizures. Immunoglobulins 2 mg/kg over 2 consecutive days have shown efficacy. Anticonvulsants, including levetiracetam, valproic acid, clobazam, lamotrigine, and clonazepam, may be helpful.

Acquired Epileptiform Opercular Syndrome

This syndrome is distinct from acquired epileptiform aphasia but may represent a spectrum of the same underlying disease process.

Clinical features. Onset is before the age of 10 years. Brief nocturnal seizures occur that mainly affect the face and mouth, but may become secondarily generalized. Oral dysphasia, inability to initiate complex facial movements (blowing out a candle), speech and lingual dyspraxia, and drooling develop concurrently with seizure onset. Cognitive dysfunction is associated.

Diagnosis. The EEG shows centrotemporal discharges or electrical status epilepticus of sleep (ESES).

Management. The dysphasia often does not respond to anticonvulsant drugs. Valproic acid, lamotrigine, clobazam, and benzodiazepines may be used. Consider high-dose steroids or other immune modulators.

Autosomal Dominant Sleep-Related Hypermotor Epilepsy

This disorder was previously known as autosomal dominant nocturnal frontal lobe epilepsy. Bizarre behavior and motor features during sleep are the characteristics of this epilepsy syndrome, often misdiagnosed as a sleep or psychiatric disorder. It is associated with mutations of *CHRNA4, CHRNB2,* and *CHRNA2* which, respectively, affect alpha 4, beta 2, and alpha 2 subunits of the nACh receptor. Other associated mutations include *CABP4, CRH, DEPDC5, KCNT1, NPRL2, NPRL3,* and *STX1B*.[80]

Clinical features. Seizures begin in childhood and usually persist into adult life. The seizures occur in NREM sleep with sudden awakenings associated with brief hyperkinetic or tonic manifestations. Patients frequently remain conscious and often report auras of shivering, tingling, epigastric, or thoracic sensations, as well as other sensory and psychic phenomena.

Clusters of seizures, each lasting less than a minute, occur in one night. Interictal EEG is often normal. Video-EEG recordings demonstrate partial seizures originating in the frontal lobe. A vocalization, usually a gasp or grunt that awakens the child, is common. Other auras include sensory sensations, psychic phenomena (fear, malaise, etc.), shivering, and difficulty breathing. Thrashing or tonic stiffening with superimposed clonic jerks follows. The eyes are open, and the individual is often aware of what is happening; many sit up and try to grab onto a bed part.

Most patients have normal neurological exams, and the presence of intellectual or developmental disabilities should prompt reevaluation of the diagnosis; however, cognitive deficits and psychiatric symptoms may occur.

Diagnosis. The family history is important to the diagnosis but many family members may not realize that their own attacks are seizures, and phenotypes vary significantly within families. The interictal EEG is usually normal, and concurrent video-EEG is often required to capture the event, which reveals rapidly generalized discharges with diffuse distribution. Often, movement artifact obscures the initial ictal EEG. The disorder is challenging to diagnose; obtain genetic testing whenever possible. Brain MRI is normal.

Children who have seizures characterized by tonic posturing of arms or legs without loss of consciousness may have supplementary sensorimotor seizures. Sensory auras are common in children who have daytime seizures.[81]

Management. Any of the anticonvulsant agents except for ethosuximide may be effective. Many of these patients achieve only partial control with monotherapy and most require polypharmacy. In our experience carbamazepine or oxcarbazepine is the most effective agent for this epilepsy type.

Childhood Epilepsy With Occipital Paroxysms

Two self-limited occipital epilepsies with distinct phenotypes present in school-age children.

Late-onset/idiopathic childhood occipital epilepsy, gastaut type. Although presumed to be genetic, no specific variants have been identified as the cause of idiopathic childhood occipital epilepsy, Gastaut type (ICOE-G). It is clinically distinct from the other genetic occipital epilepsy, Panayiotopoulos syndrome (discussed in the following section). Both epilepsies are commonly associated with migraine.

Clinical features. Peak age at onset is around 8 years but the disorder can present in adolescents. One-third of patients have a family history of epilepsy, frequently another type of self-limited focal epilepsy. The initial seizure manifestations typically comprise: (1) unformed visual hallucinations, usually flashing lights or spots occurring multiple times daily, (2) ictal blindness, hemianopia, or complete amaurosis, (3) visual illusions, such as micropsia, macropsia, or metamorphopsia, or (4) loss of consciousness or awareness. More than one feature may occur simultaneously. Unilateral clonic seizures or secondary generalized tonic-clonic seizures may follow the visual aura. Afterward, the child complains of migraine-like headaches and nausea. Attacks occur when the child is awake or asleep, but the greatest frequency is at the transition from wakefulness to sleep. Photic stimulation may induce seizures in some patients.

Diagnosis. The results of the neurological examination, CT, and MRI are normal. As with other self-limited or "benign" childhood epilepsies, development is normal overall but the child often displays deficits in memory or attention. The interictal EEG shows unilateral or bilateral independent high-amplitude, occipital spike-wave discharges. Discharges demonstrate fixation-off sensitivity, meaning that eye opening with fixation suppresses the discharges, while eye closure or eye opening with inhibited fixation by any means enhances them.[82] During a seizure, rapid firing of spike discharges occurs in one or both occipital lobes.

Management. Standard anticonvulsant drugs usually provide complete seizure control. Typical seizures never persist beyond 12 years of age. However, not all children with occipital discharges have a self-limited epilepsy syndrome. Persistent or hard-to-control seizures raise the question of a structural abnormality in the occipital lobe, and require MRI examination.

Early-onset childhood occipital epilepsy (Panayiotopoulos syndrome).

Clinical features. The age at onset of Panayiotopoulos syndrome is 3–6 years, but the range extends from 1 to 14 years. Seizures usually occur in sleep and autonomic and behavioral features predominate. These include vomiting, pallor, sweating, irritability, and tonic eye deviation. The seizures are often prolonged, lasting from 1 to 30 minutes and sometimes up to 2 hours, and may be mistaken for other disorders, including cyclic vomiting syndrome or complicated migraine. Seizures are infrequent and the overall prognosis is good with remission occurring in 1–2 years.

Diagnosis. The interictal EEG shows runs of high-amplitude 2–3 Hz sharp and slow wave complexes in the posterior quadrants. Many children may have centrotemporal or frontal spikes. Paroxysmal posterior slowing characterizes the ictal EEG.

Management. Standard anticonvulsant drugs usually accomplish seizure control.

Idiopathic Occipital Epilepsy With Photosensitivity

Idiopathic occipital epilepsy with photosensitivity is a poorly understood subtype of occipital epilepsies, but in contrast to others discussed in this chapter it is often not self-limited.

Clinical features. Children present between 5 and 17 years of age with seizures induced by photic stimulation.[83] The seizures begin with colorful, moving spots in the peripheral field of vision. With the progression of the seizure, tonic head and eye movement develops with blurred vision, nausea, vomiting, sharp pain in the head or orbit, and unresponsiveness. Cognitive status, the neurological examination, and brain imaging are normal.

Diagnosis. Interictal EEG shows bilateral synchronous or asynchronous occipital spikes and spike-wave complexes. Intermittent photic stimulation may induce an occipital photoparyoxysmal response and generalized discharges. The ictal EEG shows occipital epileptiform activity, which may shift from one side to the other. This epilepsy requires distinction from idiopathic generalized epilepsy with photosensitivity, and there may be an overlap between the two disorders.

Management. Due to the clinical overlap with primary generalized epilepsy with photosensitivity, it is prudent to treat with broad-spectrum anticonvulsants.

Self-Limited Childhood Epilepsy With Centrotemporal Spikes

Benign rolandic epilepsy is the original name for self-limited childhood epilepsy with centrotemporal spikes (SLECTS). Genetic transmission is an autosomal dominant trait. Forty percent of close relatives have a history of febrile seizures or epilepsy.

Clinical features. The age at onset is between 3 and 13 years, with a peak at 7–8 years. Seizures usually stop spontaneously by the age of 13–15 years. This epilepsy is not always benign. In fact, some children have their seizures only partially controlled with polypharmacy. Observations such as "incomplete phenotype penetrance," the incidence of seizures, and the response to treatment may be incorrect by the "incomplete observation" in children that may have only mild seizures when everybody is sleeping. Seventy percent of children have seizures only while asleep, 15% only when awake, and 15% both awake and asleep.

The typical seizure wakes the child from sleep. Paresthesias occur on one side of the mouth, followed by ipsilateral twitching of the face, mouth, and pharynx, resulting in speech arrest (if dominant hemisphere) or dysarthria (if nondominant hemisphere), and drooling. Consciousness is often preserved. The seizure lasts for 1 or 2 minutes. Daytime seizures typically do not generalize, but nocturnal seizures in children younger than 5 years old often spread to the arm or evolve into a bilateral tonic-clonic seizure. Some children with SLECTS have cognitive or behavioral problems, particularly difficulty with sustained attention, reading, and language processing.[84]

Diagnosis. When evaluating a child for a first nocturnal, generalized tonic-clonic seizure, ask the parents if the child's mouth was "twisted." If they answer affirmatively, the child probably has SLECTS.

Results of neurological examination and brain imaging studies, if obtained, are normal. Interictal EEG shows unilateral or bilateral spike discharges in the central or centrotemporal region. The spikes are typically of high voltage and activated by drowsiness and sleep. The frequency of spike discharges, particularly during NREM sleep, can indicate an increased risk of long-term neuropsychiatric, developmental, and educational problems. For this reason SLECTS is sometimes considered the milder end of a spectrum of disease that ranges from brief, infrequent nocturnal seizures all the way to an epileptic encephalopathy with aphasia.[85] Children with both typical clinical seizures and typical EEG abnormalities, especially with a positive family history, do not necessarily require neuroimaging although it is frequently obtained. However, those with atypical features or hard-to-control seizures warrant MRI to exclude structural abnormalities.

Management. Most anticonvulsant drugs are effective. We often prescribe levetiracetam or oxcarbazepine in these children. Most children eventually stop having seizures whether they are treated or not, but there is evidence that children with daytime seizures and a high burden of nocturnal interictal abnormalities suffer from significantly more cognitive and behavioral deficits.[86] Treatment may reduce the burden of epileptiform discharges and improve cognitive outcomes, provided that the medication chosen does not have significant cognitive side effects.

Electrical Status Epilepticus During Slow Wave Sleep

In electrical status epilepticus during slow wave sleep (ESES), sleep induces paroxysmal EEG activity and ultimately produces an epileptic encephalopathy. The paroxysms may appear continuously or discontinuously during NREM sleep. The exact threshold of spike-wave activity required for diagnosis has varied over time and among institutions, but is typically 50%–85%. Importantly, epileptiform discharges during wakefulness should be relatively infrequent. If a child has a high spike burden during wakefulness, she will naturally have a very high burden during sleep due to typical sleep activation of epileptiform discharges—this is worrisome in its own right but does not represent ESES. Spike-wave discharges are usually bilateral, but sometimes strictly unilateral or with unilateral predominance.

Clinical features. Age at onset is 3–14 years. Seizures during wakefulness are usually rare and include atypical absence, myoclonic, or akinetic seizures. A minority of children never have clinical seizures. Neuropsychological impairment and behavioral disorders are common. Hyperactivity, learning disabilities, and in some instances, psychotic episodes may persist even after ESES has ceased.

Diagnosis. The most typical paroxysmal discharges of EEG are spike-waves of 1.5 and 3.5 Hz, sometimes associated with polyspikes, or polyspikes and waves. The majority of epileptiform discharges occur in NREM sleep and can be entirely missed on a routine awake or drowsy EEG. Multiple genes have been implicated in the etiology of ESES, but *GRIN2A* is the most common. Copy number variants may cause ESES, including 15q11 duplication, Xp22.12 deletion, 16p13 deletion, and others.[87]

Treatment. Standard anticonvulsant drugs are rarely effective. High-dose steroids, ACTH, high-dose benzodiazepines, levetiracetam, and IV immunoglobulin have all reported some success.

Epilepsia Partialis Continua

Focal motor seizures that do not stop spontaneously are termed *epilepsia partialis continua*. This is an ominous symptom and usually indicates an underlying cerebral disorder. Possible causes include infarction, hemorrhage, tumor, hyperglycemia, Rasmussen encephalitis, and inflammation. Make every effort to stop the seizures with IV antiepileptic drugs (see later section on Treatment of Status Epilepticus). The response to anticonvulsant drugs and the outcome depend on the underlying cause.

Hemiconvulsions-Hemiplegia Syndrome (Rasmussen Syndrome)

Rasmussen syndrome is a poorly understood and fortunately rare disorder. The incidence is around 1 to 7 cases per 10,000,000 below the age of 18. While originally described as a form of focal viral encephalitis, an infectious etiology is not established. It is believed to be caused by initial T-cell response to antigenic epitopes with potential subsequent contribution of autoantibodies.[88]

Clinical features. Focal jerking frequently begins around age 6 years. It begins in one body part, usually one side of the face or one hand, and then spreads to contiguous parts. Trunk muscles are rarely affected. The rate and intensity of the seizures vary at first, but then become more regular and persist during sleep. Refractory motor seizures develop in all affected individuals only 4 months after the onset of the initial symptom.[89] Fifty percent of patients develop epilepsia partialis continua.[90] The seizures defy treatment and progress to affect first both limbs on one side of the body and then the limbs on the other side. Progressive hemiplegia develops and remains after seizures have stopped.

Diagnosis. EEG and MRI are initially normal and then the EEG shows continuous spike discharges originating in one portion of the cortex, with spread to contiguous areas of the cortex and to a mirror focus on the other side. Secondary generalization may occur. Repeated MRI shows rapidly progressive hemiatrophy with ex vacuo dilation of the ipsilateral ventricle. Positron emission tomography (PET) shows widespread hypometabolism of the affected hemisphere at a time when the spike discharges remain localized. The CSF is usually normal, although a few monocytes may be present.

Management. The treatment of Rasmussen syndrome is especially difficult. Standard antiepileptic therapy is not effective for stopping seizures or the progressive hemiplegia. The use of immunosuppressive therapy is recommended by some, but seems to only slow the progression. These medical approaches are rarely successful. Early hemispherectomy is the treatment of choice; however, there are inevitable functional compromises. Most patients are able to recover functional ambulation, but have poor function of the affected hand.

Reading Epilepsy

There was a belief that reading epilepsy and JME were variants because many children with reading epilepsy experience myoclonic jerks of the limbs shortly after arising in the morning. However, recent studies indicate that reading epilepsy is a reflex epilepsy originating from the dominant (usually left) posterior temporo-occipital junction. The myoclonic variant may have bilateral discharges with a left temporal predominance. [91]

Clinical features. Age at onset is usually in the second decade. Myoclonic jerks involving orofacial and jaw muscles develop while reading. Reading time before seizure onset is variable. The initial seizure is usually in the jaw and is described as "jaws locking or clicking." Other initial features are quivering of the lips, choking in the throat, or difficulty speaking. Most patients experience ictal alexia (inability to read). Myoclonic jerks of the limbs may follow, and some children experience a generalized tonic-clonic seizure if they continue reading. Generalized tonic-clonic seizures may also occur at other times.

Diagnosis. The history of myoclonic jerks during reading and other processes requiring higher cognitive function is critical to the diagnosis. The interictal EEG usually shows generalized discharges, and brief spike-wave complexes, simultaneous with jaw jerks, can be provoked by reading.

Management. Some patients claim to control their seizures without the use of anticonvulsant drugs by quitting reading at the first sign of orofacial or jaw jerks. This seems an impractical approach and an impediment to education. Levetiracetam and lamotrigine are good treatment options.

Temporal Lobe Epilepsy

Temporal lobe epilepsy in children may be primary or secondary. Inheritance of primary temporal lobe epilepsy is often an autosomal dominant trait. Among children with secondary temporal lobe epilepsy, 30% give a history of an antecedent illness or event, and 40% show MRI evidence of a structural abnormality.

Clinical features. Seizure onset in primary temporal lobe epilepsy typically occurs in adolescence or later. The seizures consist of simple psychic (déjà vu, cognitive disturbances, illusions, and hallucinations) or autonomic (nausea, tachycardia, and sweating) symptoms. Secondary generalization is unusual. Seizure onset in secondary temporal lobe epilepsy is during the first decade and often occurs during an acute illness. The seizures are usually complex partial in type, and secondary generalization is more common.

Diagnosis. A single EEG in children with primary temporal lobe epilepsy is likely to be normal. The frequency of interictal temporal lobe spikes is low, and diagnosis requires prolonged video-EEG monitoring. The incidence of focal interictal temporal lobe spikes is higher in children with secondary temporal lobe epilepsy, but detection may require several standard or prolonged EEG studies.

Management. Monotherapy with oxcarbazepine, levetiracetam, lamotrigine, or topiramate is usually satisfactory for seizure control in both types. Other anticonvulsants such as phenytoin, carbamazepine, and valproate have similar efficacy. We choose medications based on safety, tolerability, potential side effects, and cost.

Generalized Seizures

Generalized tonic-clonic seizures are the most common seizures of childhood. They are dramatic and frightening events that invariably demand medical attention. Seizures that are prolonged or repeated without recovery are termed *status epilepticus*. Many children with generalized tonic-clonic seizures have a history of febrile seizures during infancy. Some of these represent

> ### BOX 1.10 Diagnostic Considerations for a First Nonfebrile Tonic-Clonic Seizure After 2 Years of Age
>
> - Acute encephalopathy or encephalitis (see Chapter 2)
> - Isolated unexplained seizure
> - Partial seizure of any cause with secondary generalization
> - Primary generalized epilepsy
> - Progressive disorder of the nervous system (see Chapter 5)

a distinct autosomal dominant disorder. Box 1.10 summarizes the diagnostic considerations in a child who has had a generalized tonic-clonic seizure.

Clinical features. The onset may occur any time after the neonatal period, but the onset of primary generalized epilepsy without absence is usually during the second decade. With absence, the age at onset shifts to the first decade.

Sudden loss of consciousness is the initial feature. The child falls to the floor, and the body stiffens (tonic phase). Repetitive jerking movements of the limbs follow (clonic phase); these movements at first are rapid and rhythmic and then become slower and more irregular as the seizure ends. The eyes roll backward in the orbits; breathing is rapid and deep, causing saliva to froth at the lips; and urinary and fecal incontinence may occur. A postictal sleep follows the seizure from which arousal is difficult. Afterward, the child appears normal but may have sore limb muscles and a painful tongue, bitten during the seizure.

Diagnosis. A first generalized tonic-clonic seizure requires laboratory evaluation. Individualize the evaluation. Important determining factors include neurological findings, family history, and known precipitating factors. An eyewitness report of focal features at the onset of the seizure, or the recollection of an aura, indicates a partial seizure with secondary generalization.

During the seizure, the EEG shows generalized repetitive spikes in the tonic phase and then periodic bursts of spikes in the clonic phase. Movement artifact usually obscures the clonic portion. As the seizure ends, the background rhythms are slow and the amplitude attenuates.

Between seizures, brief generalized spike or spike-wave discharges that are polymorphic in appearance may occur. Discharge frequency sometimes increases with drowsiness and light sleep. The presence of focal discharges indicates a secondary generalization of the tonic-clonic seizure.

The CSF is normal following a brief tonic-clonic seizure due to primary epilepsy. However, prolonged or repeated seizures may cause a leukocytosis, as many as 80 cells/mm^3 with a polymorphonuclear predominance. The protein concentration can be mildly elevated, but the glucose concentration is normal.

Management. We do not start prophylactic antiepileptic therapy in an otherwise normal child who has had a single unexplained seizure unless the EEG is clearly abnormal. The recurrence rate is probably less than 50% after 1 year. Several drugs are equally effective in children with recurrent seizures that require treatment. Offer all families an emergency seizure medication (intranasal diazepam or midazolam, or rectal diazepam) and provide education regarding seizure precautions and first aid.

Epilepsy With Generalized Tonic-Clonic Seizures Alone

EGTCS, previously called epilepsy with generalized tonic-clonic seizures on awakening, is a familial syndrome distinct from JME. The mode of inheritance is not clear. A minority of patients demonstrate pathogenic mutations on *CLCN2*.[92] Some patients (10%–20%) report a family history of epilepsy or a personal history of febrile seizures, but many times the history is negative.

Clinical features. Onset occurs in the second decade, and 90% of seizures occur on awakening, regardless of the time of day. Seizures also occur with relaxation in the evening. Absence and myoclonic seizures may occur.

Diagnosis. The EEG shows a pattern of idiopathic generalized epilepsies.

Management. Treatment is similar to that of JME with levetiracetam, valproate, lamotrigine, and topiramate. Perampanel is also helpful with this seizure type.

Psychogenic Nonepileptic Spells/Pseudoseizures

Psychogenic nonepileptic spells (PNES) are common in the pediatric (especially adolescent) population. PNES and other psychogenic symptoms will be discussed in Chapter 19.

MANAGING SEIZURES

Antiepileptic Drug Therapy

Proper epilepsy treatment involves caring for the child's neurological, behavioral, and cognitive health in between seizures, not simply stopping attacks. We often describe this to our patients as "walking a tightrope" to find the optimal balance between our goal of seizure freedom and our responsibility to minimize medication side effects. In other words, we attempt to achieve maximal functionality by balancing seizure control against drug toxicity. We are able to achieve seizure freedom in about 70% of localization-related epilepsies. Genetic generalized epilepsies have more variable outcomes depending on the causative mutation.

Indications for Starting Therapy

Consider initiating therapy in children with preexisting neurological deficits (symptomatic epilepsy) after the first seizure, because more seizures are expected. Conversely, less than half of typically developing children will have a second seizure after a first-time unexplained and untreated generalized ton-clonic seizure. It is reasonable to delay therapy if the child is not operating a motor vehicle. Always treat JME and absence epilepsy, not only because of expected seizure recurrence, but also because uncontrolled absence impairs education and carries higher risks of trauma.

Discontinuing Therapy

Antiepileptic drug therapy is required in children who experience seizures during an acute encephalopathy, for example, anoxia, head trauma, encephalitis. However, it is reasonable to stop therapy when the acute encephalopathy is over and seizures have stopped, if there are no significant residual deficits.

Pooled data on epilepsy in children suggest that discontinuing antiepileptic therapy is successful after 2 years of complete control. We note that pooled data are worthless when applied to the individual child. It is thought that many otherwise normal children started on antiepileptic medication after a first seizure who then remain seizure free for 2 years should not have received medication in the first place. The decision to stop therapy, like the decision to start therapy, requires an individualized approach to the child and the cause of the epilepsy. Children with neurological deficits and those with specific epileptic syndromes that are known to

persist into adult life are likely to have recurrences, while some cryptogenic cases have a low incidence of recurrence after the first or second seizure. Three-quarters of relapses occur during the withdrawal phase and in the 2 years thereafter. Contrary to popular belief, the rapid withdrawal of antiepileptic drugs in a person who does not need therapy does not provoke seizures, with the probable exception of high-dose benzodiazepines and oxcarbazepine. However, all parents *know* that seizure medication is never abruptly withdrawn and it is foolish to suggest otherwise. Attempt to stop antiepileptic therapy 1 year before driving age in children who are seizure free and neurologically normal, provided they do not have evidence of a lifelong epileptic tendency.

Principles of Therapy

Start therapy with a single drug. About 50% of patients with epilepsy achieve complete seizure control with monotherapy when using the first and correct drug for the seizure type. An additional 10% becomes controlled with the second medication tried.[93] Even patients whose seizures are never controlled are likely to do better on the smallest number of drugs.

Polypharmacy poses several problems: (1) drugs compete with each other for protein-binding sites, (2) one drug can increase the rate and pathway of metabolism of a second drug, (3) drugs have cumulative toxicity, and (4) compliance is more difficult. Polypharmacy may also reduce toxicity by targeting different mechanisms of action with effective but not toxic dosing. Most chronic and difficult-to-control conditions in medicine, such as hypertension, often benefit from this approach.

When using more than one drug, change only one drug at a time. When making several changes simultaneously, it is impossible to determine which drug is responsible for a beneficial or an adverse effect.

Administer anticonvulsant drugs no more than twice a day if at all possible (preferably once daily) and urge families to buy pillboxes marked with the 7 days of the week. Encourage older children and adolescents to set a reminder alarm on their cell phones. It is difficult to remember to take medicine when you are not in pain to prevent an event that you will not recall. If you ask people if they ever miss their doses, the answer is often "no," as it is impossible to remember what you forgot!

Blood concentrations. The development of techniques to measure blood concentrations of antiepileptic drugs was an important advance in the treatment of epilepsy. However, reference values of drug concentrations are guidelines. Some patients are seizure free with concentrations that are below the reference value, and others are unaffected by what are labeled as "toxic concentrations." We rely more on patient response than on blood concentration. Fortunately, for children many of the newer drugs (e.g., lamotrigine and levetiracetam) do not require the measurement of blood concentrations, although levels may be helpful in some situations.

Measuring total drug concentrations, protein-bound and free fractions, is customary even though the free fraction is responsible for efficacy and toxicity. While the ratio of free-to-bound fractions is relatively constant, some drugs have a greater affinity for binding protein than other drugs and displace them when used together.

The free fraction of the displaced drug increases and causes toxicity even though the measured total drug concentration is "therapeutic."

Most antiepileptic drugs follow first-order kinetics (i.e., blood levels increase proportionately with increases in the oral dose). The main exception is phenytoin, whose metabolism changes from first-order to zero-order kinetics when the enzyme system responsible for its metabolism saturates. Then a small increment in oral dose produces large increments in blood concentration.

The half-lives of the antiepileptic drugs listed in Table 1.2 are at a steady state. Half-lives are generally longer when therapy with a new drug begins. Achieving a steady state usually requires five half-lives. Similarly, five half-lives are required to eliminate

Drug	Initial Dose (mg/kg/day)	Target Dose (mg/kg/day)	Therapeutic Blood Concentration (mg/mL)	Half-Life (h)
Cannabidiol	5	10–20	a	56–61
Carbamazepine	10	20–30	4–12	10–20
Clobazam	0.25	0.5–1	a	Active metabolite 71–82
Clonazepam	0.02	0.5–1	a	20–40
Ethosuximide	20	20–60	50–120	30–40
Felbamate	15	45	40–80	20–23
Gabapentin	10	20–60	a	5–7
Lamotrigine (low with valproate, high with enzyme inducers)	0.15–0.6	5–15	2–20	25 (monotherapy)
Levetiracetam	20	20–60	10–40	6–8
Oxcarbazepine	10	20–60	10–40	9
Perampanel	2	4–12	a	105
Phenobarbital	3–5	5–10	15–40	50–200
Phenytoin	5–10	5–10	10–25	24
Pregabalin	2	4–10	a	6
Primidone	5	10–25	8–12	8–22
Rufinamide	15	45	a	6–10
Tiagabine	0.2	1–1.5	a	7–9
Topiramate	1–3	10–15	a	18–30
Valproate	20	20–60	50–100	6–15
Vigabatrin	50	150–200	a	5–7, but effect lasts days
Zonisamide	2	10	a	63

[a]Not established.

a drug after discontinuing administration. Drug half-lives vary from individual to individual and may be shortened or increased by the concurrent use of other anticonvulsants or other medications. This is one reason that children with epilepsy may have a toxic response to a drug or increased seizures at the time of a febrile illness.

Some anticonvulsants have active metabolites. With the exception of phenobarbital derived from primidone and S-licarbazepine/R-licarbazepine (monohydroxy-derivative) derived from oxcarbazepine, these metabolites are not usually measured. Active metabolites may provide seizure control or have toxic effects when the blood concentration of the parent compound is low.

Adverse reactions. Some anticonvulsant drugs irritate the gastric mucosa and cause nausea and vomiting. When this occurs, taking smaller doses at shorter intervals, using enteric-coated preparations, and administering the drug after meals may relieve symptoms.

Toxic adverse reactions are dose related. Almost all anticonvulsant drugs cause sedation when blood concentrations are excessive. Subtle cognitive and behavioral disturbances, recognizable only by the patient or family, often occur at low blood concentrations. Never discount the patient's observation of a toxic effect because the blood concentration is within the "therapeutic range." As doses are increased, attention span, memory, and interpersonal relations may become seriously impaired. This is especially common with barbiturates but can occur with any drug.

Idiosyncratic reactions are not dose related. They may occur as hypersensitivity reactions (usually manifest as rash, fever, and lymphadenopathy) or because of toxic metabolites. Idiosyncratic reactions are not always predictable, and respecting the patient's observation is essential. Notwithstanding package inserts and threats of litigation, routine laboratory studies of blood counts and organ function in a healthy child are neither cost-effective nor helpful for the majority of anticonvulsant drugs (certain notable exceptions are detailed below). It is preferable to do studies based on clinical features.

Selection of an Antiepileptic Drug

The use of generic drugs is difficult to avoid in managed healthcare programs. Unfortunately, several different manufacturers provide generic versions of each drug; the bioavailability and half-life of these products vary considerably, and maintaining a predictable blood concentration may be difficult. We usually increase the dose of patients partially controlled when they have a breakthrough seizure by 10% and decrease the dose by 10% when they experience side effects. A variation of 10% up and down from one refill to the next when changing between brands and multiple generics is not trivial. These changes may result in loss of seizure control or side effects.

Common reasons for loss of seizure control in children who were previously seizure free are nonadherence and changing from the brand name to a generic drug, or from one generic to another. Patients should be told when their medication is being changed from brand to generic, generic to brand, or generic to different generic.

For the most part, the basis of drug selection is the neurologist's comfort with using a specific drug, other health conditions and drug use in the patient, the available preparations with respect to the child's age, and the spectrum of antiepileptic activity of the drug. Clobazam, levetiracetam, lamotrigine, perampanel, topiramate, valproate, zonisamide, rufinamide, and felbamate are drugs with a broad spectrum of efficacy against many different seizure types. The basis of the following comments is personal experience and published reports. Patent extensions granted by the FDA, when research in children is completed, have helped tremendously in the acquisition of knowledge of the use of anticonvulsants in children.

Brivaracetam (Briviact, UCB Pharma)

Indications. Brivaracetam is similar to levetiracetam in that it most likely modulates neurotransmission by binding to the presynaptic vesicle glycoprotein A2. However, it binds with a 20-fold greater affinity than levetiracetam; it also has no calcium channel or AMPA (alpha-amino-2-hydroxy-5-methyl-4-isoxazolepropionic acid) receptor effect. It has proven efficacy in focal epilepsies, but it is believed to have a wide spectrum of efficacy.

Administration. Brivaracetam is available as a 10, 25, 50, 75, and 100 mg tablet, an IV solution of 50 mg/5 mL, and an oral suspension of 10 mg/mL. The half-life is 9 hours, but the duration of efficacy is longer likely due to its high affinity for the site of action. Twice daily oral dosing is required. The initial dose in adolescents older than 16 years is 50 mg bid for 1 week and may be raised to 100 mg bid.

Adverse effects. Adverse effects are similar to levetiracetam, but some studies suggest overall greater tolerability with fewer behavioral or mood side effects.

Cannabidiol (Epidiolex, Jazz Pharmaceuticals)

Indications. Cannabidiol is approved for the treatment of seizures within the spectrum of Lennox-Gastaut, which includes all seizure types. In addition, it is approved for seizures associated with Dravet syndrome as well as focal seizures in the setting of tuberous sclerosis.

Administration. Start with 5 mg/kg/day divided into two doses (bid) for 1 week, and then 10 mg/kg/day divided bid. The maximum recommended dose is 20 mg/kg/day divided bid (25 mg/kg/day for tuberous sclerosis). Cannabidiol is available as a 100 mg/mL sugar-free solution. Check serum transaminases (alanine aminotransferase and aspartate aminotransferase) and bilirubin levels before starting treatment. Many insurance companies in the United States require yearly liver function tests thereafter to continue coverage.

Adverse effects. Adverse effects include somnolence, decreased appetite, diarrhea, elevation in transaminases, fatigue, and insomnia. Cannabidiol increases the serum concentration of desmethylclobazam (the active metabolite of clobazam) threefold, and patients on high doses of clobazam will likely require dose reduction to avoid sedation. Conversely, clobazam itself increases the serum concentration of cannabidiol's active metabolite by approximately 70%. Concomitant use with valproate increases the risk of transaminase elevation. Due to the risk of diarrhea, a reduction in laxatives should be considered in children who are on a daily bowel regimen.

Carbamazepine (Tegretol, Tegretol-XR, Novartis; Carbatrol, Shire Pharmaceuticals).

In our practices, oxcarbazepine has replaced carbamazepine entirely because of its better side effect profile and tolerability.

Indications. Use carbamazepine for the treatment of focal seizures and primary or secondary generalized tonic-clonic seizures. It often increases the frequency of absence and myoclonic seizures and is therefore contraindicated for those seizure types.

Administration. Approximately 85% of the drug is protein bound. Carbamazepine induces its own metabolism, and the initial dose should be 25% of the maintenance dose to prevent toxicity. The usual maintenance dosage is 15–20 mg/kg/day to provide a blood concentration of 4–12 μg/mL. However, infants often require 30 mg/kg/day. The half-life at steady state is 5–27 hours, and children usually require doses three times a day. Two long-acting preparations are available for twice a day dosing. Concurrent use of cimetidine, erythromycin, grapefruit, fluoxetine, and propoxyphene interferes with carbamazepine metabolism and causes toxicity.

Adverse effects. A depression of peripheral leukocytes is expected but is rarely sufficient (absolute neutrophil count less than 1000) to warrant discontinuation of therapy. Routine white blood cell counts each time the patient returns for a follow-up visit are not cost effective and do not allow the prediction of life-threatening events. The most informative time to repeat the white blood cell count is concurrently with a febrile illness. Screening for the *HLA-B*1502* allele is recommended before initiation of carbamazepine therapy in patients with Asian ancestry to decrease the risk of Stevens-Johnson syndrome and toxic epidermal necrolysis. The use of these tests in other ethnic groups is unclear. Cognitive disturbances may occur within the therapeutic range. Sedation, ataxia, and nystagmus occur at toxic blood concentrations.

Cenobamate (Xcopri, SK Life Sciences)

Indications. Cenobamate is indicated for the treatment of focal seizures with and without secondary generalization in patients 18 years of age and older. The precise mechanism of action is not known but is believed to be secondary to the inhibition of sodium channels and a positive allosteric modulation of the $GABA_A$ ion channel.

Administration. Cenobamate is rapidly absorbed after oral intake. Maximal plasma concentrations occur 1–4 hours after dosing. A long half-life of 50–60 hours allows for once daily dosing. Begin with 12.5 mg daily for 2 weeks, then 25 mg daily for 2 weeks, then 50 mg daily for 2 weeks, and then 100 mg daily. In our practices we continue to increase doses by 50 mg every 2 weeks for patients that remain incompletely controlled, provided they are able to tolerate higher dosing. Proactively lower the clobazam dose for patients taking high doses of clobazam. Cenobamate inhibits the metabolism of desmethylclobazam and may result in sedation when the clobazam dose is not reduced. Concomitant use of sodium channel blockers such as oxcarbazepine and lacosamide may result in dizziness; lower the dose if this occurs.

Adverse effects. The main side effects are dizziness and somnolence. If these are ignored and titration continues at the same pace you may see balance difficulties, coordination issues, nystagmus, or tremor. Drug reaction with eosinophilia and systemic symptoms (DRESS) is a class warning for all antiseizure medications. The rate of DRESS does not seem to be different for ceno-bamate when following the recommended titration schedule; however, higher rates were noted with faster titrations during clinical development.

Clobazam (Onfi, Lundbeck; Sympazan, Aquestive Therapeutics)

Indications. Clobazam is indicated for the treatment of seizures within the spectrum of Lennox-Gastaut, which includes all seizure types, even a small percentage of typical absence seizures.

Administration. For patients weighing less than 30 kg, the initial dosage is 5 mg daily titrating up to 20 mg divided twice daily, as tolerated. For patients weighing more than 30 kg, the initial dosage is 10 mg daily titrating up to 40 mg divided bid as tolerated. Some patients benefit from higher doses up to 100 mg daily.

Adverse effects. Sedation and increased drooling are common. Monitor secretions in children with dysphagia and those at risk of aspiration pneumonia. If seizure control improves but secretions are problematic, consider initiating medication to reduce drooling.

Clonazepam (Klonopin, Roche)

Indications. Clonazepam treats infantile spasms, myoclonic seizures, absence, and focal seizures.

Administration. The initial dosage is 0.025 mg/kg/day in two divided doses. Recommended increments are 0.025 mg/kg every 3–5 days as needed and tolerated. The usual maintenance dosage is 0.1 mg/kg/day in three divided doses. Most children cannot tolerate dosages of more than 0.15 mg/kg/day. The therapeutic blood concentration is 0.02–0.07 µg/mL, 47% of the drug is protein-bound, and the half-life is 20–40 hours. Rectal administration is suitable for maintenance if needed.

Adverse effects. Toxic effects with dosages within the therapeutic range include sedation, cognitive impairment, hyperactivity, and excessive salivation. Idiosyncratic reactions are unusual.

Ethosuximide (Zarontin, Pfizer)

Indications. Ethosuximide is the drug of choice for treating absence epilepsy. It is also useful for myoclonic absence.

Administration. The drug is absorbed rapidly, and peak blood concentrations appear within 4 hours. The half-life is 30 hours in children and up to 60 hours in adults. The initial dosage is 20 mg/kg/day in two divided doses after meals to avoid gastric irritation. Increase the dose at increments of 10 mg/kg/day as needed and

tolerated, to achieve seizure control without adverse effects. Levels between 50 and 120 µg/mL are usually therapeutic.

Adverse effects. Common adverse reactions are nausea and abdominal pain. These symptoms occur from gastric irritation within the therapeutic range and limit the drug's usefulness. The liquid preparation causes more irritation than the capsule. Unfortunately, gel capsules are large and some young children refuse to try this option until older. Always take the medication after eating.

Felbamate (Meda Pharmaceuticals)

Indications. Felbamate has a wide spectrum of antiepileptic activity. Its primary use is for refractory focal and generalized seizures, LGS, atypical absence, and atonic seizures.

Administration. Felbamate is rapidly absorbed after oral intake. Maximal plasma concentrations occur in 2–6 hours. The initial dosage is 15 mg/kg/day in three divided doses. Avoid nighttime doses if the drug causes insomnia. To attain seizure control, use weekly dosage increments of 15 mg/kg, as needed, to a total dose of approximately 45 mg/kg/day. Toxicity limits the total dosage. Levels between 50 and 100 µg/mL are usually therapeutic.

Adverse effects. Initial evidence suggested that adverse effects of felbamate were mild and dose related (nausea, anorexia, insomnia, and weight loss) except when in combination with other antiepileptic drugs. The addition of felbamate increases the plasma concentrations of phenytoin and valproate by as much as 30%. The carbamazepine serum concentration falls, but the concentration of its active epoxide metabolite increases by almost 50%.

Postmarketing experience showed that felbamate causes fatal liver damage and aplastic anemia in about 1 in 10,000 exposures. Regular monitoring of blood counts and liver function is required and may not help decrease these fatalities. However, this is a valuable drug in refractory epilepsy and has a place when used with caution and informed consent.

Fenfluramine (Fintepla, UCB Pharma)

Indications. Fenfluramine has a wide spectrum of antiepileptic activity and is specifically indicated for DS and LGS. The precise mechanism of action is not known but may be a novel agonist action on serotonin 5-HT2 receptors.

Administration. The initial dose is 0.1 mg/kg twice a day (0.2 mg/kg/day) for 1 week, then 0.2 mg/kg twice a day (0.4 mg/kg/day) for 1 week, then 0.35 mg/kg twice a day (0.7 mg/kg/day) as a goal dose. The maximum daily dose is 25 mg daily, unless the patient is taking stiripentol in which case it is 17 mg/day. The maximum dose for patients taking bupropion, fluoxetine, or paroxetine is 20 mg/day.

Adverse effects. Fenfluramine is only available through a risk evaluation and mitigation strategy (REMS) program in the United States, because of the known history of pulmonary hypertension and valvular heart disease when used at much higher doses for weight reduction. Patients underwent intense echocardiogram monitoring during the clinical development of Fintepla with no cardiac adverse effects seen. The most common side effects include decreased appetite and weight, somnolence, sedation, and lethargy. The REMS program requires regular cardiac monitoring.

Gabapentin (Neurontin, Pfizer)

Indications. Use gabapentin for the treatment of focal seizures with and without secondary generalization and neuropathic pain.

Administration. The usual titration dose is from 10 to 60 mg/kg/day, over 2 weeks. The mechanism of action is similar to pregabalin, but the efficacy is significantly lower.

Adverse effects. The adverse effects are sedation, edema, and increased weight.

Lacosamide (Vimpat, UCB Pharma)

Indications. Lacosamide is indicated for the treatment of focal seizures with and without secondary generalization.

Administration. The usual titration dose is from 2 to 10 mg/kg/day, over 2–4 weeks. The mechanism of action is on the sodium channel but different from the traditional sodium channel anticonvulsants.

Adverse effects. The adverse effects are sedation, ataxia, and dizziness.

Lamotrigine (Lamictal and Lamictal XR, Glaxo-SmithKline)

Indications. Lamotrigine is useful in the absence of epilepsy, atonic seizures, JME, LGS, focal epilepsies, and primary generalized tonic-clonic seizures. The spectrum of activity is similar to that of valproate.

Administration. The initial dose depends on whether the medication is used as monotherapy, combined with liver enzyme-inducing drugs, or combined with valproate. If used as monotherapy, give an initial dose of 0.3 mg/kg/day, then double the dose for 2 weeks

before increasing by the same amount weekly for a goal dose of 5–7 mg/kg/day. If using enzyme-inducing drugs, begin with 0.6 mg/kg/day and follow the same titration schedule to a goal dose of 5–15 mg/kg/day. When combined with valproate, the initial dose is 0.15 mg/kg/day with a goal dose of 1–3 mg/kg/day.

Plasma concentrations between 2 and 20 µg/mL are considered therapeutic.

Adverse effects. The main adverse reaction is a rash, which is more likely with titrations faster than recommended and can result in serious illness, including Steven-Johnson syndrome and toxic epidermal necrolysis. Other adverse effects are dizziness, ataxia, diplopia, insomnia, and headache. Female patients of childbearing age must be informed that lamotrigine can interact with hormonal contraceptives. Oral contraceptive pills may lower the level of lamotrigine and lamotrigine, in turn, may decrease the efficacy of contraceptives. Likewise, if a female patient becomes pregnant serum concentrations of lamotrigine can change quickly and drastically, requiring frequent monitoring and dose adjustments.

Levetiracetam (Keppra and Keppra XR, UCB Pharma)

Indications. Levetiracetam has a broad spectrum of activity and is useful for most seizure types. It is especially effective in the treatment of JME.[94] Its broad spectrum of activity, overall safety, and lack of drug-drug interactions make it an excellent first-line choice for most epilepsies.

Administration. Levetiracetam is available as a tablet, a suspension, and a solution for IV administration. The half-life is short, but the duration of efficacy is longer. Twice daily oral dosing is required unless using the extended-release version. The initial dose in children is 20 mg/kg/day, and the target dose is 20–80 mg/kg/day. A small number of children respond better to very high doses, and we treat a few children who seem to do best on doses close to 100 mg/kg/day.

Adverse effects. Levetiracetam is minimally liver metabolized. Metabolism occurs in the blood and excretion in the urine. It does not interfere with the metabolism of other drugs and has no life-threatening side effects. It frequently causes minor crankiness, but at times may cause more severe behavioral or mood disturbances. This was a rare event in the initial studies on the drug, but the incidence approaches 10%. The concomitant use of a small dose of pyridoxine 50–100 mg a day seems to relieve the irritability in some children, most likely via a GABA-mediated effect.

Oxcarbazepine (Trileptal, Novartis and Oxtellar, Supernus and Aptiom, Sunovion)

Indications. Oxcarbazepine is indicated for the treatment of focal seizures with and without secondary generalization, and has an almost identical chemical structure to carbamazepine with the addition of an O_2 molecule. This simple addition of the O_2 makes the molecule as different as water and hydrogen peroxide. It has the same therapeutic profile as carbamazepine but much better tolerability and adverse effect profile. The oxcarbazepine is further metabolized into S-licarbazepine (80%) and R-licarbazepine (20%). Aptiom is S-licarbazepine that is metabolized into a small amount of oxcarbazepine, 95% S-licarbazepine, and 5% R-licarbazepine. Both enantiomers are active and responsible for the anticonvulsant and side effects of these drugs. Oxtellar is the only extended-release formulation that decreases the fluctuation between peak and trough levels and therefore accommodates a once-a-day regimen. Aptiom has a larger peak-to-trough difference than the immediate-release oxcarbazepine but is also approved for once daily dosing.

Administration. Oxcarbazepine is available as a tablet (150, 300, and 600 mg) and as a suspension (300 mg/5 mL). Twice daily dosing is required for the immediate-release formulation. The initial dose is 10 mg/kg/day and then incrementally increased, as needed, to a total dose of 20–60 mg/kg/day in two divided doses. Oxtellar is available as 150, 300, and 600 mg tablets, and Aptiom as tablets 200, 400, 600, and 800 mg.

Adverse effects. The main adverse effect is drowsiness, but this is not as severe as with carbamazepine. Hyponatremia is a potential problem mainly in older populations or patients taking diuretics and SSRIs, or in medically fragile children with multiple comorbidities. Anecdotally, we note that some patients report constipation and weight gain.

Perampanel (Fycompa, Catalyst)

Indications. Parampanel is used to treat focal seizures with and without secondary generalization and primary generalized tonic-clonic seizures.

Administration. The usual titration dose is from 2 to 12 mg/day, over 5–15 weeks. The mechanism of action is the noncompetitive inhibition of glutaminergic AMPA receptors. The half-life is 105 hours and the dose should be increased from 2 mg daily by 2 mg every 2–3 weeks to the desired target.

Adverse effects. The adverse effects are sedation, ataxia, and irritability.

Phenobarbital

Indications. Phenobarbital is effective for focal and generalized tonic-clonic seizures. It is especially useful to treat status epilepticus.

Administration. Oral absorption is slow and once daily dosing is best when given with the evening meal rather than at bedtime if seizures are hypnagogic. Since intramuscular absorption requires 1–2 hours, the intramuscular route is useless for rapid loading (see the section on Management of Status Epilepticus); 50% of the drug is protein-bound, and 50% is free.

Initial and maintenance dosages are 3–5 mg/kg/day. The half-life is 50–140 hours in adults, 35–70 hours in children, and 50–200 hours in term newborns. Because of the very long half-life at all ages, once-a-day doses are usually satisfactory, achieving steady-state blood concentrations after 2 weeks of therapy. Therapeutic blood concentrations are 15–40 µg/mL.

Adverse effects. Hyperactivity is the most common and limiting side effect in children. Adverse behavioral changes occur in half of children between ages 2 and 10 years. Cognitive impairment is common. Hyperactivity and behavioral changes are both idiosyncratic and dose related.

Stevens-Johnson syndrome is more likely when compared with other anticonvulsant agents. Drowsiness and cognitive dysfunction, rather than hyperactivity, are the usual adverse effects after 10 years of age. Allergic rash is the main idiosyncratic reaction.

Phenytoin (Dilantin, Pfizer US Pharmaceuticals)

Indications. Phenytoin treats tonic-clonic and focal seizures.

Administration. Oral absorption is slow and unpredictable in newborns, erratic in infants, and probably not reliable until 3–5 years of age. Even in adults, considerable individual variability exists. Once absorbed, phenytoin is 70%–95% protein bound. A typical maintenance dosage is 7 mg/kg/day in children. The half-life is up to 60 hours in term newborns, up to 140 hours in premature infants, 5–14 hours in children, and 10–34 hours in adults. Capsules usually require two divided doses, but tablets are more rapidly absorbed and may require three divided doses a day. Administration of three times the maintenance dose achieves rapid oral loading. Fosphenytoin sodium has replaced parenteral phenytoin (see discussion of Status Epilepticus).

Adverse effects. The major adverse reactions are hypersensitivity, gum hypertrophy, and hirsutism.

Hypersensitivity reactions usually occur within 6 weeks of the initiation of therapy. Rash, fever, and lymphadenopathy are characteristic. Once such a reaction has occurred, discontinue the drug. Concurrent use of antihistamines is not appropriate management. Continued use of the drug may produce a Stevens-Johnson syndrome or a lupus-like disorder.

The cause of gum hypertrophy is a combination of phenytoin metabolites and plaque on the teeth. Persons with good oral hygiene are unlikely to have gum hypertrophy. Discuss the importance of good oral hygiene at the onset of therapy. Hirsutism is rarely a problem, but discontinues the drug when it occurs. Memory impairment, decreased attention span, and personality change may occur at therapeutic concentrations, but they occur less often and are less severe than with phenobarbital.

Pregabalin (Lyrica, Pfizer)
Indications. Pregabalin is indicated for the treatment of focal seizures with and without secondary generalization, and neuropathic pain.

Administration. The usual titration dose is from 2 to 10 mg/kg/day over 2 weeks. The mechanism of action is similar to gabapentin, but the efficacy is significantly higher.

Adverse effects. The adverse effects are sedation, edema, and increased weight.

Primidone (Mysoline, Valeant Pharmaceuticals)
Indications. Mysoline treats tonic-clonic and focal seizures.

Administration. Primidone metabolizes to at least two active metabolites: phenobarbital and phenylethylmalonamide (PEMA). The half-life of primidone is 6–12 hours, and that of PEMA is 20 hours. The usual maintenance dosage is 10–25 mg/kg/day, but the initial dosage should be 25% of the maintenance dosage or intolerable sedation will occur. A therapeutic blood concentration of primidone is 8–12 µg/mL. The blood concentration of phenobarbital derived from primidone is generally four times greater, but this ratio alters with concurrent administration of other antiepileptic drugs.

Adverse effects. The adverse effects are the same as for phenobarbital, except that the risk of intolerable sedation from the first tablet is greater.

Rufinamide (Banzel, Eisai)
Indications. Use rufinamide for the treatment of seizures within the spectrum of Lennox-Gastaut, which includes all seizure types.

Administration. The initial dosage is 15 mg/kg/day divided twice a day, titrating up to 45 mg/kg/day over 2 weeks. Valproic acid may decrease the metabolism by 15%–70%. Lower dosing and slower titration are recommended when using rufinamide and valproate concurrently.

Adverse effects. Sedation, emesis, and gastrointestinal symptoms may occur.

Stiripentol (Diacomit, Bicodex)
Indications. Approved for the treatment of seizures in DS as an adjunctive therapy to clobazam. The inhibition of CYP3A4 and 2C19 results in increasing levels of clobazam and norclobazam.

Administration. The recommended dose is 50 mg/kg/day, maximum dose 3 g/day, divided into two or three doses. Stiripentol is available as 250- and 500-mg capsules, and 250- or 500-mg powder sachets that are mixed with water and immediately administered. The possible mechanism of action is an effect on $GABA_A$ receptors and inhibition of cytochrome P450, resulting in increased levels of clobazam. The half-life is 4.5–13 hours and increases with dosage between 500 and 2000 mg daily.

Adverse effects. The adverse effects reported include decreased appetite and weight, drowsiness, ataxia, low muscle tone, dystonia, neutropenia, aggression, irritability, insomnia, and elevation of gamma-glutamyltransferase.

Tiagabine (Gabitril, Cephalon Inc.)
Indications. Tiagabine is indicated for use as adjunctive therapy for focal and generalized seizures.

Administration. The initial single-day dose is 0.2 mg/kg. Increase every 2 weeks by 0.2 mg/kg until achieving optimal benefit or adverse reactions occur.

Adverse effects. The most common adverse effects are somnolence and difficulty concentrating.

Topiramate (Topamax, Ortho McNeil)
Indications. Topiramate is used for focal and generalized epilepsies, especially LGS. It is also effective for migraine prophylaxis and a reasonable choice in children with both headaches and epilepsy.

Administration. The initial dose is 1–2 mg/kg/day, increased incrementally to up to 10–15 mg/kg/day divided into two doses.

Adverse effects. Weight loss may occur at therapeutic dosages. Cognitive impairment is common and often detected by relatives rather than the patient. Fatigue and altered mental status occur at toxic dosages. Glaucoma is a rare idiosyncratic reaction. Oligohydrosis is common, and the physician should advise patients to avoid overheating.

Valproate (Depakene, Depakote, and Depacon, Abbott Pharmaceutical)

Indications. Use mainly for generalized seizures. It is especially useful for mixed seizure disorders. Included are myoclonic seizures, simple absence, myoclonic absence, myoclonus, and tonic-clonic seizures.

Administration. Oral absorption is rapid, and the half-life is 6–15 hours. Three times a day dosing of the liquid achieves constant blood concentrations. An enteric-coated capsule (Depakote ER and Depakote sprinkles) slows absorption and allows twice daily dosing in children.

The initial dosage is 20 mg/kg/day. Increase in increments of 10 mg/kg/day to a goal dose of 60 mg/kg/day will provide a blood concentration of 50–100 μg/mL. Blood concentrations of 80–120 μg/mL are often required to achieve seizure control and are acceptable provided the patient is not experiencing adverse effects. Protein binding is 95% at blood concentrations of 50 μg/mL and 80% at 100 μg/mL. Therefore doubling the blood concentration increases the free fraction eightfold. Valproate has a strong affinity for plasma proteins and displaces other antiepileptic drugs.

Valproate is available for IV use. A dose of 25 mg/kg IV leads to a serum level of 100 μg/mL. Maintenance should start 1–3 hours after loading at 20 mg/kg/day divided into two doses.

Adverse effects. Valproate has dose-related and idiosyncratic hepatotoxicity. Dose-related hepatotoxicity is harmless (provided it is detected) and characterized by increased serum concentrations of transaminases. Important dose-related effects are a reduction in the platelet count, pancreatitis, and hyperammonemia. Thrombocytopenia may result in serious bleeding after trivial injury, whereas pancreatitis and hepatitis are both associated with nausea and vomiting.

Hyperammonemia causes cognitive disturbances and nausea. These adverse reactions are reversible by reducing the daily dose. Reduced plasma carnitine concentrations occur in children taking valproate, and some believe that carnitine supplementation helps relieve cognitive impairment.

The major idiosyncratic reaction is fatal liver necrosis attributed to the production of an aberrant and toxic metabolite. The major risk (1:800) is in children younger than 2 years of age who are receiving polytherapy. Many such cases may result from the combination of valproate on an underlying inborn error of metabolism. Fatal hepatotoxicity is unlikely to occur in children over 10 years of age treated with valproate alone.

The clinical manifestations of idiosyncratic hepatotoxicity are similar to those of Reye syndrome (see Chapter 2). They may begin after 1 day of therapy or may not appear for months or even years. No reliable way exists to monitor patients for idiosyncratic hepatotoxicity or to predict its occurrence, although routine monitoring of liver enzymes and platelet counts may allow earlier discovery of adverse reactions.

Vigabatrin (Sabril, Lundbeck)

Indications. Vigabatrin is indicated in the treatment of infantile spasms, particularly those associated with tuberous sclerosis, and focal seizures.

Administration. Vigabatrin is a very long-acting drug and needs only single-day dosing, but twice daily dosing is preferable to reduce adverse effects. The initial dose is 50 mg/kg/day, which increases incrementally, as needed, to 200–250 mg/kg/day. It is available in a powder sachet that can be mixed with water, as well as in tablet form.

Adverse effects. Peripheral loss of vision is the main serious adverse event, but the incidence seems to be much lower than when first labeled by the FDA. The defect is rare and consists of circumferential field constriction with nasal sparing. Behavioral problems, fatigue, confusion, and gastrointestinal upset are usually mild and dose related.

Zonisamide (Zonegran, Eisai Inc.)

Indications. Like levetiracetam, zonisamide has a broad spectrum of activity. It is effective against both primary generalized and focal epilepsies and is one of the most effective drugs in myoclonic epilepsies.

Administration. Zonisamide is a long-acting drug and should be given once at bedtime. The initial dose in children is 2 mg/kg/day. The maximum dose is around 15 mg/kg/day.

Adverse effects. Common adverse effects are drowsiness and anorexia. Of greater concern is the possibility of oligohydrosis and hyperthermia. Advise parents to monitor for decreased sweating and educate them regarding signs of hyperthermia. This is particularly important in warm climates.

Management of Status Epilepticus

The definition of status epilepticus is a prolonged single seizure (longer than 5–15 minutes , depending on seizure type) or repeated seizures without interictal recovery. Generalized tonic-clonic status is life-threatening and the most common emergency in pediatric neurology. The prognosis after status epilepticus in newborns is poor,[95] but is variable in other age groups depending on etiology. The causes of status epilepticus are the following: (1) a new acute illness such as encephalitis, (2) a progressive neurological disease, (3) loss of seizure control in a known epileptic, or (4) a prolonged febrile seizure in an otherwise normal child. The cause is the main determinant of outcome. Recurrence of status epilepticus is most likely in children who are neurologically abnormal and is rare in children with febrile seizures. The assessment of status epilepticus in children is the subject of a Practice Parameter of the Child Neurology Society.[96]

Absence status and complex partial status are often difficult to identify as status epilepticus. The child may appear to be in a confusional state.

Management of Seizure Emergencies in the Home

Home management of prolonged seizures or seizure clusters in children with known epilepsy is possible using the medications discussed later to prevent or abort status epilepticus. If the initial dose fails to stop the seizures, a second dose is recommended 10 minutes after the first dose and the family should activate emergency medical services who can treat in the field and while transporting the child to the hospital. Educate all caregivers regarding seizure first aid and when and how to utilize rescue medications. Many pictographs are available that provide easy-to-follow, step-by-step instructions for seizure management; we recommend families keep these displayed in the home in a clearly visible location. Most families need multiple doses of rescue medicines: one to keep at home, one for school, one to keep at the babysitter's house, etc.

Initial Hospital Management

Status epilepticus is a medical emergency requiring prompt attention. Initial assessment should be rapid and includes a cardiorespiratory assessment, a history leading up to the seizure, and a neurological examination. Most cases of convulsive status epilepticus require the establishment of a controlled airway and mechanical ventilation. Next, establish venous access. Measures of blood glucose, electrolytes, and anticonvulsant drug concentrations in children with known epilepsy are required.

Perform other tests, that is, toxic and/or infectious screen, as indicated. Once blood is drawn, start an IV infusion of saline solution for the administration of anticonvulsant drugs and the administration of an IV bolus. *Do not give IV fluids containing glucose to children who are on the ketogenic diet, as this can exacerbate seizures.*

Medications for Treatment of Seizure Clusters

Some children consistently experience seizure clusters during illness or with other exacerbating conditions. "Seizure cluster" is a poorly defined term and is also referred to as acute repetitive seizures and seizure flurries. It has been defined in various ways but is most commonly understood as three or more seizures within 24 hours, or seizures occurring at three times the normal baseline. Several medications have been approved to treat seizure clusters in the United States, including rectal diazepam, intranasal diazepam, and intranasal midazolam. During the clinical development of these drugs, the abortive benefits for prolonged (continuous) seizures were discovered in the secondary objectives.

In our practices we recommend rescue medications immediately on seizure onset in patients who are known to experience frequent clustering. Most convulsive seizures last no more than 2 minutes, and a rescue medication's abortive benefit should be considered after 3 minutes of convulsive activity. Rescue medications are clearly cost-effective, and multiple studies have confirmed that they reduce morbidity and mortality from seizures as well as reduce the need for emergency or intensive care unit (ICU) care.

Diazepam (Diastat, Valiant; Valtoco, Neurelis)

We use rectal diazepam (Diastat) for patients under 6 years of age. Diazepam is fat distributed and the dose varies by age: use 0.5 mg/kg for children aged 2–5 years. Rectal diazepam can be given to older children and adolescents although we prefer to use intranasal formulations when possible, which are equally efficacious while being easier to administer. Use 0.3 mg/kg rectal diazepam for children aged 6–11 years, and 0.2 mg/kg for children and adolescents aged 12 years and up with a maximum dose of 20 mg.

Intranasal diazepam (Valtoco) is used for patients older than 6 years. The dosing is the same as for the rectal formulation: use 0.3 mg/kg for children aged 6–11 years and 0.2 mg/kg for children aged 12 years and up, with a maximum dose of 20 mg.

Midazolam (Nayzilam, UCB Pharma)

Intranasal midazolam is approved for patients older than 12 years. The dose is 5 mg given intranasally. As with intranasal and rectal diazepam, the dose can be repeated after 10 minutes if necessary.

Adverse Effects

Benzodiazepines administered as rescue medications may cause sedation, lethargy, or somnolence. Families are frequently concerned about the possibility of respiratory depression, but in clinical trials the incidence was low. The risk of respiratory failure is far higher if the seizure is allowed to continue.

Hospital-Based Treatment of Status Epilepticus

Status epilepticus is a medical emergency requiring prompt attention. Initial assessment should be rapid and includes a cardiorespiratory assessment, a history leading up to the seizure, and a neurological examination. Most cases of convulsive status epilepticus require the establishment of a controlled airway and mechanical ventilation. Next, establish venous access. Measures of blood glucose, electrolytes, and anticonvulsant drug concentrations in children with known epilepsy are required. Perform toxic and infectious screens as indicated. Once blood is drawn, start an IV infusion of saline solution for the administration of anticonvulsant drugs and the administration of an IV bolus. *Do not give IV fluids containing glucose to children who are on the ketogenic diet, as this can exacerbate seizures.*

The ideal drug for treating status epilepticus is one that acts rapidly, has a long duration of action, and produces minimal or quickly resolving sedation. The use of benzodiazepines (diazepam and lorazepam) for this purpose is common. However, they are inadequate by themselves because their duration of action is brief. In addition, children given IV benzodiazepines after a prior load of barbiturate often have respiratory depression. The dose of diazepam is 0.2 mg/kg, not to exceed 10 mg at a rate of 1 mg/min. Lorazepam may be preferable to diazepam because of its longer duration of action. The usual dosage in children 12 years of age or younger is 0.1 mg/kg. After age 12 years, it is 0.07 mg/kg.

IV fosphenytoin is an ideal agent because it has a long duration of action, does not produce respiratory depression, and does not impair consciousness. The initial dose is 20 mg/kg (calculated as phenytoin equivalents).

Administration can be IV or intramuscular, but the IV route is greatly preferred. Unlike phenytoin, which requires slow infusions (0.5 mg/kg/min) to avoid cardiac toxicity, fosphenytoin infusions are rapid and often obviate the need for prior benzodiazepine therapy. Infants generally require 30 mg/kg. Fosphenytoin is usually effective unless a severe, acute encephalopathy is the cause of status. Children who fail to wake up at an expected time after the clinical signs of status have stopped require an EEG to exclude the possibility of electrical status epilepticus.

IV valproate can be infused rapidly with loading doses of 20–40 mg/kg. It is likely more efficacious than IV fosphenytoin, levetiracetam, or phenobarbital and has a wide spectrum of action, including modulation of sodium channels, calcium channels, and GABA. Many institutions use IV valproate as their preferred second-line agent rather than fosphenytoin. Valproate may cause hepatotoxicity particularly in patients under the age of 2 and in those with suspected mitochondrial or metabolic disease.

IV levetiracetam 20–60 mg/kg is safe, readily available, does not require hepatic metabolism, has minimal interactions, is not cardiotoxic, and can be infused faster; however, it has not undergone the testing to be universally accepted in status protocols. The maximum single dose is 2 g. Many emergency departments routinely give IV levetiracetam despite the lack of clear evidence for use in status epilepticus.

IV lacosamide at a loading dose of 10 mg/kg has promising initial evidence regarding use in both focal and generalized convulsive status epilepticus in children.[97] It does not have significant interactions with other medications and can be given rapidly via the IV route and uptitrated quickly. The main adverse effects were similar to fosphenytoin, consisting of diplopia, ataxia, and dizziness.

IV phenobarbital has long been used as a treatment for status epilepticus. It does cause significant sedation, which makes it difficult to obtain an accurate neurologic examination; other potentially serious side effects include respiratory depression and hypotension. We prefer not to use phenobarbital boluses unless other treatments such as IV valproate, fosphenytoin, and lacosamide have failed. However, it does have its place in the treatment of status epilepticus. Loading doses are typically 20–40 mg/kg with additional boluses of 10–20 mg/kg if needed. In general, the physician must secure the patient's airway before giving large doses of phenobarbital due to the risk of respiratory depression.

When all else fails, consider initiating continuous infusions of midazolam or pentobarbital. Transfer the patient from the emergency department to an ICU. Intubation and mechanical ventilation must be in place. After placing an arterial line, monitor the patient's blood pressure, cardiac rhythm, body temperature, and blood oxygen saturation as well as their continuous EEG tracing (video EEG preferred).

For pentobarbital, infuse 10 mg/kg boluses until a burst-suppression pattern appears on the EEG (Fig. 1.4); a minimum of 30 mg/kg is generally required. Hypotension is the most serious complication and requires treatment with vasopressors. It generally does not occur until after the administration of 40–60 mg/kg. Barbiturates tend to accumulate, and the usual dosage needed to maintain pentobarbital coma is 3 mg/kg/h. Maintaining a coma for several days may be necessary and has a relatively low-risk profile. Continuous EEG recording indicates a burst-suppression pattern. Slow or

stop the barbiturate infusion every 24–48 hours to see if coma is still required to prevent seizure discharges. Pentobarbital may produce an "emergence pattern" on EEG during which the former bursts become more epileptiform-appearing and prolonged. This often leads to concern that the patient is about to experience a recurrence of status epilepticus. In our practice we try to continue with the planned wean unless the patient has clear clinical or electrographic seizures. The EEG pattern typically becomes more reassuring as the wean continues.

The Ketogenic Diet

The Bible mentions fasting and praying as a treatment for epilepsy. The introduction of diet-induced ketosis to mimic fasting dates to 1921, when barbiturates and bromides were the only available antiepileptic drugs. This method became less popular with the introduction of effective pharmacotherapy. However, it remains an effective method to treat children with seizures refractory to antiepileptic drugs at nontoxic levels. The diet is

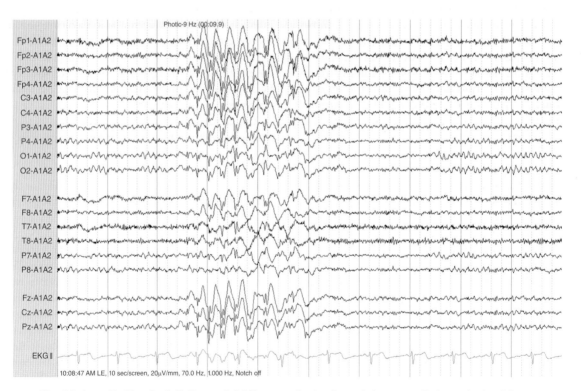

Fig. 1.4 Juvenile Myoclonic Epilepsy. A 4.7 Hz generalized spike and slow wave discharge lasting 2.5 seconds during photic stimulation.

most effective in infants and young children. A diet that consists of 60% medium-chain triglycerides, 11% long-chain saturated fat, 10% protein, and 19% carbohydrate is commonly used. The main side effects are abdominal pain and diarrhea.[98]

The ketogenic diet causes a prompt elevation in plasma ketone bodies that the brain uses as an energy source. The exact mechanism of action is not established. The ketogenic diet is most effective for the control of myoclonic seizures, infantile spasms, atonic/akinetic seizures, and mixed seizures of the LGS. *The ketogenic diet is not a "natural" treatment for epilepsy.* Side effects are common and alterations in blood chemistries are more significant than with the use of medications; however, it is a good alternative when epilepsy is not controlled or medications are not tolerated.

Vagal Nerve Stimulation

Vagal nerve stimulation (VNS) is a treatment for refractory seizures that uses a programmed stimulus from a chest-implanted generator via coiled electrodes tunneled to the left cervical vagus nerve. Current indications for VNS are for adjunctive treatment of refractory partial seizures. The main adverse effects are voice changes or hoarseness; some patients report a tickling sensation in the throat that causes coughing. The ketogenic diet is preferable to VNS in children less than 12 years of age.[99] However, VNS is a reasonable adjunctive treatment in children with refractory epilepsy. Many patients seem to have shorter postictal periods and improved mood with this therapy, and a small but important minority finds that swiping the magnet (which delivers an extra burst of stimulation) helps abort their seizures more quickly. A 30%–40% reduction in seizures is, in general, a realistic expectation. Seizure freedom should not be expected or promised.

Surgical Approaches to Childhood Epilepsy

Epilepsy surgery is an excellent option for selected children with intractable epilepsy, and surgical options and techniques have made great strides forward within the past 10 years. However, this also means that much of the discussion of epilepsy surgery is beyond the scope of this book. Surgery is never a substitute for good medical therapy, and antiepileptic drug therapy often continues after surgery. Lesionectomy, hemispherectomy, interhemispheric commissurotomy, and temporal lobectomy or hippocampectomy are appropriate for different situations. None of these procedures are new, and all have gone through phases of greater or lesser popularity since their introduction. Newer surgical techniques include the use of laser ablation to eliminate focal lesions with clearly defined boundaries and the emerging use of DBS to treat some refractory generalized epilepsies. The use of functional MRI, Wada test, single-photon emission CT, PET, and magnetoencephalography, when indicated, improves the localization of the epileptogenic foci and the surgical outcomes. Invasive monitoring techniques such as stereotactic EEG are standard in cases in which the exact anatomical location of the seizure focus is uncertain; invasive monitoring also allows for cortical mapping to minimize surgery-related deficits.

Lesionectomy, Temporal Lobectomy, or Hippocampectomy

The resection of an epileptogenic lesion may be needed for diagnosis when neoplasms are suspected. Lesionectomy is often an excellent treatment choice for epilepsies resistant to medical treatment when the MRI shows an underlying structural abnormality in the focus of seizures. Around 80% of patients with well-circumscribed unifocal epilepsies associated with lesions may remain seizure free after surgical resections. The hippocampus or the temporal lobe is often the target of a potential epilepsy surgery. The success rate decreases in cases where the MRI shows no underlying abnormality or the patient has multiple seizure semiologies and multifocal epilepsies. Laser ablation of hippocampal sclerosis offers a newer, less invasive means of lesion removal although we note that it works best in cases in which the lesion is clearly defined.

Hemispherectomy

The use of hemispherectomy, or more correctly hemidecortication, is exclusively for children with intractable epilepsy and hemiplegia. The hemiplegia may be preexisting (as in children with large unilateral perinatal strokes) or inevitable (as in children with Rasmussen's encephalitis). The original procedure consisted of removing the cortex of one hemisphere along with a variable portion of the underlying basal ganglia. The extent of surgery depended partly on the underlying disease. The resulting cavity communicated with the third ventricle and developed a subdural membrane lining. The immediate results were good. Seizures were relieved in about 80% of children, and behavior and spasticity improved without deterioration of intellectual function or motor function in the hemiparetic limbs.

However, late complications of hemorrhage, hydrocephalus, and hemosiderosis occurred in up to 35% of children and were sometimes fatal. The subdural membrane repeatedly tore, bleeding into the ventricular system and staining the ependymal lining and the pia arachnoid with iron.

Because of these complications, less radical alternatives are generally preferred. These alternatives are the Montreal-type hemispherectomy and interhemispheric commissurotomy. The Montreal-type hemispherectomy is a modified procedure with the removal of most of the damaged hemisphere, with portions of the frontal and occipital lobes left in place, but disconnected from the other hemisphere and brainstem. The best results are in children with diseases affecting only one hemisphere, Sturge-Weber syndrome, and Rasmussen encephalitis.

Interhemispheric Commissurotomy (Corpus Callosotomy)

Disconnecting the hemispheres from each other and the brainstem is an alternative to hemispherectomy in children with intractable epilepsy and hemiplegia. Another use of this procedure is to decrease the occurrence of secondary generalized tonic-clonic seizures from partial or minor generalized seizures. The efficacy of commissurotomy and hemispherectomy in children with infantile hemiplegia is probably comparable, but the efficacy of commissurotomy in other forms of epilepsy is unknown.

Complete and partial commissurotomies are in use. Complete commissurotomy entails the division of the entire corpus callosum, anterior commissure, one fornix, and the hippocampal commissure. Complete commissurotomies may be one- or two-stage procedures. Partial commissurotomies vary from division of the corpus callosum and hippocampal commissure to division of only the anterior portion of the corpus callosum.

Two immediate, but transitory, postoperative complications may follow interhemispheric commissurotomy: (1) a syndrome of mutism, nondominant arm and leg apraxia, and urinary incontinence and (2) hemiparesis. They are both more common after one-stage, complete commissurotomy than after two-stage procedures or partial commissurotomy and probably caused by prolonged retraction of one hemisphere during surgery. Long-term complications may include stuttering and poorly coordinated movements of the hands.

REFERENCES

1. Silverstein FS, Jensen FE. Neonatal seizures. *Annals of Neurology*. 2007;62:112-120.
2. Ronen GM, Buckley D, Penney S, et al. Long-term prognosis in children with neonatal seizures. A population study. *Neurology*. 2007;69:1816-1822.
3. Hudak ML, et al. Neonatal drug withdrawal. *Pediatrics*. 2012;129:e540-e560.
4. Millevert C, Weckhuysen S. ILAE Genetics Commission ILAE Genetic Literacy Series: self-limited familial epilepsy syndromes with onset in neonatal age and infancy. *Epileptic Disorders*. 2023;25:445-453. https://doi.org/10.1002/epd2.20026. PMID: 36939707.
5. McDonald-McGinn DM, Hain HS, Emanuel BS, et al. 22q11.2 Deletion syndromeSep 23, 1999 [Updated Feb 27, 2020]. In: Adam MP, Mirzaa GM, Pagon RA, et al., eds. *GeneReviews®*. University of Washington; 1993–2023. https://www.ncbi.nlm.nih.gov/books/NBK1523/.
6. Burn J. Closing time for CATCH22. *Journal of Medical Genetics*. 1999;36:737-738.
7. Miller SP, Ramaswamy V, Michelson D, et al. Patterns of brain injury in term neonatal encephalopathy. *Journal of Pediatrics*. 2005;146:453-460.
8. Committee on Fetus and Newborn Hypothermia and neonatal encephalopathy. *Pediatrics*. 2014;133(6):1146-1150. https://doi.org/10.1542/peds.2014-0899.
9. McHugh DC, Lancaster S, Manganas LN. A systematic review of the efficacy of levetiracetam in neonatal seizures. *Neuropediatrics*. 2018;49(1):12-17. https://doi.org/10.1055/s-0037-1608653. Epub 2017 Nov 27, 2017. PMID: 29179233.
10. Bamgbose O, Boyle F, Kean AC, Stefanescu BM, Wing S. Tolerability and safety of lacosamide in neonatal population. *Journal of Child Neurology*. 2023;38(3-4):137-141. https://doi.org/10.1177/08830738231164835. PMID: 36972493.
11. Lynch NE, Stevenson NJ, Livingstone V, Murphy BP, Rennie JM, Boylan GB. The temporal evolution of electrographic seizure burden in neonatal hypoxic ischemic encephalopathy. *Epilepsia*. 2012;53(3):549-557. https://doi.org/10.1111/j.1528-1167.2011.03401.x. Epub 2012 Feb 6. PMID: 22309206.
12. Seashore M. Organic acidemias: an overview. In: *GeneClinics: Medical Genetics Knowledge Base [database online]*. University of Washington; 2009. http://www.geneclinics.org. PMID: 20301313. Last updated Dec 22.
13. Van Hove JLK, Coughlin II C, Swanson M, et al. Nonketotic hyperglycinemia. (Nov 14, 2002). In: Adam MP, Mirzaa GM, Pagon RA, et al., eds. *GeneReviews®*. University of Washington; 1993–2023:[Updated May 23, 2019] https://www.ncbi.nlm.nih.gov/books/NBK1357/.

14. Bjoraker KJ, et al. Neurodevelopmental outcome and treatment efficacy of benzoate and dextromethorphan in siblings with attenuated nonketotic hyperglycinemia. *Journal of Pediatrics*. 2016;170:234-239.

15. Strauss KA, Puffenberger EG, Carson VJ. Maple syrup urine disease. Jan 30, 2006 [Updated Apr 23, 2020]. In: Adam MP, Mirzaa GM, Pagon RA, et al., eds. *GeneReviews®*. University of Washington; 1993–2023. https://www.ncbi.nlm.nih.gov/books/NBK1319/.

16. Grünert SC, Wendel U, Lindner M, et al. Clinical and neurocognitive outcome in symptomatic isovaleric acidemia. *Orphanet Journal of Rare Diseases*. 2012;7:9. https://doi.org/10.1186/1750-1172-7-9. PMID: 22277694; PMCID: PMC3292949.

17. Manoli I, Sloan JL, Venditti CP. Isolated methylmalonic acidemia. Aug 16, 2005 [updated Sep 8, 2022]. In: Adam MP, Mirzaa GM, Pagon RA, eds, et al. *GeneReviews®*. University of Washington; 1993–2023.PMID: 20301409.

18. Shchelochkov OA, Carrillo N, Venditti C. Propionic acidemia. May 17, 2012 [Updated Oct 6, 2016]. In: Adam MP, Mirzaa GM, Pagon RA, et al., eds. *GeneReviews®*. University of Washington; 1993–2023. https://www.ncbi.nlm.nih.gov/books/NBK92946/.

19. Gospe Jr SM. Pyridoxine-dependent epilepsy – ALDH7A1. Dec 7, 2001 [Updated Sep 22, 2022]. In: Adam MP, Mirzaa GM, Pagon RA, et al., eds. *GeneReviews®*. University of Washington; 1993–2023. https://www.ncbi.nlm.nih.gov/books/NBK1486/.

20. Coughlin II CR, Tseng LA, Abdenur JE, et al. Consensus guidelines for the diagnosis and management of pyridoxine-dependent epilepsy due to α-aminoadipic semialdehyde dehydrogenase deficiency. *Journal of Inherited Metabolic Disease*. 2021;44(1):178-192. https://doi.org/10.1002/jimd.12332. Epub Dec 1, 2020. PMID: 33200442.

21. Tso WWY, Kwong AKY, Fung CW, et al. Folinic acid responsive epilepsy in Ohtahara syndrome caused by STXBP1 mutation. *Pediatric Neurology*. 2014;50(2):177-180.

22. Al-Baradie RS, Chaudhary MW. Diagnosis and management of cerebral folate deficiency. A form of folinic acid-responsive seizures. *Neuroscience (Riyadh)*. 2014;19(4):312-316. PMID: 25274592; . PMCID: PMC4727671.

23. Freed GE, Martinez F. Atypical seizures as the cause of apnea in a six-month old child. *Clinical Pediatrics*. 2001;40:283-285.

24. Yang JY, Chan AK, Callen DJ, Paes BA. Neonatal cerebral sinovenous thrombosis: sifting the evidence for a diagnostic plan and treatment strategy. *Pediatrics*. 2010;126:e693-e700.

25. Scheuerle AE, Ursini MV. Incontinentia pigmenti. Jun 8, 1999 [Updated Dec 21, 2017]. In: Adam MP, Mirzaa GM, Pagon RA, et al., eds. *GeneReviews®*. University of Washington; 1993–2023. https://www.ncbi.nlm.nih.gov/books/NBK1472/.

26. Painter MJ. Phenobarbital compared with phenytoin for the treatment of neonatal seizures. *New England Journal of Medicine*. 1999;341:485.

27. Pina-Garza JE, Espinoza R, Nordli D, et al. Oxcarbazepine adjunctive therapy in infants and young children with partial seizures. *Neurology*. 2005;65:1370-1375.

28. Pina-Garza JE, Levinson P, Gucuyener K, et al. Adjunctive lamotrigine for partial seizures in patients ages 1 to 24 months old. *Neurology*. 2008;70(22, pt 2):2099-2108.

29. Pina-Garza JE, Elterman RD, Ayala R, et al. Long term tolerability and efficacy of lamotrigine in infants 1 to 24 months old. *Journal of Child Neurology*. 2008;23(8):853-861.

30. Pina-Garza JE, Nordli D, Rating D, et al. Adjunctive levetiracetam in infants and young children with refractory partial-onset seizures. *Epilepsia*. 2009;50(5):1141-1149.

31. Pina-Garza JE, Schiemann-Delgado J, Yang H, Duncan B. Adjunctive levetiracetam in patients age 1 month to <4 years with partial onset seizures; an open label long term follow-up. *Clinical Therapeutics*. 2010;32:1935-1950.

32. Shoaib A, Dolce A, Machie M, Thomas J. Use of Lacosamide in neonatal seizures (P6-5.001). *Neurology*. 2022;98(suppl 18):693.

33. McHarg ML, Shinnar S, Rascoff H, Walsh CA. Syncope in childhood. *Pediatric Cardiology*. 1997;18(5):367-371. https://doi.org/10.1007/s002469900202. PMID: 9270107.

34. Balint B, Thomas R. Hereditary hyperekplexia overviewJul 31, 2007 [Updated Dec 19, 2019]. In: Adam MP, Mirzaa GM, Pagon RA, et al., eds. *GeneReviews®*. University of Washington; 1993–2023. https://www.ncbi.nlm.nih.gov/books/NBK1260/.

35. Rhys HT, et al. Genotype-phenotype correlations in hyperekplexia: apnoeas, learning difficulties and speech delay. *Brain*. 2013;136:3085-3095.

36. Tarkka R, Paakko E, Pyhtinen J, et al. Febrile seizures and mesial temporal sclerosis. No association in a long-term follow-up study. *Neurology*. 2003;60:215-218.

37. Striano P, Coppola A, Pezzella M, et al. An open-label trial of levetiracetam in severe myoclonic epilepsy of infancy. *Neurology*. 2007;69:250-254.

38. Lagae L, Sullivan J, Knupp K, et al. Fenfluramine hydrochloride for the treatment of seizures in Dravet syndrome: a randomised, double-blind, placebo-controlled trial. *Lancet*. 2019;394(10216):2243-2254. https://doi.org/10.1016/S0140-6736(19)32500-0. Epub Dec 17, 2019. PMID: 31862249.

39. Camfield P, Camfield C. Febrile seizures and genetic epilepsy with febrile seizures plus (GEFS+). *Epileptic*

Disorders. 2015;17(2):124-133. https://doi.org/10.1684/epd.2015.0737. PMID: 25917466.

40. Shinnar S, Berg AT, Moshe SL, et al. The risk of seizure recurrence after a first unprovoked afebrile seizure in childhood: an extended follow-up. *Pediatrics.* 1996; 98(2 Pt 1):216-225. PMID: 8692621.

41. Mizorogi S, Kanemura H, Sano F, Sugita K, Aihara M. Risk factors for seizure recurrence in children after first unprovoked seizure. *Pediatrics International.* 2015;57(4):665-669. https://doi.org/10.1111/ped.12600. Epub Apr 28, 2015. PMID: 25676481.

42. Sutton VR, Van den Veyver IB. Aicardi syndrome. Jun 30, 2006 [Updated Nov 12, 2020]. In: Adam MP, Mirzaa GM, Pagon RA, et al., eds. *GeneReviews®.* University of Washington; 1993–2023. https://www.ncbi.nlm.nih.gov/books/NBK1381/.

43. Mackay MT, Weiss SK, Adams-Webber T, et al. Practice parameter: medical treatment of infantile spasms. Report of the American Academy of Neurology and the Child Neurology Society. *Neurology.* 2004;62:1668-1681.

44. Hussain SA, Shinnar S, Kwong G, et al. Treatment of infantile spasms with very high dose prednisolone before high dose adrenocorticotropic hormone. *Epilepsia.* 2014;55(1):103-107. https://doi.org/10.1111/epi.12460. Epub 2013 Nov 8. PMID: 24446954; PMCID: PMC3904676.

45. Gümüş H, Kumandas S, Per H. Levetiracetam monotherapy in newly diagnosed cryptogenic West syndrome. *Pediatric Neurology.* 2007;37:350-353.

46. Mikati MA, El Bannan D, Sinno D, et al. Response of infantile spasms to levetiracetam. *Neurology.* 2008;70: 574-575.

47. Lotze TE, Wilfong AA. Zonisamide treatment for symptomatic infantile spasms. *Neurology.* 2004;62:296-298.

48. Glausser TA, Nigro M, Sachdeo R, et al. Adjunctive therapy with oxcarbazepine in children with partial seizures. *Neurology.* 2000;54(12):2237-2244.

49. Parisi P, Bombardieri R, Curatolo P. Current role of vigabatrin infantile spasms. *European Journal of Paediatric Neurology.* 2007;11:331-336.

50. Campostrini G, DiFrancesco JC, Castellotti B, et al. A loss-of-function *HCN4* mutation associated with familial benign myoclonic epilepsy in infancy causes increased neuronal excitability. *Frontiers in Molecular Neuroscience.* 2018;11:269. https://doi.org/10.3389/fnmol.2018.00269. PMID: 30127718; PMCID: PMC6089338.

51. Dulac O. Epileptic encephalopathy. *Epilepsia.* 2001;92(3): 23-26.

52. Wolf B. Biotinidase deficiency. Mar 24, 2000 [Updated Jun 9, 2016]. In: Adam MP, Mirzaa GM, Pagon RA, et al., eds. *GeneReviews®.* University of Washington;

1993–2023. https://www.ncbi.nlm.nih.gov/sites/books/NBK1322/.

53. Minewer M. New evidence for a genetic link between epilepsy and migraine. *Neurology.* 2007;68:1969-1970.

54. Ebrahimi-Fakhari D, El Achkar CM, Klein C. PRRT2-associated paroxysmal movement disorders. Jan 11, 2018. In: Adam MP, Mirzaa GM, Pagon RA, et al., eds. *GeneReviews®.* University of Washington; 1993–2023. https://www.ncbi.nlm.nih.gov/sites/books/NBK475803/.

55. Erro R. Familial paroxysmal nonkinesigenic dyskinesia. Jun 24, 2005 [Updated Apr 4, 2019]. In: Adam MP, Mirzaa GM, Pagon RA, et al., eds. *GeneReviews®.* University of Washington; 1993–2023. https://www.ncbi.nlm.nih.gov/books/NBK1221/.

56. Hisama FM, Friedman J, Raskind WH, et al. ADCY5 dyskinesia. Dec 18, 2014 [Updated Jul 30, 2020]. In: Adam MP, Mirzaa GM, Pagon RA, et al., eds. *GeneReviews®.* University of Washington; 1993–2023. https://www.ncbi.nlm.nih.gov/sites/books/NBK263441/.

57. Suls A, Dedeken P, Goffin K, et al. Paroxysmal exercise-induced dyskinesia and epilepsy is due to mutations in SLC2A1, encoding the glucose transporter GLUT1. *Brain.* 2008 Jul;131(Pt 7):1831-1844. https://doi.org/10.1093/brain/awn113. Epub Jun 24, 2008. PMID: 18577546; PMCID: PMC2442425.

58. Scammell TE. The neurobiology, diagnosis, and treatment of narcolepsy. *Annals of Neurology.* 2003;53: 154-160.

59. Nishino S. Clinical and neurobiological aspects of narcolepsy. *Sleep Medicine.* 2007;8:373-399.

60. Plazzi G, Ruoff C, Lecendreux M, et al. Treatment of paediatric narcolepsy with sodium oxybate: a double-blind, placebo-controlled, randomised-withdrawal multicentre study and open-label investigation. *Lancet Child & Adolescent Health.* 2018;2(7):483-494. https://doi.org/10.1016/S2352-4642(18)30133-0. Epub May 21, 2018. PMID: 30169321.

61. Guilleminault C, Palombini L, Pelayo R, et al. Sleepwalking and sleep terrors in prepubertal children: what triggers them? *Pediatrics.* 2003;111:e17-e25.

62. Norcliffe-Kaufman IJ, Kaufman H, Hainsworth R. Enhanced vascular response to hypocapnia in neutrally mediated syncope. *Annals of Neurology.* 2008;63:288-294.

63. Vernino S, Bourne KM, Stiles LE, et al. Postural orthostatic tachycardia syndrome (POTS): state of the science and clinical care from a 2019 National Institutes of Health Expert Consensus Meeting - Part 1. *Autonomic Neuroscience.* 2021 Nov;235:102828. https://doi.org/10.1016/j.autneu.2021.102828. Epub Jun 5, 2021. PMID: 34144933; PMCID: PMC8455420.

64. Glausser TA, Cnan A, et al. Ethosuximide, valproic acid, and lamotrigine in childhood absence epilepsy. *New England Journal of Medicine*. 2010;362:790-799.

65. Pina-Garza JE, Schwarzman L, et al. A pilot study of topiramate in childhood absence epilepsy. *Acta Neurologica Scandinavica*. 2011;123(1):54-59.

66. Vrielynck P. Current and emerging treatments for absence seizures in young patients. *Neuropsychiatric Disease and Treatment*. 2013;9:963-975. https://doi.org/10.2147/NDT.S30991. Epub Jul 15, 2013. PMID: 23885176; PMCID: PMC3716601.

67. Valentín A, Navarrete EG, Chelvarajah R, et al. Deep brain stimulation of the centromedian thalamic nucleus for the treatment of generalized and frontal epilepsies. *Epilepsia*. 2013 Oct;54(10):1823-1833. https://doi.org/10.1111/epi.12352. Epub Sep 13, 2013. PMID: 24032641.

68. Giraldez BG, Serratosa JM. Jeavons syndrome as an occipital cortex initiated generalized epilepsy: further evidence from a patient with a photic induced occipital seizure. *Seizure*. 2015;32:72-74.

69. Tang S, Addis L, Smith A, et al. Phenotypic and genetic spectrum of epilepsy with myoclonic atonic seizures. *Epilepsia*. 2020;61(5):995-1007. https://doi.org/10.1111/epi.16508. Epub May 29, 2020. PMID: 32469098.

70. Wheless JW, Kim HL. Adolescent seizures and epilepsy syndromes. *Epilepsia*. 2002;43:33-52.

71. Sharpe DV, Patel AD, Abou-Khalil B, et al. Levetiracetam monotherapy in juvenile myoclonic epilepsy. *Seizure*. 2008;17:64-68.

72. Knupp KG, Scheffer IE, Ceulemans B, et al. Efficacy and safety of Fenfluramine for the treatment of seizures associated with Lennox-Gastaut syndrome: a randomized clinical trial. *JAMA Neurology*. 2022;79(6):554-564. https://doi.org/10.1001/jamaneurol.2022.0829.

73. Jansen AC, Andermann E. Progressive myoclonus epilepsy, Lafora type. Dec 28, 2007 [Updated Feb 21, 2019]. In: Adam MP, Mirzaa GM, Pagon RA, et al., eds. *GeneReviews®*. University of Washington; 1993–2023. https://www.ncbi.nlm.nih.gov/books/NBK1389/.

74. Lehesjoki AE, Kälviäinen R. Progressive myoclonic epilepsy type 1. Jun 24, 2004 [Updated Jul 2, 2020]. In: Adam MP, Mirzaa GM, Pagon RA, et al., eds. *GeneReviews®*. University of Washington; 1993–2023. https://www.ncbi.nlm.nih.gov/books/NBK1142/.

75. Mastrangelo M, Caputi C, Esposito D, et al. PRICKLE1-related disorders. Sep 8, 2009 [Updated Apr 21, 2022]. In: Adam MP, Mirzaa GM, Pagon RA, eds. *GeneReviews®*. University of Washington; 1993–2023. https://www.ncbi.nlm.nih.gov/books/NBK9674/.

76. Porter BE, Judkins AR, Clancy RR, et al. Dysplasia. A common finding in intractable pediatric temporal lobe epilepsy. *Neurology*. 2003;61:365-368.

77. Carpio A, Hauser WA. Prognosis for seizure recurrence in patients with newly diagnosed neurocysticercosis. *Neurology*. 2002;59:1730-1734.

78. Camfield P, Camfield C. Epileptic syndromes in childhood: clinical features, outcomes, and treatment. *Epilepsia*. 2002;43:27-32.

79. Lesca G, Møller RS, Rudolf G, Hirsch E, Hjalgrim H, Szepetowski P. Update on the genetics of the epilepsy-aphasia spectrum and role of GRIN2A mutations. *Epileptic Disorders*. 2019;21(suppl 1):41-47. https://doi.org/10.1684/epd.2019.1056. PMID: 31149903.

80. Kurahashi H., Hirose S. Autosomal dominant sleep-related hypermotor (hyperkinetic) epilepsy. May 16, 2002 [Updated Mar 23, 2023]. In: Adam MP, Mirzaa GM, Pagon RA, et al., eds. *GeneReviews®*. University of Washington. 1993–2023. https://www.ncbi.nlm.nih.gov/books/NBK1169/

81. Connolly MB, Langill L, Wong PKH, et al. Seizures involving the supplementary sensorimotor area in children: a video-EEG analysis. *Epilepsia*. 1995;36:1025-1032.

82. Rots ML, De Vos CC, Smeets-Schouten JS, Portier R, van Putten MJ. Suppressors of interictal discharges in idiopathic childhood occipital epilepsy of Gastaut. *Epilepsy & Behavior*. 2012 Oct;25(2):189-191. https://doi.org/10.1016/j.yebeh.2012.06.026. Epub 2012 Sep 30. PMID: 23032130.

83. Politi-Elishkevich K, Kivity S, Shuper A, Levine H, Goldberg-Stern H. Idiopathic photosensitive occipital epilepsy: clinical and electroencephalographic (EEG) features. *Journal of Child Neurology*. 2014;29(3):307-311. https://doi.org/10.1177/0883073812473366. Epub 2013 Jan 17. PMID: 23334080.

84. Nicolai J, Aldenkamp AP, Arends J, et al. Cognitive and behavioral effects of nocturnal epileptiform discharges in children with benign childhood epilepsy with centrotemporal spikes. *Epilepsy & Behavior*. 2006;8:56-70.

85. Lesca G, Møller RS, Rudolf G, Hirsch E, Hjalgrim H, Szepetowski P. Update on the genetics of the epilepsy-aphasia spectrum and role of GRIN2A mutations. *Epileptic Disorders*. 2019;21(suppl 1):41-47. https://doi.org/10.1684/epd.2019.1056. PMID: 31149903.

86. Filippini M, Boni A, Giannotta M, Gobbi G. Neuropsychological development in children belonging to BECTS spectrum: long-term effect of epileptiform activity. *Epilepsy & Behavior*. 2013 Sep;28(3):504-511. https://doi.org/10.1016/j.yebeh.2013.06.016. Epub 2013 Jul 27. PMID: 23896351.

87. Samanta D, Al Khalili Y. *Electrical status epilepticus in sleep* [Updated Jul 21, 2022]. In: *StatPearls [Internet]*. StatPearls Publishing; 2023. https://www.ncbi.nlm.nih.gov/books/NBK553167/.

88. Granata T, Fusco L, Gobbi G, et al. Experience with immunomodulating treatments in Rasmussen's encephalitis. *Neurology.* 2003;61:1807-1810.

89. Granata T, Gobbi G, Spreaficio Rasmussen's encephalitis. Early characteristics allows diagnosis. *Neurology.* 2003;60:422-425.

90. Kossoff EH, Vining EPG, Pillas DJ, et al. Hemispherectomy for intractable unihemispheric epilepsy. Etiology vs outcome. *Neurology.* 2003;61:887-890.

91. Archer JS, Briellmann RS, Syngeniotis A, et al. Spike-triggered fMRI in reading epilepsy. Involvement of left frontal cortex working memory area. *Neurology.* 2003;60:415-421.

92. Kleefuss-Lie A, Friedl W, Cichon S, et al. CLCN2 variants in idiopathic generalized epilepsy. *Nature Genetics.* 2009 Sep;41(9):954-955. https://doi.org/10.1038/ng0909-954. PMID: 19710712.

93. Brodie MJ, Barry SJE, et al. Patterns of treatment response in newly diagnosed epilepsy. *Neurology.* 2012;78(20):1548-1554.

94. Noachtar S, Andermann E, Meyvisch P, et al. Levetiracetam for the treatment of idiopathic generalized epilepsy with myoclonic seizures. *Neurology.* 2008;70:607-616.

95. Pisani F, Cerminara C, Fuscio C, et al. Neonatal status epilepticus vs. recurrent neonatal seizures. Clinical findings and outcome. *Neurology.* 2007;69:2177-2185.

96. Rivello JJ, Ashwal S, Hirtz D, et al. Practice parameter: diagnostic assessment of the child with status epilepticus (an evidence based review). Report of the Quality Standards Subcommittee of the American Academy of Neurology and the Child Neurology Society. *Neurology.* 2006;67:1542-1550.

97. Poddar K, Sharma R, Ng YT. Intravenous Lacosamide in pediatric status epilepticus: an open-label efficacy and safety study. *Pediatric Neurology.* 2016;61:83-86. https://doi.org/10.1016/j.pediatrneurol.2016.03.021. Epub 2016 Apr 24. PMID: 27241232.

98. Nordli D. The ketogenic diet, uses and abuses. *Neurology.* 2002;58(7):S21-S23.

99. Wheless JW, Maggio V. Vagus nerve stimulation therapy in patients younger than 18 years. *Neurology.* 2002;59(4):S21-S25.

2

Altered States of Consciousness

OUTLINE

Diagnostic Approach to Delirium, 64
  History and Physical Examination, 64
  Laboratory Investigations, 65
Diagnostic Approach to Lethargy and Coma, 65
  History and Physical Examination, 65
  Laboratory Investigations, 66
Hypoxia and Ischemia, 66
  Prolonged Hypoxia, 66
  Acute Anoxia and Ischemia, 67
  Persistent Vegetative State or Unresponsive
    Wakefulness Syndrome, 68
Brain Death, 68
Infectious Disorders, 68
  Bacterial Infections, 68
Autoimmune Encephalopathies, 76
  Rhombencephalitis (Bickerstaff Encephalitis), 76
  Acute Disseminated Encephalomyelitis, 76
  Hashimoto encephalopathy, 77
  Systemic Lupus Erythematosus, 78
  Anti-N-Methyl-d-Aspartate Receptor Antibody
    Encephalopathy, 78
  Reye Syndrome, 79
Postimmunization Encephalopathy, 80

Metabolic and Systemic Disorders, 80
  Disorders of Osmolality, 80
  Endocrine Causes of Encephalopathy, 82
  Hepatic Encephalopathy, 82
  Inborn Errors of Metabolism, 83
  Renal Disorders, 84
  Other Metabolic Encephalopathies, 85
  Migraine Coma, 86
Psychological Disorders, 86
  Panic Disorder, 87
  Schizophrenia, 87
Toxic Encephalopathies, 87
  Immunosuppressive Drugs, 87
  Corticosteroid Psychosis, 87
  Calcineurin Inhibitor Encephalopathy, 87
  OKT3 Meningoencephalitis, 88
  Prescription Drug Overdoses, 88
  Poisoning, 89
  Substance Abuse, 89
Trauma, 89
  Concussion, 90
  Severe Head Injuries, 90
References, 92

Encephalopathy is a nonspecific term encompassing a diffuse disturbance of brain activity with resultant alterations in behavior or alertness. Encephalopathy has a host of potential etiologies with clinical symptoms ranging from relatively minor changes in personality to seizures, lethargy, and coma. Hypoxia, ischemia, head trauma, and concussion produce encephalopathy of varying degrees, while infectious or autoimmune disorders result in encephalitis, meningoencephalitis, or encephalomyelitis. Metabolic derangements such as disruptions in glucose or sodium cause encephalopathy, as can various other toxic-metabolic processes. Treatment depends on the underlying cause and level of severity.

The terms used to describe states of decreased consciousness are listed in Table 2.1. With the exception of *coma*, these definitions are not standard. However, they are more precise and therefore more useful than such terms as *semicomatose* and *semistuporous*. The term *encephalopathy* describes a diffuse disorder of the brain in which altered states of consciousness, altered cognition or personality, and seizures may occur. *Encephalitis* is an encephalopathy accompanied by inflammation, seizures, and usually cerebrospinal fluid (CSF) pleocytosis.

A lack of responsiveness is not always a lack of consciousness. For example, infants with botulism (see Chapter 6) may have such severe hypotonia and ptosis

that they cannot move their limbs or eyelids in response to stimulation. They appear to be in a coma or stupor but are actually alert. The *locked-in syndrome* (a brainstem disorder in which the individual can process information but cannot respond due to paralysis) and catatonia are other examples of diminished responsiveness in the alert state. Lack of responsiveness is also common in psychogenic spells, and a transient lack of responsiveness may be seen in children with inattentiveness or obsessive-compulsive traits.

Either increased or decreased neuronal excitability may characterize the progression from consciousness to coma. Patients with increased neuronal excitability (the *high road to coma*) become restless and then confused; next, tremor, hallucinations, and delirium (an agitated confusional state) develop. Myoclonic jerks may occur.

TABLE 2.1   States of Decreased Consciousness

Term	Definition
Lethargy	Difficult to maintain the aroused state
Obtundation	Responsive to stimulation other than pain[a]
Stupor	Responsive only to pain[a]
Coma	Unresponsive to pain

[a]Responsive indicates cerebral alerting, not just reflex withdrawal.

BOX 2.1   Causes of Agitation and Confusion

Epileptic
- Absence status[a] (see Chapter 1)
- Focal seizure with impaired awareness[a] (see Chapter 1)
- Epileptic encephalopathies[a]

Infectious Disorders
- Bacterial infections
  - Cat-scratch disease[a]
  - Meningitis[a] (see Chapter 4)
- Rickettsial infections
  - Lyme disease[a]
  - Rocky Mountain spotted fever[a]
- Viral infections
  - Arboviruses
  - Aseptic meningitis
  - Herpes simplex encephalitis[a]
  - Measles encephalitis
  - Enteroviruses
  - Human parechovirus

Metabolic and Systemic Disorders
- Disorders of osmolality
  - Hypoglycemia[a]
  - Hyponatremia[a]
- Endocrine disorders
  - Adrenal insufficiency[a]
  - Hypoparathyroidism[a]
  - Thyroid disorders[a]
- Hepatic encephalopathy
- Inborn errors of metabolism
  - Disorders of pyruvate metabolism (see Chapter 5)

- Medium-chain acyl-coenzyme A dehydrogenase deficiency
- Respiratory chain disorders (see Chapters 5, 6, 8, and 10)
- Urea cycle disorder, heterozygote (see Chapter 1)
- Renal disease
  - Hypertensive encephalopathy[a]
  - Uremic encephalopathy[a]

Migraine
- Acute confusional[a]
- Aphasic[a]

Psychological
- Panic disorder[a]
- Schizophrenia

Toxic
- Immunosuppressive drugs[a]
- Prescription drugs[a]
- Substance abuse[a]
- Toxins[a]

Vascular
- Congestive heart failure[a]
- Embolism[a]
- Hypertensive encephalopathy[a]
- Subarachnoid hemorrhage[a]
- Vasculitis[a]

Autoimmune
- Anti-NMDAR antibody encephalitis[a]
- Lupus erythematosus[a]
- Bickerstaff encephalitis[a]

[a]The most common conditions and the ones with disease-modifying treatments.

NMDAR, *N*-Methyl-D-aspartate receptor.

Seizures herald the end of delirium, and stupor or coma follows. Box 2.1 summarizes the differential diagnosis of the high road to coma. Tumors and other mass lesions are not expected causes. Instead, metabolic, toxic, and inflammatory disorders are likely.

Decreased neuronal excitability (the *low road to coma*) lacks an agitated stage. Instead, awareness progressively deteriorates from lethargy to obtundation, to stupor, and to coma. The differential diagnosis is considerably larger than that with the high road and includes mass lesions and other causes of increased intracranial pressure (ICP) (Box 2.2). Box 2.3 lists conditions that cause recurrent encephalopathies. A comparison of Boxes 2.1 and 2.2 shows considerable overlap between conditions whose initial features are agitation and confusion and those that begin with lethargy and coma; therefore the disorders responsible for each are described together to prevent repetition.

BOX 2.2 Causes of Lethargy and Coma

Epilepsy
- Epileptic encephalopathies
- Postictal state (see Chapter 1)
- Status epilepticus (see Chapter 1)

Hypoxia-Ischemia
- Cardiac arrest
- Cardiac arrhythmia
- Congestive heart failure
- Hypotension
  - Autonomic dysfunction
  - Dehydration
  - Hemorrhage
  - Pulmonary embolism
- Near drowning
- Neonatal (see Chapter 1)

Increased Intracranial Pressure
- Cerebral abscess (see Chapter 4)
- Cerebral edema (see Chapter 4)
- Cerebral tumor (see Chapters 4 and 10)
- Herniation syndromes (see Chapter 4)
- Hydrocephalus (see Chapters 4 and 18)
- Intracranial hemorrhage
  - Spontaneous (see Chapter 4)
  - Traumatic

Infectious Disorders
- Bacterial infections
  - Cat-scratch disease[a]
  - Gram-negative sepsis[a]
  - Hemorrhagic shock and encephalopathy syndrome[a]
  - Meningitis[a] (see Chapter 4)
  - Toxic shock syndrome
- Postimmunization encephalopathy
- Rickettsial infections
  - Lyme disease[a]
  - Rocky Mountain spotted fever[a]
- Viral infections

- Arboviruses
- Aseptic meningitis
- Herpes simplex encephalitis
- Human parechovirus
- Enteroviruses
- Measles encephalitis
- Postinfectious encephalomyelitis
- Reye syndrome

Metabolic and Systemic Disorders
- Disorders of osmolality
  - Diabetic ketoacidosis (hyperglycemia)
  - Hypoglycemia
  - Hypernatremia
  - Hyponatremia
- Endocrine disorders
  - Adrenal insufficiency
  - Hypoparathyroidism
  - Thyroid disorders
- Hepatic encephalopathy
- Inborn errors of metabolism
  - Disorders of pyruvate metabolism (see Chapter 5)
  - Glycogen storage disorders (see Chapter 1)
  - Medium-chain acyl-coenzyme A dehydrogenase deficiency
  - Respiratory chain disorders (see Chapters 5, 6, 8, and 10)
  - Urea cycle disorder, heterozygote (see Chapter 1)
- Renal disorders
  - Acute uremic encephalopathy
  - Chronic uremic encephalopathy
  - Dialysis encephalopathy
  - Hypertensive encephalopathy
- Other metabolic disorders
  - Burn encephalopathy
  - Hypomagnesemia
  - Parenteral hyperalimentation
  - Vitamin B complex deficiency
- Migraine coma
- Toxic

(Continued)

BOX 2.2   Causes of Lethargy and Coma—cont'd

- Immunosuppressive drugs[a]
- Prescription drugs[a]
- Substance abuse[a]
- Toxins[a]
- Trauma
  - Epidural hematoma
  - Subdural hematoma
  - Intracerebral hemorrhage
  - Concussion
  - Contusion
- Intracranial hemorrhage
- Neonatal (see Chapter 1)
- Vascular
  - Hypertensive encephalopathy[a]
  - Intracranial hemorrhage, nontraumatic[a] (see Chapter 4)
  - Lupus erythematosus[a] (see Chapter 11)
  - Neonatal idiopathic cerebral venous thrombosis (see Chapter 1)
  - Vasculitis[a] (see Chapter 11)

[a]The most common conditions and the ones with disease-modifying treatments.

BOX 2.3   Causes of Recurrent Encephalopathy

- Burn encephalopathy
- Epileptic encephalopathies[a]
- Hashimoto encephalopathy[a]
- Hypoglycemia[a]
- Increased intracranial pressure[a] (recurrent)
- Recurrent acute demyelinating encephalomyelitis[a] (ADEM)
- Medium-chain acyl-coenzyme A dehydrogenase deficiency
- Psychiatric disorders
- Migraine
- Mitochondrial disorders
- Pyruvate metabolism disorders
- Substance abuse
- Urea cycle disorder

[a]The most common conditions and the ones with disease-modifying treatments.

ADEM, Acute disseminated encephalomyelitis.

DIAGNOSTIC APPROACH TO DELIRIUM

The term "altered mental status" is nonspecific; in this section we refer to altered mental status with delirium characterized by diffuse cognitive dysfunction, altered sleep-wake cycle, perceptual disturbances, thought and language disturbance, and altered mood and affect. The symptom onset is characteristically acute, and the intensity of symptoms fluctuates for the duration of the delirium.[1]

Assume that any child with the acute behavioral changes of delirium (agitation, confusion, delusions, or hallucinations) has an organic encephalopathy until proven otherwise. Some of the most frequent etiologies include central nervous system (CNS) infection, medication-induced (anticholinergics, opioids, etc.), autoimmune disease (anti-*N*-methyl-D-aspartate receptor [NMDAR], lupus, polyarteritis nodosa), CNS neoplasm, organ failure (respiratory, cardiac, kidney, liver) following transplant or surgery, sepsis, illicit drugs, and trauma. The usual causes of delirium are toxic or metabolic disorders diffusely affecting both cerebral hemispheres.

Schizophrenia should not be considered in a prepubertal child with acute delirium. Fixed beliefs, unalterable by reason, are *delusions.* The paranoid delusions of schizophrenia are logical to the patient and frequently part of an elaborate system of irrational thinking in which the patient feels menaced. Delusions associated with organic encephalopathy are less logical, not systematized, and tend to be stereotyped.

Hallucination is the perception of sensory stimuli that is not present. Organic encephalopathies usually cause nonformed visual hallucinations more often than auditory hallucinations, whereas psychiatric illness usually causes formed auditory hallucinations more often than visual hallucinations, especially if the voices are accusatory. Stereotyped auditory hallucinations that represent a recurring memory are an exception and suggest temporal lobe seizures.

History and Physical Examination

Delirious children, even with stable vital functions, require rapid assessment because the potential for deterioration to a state of diminished consciousness is real. Mortality is significant. Obtain a careful history of the following: (1) the events leading to the behavioral change; (2) drug or toxic exposure (prescription drugs are more often at fault than substances of abuse, and a medicine cabinet inspection should be ordered in every home the child has visited); (3) a personal or family history of migraine or epilepsy; (4) recent or concurrent fever, infectious disease, or systemic illness; and (5) a previous personal or family history of encephalopathy.

Examination of the eyes, in addition to determining the presence or absence of disk edema, provides other etiological clues. Small or large pupils that respond poorly to light, nystagmus, or impaired eye movements suggest a drug or toxic exposure. Fixed deviation of the eyes in one lateral direction may indicate seizure or a significant loss of function in one hemisphere. The general and neurological examinations should specifically include a search for evidence of trauma, needle marks on the limbs, meningismus, lymphadenopathy, and cardiac disease.

Laboratory Investigations

Individualize laboratory evaluation; not every test is essential for each clinical situation. Studies of potential interest include blood, urine, and CSF cultures; complete blood count; sedimentation rate; C-reactive protein; fingerstick glucose; a complete metabolic panel; thyroid-stimulating hormone and free T4; urine drug screen; blood alcohol level; and autoimmune antibodies. If possible, obtain computed tomography (CT) or rapid-sequence magnetic resonance imaging (MRI) while the results of these tests are pending. If sedation is required to perform the study, a short-acting benzodiazepine is preferred. Nondiagnostic blood studies and normal imaging results are an indication for lumbar puncture to look for infection, inflammation, or increased ICP. A manometer should always be available to measure CSF pressure.

An electroencephalogram (EEG) is useful in the evaluation of altered mentation. Acute organic encephalopathies will show a slow or absent occipital dominant rhythm during the waking state. EEG is often normal in psychiatric illnesses. Diffuse theta and delta activity, absence of faster frequencies, and intermittent rhythmic delta activity are characteristic of severe encephalopathies. Specific abnormalities may include epileptiform activity consistent with absence or complex partial status; triphasic waves indicating hepatic, uremic, or other toxic encephalopathy; and periodic lateralizing epileptiform discharges in one temporal lobe, suggesting herpes encephalitis.

DIAGNOSTIC APPROACH TO LETHARGY AND COMA

The diagnostic approach to states of diminished consciousness in children is similar to that suggested for delirium, except with greater urgency. The causes of progressive decline in the state of consciousness are diffuse or multifocal disturbances of the cerebral hemispheres or focal injury to the brainstem. Physical examination often reveals the anatomical site of abnormality in the brain.

History and Physical Examination

Obtain the same historical data as for delirium, except that mass lesions are an important consideration. Inquire further concerning trauma or preceding symptoms of increasing ICP. Direct the physical examination to determine both the anatomical site of disturbed cerebral function and its cause. The important variables in locating the site of abnormality are state of consciousness, pattern of breathing, pupillary size and reactivity, eye movements, and motor responses. The cause of lethargy and obtundation is usually mild depression of hemispheric function. Stupor and coma are characteristic of much more extensive disturbance of hemispheric function, or involvement of the diencephalon and upper brainstem. Derangements of the dominant hemisphere may have a greater effect on consciousness than derangements of the nondominant hemisphere.

Cheyne-Stokes respiration, in which periods of hyperpnea alternate with periods of apnea, is usually caused by bilateral hemispheric or diencephalic injuries, but can result from bilateral damage anywhere along the descending pathway between the forebrain and upper pons. Alertness, pupillary size, and heart rhythm may vary during Cheyne-Stokes respiration. Alertness is greater during the waxing portion of breathing. Lesions just ventral to the aqueduct or fourth ventricle cause a sustained, rapid, deep hyperventilation (central neurogenic hyperventilation). Abnormalities within the medulla and pons affect the respiratory centers and cause three different patterns of respiratory control: (1) *apneustic breathing*, a pause at full inspiration; (2) *ataxic breathing*, haphazard breaths and pauses without a predictable pattern; and (3) *Ondine curse* (central hypoventilation syndrome), a failure of automatic breathing when asleep.

Children usually retain the pupillary light reflex in metabolic encephalopathies. Absence of the pupillary reflex in a comatose patient indicates a structural abnormality. The major exception is drugs; the cause of fixed dilation of pupils in an alert patient is the topical administration of mydriatics. In comatose patients, hypothalamic damage causes unilateral pupillary constriction and Horner syndrome; midbrain lesions cause mid-position fixed pupils; pontine lesions cause small but reactive pupils; and lateral medullary lesions cause Horner syndrome.

Tonic lateral deviation of both eyes indicates a seizure originating in the frontal lobe opposite to the direction of gaze (saccade center); the parietal lobe ipsilateral to the direction of gaze (pursuit center); or the presence of a destructive lesion present in the ipsilateral frontal lobe in the direction of gaze. The assessment of ocular motility in comatose patients is the instillation of ice water sequentially 15 minutes apart in each ear to chill the tympanic membrane. Ice water in the right ear causes both eyes to deviate rapidly to the right and then slowly return to the midline. The rapid movement to the right is a brainstem reflex, and its presence indicates that much of the brainstem is intact. Abduction of the right eye with failure of left eye adduction indicates a lesion in the medial longitudinal fasciculus (see Chapter 15). The slow movement that returns the eyes to the left requires a cortico-pontine pathway originating in the right hemisphere and terminating in the left pontine lateral gaze center. Its presence indicates unilateral hemispheric function. Skew deviation, the deviation of one eye above the other (hypertropia), usually indicates a lesion of the brainstem or cerebellum.

Carefully observe trunk and limb positions at rest, spontaneous movements, and response to noxious stimuli. Spontaneous movement of all limbs generally indicates a mild depression of hemispheric function without structural disturbance. Monoplegia or hemiplegia suggests a structural disturbance of the contralateral hemisphere, except when in the postictal state. An extensor response of the trunk and limbs to a noxious stimulus is termed *decerebrate rigidity*. The most severe form is *opisthotonos*. The neck is hyperextended, and the teeth clenched; the arms adducted, hyperextended, and hyperpronated; and the legs extended with the feet plantar flexed. Decerebrate rigidity indicates brainstem compression and is considered an ominous sign whether present at rest or in response to noxious stimuli. Flexion of the arms and extension of the legs are termed *decorticate rigidity*. It is uncommon in children except following head injury and indicates hemispheric dysfunction with brainstem integrity.

Laboratory Investigations

Laboratory investigations are similar to those described for the evaluation of delirium. Perform head CT with contrast enhancement promptly in order to exclude the possibility of a mass lesion and herniation. It is a great error to send a child, whose condition is uncertain, for CT without someone in attendance who knows how to monitor deterioration and intervene appropriately.

HYPOXIA AND ISCHEMIA

Hypoxia and ischemia usually occur together. Prolonged hypoxia causes personality change first and then loss of consciousness, while acute anoxia results in immediate loss of consciousness.

Prolonged Hypoxia

Clinical features. Prolonged hypoxia can result from severe anemia (oxygen-carrying capacity reduced by at least half), congestive heart failure, chronic lung disease, and neuromuscular disorders. The best-studied model of prolonged, mild hypoxia involves ascent to high altitudes. Mild hypoxia causes impaired memory and judgment, confusion, and decreased motor performance. Greater degrees of hypoxia result in obtundation, multifocal myoclonus, and sometimes focal neurological signs such as monoplegia and hemiplegia. Children with chronic cardiopulmonary disease may have an insidious alteration in behavioral state as the arterial oxygen concentration slowly declines.

The neurological complications of cystic fibrosis result from chronic hypoxia and hypercapnia leading to lethargy, somnolence, and sometimes coma. Neuromuscular disorders that weaken respiratory muscles, such as muscular dystrophy, often produce nocturnal hypoventilation as a first symptom of respiratory insufficiency. Frequent awakenings and fear of sleeping are characteristic (see Chapter 7).

Diagnosis. Consider chronic hypoxia in children with chronic cardiopulmonary disorders who become depressed or undergo personality change. Arterial oxygen pressure (P_aO_2) values below 40 mm Hg are regularly associated with obvious neurological disturbances, but minor mental disturbances may occur at P_aO_2 concentrations of 60 mm Hg, especially when hypoxia is chronic.

Management. Encephalopathy usually reverses when P_aO_2 is increased, but persistent cerebral dysfunction may occur in mountain climbers after returning to sea level, and permanent cerebral dysfunction may develop in children with chronic hypoxia. As a group, children with chronic hypoxia from congenital heart disease have a lower IQ than nonhypoxic children. The severity of mental decline relates to the duration of hypoxia. Treat children with neuromuscular disorders who develop symptoms during sleep with overnight, intermittent positive-pressure ventilation (see Chapter 7).

Acute Anoxia and Ischemia

The usual circumstance in which acute anoxia and ischemia occur is cardiac arrest or sudden hypotension. Anoxia without ischemia occurs with suffocation (near drowning, choking). Prolonged anoxia leads to bradycardia and cardiac arrest. In adults, hippocampal and Purkinje cells begin to die after 4 minutes of total anoxia and ischemia. Exact timing may be difficult in clinical situations when ill-defined intervals of anoxia and hypoxia occur. Remarkable survivals are sometimes associated with near drowning in water cold enough to lower cerebral temperature and metabolism. The pattern of hypoxic-ischemic brain injury in newborns is different and depends largely on brain maturity (see Chapter 1).

Clinical features. Consciousness is lost within 8 seconds of cerebral circulatory failure, but the loss may take longer when anoxia occurs without ischemia. Presyncopal symptoms of light-headedness and visual disturbances sometimes precede loss of consciousness. Initially, myoclonic movements due to a lack of cortical spinal inhibition may occur. Seizures may follow.

Prediction of outcome after hypoxic-ischemic events depends on age and circumstances. The majority of adults who have had a cardiac arrest do not regain independent function in the first year after arrest. The outcome in children is somewhat better because the incidence of preexisting cardiopulmonary disease is lower. Absence of pupillary responses on initial examination is an ominous sign; such patients are less likely to recover independent function. Twenty-four hours after arrest, lack of motor responses in the limbs and eyes identifies patients with a poor prognosis. Persistent early-onset myoclonus is a negative prognostic sign.[2] In contrast, a favorable outcome is predictable for patients who rapidly recover roving or conjugate eye movements and limb withdrawal from pain. Children who are unconscious for longer than 60 days are very unlikely to regain language skills or the ability to walk.

Two delayed syndromes of neurological deterioration follow anoxia. The first is *delayed postanoxic encephalopathy*, the appearance of apathy or confusion 1–2 weeks after apparent recovery. Motor symptoms follow, usually rigidity or spasticity, and may progress to coma or death. Demyelination is the suggested mechanism. Diffuse restricted diffusion-weighted signal in all white matter extending to subcortical regions with sparing of U-fibers is a common finding.[3] The other syndrome is *postanoxic action myoclonus*. This usually follows a severe episode of anoxia and ischemia caused by cardiac arrest. All voluntary activity initiates disabling myoclonus (see Chapter 14). Symptoms of cerebellar dysfunction are also present.

Diagnosis. Cerebral edema is prominent during the first 72 hours after severe hypoxia. CT during that time shows decreased density with loss of the differentiation between gray and white matters. Severe, generalized loss of density on the CT correlates with a poor outcome. An EEG that shows a burst-suppression pattern or absence of activity is associated with a poor neurological outcome or death; lesser abnormalities typically are not useful in predicting the prognosis. MRI is a more sensitive imaging modality that shows the extent of hypoxia very well in diffusion-weighted T_2 and fluid-attenuated inversion recovery (FLAIR) images; however, some of the changes noted with this technique may be reversible.

Management. The principles of treating patients who have sustained hypoxic-ischemic encephalopathy do not differ substantially from the principles of caring for other comatose patients. Maintaining oxygenation, circulation, and blood glucose concentration is essential. Regulate ICP to levels that allow satisfactory cerebral perfusion (see Chapter 4). Anticonvulsant drugs manage seizures (see Chapter 1). Anoxia is invariably associated with lactic acidosis. Restoration of acid-base balance is essential.

The use of barbiturate coma to slow cerebral metabolism is common practice, but neither clinical nor experimental evidence indicates a beneficial effect following cardiac arrest or near drowning (its use in traumatic brain injury is mainly for lowering ICP). Hypothermia prevents brain damage during the time of hypoxia and ischemia, and it has some value after the event. Whole body and head cooling are now the standard of care for perinatal hypoxic-ischemic encephalopathy. Corticosteroids do not improve neurological recovery in patients with global ischemia following cardiac arrest. Postanoxic action myoclonus sometimes responds to levetiracetam, zonisamide, or valproate.

Persistent Vegetative State or Unresponsive Wakefulness Syndrome

The term *persistent vegetative state* (PVS) or *unresponsive wakefulness syndrome* describes patients who, after recovery from coma, return to a state of wakefulness without signs of awareness of the self or the environment. PVS is a form of eyes-open permanent unconsciousness with loss of cognitive function and awareness of the environment but preservation of sleep-wake cycles and vegetative function. Survival is indefinite with good nursing care. The usual causes, in order of frequency, are anoxia and ischemia, metabolic or encephalitic coma, and head trauma. Anoxia-ischemia has the worst prognosis. Children who remain in a PVS for 3 months virtually never regain functional skills.

The American Academy of Neurology has adopted the policy that discontinuing medical treatment, including the provision of nutrition and hydration, is ethical in a patient whose diagnosed condition is PVS when the patient would not want maintenance in this state, and the family agrees to discontinue therapy.

BRAIN DEATH

The guidelines for brain death suggested by the American Association of Pediatrics (1987, reviewed in 2011[4]) are generally accepted. Box 2.4 summarizes the important features of the report. The absence of cerebral blood flow is the earliest and most definitive proof of brain death.

Determination of brain death in term newborns (>37 weeks' gestational age), infants, and children is a clinical diagnosis based on the absence of neurological function with a known irreversible cause of coma. Hypotension, hypothermia, and metabolic disturbances should be corrected, and medications that can interfere with the neurological examination and apnea testing should be discontinued allowing for adequate clearance before proceeding with these evaluations. Two exams including an apnea test by

---

BOX 2.4 Diagnostic Criteria for the Clinical Diagnosis of Brain Death

Prerequisites
- Cessation of all brain function
- Proximate cause of brain death is known
- Condition is irreversible

Cardinal Features
- Coma
  - Absent brainstem reflexes
  - Pupillary light reflex
  - Corneal reflex
  - Oculocephalic reflex
  - Oculovestibular reflex
  - Oropharyngeal reflex
- Apnea (established by formal apnea test)

Confirmatory Tests (Optional)
- Cerebral angiography
- Electroencephalography
- Radioisotope cerebral blood flow study
- Transcranial Doppler ultrasonography

---

different attending physicians separated by an observation period are required. Apnea testing may be performed by the same physician. An observation period of 24 hours for term newborns up to age 30 days and 12 hours for infants and children up to 18 years is recommended. Apnea testing requires documentation of an arterial $PaCO_2$ 20 mm Hg above the baseline and >60 mm Hg with no respiratory effort during the testing period. Ancillary testing is required (EEG, radionucleotide cerebral blood flow) if an apnea test cannot be safely completed, if the observation period needs to be abbreviated, if the clinical findings are uncertain, or if a medication effect may be present.[5]

INFECTIOUS DISORDERS

Bacterial Infections
Cat-Scratch Disease

The causative agent of cat-scratch disease is *Bartonella* (*Rochalimaea*) *henselae*, a gram-negative bacillus transmitted by a cat scratch or cat bite contaminated by flea feces, or less frequently ticks may act as vectors. It is the most common cause of chronic benign lymphadenopathy in children and young adults. The estimated incidence in the United States is highest in the southern states where it is 6.4 per 100,000.[6] The majority of cases occur in children less than 12 years.

Clinical features. The major feature is lymphadenopathy proximal to the site of the scratch. Fever is present in only 60% of cases. The disease is usually benign and self-limited. Unusual systemic manifestations are oculoglandular disease, erythema nodosum, osteolytic lesions, and thrombocytopenic purpura. The most common neurological manifestation is encephalopathy. Transverse myelitis, radiculitis, cerebellar ataxia, and neuroretinitis are rare manifestations. Neurological manifestations, when present, occur 2 or 3 weeks after the onset of lymphadenopathy.

Neurological symptoms occur in 2% of cases of cat-scratch disease, and 90% of them manifest as encephalopathy. The mechanism is unknown, but the cause may be either a direct infection or vasculitis. The male-to-female ratio is 2:1. Only 17% of cases complicated by encephalitis occur in children less than 12 years old, and 15% occur in children aged 12–18 years old. The frequency of fever and the site of the scratch are the same in patients with encephalitis compared to those without encephalitis. The initial and most prominent feature is a decreased state of consciousness ranging from lethargy to coma. Seizures occur in 46%–80% of cases and combative behavior in 40%. Focal findings are rare,[7] but neuroretinitis, Guillain-Barré syndrome (GBS), and transverse myelitis can be seen.

Diagnosis. The diagnosis requires local lymphadenopathy, contact with a cat, and an identifiable site of inoculation. Confirmatory testing consists of serologies, PCR, and culture. CSF is normal in 70% of cases. Lymphocytosis in the CSF, when present, does not exceed 30 cells/mm. The EEG is diffusely slow. Only 19% of patients have abnormal findings on CT scans or MRI of the brain, and these include lesions of the cerebral white matter, basal ganglia, thalamus, and gray matter.

Management. Most children recover without the need for intervention, although lymphadenopathy may be prolonged, lasting 2–4 months. For children with mild complications (such as local skin infection), prescribe oral azithromycin. Treat patients with severe complications such as neuroretinitis, encephalitis, or endocarditis with 4–6 weeks of doxycycline and rifampin. Current literature suggests adjunctive use of corticosteroids to decrease inflammation.[8]

Gram-Negative Sepsis

Clinical features. The onset of symptoms in gram-negative sepsis may be explosive and characterized by fever or hypothermia, chills, hyperventilation, hemodynamic instability, and mental changes (irritability, delirium, or coma). Neurological features may include asterixis, tremor, and multifocal myoclonus. Multiple organ failure follows: (1) renal shutdown caused by hypotension; (2) hypoprothrombinemia caused by vitamin K deficiency; (3) thrombocytopenia caused by nonspecific binding of immunoglobulin; (4) disseminated intravascular coagulation with infarction or hemorrhage in several organs; and (5) progressive respiratory failure.

Diagnosis. Always consider sepsis in the differential diagnosis of shock and obtain blood cultures. When shock is the initial feature, gram-negative sepsis is the likely diagnosis. In *Staphylococcus aureus* infections shock is more likely to occur later in the infection and not as an initial feature. The CSF is usually normal or may have an elevated concentration of protein. MRI or CT of the brain is normal early in the course and subsequently shows edema.

Management. Septic shock is a medical emergency. Promptly initiate antibiotic therapy at maximal doses (see Chapter 4). Treat hypotension by restoration of intravascular volume, and address each factor contributing to coagulopathy. Mortality is high even with optimal treatment.

Hemorrhagic Shock and Encephalopathy Syndrome

Hemorrhagic shock and encephalopathy syndrome is a rare and devastating disorder affecting young children, presumably caused by bacterial sepsis.

Clinical features. Most affected children are younger than 1 year, but cases can occur in children up to 26 months. Half have mild prodromal symptoms of a viral gastroenteritis or respiratory illness. In the rest, the onset is explosive; a previously well child is found unresponsive and seizing. Fever of 38°C or higher is a constant feature. Although not all children are in shock at the initial presentation, it develops quickly in all cases. Refractory metabolic acidosis is a key finding; other cardinal features include elevated creatine kinase, transaminitis, and hypotension.[9] Disseminated intravascular coagulopathy develops, and bleeding occurs from every venipuncture site. The mortality rate is 50%; the survivors have cognitive and motor impairment.

Diagnosis. The syndrome resembles toxic shock syndrome, gram-negative sepsis, heat stroke, and Reye syndrome. Abnormal renal function occurs in every case, but serum ammonia concentrations remain normal, hypoglycemia is unusual, and blood cultures yield no growth.

CSF is normal except for increased pressure. CT shows small ventricles and loss of sulcal marking caused by cerebral edema. The initial EEG background is diffusely slow and may be isoelectric. A striking pattern evolves over the first hours or days, characterized by runs of spikes, sharp waves, or rhythmic slow waves that fluctuate in frequency, amplitude, and location.

Management. Affected children require intensive care with ventilatory support, volume replacement, correction of acid-base and coagulation disturbances, anticonvulsant therapy, and control of cerebral edema.

Rickettsial Infections

Lyme disease. A spirochete (*Borrelia burgdorferi*) causes Lyme disease. The vector is hard-shelled deer ticks: *Ixodes dammini* in the eastern United States, *Ixodes pacificus* in the western United States, and *Ixodes ricinus* in Europe. Lyme disease is now the most common vector-borne infection in the United States. Northeastern states account for the majority of cases.

Clinical features. The neurological consequences of Lyme disease vary, and some are controversial. Those associated with the early stages of disease enjoy the greatest acceptance. The first symptom (stage 1) in 60%–80% of patients is a skin lesion of the thigh, groin, or axillae (erythema chronicum migrans), which may be associated with fever, regional lymphadenopathy, and arthralgia. The rash begins as a red macule at the site of the tick bite and then spreads to form a red annular lesion with partial clearing, sometimes appearing as alternating rings of rash and clearing.

Neurological involvement (neuroborreliosis) develops weeks or months later when the infection disseminates (stage 2).[10] Most children only have a headache, which clears completely within 6 weeks; the cause may be mild aseptic meningitis or encephalitis. Fever may not occur. Facial palsy, sleep disturbances, and papilledema are rare. Polyneuropathies are uncommon in children. Transitory cardiac involvement (myopericarditis and atrioventricular block) may occur in stage 2.

A year or more of continual migratory arthritis begins weeks to years after the onset of neurological features (stage 3). Only one joint, often the knee, or a few large joints are affected. During stage 3, the patient feels ill. Encephalopathy with memory or cognitive abnormalities and confusional states, with normal CSF results, may occur. Other psychiatric or fatigue syndromes appear less likely to be causally related.

Diagnosis. The spirochete grows on cultures from the skin rash during stage 1 of the disease. At the time of meningitis, CSF may be normal at first but then shows lymphocytic pleocytosis (about 100 cells/mm), an elevated protein concentration, and a normal glucose concentration. *B. burgdorferi* grows on culture from the CSF during meningitis. A two-test approach establishes the diagnosis of neuroborreliosis. The first step is to show the production of specific IgG and IgM antibodies in CSF. Antibody production begins 2 weeks after infection, and IgG is always detectable at 6 weeks. The second step, used when the first is inconclusive, is PCR to detect the organism.

Management. Use intravenous ceftriaxone or penicillin G to treat encephalitis. Examine the CSF toward the end of the 2- to 4-week treatment course to assess the need for continuing treatment and again 6 months after the conclusion of therapy. Intrathecal antibody production may persist for years following successful treatment, and in isolation it does not indicate active disease. Patients in whom CSF pleocytosis fails to resolve within 6 months, however, should be retreated.

The treatment of peripheral or cranial nerve involvement without CSF abnormalities is with oral amoxicillin, doxycycline, cefuroxime, or azithromycin. The American Association of Pediatrics has published guidelines for the treatment of Lyme disease in children.[11]

Rocky mountain spotted fever. Rocky Mountain spotted fever is an acute tick-borne disorder caused by *Rickettsia rickettsii*. Its geographic name is a misnomer; the disease is present in the northwestern and eastern United States, Canada, Mexico, Colombia, and Brazil.

Clinical features. Fever, myalgia, and rash are constant symptoms and begin 2–14 days after a tick bite. The rash first appears around the wrist and ankles 3–5 days after the onset of illness and spreads to the soles of the feet and forearms. It may be maculopapular, petechial, or both. Headache is present in 66% of affected individuals, meningitis or meningoencephalitis in 33%, focal neurological signs in 14%, and seizures in 6%. The focal abnormalities result from microinfarcts.

Diagnosis. *R. rickettsii* is demonstrable by direct immunofluorescence or immunoperoxidase staining of a skin biopsy specimen of the rash. Other laboratory tests may indicate anemia, thrombocytopenia, coagulopathy, hyponatremia, and muscle tissue breakdown. Serology retrospectively confirms the diagnosis. The CSF shows mild pleocytosis.

Management. Initiate treatment when the diagnosis is first suspected. Delayed treatment results in increased mortality. Doxycycline is the mainstay of treatment for all tick-borne diseases in adults and children, including children under age 8, as recommended by the Centers for Disease Control and Prevention (CDC) and the American Association of Pediatrics. The dose for children <45 kg is 2.2 mg/kg given twice a day for a minimum of 5–7 days; treatment should continue until the patient is afebrile for at least 3 days. The adult dose is 100 mg given every 12 hours.

Toxic Shock Syndrome

Toxic shock syndrome is a potentially lethal illness caused by infection or colonization with some strains of *S. aureus*.

Clinical features. The onset is abrupt. High fever, hypotension, vomiting, diarrhea, myalgia, headache, and a desquamating rash characterize the onset. Multiple organ failure may occur during desquamation. Serious complications include cardiac arrhythmia, pulmonary edema, and oliguric renal failure. Initial encephalopathic features include agitation and confusion. These may be followed by lethargy, obtundation, and generalized tonic-clonic seizures.

Many pediatric cases have occurred in menstruating girls who use tampons, but they may also occur in children with occlusive dressings after burns or surgery and as a complication of influenza and influenza-like illness in children with staphylococcal colonization of the respiratory tract.

Diagnosis. The basis for diagnosis is the typical clinical and laboratory findings. Over half of the patients have sterile pyuria, immature granulocytic leukocytes, coagulation abnormalities, hypocalcemia, low serum albumin and total protein concentrations, and elevated concentrations of blood urea nitrogen, transaminase, bilirubin, and creatine kinase. Cultures of specimens from infected areas yield *S. aureus*.

Management. Hypotension usually responds to volume restoration with physiological saline solutions. Some patients require vasopressors or fresh-frozen plasma. Initiate antibiotic therapy promptly with an agent effective against *S. aureus*.

Viral Encephalitis

Historically, viral causes of encephalitis have been nebulous and difficult to diagnose. Although diagnostic challenges remain, infectious disease researchers have made significant advances in the detection and diagnosis of specific viruses. Unfortunately, treatment options remain limited, and outcomes depend largely upon the specific viral etiology and various immutable host factors, such as age and immune status.

Viruses are the most common cause of infectious encephalitis, comprising approximately 70% of confirmed encephalitis cases. Viral encephalitis is vastly more common than bacterial encephalitis, and in most cases has a better outcome (with some notable exceptions that we will discuss later). The most common causes of viral encephalitis in the United States are herpes viruses, enteroviruses, and West Nile virus, with an incidence of 3.5–7.5 per 100,000 people; children and the elderly are especially at risk. In this section, we will discuss the most significant viruses affecting children. This should not be considered an exhaustive review.

Viruses typically spread to the CNS hematogenously with the notable exceptions of rabies, varicella-zoster virus, and herpes viruses which spread retrograde through nerve endings. Once established in the brain parenchyma, the virus causes a host inflammatory response with cerebral edema, hemorrhage, and lymphocytic and microglial perivascular infiltration.

Since diagnostic testing remains inconclusive in many patients, the clinician must be sure to take a thorough history. This includes factors such as geographic location, season, exposure to animals and insects, immune competence, vaccination status, and travel history. Some viruses present with unique symptoms and findings that aid in diagnosis.

Diagnostic Evaluation of Viral Encephalitis

Viral encephalitis presents with nonspecific symptoms of headache, malaise, fever, altered mental status, and sometimes seizures. The initial differential diagnosis will be broad, and testing recommendations reflect that fact.

Elevated ICP may occur, and head imaging must be obtained prior to lumbar puncture. During the lumbar puncture, measure the opening pressure and obtain CSF glucose, protein, cell count, and bacterial culture. Send PCR for herpes simplex virus-1 (HSV-1), HSV-2, and enteroviruses. Additional diagnostic panels are available that can rapidly identify other common causes of viral encephalitis. For certain viruses such as arboviruses and rabies, confirmatory testing may be required through the local health department or CDC. Note that initial presentation has considerable overlap with autoimmune encephalitis; we recommend considering an autoimmune workup for all patients.

CSF is normal in 10% of cases. For the remainder, the most common abnormalities are moderately elevated protein and moderate leukocytosis. CSF glucose is normal. Viruses notoriously do not grow well in culture, and viral culture is almost never helpful.

Some viruses produce specific changes on MRI. For example, HSV-1 and HSV-2 produce focal necrosis particularly in the frontal and bilateral temporal lobes (see Fig. 2.1). Human parechovirus leads to widespread restricted diffusion in infants. Arboviruses often produce changes in the basal ganglia; Japanese encephalitis (JE) and Eastern equine encephalitis (EEE) can cause devasting and extensive necrosis throughout the brain.

Management. All patients with symptoms of encephalitis require broad-spectrum treatment pending a more definitive diagnosis. In addition to basic supportive care, begin broad-spectrum antibiotics and acyclovir 10 mg/kg IV every 8 hours. Consider infectious disease and rheumatology consultation. Respiratory support and admission to the intensive care unit are needed in some cases, and many children require long-term rehabilitation services on an inpatient or outpatient basis. Serial ICP measurements should be performed in children that remain profoundly encephalopathic; elevated ICP heralds a poor prognosis. Seizures are common and should be treated with anticonvulsants. Continuous EEG monitoring may be required.

Herpes Simplex Virus Encephalitis

HSV-1 and HSV-2 cause HSV encephalitis, a potentially devastating encephalitis preferentially affecting the bilateral temporal and frontal lobes. Psychiatric symptoms, aphasia, and memory problems are common presenting symptoms in older children and adolescents. Most patients have seizures, which are often medically intractable and persist for life. MRI of the brain shows necrosis of the temporal and frontal lobes. Newborns acquire HSV-1 or HSV-2 during vaginal delivery when the mother has active genital lesions (see Chapter 1). In older children and adolescents, encephalitis represents the reactivation of latent virus with retrograde spread through nerve endings into the CNS.

HSV encephalitis is the only viral encephalitis with clear pharmacologic treatment, consisting of acyclovir 10 mg/kg IV given every 8 hours for 14–21 days. Nevertheless, survivors may have persistent neurologic deficits and epilepsy.

Human Parechovirus Encephalitis

Human parechovirus is a rare but catastrophic cause of encephalitis in neonates and infants. Seizures and

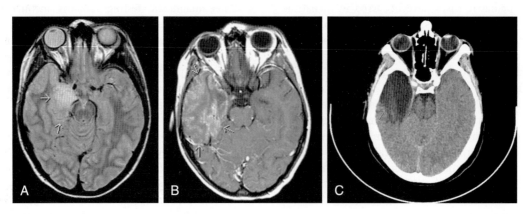

Fig. 2.1 Herpes Encephalitis (Same Patient Over Time). (A) Axial T$_2$ magnetic resonance imaging (MRI) shows high signal in mesial temporal region in early encephalitis. (B) Axial T$_2$ MRI shows involvement of the whole temporal lobe. (C) Computed tomography scan shows residual encephalomalacia of the temporal lobe.

significant neurologic sequelae are common, including gross motor developmental delays, quadriplegia, and cortical visual impairment.[12] MRI of the brain shows extensive restricted diffusion of the white matter. CSF is often normal or shows only moderately elevated protein without pleocytosis. Treatment is supportive.

Enterovirus Encephalitis

Over 100 different serotypes of enterovirus exist, and several cause encephalitis in infants and children. The illness typically begins with diarrhea or a mild upper respiratory infection, and outbreaks follow seasonal trends with most occurring in summer and autumn in temperate climates. Most cases are mild or asymptomatic with full recovery, but significant exceptions exist as discussed here.

Coxsackievirus B encephalitis mostly affects neonates and infants. It is associated with myocarditis, meningitis, and encephalitis with a mortality rate as high as 10%.

EV71 is an aggressive neurotrophic enterovirus that causes encephalitis associated with outbreaks of hand-foot-mouth disease. Poor outcomes are most common in children under the age of 4 with skin rash, significant leukocytosis, and myoclonus. EB71 is particularly devastating in children under three in whom the virus directly attacks the brainstem (Bickerstaff encephalitis [BEE], discussed later in this chapter), causing rapidly progressive sympathetic hyperactivity, neurogenic pulmonary edema, and cardiopulmonary collapse. MRI may demonstrate lesions in the posterior medulla and pons.

There are no specific treatments for enterovirus encephalitis, but ribavirin and intravenous immunoglobulins (IVIGs) are helpful in some cases.[13] Other treatments are in development.

Rabies Encephalitis

Rabies is a neurotrophic virus transmitted through the saliva (bite) of an infected animal which then travels retrogradely through peripheral nerves to reach the CNS. It is uniformly fatal.

Globally, dogs are the most common vector transmitting rabies to humans. Animal vaccination programs have reduced the incidence of canine rabies in the United States, and bats are now the most common vector. Children should be taught to avoid contact with wild animals, particularly bats. Small bats inflict bites that are barely visible and may not be severe enough for the child to report to his parents. The incubation period is anywhere from a few days to several months, which can complicate efforts to identify the source.

The World Health Organization recommends fluorescent antibody testing as the reference method for diagnosis. RT-PCR is available for clinical testing but is most sensitive and specific for brain tissue; reliability declines when CSF or serum is tested. Cerebral inclusion bodies called Negri bodies are pathognomonic for rabies but are not always present. The local health department or CDC should be involved with all suspected cases of human rabies encephalitis.

Initial symptoms include tingling at the site of the bite, followed by nausea, vomiting, fever, agitated delirium, aggression, excessive salivation, inability to swallow, and hydrophobia. The level of consciousness declines rapidly, and coma and death follow within 2–10 days of initial symptoms. Treatment is palliative.

Arbovirus-Associated Encephalitis

The arboviruses are a group of viruses transmitted via ticks, mosquitos, or other insect bites. Most are not neurotrophic, but those that are include EEE, Western equine encephalitis (WEE), St. Louis encephalitis, La Crosse-California encephalitis, Colorado tick fever virus, and West Nile encephalitis in the United States. Globally, JE, Venezuela equine encephalitis (VEE), Dengue, Zika, and Chikungunya viruses are also common.

Outbreaks are seasonal and geographic, usually occurring in spring or summer when insects are most active. Exposure and travel history are particularly important for diagnosis. West Nile virus is the most common cause of arbovirus-associated encephalitis in the United States.

Presenting symptoms are similar but some distinguishing features exist. EEE causes significant brain necrosis and profound neurologic sequelae including paralysis and epilepsy. JE causes similarly severe necrosis and poor outcomes; a vaccine is available but not widely administered outside of endemic areas of Asia. WEE is milder but causes marked behavioral changes and seizures. St. Louis encephalitis causes hyponatremia and syndrome of inappropriate antidiuretic hormone secretion (SIADH). In general, patients suffering from arbovirus-related encephalitis typically have motor and movement disorders; children often develop brain calcifications postinfection. The summary of arboviruses is shown in Box 2.5.[14]

BOX 2.5	Arbovirus Families: Vectors, Geographical Distribution, and the Illnesses They Cause				
Family	Virus	Vector	Geographical Distribution	Systemic Illnesses	Neurologic Diseases
Togaviridae	EEEV	Mosquito (Culiseta, Aedes)	Eastern and Gulf coasts of the United States, Caribbean islands, Central America, northeast South America	Flu-like illness with nausea and vomiting	Meningoencephalitis, coma
	WEEV	Mosquito (Culiseta, Culex)	Mid-west and western USA, Canada	Febrile illness	Encephalitis
	VEEV	Mosquito (Culex, Aedes)	South and Central Americas, southeast and southwest USA	Flu-like illness	Encephalitis
	CHIKV	Mosquito (Aedes)	Africa, India, Southeast Asia, Caribbean islands, southeast USA	Fever, rash, arthralgias, myalgias	Rare encephalitis, GBS
Flaviviridae	SLEV	Mosquito (Culex)	North, Central, and South America	Flu-like illness with nausea	Meningitis, encephalitis, coma
	JEV	Mosquito (Culex)	Japan, Northeast, Southeast, and Central Asia, Indian subcontinent	–	Meningoencephalitis with seizures
	WNV	Mosquito (Culex)	Africa, the Mediterranean region, Central Asia, India, Europe, North, Central, and South Americas	Flu-like illness	Meningitis, flaccid paralysis, encephalitis
	ZIKV	Mosquito (Aedes), sexual transmission	Africa, India, Southeast Asia, Caribbean islands, Central, North, and South Americas	Flu-like illness with arthralgias, conjunctivitis	Meningoencephalitis, ADEM, GBS, IUGR, microcephaly (if contracted in utero)
	DENV	Mosquito (Aedes)	Asia, tropical and subtropical regions of the world	Fever, rash, headache, myalgias, hemorrhagic fever	Encephalopathy, rare encephalitis
	MVEV	Mosquito (Culex, Aedes)	Australia, New Zealand, New Guinea	Flu-like illness with nausea	Encephalitis
Bunyaviridae	CEV	Mosquito (Aedes)	Western USA	Flu-like illness with nausea and vomiting	Meningoencephalitis with seizures
	LACV	Mosquito (Aedes)	Mid-west and eastern USA	–	Meningoencephalitis with seizures
	TOSV	Sandfly (Phlebotomus)	Europe, North Africa	–	Meningitis
	RVFV	Mosquito (Culex, Aedes)	East and South Africa, Saudi Arabia	Fever, hepatitis, hemorrhagic fever	Encephalitis
Reoviridae	CTFV	Ticks (Dermacentor)	Rocky Mountains of the United States	Flu-like illness with nausea, vomiting, hepatitis, rash, hemorrhagic fever	Meningitis, encephalitis

ADEM, Acute demyelinating encephalomyelitis; *CEV*, California encephalitis virus; *CHIKV*, chikungunya virus; *CTFV*, Colorado tick fever virus; *DENV*, dengue virus; *EEEV*, eastern equine encephalitis virus; *GBS*, Guillain-Barré syndrome; *IUGR*, intrauterine growth retardation; *JEV*, Japanese encephalitis virus; *LACV*, La Crosse virus; *MVEV*, Murray Valley encephalitis virus; *RVFV*, Rift Valley fever virus; *SLEV*, Saint Louis encephalitis virus; *TOSV*, Toscana virus; *VEEV*, Venezuelan

Diagnosis depends on the identification of virus-specific and neutralizing antibodies in serum and CSF. Treatment is supportive, although several new treatment options are being investigated.

COVID-19 Encephalitis

Neurological symptoms are common during infection with SARS-CoV-2 (the coronavirus that causes COVID-19 disease), occurring in up to 35% of patients and including headache, dizziness, confusion, anosmia, and decreased level of consciousness. Most neurological symptoms represent encephalopathy related to hypoxia or other organ dysfunction. However, a small number of severely or critically ill patients may suffer from COVID-19 encephalitis. This is a rare complication, and it is not known how often it affects infants or children.

The exact incidence and mechanism of COVID-19 neurotropism remains unclear. SARS-CoV-2 is virtually never isolated from CSF, although it has been documented in a small number of cases. Some cases of encephalitis are autoimmune in nature, with the presumption that COVID-19 infection triggered the abnormal immune response.[15] MRI may demonstrate cortical and subcortical T2/FLAIR abnormalities, and CSF shows pleocytosis. The prognosis is poor.[16] All patients with encephalitis were hospitalized with severe respiratory symptoms, and most were critically ill; there are no reports of COVID-19 encephalitis resulting from mild or asymptomatic infections.[17] Management consists of treatment of the COVID-19 infection and supportive care.

Vaccine-Preventable Encephalitis

The types of viral encephalitis have changed over time. Many previously frequent causes of viral encephalitis became less common with widespread vaccination; unfortunately, some of these viruses are resurgent due to antivaccine sentiment. The most significant vaccine-preventable causes of encephalitis include measles, mumps, and varicella-zoster virus.

Measles can cause several different forms of encephalitis including primary measles encephalitis, acute postmeasles encephalitis, measles inclusion body encephalitis, and a chronic form known as subacute sclerosing panencephalitis (discussed in Chapter 5). It is a neurotropic virus and EEG abnormalities are often present even without clinical symptoms of encephalopathy. Symptoms of encephalitis usually begin 1–8 days after the appearance of rash but may be delayed for up to 3 weeks. The onset is usually abrupt and characterized by lethargy or obtundation that rapidly progresses to coma. Generalized seizures occur in half of children. The spectrum of neurological disturbances includes hemiplegia, ataxia, and involuntary movement disorders. Acute transverse myelitis may occur as well (see Chapter 12). The incidence of neurological morbidity (cognitive impairment, epilepsy, and paralysis) is high, but does not correlate with the severity of acute encephalitis. Treatment is supportive; the only way to prevent the disease is through routine vaccination.

Mumps encephalitis and varicella-zoster encephalitis are mainly diseases of adults, rarely seen in children. Varicella-zoster virus causes cerebellitis in young children.

Aseptic Meningitis

The term *aseptic meningitis* defines a syndrome of meningismus and CSF leukocytosis without bacterial or fungal infection. Drugs or viral infections are the usual cause. Viral meningitis is usually a benign, self-limited disease from which 95% of children recover completely.

Clinical features. The onset of symptoms is abrupt and characterized by fever, headache, and stiff neck, except in infants who do not have meningismus. Irritability, lethargy, and vomiting are common. *"Encephalitic" symptoms are not part of the syndrome.* Systemic illness is uncommon, but its presence may suggest specific viral disorders. The acute illness usually lasts less than 1 week, but malaise and headache may continue for several weeks.

Diagnosis. In most cases of aseptic meningitis, the CSF contains 10–200 leukocytes/mm³, but cell counts of 1000 cells/mm³ or greater may occur with lymphocytic choriomeningitis. The response is primarily lymphocytic, but polymorphonuclear leukocytes may predominate early in the course. The protein concentration is generally between 50 and 100 mg/dL (0.5 and 1 g/L) and the glucose concentration is normal, although it may be slightly reduced in children with mumps and lymphocytic choriomeningitis.

Aseptic meningitis usually occurs in the spring or summer, and enteroviruses are responsible for most cases in children. Nonviral causes of aseptic meningitis are rare, but considerations include Lyme disease, Kawasaki disease, leukemia, systemic lupus erythematosus (SLE), and migraine.

Bacterial meningitis is a major concern when a child has meningismus. Although CSF examination provides several clues that differentiate bacterial from viral meningitis, initiate antibiotic therapy for every child with a clinical syndrome of aseptic meningitis until CSF culture is negative for bacteria (see Chapter 4). This is especially true for children who received antibiotic therapy before examination of the CSF.

Management. Treatment for herpes encephalitis with acyclovir is routine in children with viral meningitis or encephalitis until excluding that diagnosis by PCR analysis of CSF. Treatment of viral aseptic meningitis is symptomatic. Bed rest in a quiet environment and mild analgesics provide satisfactory relief of symptoms in most children.

AUTOIMMUNE ENCEPHALOPATHIES

Autoimmune encephalitis presents with a variety of symptoms, many of which overlap with infectious encephalitis. Acute disseminated encephalomyelitis (ADEM, discussed later) constitutes a subtype of autoimmune encephalitis. Consider autoimmune encephalitis in all children presenting with altered mental status and new psychiatric symptoms (including symptoms of psychosis); supporting symptoms include seizures, acute new-onset movement disorders, confusion, delirium, focal neurologic signs, and depressed level of consciousness. All children should also undergo a thorough infectious workup.

By far the most common cause of antibody-mediated autoimmune encephalitis in the pediatric population is anti-NMDAR encephalitis; multiple other antibodies can cause encephalitis, but these are rare in children. Comprehensive CSF antibody panels for pediatric autoimmune encephalitis are available commercially. ADEM is the most common cause of autoimmune encephalitis in which there is no specific antibody implicated.[18] BEE is rare but an important consideration in children with cranial nerve symptoms. Having one autoimmune disorder tends to predispose to others, and preexisting autoimmune diseases such as Hashimoto thyroiditis and SLE are risk factors for the development of encephalitis.

Rhombencephalitis (Bickerstaff Encephalitis)

BEE is characterized by the triad of ophthalmoplegia, ataxia, and decreased level of consciousness. Other than the alteration in mental status it is quite similar to Miller Fisher syndrome and is often considered as a continuum of central and peripheral postinfectious disease ranging from BEE to GBS. Many affected children have evidence of both central and peripheral nervous system pathology.

Clinical features. In addition to the classic triad, associated symptoms may include hyper- or hyporeflexia, weakness of the limbs and bulbar musculature, and pupillary abnormalities.

Diagnosis. BEE is typically an autoimmune condition, and 46% of patients are positive for anti-GQ1b antibodies (the same antibodies seen in Miller Fisher syndrome). Nerve conduction velocities are abnormal in 64%, further supporting the idea that central and peripheral postinfectious processes overlap.[19] MRI abnormalities are less common, seen in 25% of patients; these abnormalities may provide a vital diagnostic clue, as EV71 (discussed earlier) is known to cause medullary and pontine lesions and is associated with a significantly worse prognosis. Infectious causes of BBE are more likely to be associated with elevated CSF protein and pleocytosis.[20]

Management. Antibody-positive cases respond well to IVIG and plasma exchange, and most patients make a full recovery. Antibody-negative cases are treated with supportive care. EV71-positive cases have a much worse prognosis and high mortality rate.

Acute Disseminated Encephalomyelitis

ADEM is a central demyelinating disorder of childhood. The belief was that ADEM was a monophasic immunological reaction to an infectious illness because fever is an initial feature. This belief has been questioned for two reasons. First, fever may be part of ADEM and not evidence of prior infection; second, ADEM often is not monophasic, but the first attack of a recurring disorder similar to multiple sclerosis. An immune-mediated mechanism is the presumed pathophysiology.[21]

Examples of postinfectious disorders appear in several chapters of this book and include GBS (see Chapter 7), acute cerebellar ataxia (see Chapter 10), transverse myelitis (see Chapter 12), brachial neuritis (see Chapter 13), optic neuritis (see Chapter 16), and Bell palsy (see Chapter 17). The cause-and-effect relationship between viral infection and many of these syndromes is impossible to establish, especially when

30 days is the accepted latency period between viral infection and the onset of neurological dysfunction. The average school-age child has at least four to six "viral illnesses" each year, so that as many as half of children report a viral illness 30 days before the onset of any life event. This average is probably higher for preschool-age children in daycare.

Clinical features. Initial symptoms include lethargy, headache, and vomiting. Whether these systemic features are symptoms of an infectious illness or early encephalopathy is not clear. The onset of neurological symptoms is abrupt and characterized by focal motor signs and/or altered mental status. Optic neuritis, transverse myelitis, or both may precede encephalopathy (see Chapter 12). The prognosis is generally favorable, but some children experience long-term cognitive or motor deficits, and a significant minority experience repeated episodes and follow a course similar to multiple sclerosis.[22] Unlike in multiple sclerosis, the burden of white matter abnormalities on MRI correlates well with the severity of symptoms.

Diagnosis. T_2-weighted MRI reveals a marked increase in signal intensity throughout the white matter (Fig. 2.2), but also involves the gray matter. The thalami, basal ganglia, corpus callosum, and periventricular white matter are often affected. The lesions may resolve in the weeks that follow. In boys, consider the diagnosis of adrenoleukodystrophy (see Chapter 5). CSF is frequently normal or shows mild protein elevation and leukocytosis, with negative oligoclonal bands.

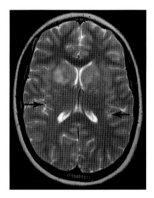

Fig. 2.2 Acute Disseminated Encephalomyelitis. T_2 axial magnetic resonance imaging shows high signal in basal ganglia and surrounding white matter. The arrows indicate perivascular inflammation.

Management. Treatment with intravenous high-dose methylprednisolone (20–30 mg/kg/day, up to 1 g) helps in about 50% of cases. IVIG (2 g/kg divided over 2–5 days) and plasma exchange may benefit children who fail to respond to corticosteroids. In very rare cases, decompressive craniectomy may be needed to treat high ICP. Early empiric treatment results in better outcomes.[23] Involve physical, occupational, and speech therapies early and continue to reassess rehabilitation needs throughout the hospitalization. Some children require inpatient rehabilitative services.

Hashimoto encephalopathy

Hashimoto encephalopathy is a steroid-responsive encephalopathy associated with high titers of antithyroid antibodies.[24] It often occurs in association with other immune-mediated disorders.

Clinical features. The progression of symptoms is variable. In some, it begins with headache and confusion that progress to stupor. In others, a progressive encephalopathy characterized by dementia occurs. Focal or generalized seizures and transitory neurological deficits (stroke-like episodes) may be an initial or a late feature. Tremulousness and/or myoclonus are often seen. Other symptoms, including cognitive decline, transient aphasia, hallucinations, sleep disturbances, and ataxia, may occur.[25] The encephalopathy lasts for days to months and often gradually disappears. Recurrent episodes are the rule and may coincide with the menstrual cycle in females.[26]

Diagnosis. Suspect Hashimoto encephalopathy in every case of recurrent or progressive encephalopathy. The CSF protein concentration is usually elevated, sometimes above 100 mg/dL (1 g/L), but the pressure and cell count are normal. Affected individuals are usually euthyroid. The diagnosis depends on the presence of antithyroid antibodies. Antibodies against thyroglobulin and the microsomal fraction are most common, but antibodies against other thyroid elements and other organs may be present as well. Thyroid peroxidase antibodies and circulating immune complexes are detectable in serum and CSF, but the titers do not correlate with clinical symptoms.[27] These antibodies are present in 10% of normal individuals, so the diagnosis is based on the history and response to steroids. MRI may show diffuse signal abnormalities in the white matter or meningeal enhancement. EEG shows diffuse slowing.[28]

Management. Corticosteroids are beneficial in ending an attack and preventing further episodes. Some cases benefit from plasma exchange or IVIG. Fifty-five percent have complete recovery.

Systemic Lupus Erythematosus

SLE is a multisystem autoimmune disease, characterized by the presence of antinuclear antibodies, especially antibodies to double-standard DNA. It accounts for 5% of patients seen in pediatric rheumatology clinics. The onset of SLE is uncommon before adolescence. In childhood, the ratio of girls affected to boys is 5:1 and 8:1 when all ages are included.

Immune complex deposition in the brain causes neurologic dysfunction, rather than vasculitis. The clinical and imaging features are consistent with diffuse encephalopathy rather than stroke.

Clinical features. CNS manifestations are the initial feature of SLE in 20% of cases and occur in half of children with SLE overall. Neuropsychiatric abnormalities occur in up to 95% of patients. Patients with CNS involvement have usually a more severe course. Other common features are recurrent headaches, cognitive disorders, and seizures. Some degree of cognitive dysfunction is measurable in most patients, but dementia is uncommon. Depression and anxiety are relatively common. It is uncertain whether depression is symptomatic of the disease or a reaction to chronic illness. Corticosteroids, which are a mainstay of treatment, may also contribute to anxiety. Frank psychosis, as defined by impaired reality testing and hallucinations, occurs in less than 15% of patients.

Diagnosis. Other criteria establish the diagnosis of SLE before the development of encephalopathy. Patients with encephalopathy usually have high serum titers of anti-DNA and lymphocytotoxic antibodies and high CSF titers of antineuronal antibodies.

Management. The usual treatment of the CNS manifestations of SLE is high-dose oral or intravenous corticosteroids after ruling out an infectious process. Second-line treatments include rituximab, cyclophosphamide, and synthetic disease-modifying antirheumatic drugs such as mycophenolate, azathioprine, and intrathecal methotrexate.

Anti–*N*-Methyl-D-Aspartate Receptor Antibody Encephalopathy

This condition was recently recognized and has become the most common cause of autoimmune encephalitis in pediatric patients. Forty percent of patients are younger than 18.

Clinical features. Most children and adolescents present with a prodrome of fever, headache, and malaise. This is followed in days or weeks by behavioral personality changes (including symptoms of depression, anxiety, or psychosis), seizures, or sleep disorders, with a lesser percentage presenting with dyskinesias or dystonias (9.5%), and speech reduction (3%). Bizarre behaviors, grandiose or hyperreligious delusions, and paranoia are common. Malignant catatonia with autonomic instability is possible. Ultimately 77% of children develop seizures, 84% stereotyped movements, and 86% autonomic instability. Ovarian teratomas are an important potential cause of the syndrome in girls (31%), but less so than in adult females (56%). Tumors are rare in males.

Diagnosis. Confirmation by ELISA of antibodies against the NR1 subunit of the NMDARs in serum or CSF is diagnostic. The titers in CSF correlate better with symptom burden and outcome. The EEG shows nonspecific slowing, beta-delta complexes (similar to delta brushes in newborns) and may capture seizures. The MRI shows abnormal T2 cortical and subcortical changes in 55% of cases.[28]

Management. When possible, tumor removal offers the best prognosis, in addition to immunosuppressant therapy. Most patients have significant or full recovery after tumor removal or immunotherapy, but up to one-quarter experience relapses. IVIG, steroids, and plasmapheresis have all been associated with improvement or resolution of symptoms.[29] Electroconvulsive therapy may be required for severe cases of malignant catatonia unresponsive to benzodiazepines.

Fever Illness Refractory Epileptic Syndrome

Fever illness refractory epileptic syndrome (FIRES) is an encephalopathy associated with fever and multifocal seizures that evolves into pharmacoresistant status epilepticus in previously normal children.

Clinical features. Patients develop profound encephalopathy and seizures in the setting of a febrile illness without a clear infectious or autoimmune etiology. The CSF shows mild pleocytosis, but no evidence of any infectious process. The MRI is initially normal, but later shows edema in the mesial temporal regions followed by atrophy.[30]

Diagnosis. Diagnosis is clinical and relies on exclusion. CSF analysis including PCR in FIRES is negative for viruses, bacteria, fungi, or parasites. Patients often undergo extensive additional testing, but CSF lactic acid, biogenic amines, amino acids, ammonia, lactic acid, carnitine, acylcarnitine, very long-chain fatty acids, vitamin B_{12}, biotin, heavy metals, copper, ceruloplasmin, homocysteine, uric acid, transferrin, urine orotic acid, organic acids, and purine/pyrimidine ratio are all found to be normal. Mitochondrial enzyme studies in muscles and fibroblasts are also normal. The known epilepsy susceptibility genes are not present in these patients. Autoimmune testing is negative, including testing for SLE, anti-NMDAR antibodies, alpha-amino-3-hydroxy-5-methylisoxazole-4-proprionic acid, $GABA_B$ receptors, voltage-gated potassium channel-associated proteins, LGi1 and contactin-associated protein-like 2, and glutamic acid decarboxylase. Testing is also negative for Wegener granulomatosis, vasculitis, Hashimoto thyroiditis and encephalitis, and celiac disease.[31]

Management. Pharmacologically induced coma is often required due to refractoriness to all antiseizure medications. The ketogenic diet has been helpful in some patients. Unfortunately, the prognosis is almost always poor, with a high mortality rate. Surviving children typically have severe neurological deficits and epilepsy that remains resistant to treatment.

Reye Syndrome

Reye syndrome is a systemic disorder of mitochondrial function that occurs during or following viral infection. The occurrence is higher with salicylate use for symptomatic relief during viral illness. Recognition of this relationship has led to decreased use of salicylates in children and a marked decline in the incidence of Reye syndrome.

Clinical features. In the United States, sporadic cases are generally associated with varicella (chickenpox) or nonspecific respiratory infections; small epidemics are associated with influenza B infection. When varicella is the precipitating infection, the initial stage of Reye syndrome occurs 3–6 days after the appearance of rash.

The clinical course is relatively predictable and divisible into five stages:

- *Stage 0*: Vomiting, but no symptoms of brain dysfunction.
- *Stage I*: Vomiting, confusion, and lethargy.
- *Stage II*: Agitation, delirium, decorticate posturing, and hyperventilation.
- *Stage III*: Coma and decerebrate posturing.
- *Stage IV*: Flaccidity, apnea, dilated, and fixed pupils.

The progression from stage I to IV may be explosive, evolving in less than 24 hours. More commonly, the period of recurrent vomiting and lethargy lasts for a day or longer. In most children with vomiting and laboratory evidence of hepatic dysfunction following varicella or respiratory infection, liver biopsy shows the features of Reye syndrome, despite normal cerebral function. The designation of this stage is Reye stage 0. Stages I and II represent metabolic dysfunction and cerebral edema. Stages III and IV indicate generalized increased ICP and herniation.

Focal neurological disturbances and meningismus are not part of the syndrome. Fever is not a prominent feature, and hepatomegaly occurs in one-half of patients late in the course. The outcome is variable, but as a rule, infants do worse than older children. Progression to stages III and IV at all ages is associated with a high death rate and with impaired neurological function in survivors.

Diagnosis. Typical blood abnormalities are hypoglycemia, hyperammonemia, and increased concentrations of hepatic enzymes. Serum bilirubin concentrations remain normal, and jaundice does not occur. Acute pancreatitis sometimes develops and is identified by increased concentrations of serum amylase. The CSF is normal except for increased pressure. The EEG shows abnormalities consistent with diffuse encephalopathy.

A liver biopsy is definitive. Light microscopy shows panlobular accumulation of small intracellular lipid droplets and depletion of succinic acid dehydrogenase in the absence of other abnormalities. Electron microscopic changes include characteristic mitochondrial abnormalities, peroxisomal proliferation, swelling, proliferation of smooth endoplasmic reticulum, and glycogen depletion.

Conditions that mimic Reye syndrome are disorders of fatty acid oxidation, ornithine transcarbamylase deficiency, and valproate hepatotoxicity. Assume an inborn error of metabolism in any child with recurrent Reye syndrome (see Box 2.3) or a family history of similar illness. Metabolic products of valproate are mitochondrial poisons that produce an experimental model of Reye syndrome.

Management. Admit all children to a pediatric intensive care unit. Treatment of children with stage I or

II disease is intravenous hypertonic (10%–15%) glucose solution at normal maintenance volumes. Stages III and IV require treatment of increased ICP (see Chapter 4) by elevation of the head, controlled mechanical ventilation, and mannitol or hypertonic saline. Corticosteroids are of limited benefit and not used routinely. Some authorities continue to advocate ICP monitors and pentobarbital coma, despite the failure to affect outcome. Fortunately, this once common and deadly disease has nearly disappeared in the United States with the discontinuation of salicylate therapy for children.

POSTIMMUNIZATION ENCEPHALOPATHY

ADEM is the most common manifestation of postimmunization encephalopathy. The converse is not true: only 5% of ADEM cases are linked to vaccines.[32] Optic neuritis, transverse myelitis, and GBS also occur. The overall risk is extremely small and clearly outweighed by the benefits of vaccination. Nevertheless, postimmunization encephalopathy should be considered when no other etiology is found.

The CDC has accessible, easy-to-read information regarding vaccines on their government website. Currently several vaccine types are in use in the United States: inactivated; live-attenuated; messenger RNA (mRNA); subunit, recombinant, conjugate, and polysaccharide; toxoid; and viral vector vaccines.

Inactivated vaccines are not as strong and require boosters or yearly dosing. Influenza and polio vaccines are examples, as is rabies, which is why standard rabies vaccination is not provided to those outside certain high-risk professions within the United States. The initial vaccine is more likely to cause postimmunization encephalopathy than booster shots.

Live-attenuated vaccines are stronger and offer lifelong immunity. In the United States standard vaccines in this group include measles, mumps, rubella; chickenpox (varicella); and rotavirus vaccines.

Subunit, recombinant, polysaccharide, and conjugate vaccines include *Haemophilus influenzae* type b, hepatitis B, human papillomavirus, the pertussis component of DTaP, and meningococcal disease.

Toxoid vaccines include diphtheria and tetanus vaccinations.

mRNA is a new technology with significant promise. It is used for vaccination against the SARS-CoV-2 virus.

METABOLIC AND SYSTEMIC DISORDERS

Disorders of Osmolality

The number of particles in a solution determines the osmolality of a solution. Sodium salts, glucose, and urea are the primary osmoles of the extracellular space, potassium salts of the intracellular space, and plasma proteins of the intravascular space. Because cell membranes are permeable to water and osmotic equilibrium is constant, the osmolality of the extracellular space determines the volume of intracellular fluid. Hypernatremia and hyperglycemia are the major causes of serum hyperosmolality, and hyponatremia is the main cause of serum hypo-osmolality.

Diabetic Ketoacidosis

The major cause of symptomatic hyperglycemia in children is diabetic ketoacidosis. Nonketotic hyperglycemic coma, associated with mild or non-insulin-requiring diabetes, is unusual in children but is sometimes seen in adolescents.

Clinical features. Diabetic ketoacidosis develops rapidly in children who have neglected to take prescribed doses of insulin or who have a superimposed infection. Initial features are polydipsia, polyuria, and fatigue. The child hyperventilates to compensate for metabolic acidosis. Lethargy rapidly progresses to coma and may be fatal without treatment. Mortality rates for diabetic ketoacidosis are 0.14%–0.3% in the United States and other resource-rich countries, but much higher in other locations.

Avoiding cerebral edema is one of the main goals of treatment. Cerebral edema develops due to the retention of intracellular osmolytes in the brain during hydration, causing a shift of water into the intracellular space. Signs of cerebral edema include agitation, confusion, lethargy, headache, emesis, and incontinence. The severity of cerebral edema correlates with changes in the level of consciousness. Other, less common, neurological complications of diabetic ketoacidosis are venous sinus thrombosis and intracerebral hemorrhage. Both are associated with focal or generalized seizures.

Diagnosis. The basis for diagnosis is the combination of a blood glucose level greater than 400 mg/dL (22 mmol/L), the presence of serum and urinary ketones, an arterial pH less than 7.25, and a serum bicarbonate concentration less than 15 mmol/L.

Management. In children with moderate-to-severe diabetic ketoacidosis, avoid the rapid administration of hypotonic fluids at a time of high serum osmolality. Replace fluid deficits evenly over 48 hours. Reduce the sodium deficit by half in the first 12 hours and the remainder over the next 36 hours. Provide bicarbonate in physiological proportions.

Hypoglycemia

Symptomatic hypoglycemia after the neonatal period is usually associated with maternal gestational diabetes. A minority of cases are caused by sepsis and inborn errors of metabolism.

Clinical features. Clinical features are not precisely predictable from the blood glucose concentration. Hypoglycemia does not usually become symptomatic until blood concentrations are less than 50 mg/dL (2.8 mmol/L). The rate of falls may be important in determining the clinical features. Dizziness and tremor may occur at blood concentrations below 60 mg/dL (3.1 mmol/L) and serve as a warning of insulin overdose. Greater declines in blood glucose concentration result in confusion, delirium, and loss of consciousness. Sudden hemiplegia, usually transitory and sometimes shifting between the two sides, is a rare feature of hypoglycemia. The mechanism is unknown, and imaging shows no evidence of infarction.

Diagnosis. Prompt measurement of glucose via fingerstick is standard of care and provides near-instantaneous results; confirm with serum glucose obtained via venipuncture. Always suspect hypoglycemia in diabetic children with altered mental status or decreased consciousness or newborns of mothers with gestational diabetes.

Management. Diabetic children should be encouraged to carry a source of sugar for use at the first symptom of hypoglycemia. Children who are comatose from hypoglycemia should receive immediate intravenous glucose replacement. Malnourished infants and children should receive thiamine to avoid acute precipitation of encephalopathy. Complete recovery is the rule when the disorder is treated promptly, but severe prolonged hypoglycemia causes permanent neurologic deficits.

Hypernatremia

The usual causes of hypernatremia are: (1) dehydration in which water loss exceeds sodium loss and (2) overhydration with hypertonic saline solutions. Hypernatremia is a medical emergency, and if not corrected promptly may lead to permanent brain damage and death.

Clinical features. Hypernatremic dehydration may be a consequence of vomiting or diarrhea, especially if water intake is restricted. Overzealous correction of hyponatremia causes iatrogenic hypernatremia. Rapid alterations in sodium concentration are much more likely to cause encephalopathy than are equivalent concentrations attained slowly. The symptoms of hypernatremia are referable to the nervous system and include irritability, lethargy progressing to coma, and seizures. The presence of focal neurological deficits suggests cerebral venous sinus thrombosis.

Diagnosis. Symptomatic hypernatremia develops at sodium concentrations greater than 160 mEq/L (160 mmol/L). EEG shows the nonspecific slowing associated with metabolic encephalopathies. Focal slowing on the EEG or focal abnormalities on examination warrants neuroimaging to look for venous sinus thrombosis.

Central diabetes insipidus (DI) causes recurrent episodes of hypernatremia and is typically seen in children with congenital brain malformations (e.g., septo-optic dysplasia sequence) or a history of extensive brain injury. This is a chronic disorder that requires lifelong surveillance.

Management. Rapid water replacement can lead to cerebral edema. The recommended approach is to correct abnormalities of intravascular volume before correcting the water deficit. For children with DI, refer to an endocrinologist who can then assist with sodium monitoring and administration of desmopressin (a synthetic form of antidiuretic hormone).

Hyponatremia

Hyponatremia may result from water retention, sodium loss, or both. The antidiuretic hormone (ADH) secretion is an important determinant of water retention. Sodium loss results from renal disease, vomiting, and diarrhea. Permanent brain damage from hyponatremia is uncommon but may occur in otherwise healthy children if the serum sodium concentration remains less than 115 mEq/L for several hours.

Syndrome of Inappropriate Antidiuretic Hormone Secretion

SIADH occurs in association with several neurological disorders, including head trauma, infections, and intracranial hemorrhage.

Clinical features. Most patients with SIADH have a preexisting loss of consciousness from their underlying neurological disorder. In such patients, hyponatremia is the only feature of SIADH. In those who are alert, lethargy develops from hyponatremia but rarely progresses to coma or seizures.

Diagnosis. The care of children with acute intracranial disorders requires vigilance for SIADH. Repeated determinations of the serum sodium concentration are required. Measure the urinary sodium concentration once documenting hyponatremia and low serum osmolality. The urine osmolality in SIADH does not always exceed the serum osmolality, but the urine is less than maximally dilute, which excludes the dilutional hyponatremia of water intoxication.

Management. SIADH responds to fluid restriction. An intake of 50%–75% of daily water maintenance is generally satisfactory.

Sodium Loss

Clinical features. The movement of water into the brain causes *hyponatremic encephalopathy.* Serum sodium concentrations below 125 mEq/L (125 mmol/L) are associated with nausea, vomiting, muscular twitching, and lethargy. Seizures and coma are associated with a further decline to less than 115 mEq/L (115 mmol/L).

Diagnosis. Hyponatremia is a potential problem in children with vomiting or diarrhea, or with renal disease. Both serum and urinary sodium concentrations are low.

Management. Infuse hypertonic sodium chloride (514 mEq/L) with the goal of increasing the serum sodium concentration to 125–130 mEq/L (125–130 mmol/L), but by no more than 25 mEq/L (25 mmol/L) in the first 48 hours. More rapid corrections are associated with seizures, hypernatremic encephalopathy, and the possibility of central pontine myelinolysis.

Endocrine Causes of Encephalopathy
Adrenal Disorders

Adrenal hypersecretion causes agitation or depression but does not produce coma. Adrenal failure may result from sepsis, abrupt withdrawal of corticosteroid therapy, or adrenal hemorrhage. Initial symptoms are nausea, vomiting, abdominal pain, and fever. Lethargy progresses to coma and is associated with hypovolemic shock. Prompt intravenous infusion of fluids, glucose, and corticosteroids is lifesaving.

Parathyroid Disorders

All the neurological features of *hyperparathyroidism* relate to hypercalcemia. Weakness and myopathy are relatively common. Alterations in mental status occur in 50% of patients and include apathy, delirium, paranoia, and dementia. Apathy and delirium occur at serum calcium concentrations greater than 11 mg/dL (2.75 mmol/L), and psychosis and dementia develop at concentrations of 16 mg/dL (4.0 mmol/L) or greater.

Seizures are the main feature of *hypoparathyroidism* and hypocalcemia. They may be generalized or focal and often preceded by tetany. Hypocalcemic seizures do not respond to anticonvulsant drugs; calcium replacement is the only treatment.

Thyroid Disorders

Hyperthyroidism causes exhilaration bordering on mania and may be associated with seizures, tremors, and chorea (see Chapter 14). Thyroid storm (crisis) is a life-threatening event characterized by restlessness, cardiac arrhythmia, vomiting, and diarrhea. Delirium is an early feature and may progress to coma.

Acquired hypothyroidism affects both the central and peripheral nervous systems. Peripheral effects include neuropathy and myopathy. Central effects are cranial nerve abnormalities, ataxia, psychoses, dementia, seizures, and coma. Delusions and hallucinations occur in more than half of patients with long-standing disease. Myxedema coma, a rare manifestation of long-standing hypothyroidism in adults, is even less common in children. A characteristic feature is a profound hypothermia without shivering.

Hashimoto thyroiditis is an autoimmune disorder that may be associated with encephalitis in some patients, as discussed earlier in this chapter.

Hepatic Encephalopathy

Children with acute hepatic failure often develop severe cerebral edema. Viral hepatitis, drugs, toxins, and Reye syndrome are the main causes of acute hepatic failure. The cause of encephalopathy is a hepatic cellular failure and the diversion of toxins from the hepatic portal vein into the systemic circulation. Severe viral hepatitis with marked elevation of the unconjugated bilirubin concentration may even lead to kernicterus in older children.

In children with chronic cholestatic liver disease, demyelination of the posterior columns and peripheral nerves may result from vitamin E deficiency. The major features are ataxia, areflexia, and gaze paresis, without evidence of encephalopathy (see Chapter 10).

Clinical features. The onset of encephalopathy can be acute or slowly evolving.[33] Malaise and fatigue are early symptoms that accompany the features of hepatic failure: jaundice, dark urine, and abnormal results of liver function tests. Nausea and vomiting occur with fulminant hepatic failure. The onset of coma may be spontaneous or induced by gastrointestinal bleeding, infection, high protein intake, and excessive use of tranquilizers or diuretics. The first features are disturbed sleep and a change in affect. Drowsiness, hyperventilation, and asterixis, a flapping tremor at the wrist with arms extended and wrists flexed, follow. Hallucinations sometimes occur during the early stages, but a continuous progression to coma is more common. Seizures and decerebrate rigidity develop as the patient becomes comatose.

Diagnosis. In hepatic coma the EEG pattern is not specific but is always abnormal and suggests a metabolic encephalopathy: loss of posterior rhythm, generalized slowing of background, and frontal *triphasic waves*. Biochemical markers of liver failure include a sharp rise in serum transaminase, increased prothrombin time, mixed hyperbilirubinemia, hyperammonemia, and a decline in serum albumin concentration.

Management. The goal of treatment is to maintain cerebral, renal, and cardiopulmonary function until liver regeneration or transplantation can occur. Cerebral function is impaired, not only by abnormal concentrations of metabolites, but also by cerebral edema.

Inborn Errors of Metabolism

The inborn errors of metabolism that cause states of decreased consciousness are usually associated with hyperammonemia, hypoglycemia, or organic aciduria. Neonatal seizures are an early feature in most of these conditions (see Chapter 1), but some may not cause symptoms until infancy or childhood. Inborn errors with a delayed onset of encephalopathy include disorders of pyruvate metabolism and respiratory chain disorders (see Chapters 5, 6, 8, and 10); hemizygotes for ornithine carbamylase deficiency and heterozygotes for carbamyl phosphate synthetase deficiency (see Chapter 1); glycogen storage diseases (see Chapter 1); and primary carnitine deficiency.

Medium-Chain Acyl-Coenzyme A Dehydrogenase Deficiency

Medium-chain acyl-coenzyme A dehydrogenase (MCAD) is one of the enzymes involved in mitochondrial fatty acid oxidation. Mitochondrial fatty acid oxidation fuels hepatic ketogenesis, a major source of energy when hepatic glycogen stores deplete during prolonged fasting and periods of higher energy demands. It is caused by biallelic pathogenic variants in the *ACADM* gene; a newborn screen identifies most cases.[34]

MCAD deficiency is the main cause of the syndrome of *primary carnitine deficiency* (Box 2.6). Carnitine has two main functions: (1) the transfer of long-chain fatty acids into the inner mitochondrial membrane to undergo β-oxidation and generate energy; and (2) the modulation of the acyl-CoA/CoA ratio and the esterification of potentially toxic acyl-CoA metabolites. The transfer of fatty acids across the mitochondrial membrane requires the conversion of acyl-CoA to acylcarnitine and the enzyme carnitine palmitoyl transferase. If the carnitine concentration is deficient, toxic levels of acyl-CoA accumulate and impair the citric acid cycle, the gluconeogenesis, the urea cycle, and the fatty acid oxidation.

BOX 2.6   Differential Diagnosis of Carnitine Deficiency

Inborn Errors of Metabolism
- Aminoacidurias
  - Glutaric aciduria
  - Isovaleric acidemia
  - Methylmalonic acidemia
  - Propionic acidemia
- Disorders of pyruvate metabolism
  - Multiple carboxylase deficiency
  - Pyruvate carboxylase deficiency
  - Pyruvate dehydrogenase deficiency
- Disorders of the respiratory chain
- Medium-chain acyl-coenzyme A dehydrogenase deficiency
- Phosphoglucomutase deficiency

Acquired Conditions
- Hemodialysis
- Malnutrition
- Pregnancy
- Reye syndrome
- Total parenteral nutrition
- Valproate hepatotoxicity

Clinical features. The characteristic features of the disorder are intolerance to prolonged fasting, recurrent episodes of hypoglycemia, and coma. Affected children are normal at birth. Recurrent attacks of nonketotic hypoglycemia, vomiting, confusion, lethargy, and coma are provoked by intercurrent illness or fasting during infancy and early childhood. Cardiorespiratory arrest and sudden infant death may occur, but MCAD is not an important cause of sudden infant death syndrome. Between attacks, the child may appear normal. In some families the deficiency causes cardiomyopathy, whereas in others it causes only mild-to-moderate proximal weakness (see Chapters 6 and 7). Deficiencies of long-chain and short-chain acyl-CoA dehydrogenase cause a similar clinical phenotype.

Diagnosis. All affected children have low or absent urinary ketones during episodes of hypoglycemia and elevated serum concentrations of aspartate aminotransferase and lactate dehydrogenase. Blood carnitine concentrations are less than 20 µmol/mg of noncollagen protein. Showing the enzyme deficiency or the genetic mutation establishes the diagnosis. An abnormal acylcarnitine profile in plasma or urine organic acids is suspicious, and the diagnosis can be confirmed with measurement of MCAD enzyme activity in fibroblasts or other tissues.

Management. The prognosis is excellent once the diagnosis is established. The institution of frequent feedings avoids prolonged periods of fasting. L-Carnitine supplementation, initially 50 mg/kg/day, and increased as tolerated (up to 800 mg/kg/day), further reduces the possibility of attacks. Adverse effects of carnitine include nausea, vomiting, diarrhea, and abdominal cramps.

During an acute attack, provide a diet rich in medium-chain triglycerides and low in long-chain triglycerides in addition to carnitine. General supportive care is required for hypoglycemia and hypoprothrombinemia.

Renal Disorders

Children with chronic renal failure are at risk for acute or chronic uremic encephalopathy, dialysis encephalopathy, hypertensive encephalopathy, and neurological complications of the immunocompromised state.

Acute Uremic Encephalopathy

Clinical features. In children with acute renal failure, symptoms of cerebral dysfunction develop over several days. Asterixis is often the initial feature. Periods of confusion and headache, sometimes progressing to delirium and then to lethargy, follow. Weakness, tremulousness, and muscle cramps develop. Myoclonic jerks and tetany may be present. If uremia continues, decreasing consciousness and seizures follow.

Hemolytic-uremic syndrome is a leading cause of acute renal failure in children younger than 5 years old. The combination of thrombocytopenia, uremia, and Coombs-negative hemolytic anemia are characteristic features. Encephalopathy is the usual initial feature, but hemiparesis and aphasia caused by thrombotic stroke can occur in the absence of seizures or altered states of consciousness. Most children recover but may have chronic hypertension. Survivors usually have normal cognitive function but may have hyperactivity and inattentiveness.

Diagnosis. The mechanism of uremic encephalopathy is multifactorial and does not correlate with concentrations of blood urea nitrogen alone. Hyperammonemia and disturbed equilibrium of ions between the intracellular and extracellular spaces are probably important factors. Late in the course, acute uremic encephalopathy may be confused with hypertensive encephalopathy. A distinguishing feature is that increased ICP is an early feature of hypertensive encephalopathy, but not of acute uremic encephalopathy. Early in the course, the EEG shows the slowing of the background rhythms and periodic triphasic waves.[35]

Management. Hemodialysis reverses the encephalopathy and should be accomplished as quickly as possible after diagnosis.

Chronic Uremic Encephalopathy

Clinical features. Congenital renal hypoplasia is the usual cause of chronic uremic encephalopathy. Renal failure begins during the first year, and encephalopathy occurs between 1 and 9 years of age. Growth failure precedes the onset of encephalopathy. Three stages of disease occur sequentially.

Stage 1 consists of delayed motor development, dysmetria and tremor, or ataxia. Examination during this stage shows hyperreflexia, mild hypotonia, and extensor plantar responses. Within 6–12 months, the disease progresses to stage 2.

Stage 2 includes myoclonus of the face and limbs, partial motor seizures, dementia, and then generalized seizures. Facial myoclonus and lingual apraxia make speech and feeding difficult, and limb myoclonus interferes with ambulation. The duration of stage 2 is variable and maybe months to years.

Stage 3 consists of progressive bulbar failure, a vegetative state, and death.

Diagnosis. The basis for diagnosis is the clinical findings. Serial EEG shows progressive slowing and then superimposed epileptiform activity; serial MRI or CT shows progressive cerebral atrophy. Hyperparathyroidism with hypercalcemia occurs in some children with chronic uremic encephalopathy, but parathyroidectomy does not reverse the process.

Management. Hemodialysis and renal transplantation.

Dialysis Encephalopathy

Long-term dialysis may be associated with acute, transitory neurological disturbances attributed to the rapid shift of fluids and electrolytes between intracellular and extracellular spaces (*dialysis disequilibrium syndrome*). The most common are headaches, irritability, muscle cramps, and seizures. Seizures usually occur toward the end of dialysis or up to 24 hours later. Lethargy or delirium may precede the seizures.

Progressive encephalopathies associated with dialysis are often fatal. Two important causes exist: (1) opportunistic infections in the immunodeficient host, usually caused by cytomegalovirus and mycoses in children; and (2) the dialysis dementia syndrome (related to aluminum toxicity and now quite rare).

Hypertensive Encephalopathy

Hypertensive encephalopathy occurs when increases in systemic blood pressure exceed the limits of cerebral autoregulation. The result is damage to small arterioles, which leads to patchy areas of ischemia and edema. Therefore focal neurological deficits are relatively common.

Clinical features. The initial features are transitory attacks of cerebral ischemia and headache. Misinterpretation of such symptoms as part of uremic encephalopathy is common, despite the warning signs of focal neurological deficits. The headache persists and is accompanied by visual disturbances and vomiting. Seizures and diminished consciousness follow. The seizures are frequently focal at onset and then generalized. Examination reveals papilledema and retinal hemorrhages.

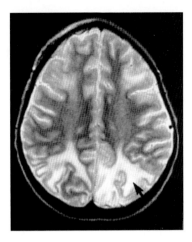

Fig. 2.3 Magnetic Resonance Imaging in Hypertensive Encephalopathy. The *arrow* points to increased signal intensity in both occipital lobes.

Diagnosis. Because the syndrome occurs in children receiving long-term renal dialysis while awaiting transplantation, the differential diagnosis includes disorders of osmolality, uremic encephalopathy, and dialysis encephalopathy. A posterior cerebral edema syndrome associated with hypertensive encephalopathy is evident on MRI (Fig. 2.3). This syndrome, otherwise known as posterior reversible encephalopathy syndrome (PRES), has been described with hypertension, immunosuppressants, renal failure, and eclampsia.[36] Hypertensive encephalopathy is distinguishable from other encephalopathies associated with renal disease by the greater elevation of blood pressure and the presence of focal neurological disturbances.

Management. Hypertensive encephalopathy is a medical emergency. Treatment consists of anticonvulsant therapy and aggressive efforts to reduce hypertension. Measures to reduce cerebral edema are required in some patients.

Other Metabolic Encephalopathies

Box 2.2 lists several less common causes of metabolic encephalopathy. Some are attributable to derangements of a single substance, but most are multifactorial.

A small number of children with burns covering >30% of the body surface develop an encephalopathy in an intermittent course (burn encephalopathy). The onset is days to weeks after the burn. Altered mental states (delirium or coma) and seizures (generalized or focal) are the major features. The encephalopathy is not attributable to a single factor.

Encephalopathies that occur during total parenteral hyperalimentation are generally due to hyperammonemia caused by excessive loads of amino acids. The causes of hypomagnesemia in infancy include prematurity, maternal deficiency, maternal or infant hypoparathyroidism, a high phosphorus diet, exchange transfusion, intestinal disorders, and specific defects in magnesium absorption. These conditions are often associated with hypocalcemia. Excessive use of diuretics causes hypomagnesemia in older children. Symptoms develop when plasma magnesium concentrations are less than 1.2 mg/dL (0.5 mmol/L), and include jitteriness, hyperirritability, and seizures. Further decline in serum magnesium concentrations leads to obtundation and coma.

Deficiency of one or more B vitamins may be associated with lethargy or delirium, but only thiamine deficiency causes coma. Thiamine deficiency is relatively common in alcoholic adults and produces Wernicke encephalopathy but is uncommon in children. Subacute necrotizing encephalopathy (Leigh disease) is a thiamine deficiency-like state in children (see Chapters 5 and 10).

Acute Confusional Migraine

Clinical features. Acute confusional migraine (ACM) was previously considered part of the spectrum of migraine, but more recent literature suggests that it is a distinct clinical entity.[37] The child may complain of a headache prodrome, then becomes acutely confused and agitated, often with speech difficulty and memory impairment. Some patients experience additional symptoms, including scotoma, transient blindness, numbness, and paresthesia. ACM is more common in the pediatric population and most cases occur between the ages of 5 and 17, with a slight male predominance. Attacks typically last less than 24 hours, although longer attacks have been reported.

Diagnosis. Migraine is always a clinical diagnosis and other possibilities require exclusion. The diagnosis relies heavily on a family history of migraine, but not necessarily of confusional migraine. During or shortly after a confusional attack the EEG may show unilateral temporal or occipital slowing.

Management. Most individuals experiencing a first attack attend for emergency treatment. Evidence-based treatment protocols are lacking, but there are some reports that valproic acid or prochlorperazine can shorten attacks. After the end of the attack, suggest a prophylactic agent to prevent further episodes (see Chapter 3).

Migraine Coma

Migraine coma is a rare condition in which patients with familial hemiplegic migraine experience recurrent episodes of loss of consciousness and coma following only minor head trauma. Pathogenic mutations in *CACNA1A* and *ATP1A2* cause familial hemiplegic migraine, and certain specific variants have been implicated in migraine coma.[38]

Clinical features. The major features of migraine coma are: (1) recurrent episodes of coma precipitated by trivial head injury and (2) apparent meningitis associated with life-threatening cerebral edema. Migraine coma occurs in kindred with familial hemiplegic migraine (see Chapter 11), but a similar syndrome may also occur in sporadic cases. Coma associated with fever follows a transient lucid state after a trivial head injury. Cerebral edema causes increased ICP. States of decreased consciousness may last for several days. Recovery is then complete, but fatalities due to cerebral edema and increased ICP may occur.

Diagnosis. Coma following even trivial head injury causes concern for intracranial hemorrhage. The initial CT scan may be normal, especially if obtained early in the course. Scans obtained between 24 and 72 hours show either generalized or focal edema. Examination of the CSF reveals increased pressure and pleocytosis (up to 100 cells/mm^3). The combination of fever, coma, and CSF pleocytosis suggests viral encephalitis, and herpes is a possibility if edema localizes to one temporal lobe.

Management. Treat children who have experienced migraine coma with a prophylactic agent to prevent further attacks (see Chapter 3). The major treatment goal during the acute attack is to decrease ICP by reducing cerebral edema (see Chapter 4).

PSYCHOLOGICAL DISORDERS

Panic disorders and schizophrenia may have an acute onset of symptoms suggesting delirium or confusion and must be distinguished from acute organic encephalopathies.

Panic Disorder

Clinical features. A panic attack is an agitated state caused by anxiety. Principal features are paroxysmal fear, dizziness, pallor, tachycardia, headache, and dyspnea. Hyperventilation often occurs and results in further dizziness, paresthesias, and light-headedness. The attacks are usually unprovoked, but some factors, such as phobias or situational anxieties, may provoke them. They can last for minutes to hours and recur daily. Patients feel drained or exhausted afterward but this is distinct from the confusion and psychomotor slowing noted after a seizure.

Diagnosis. Panic attacks simulate cardiac, pulmonary, or neurological disease, and many children undergo extensive and unnecessary medical evaluation or treatments before a correct diagnosis is reached. Suspect panic disorder in children with recurrent attacks of hyperventilation, dizziness, or dyspnea. The attacks are self-limited but can be profoundly debilitating.

Management. Selective serotonin reuptake inhibitors decrease anxiety and the occurrence of panic attacks. Citalopram at doses between 5 and 20 mg/day and escitalopram at doses of 2.5–10 mg/day are our first line of treatment. Buspirone is a helpful adjunctive treatment for persistent anxiety or panic disorder. Older children and adolescents can be taught more appropriate coping mechanisms using mindfulness techniques, grounding, breathing exercises, and meditation. Even very young children can benefit from breathing exercises.

Schizophrenia

Clinical features. Schizophrenia is a disorder of adolescence or early adult life and is almost never seen in prepubertal children. Schizophrenic individuals do not have an antecedent history of an affective disorder. An initial feature is often declining work or school performance simulating dementia. Intermittent depersonalization (not knowing where or who one is) may occur early in the course and suggests complex partial seizures.

Thoughts move with loose association from one idea to another until they become incoherent. Delusions and hallucinations are common and usually have paranoid features. Motor activity is either lacking or excessive and purposeless. This combination of symptoms in an adolescent may be difficult to distinguish clinically from drug encephalopathy.

Diagnosis. The neurologist's role is to rule out other neurologic diseases. All adolescents with psychosis need brain MRI and EEG; if onset is acute the clinician must also rule out autoimmune or infectious encephalitis and toxic or metabolic derangements. If these investigations are negative and the clinical history is consistent, the patient should be referred to child and adolescent psychiatry to formally establish the diagnosis. A family history of mental illness is common.

Management. Antipsychotic drugs may alleviate many of the symptoms.

TOXIC ENCEPHALOPATHIES

Accidental poisoning with drugs and chemicals is relatively common in children from ages 1 to 4 years. Between the ages 4 and 10, a trough occurs in the frequency of poisoning, followed by increasing frequency of intentional and accidental poisoning with substances of abuse and prescription drugs in adolescents.

Immunosuppressive Drugs

Immunosuppressive drugs are in extensive use for children undergoing organ transplantation. The drugs themselves, secondary metabolic disturbances, and cerebral infection may cause encephalopathy at times of immunosuppression. Children treated with amphotericin B for aspergillosis or mucormycosis posttransplant infections have been reported to develop a severe encephalopathy with parkinsonian features.

Corticosteroid Psychosis

Daily use of corticosteroids at doses lower than 1 mg/kg may cause hyperactivity, insomnia, and anxiety. The higher dosages used for immunosuppression, generally >2 mg/kg/day, may precipitate a psychosis similar to schizophrenia or delirium. Stopping the drug reverses the symptoms.

Calcineurin Inhibitor Encephalopathy

Tacrolimus and cyclosporine are calcineurin inhibitors frequently used to prevent organ rejection. Both mild and severe neurotoxicity may occur with use. Blood concentrations do not clearly correlate with the severity of neurological complications.

Minor effects include tremor, visual disturbance, headache, paresthesia, insomnia, and mood changes; these are quite common, occurring in up to 40%

of recipients. The most common major effect is the posterior reversible leukoencephalopathy syndrome (PRES), characterized by widespread edema and leukoencephalopathy more prominent in the posterior regions. Seizures, toxic encephalopathy, and akinetic mutism can also occur.[39] In children with the syndrome of visual disturbances and encephalopathy, the most intense disturbances are in the occipital lobes (see Fig. 2.3).

Neurotoxicity does not clearly correlate with serum drug levels, and it is important to recognize early signs so the regimen can be adjusted before progressing to the more severe effects. The offending drug should be reduced or stopped; using a lower dose in conjunction with other immune suppressants may reduce the incidence of neurotoxicity. Rare cases of irreversible neurological damage, coma, and death have been reported.

OKT3 Meningoencephalitis

Muromonab-CD3 (OKT3) is an anti-T-cell monoclonal antibody used to initiate immunosuppression and to treat rejection. Up to 14% of patients develop fever and sterile meningitis 24–72 hours after the first injection, and up to 10% develop encephalopathy within 4 days. The encephalopathy slowly resolves over the next 2 weeks, even when the drug is continued. This toxicity is also associated with PRES.

Prescription Drug Overdoses

Most deaths due to overdose in the United States involve pharmaceuticals (57.7%) because they are readily available. Most are unintentional (74.3%), and some are suicides (17.1%). The most common pharmaceuticals leading to fatal overdose are opioids (75.2%), benzodiazepines (29.4%), antidepressants (17.6%), antiepileptic and antiparkinsonian drugs (7.8%) alone, or in combination.[40] Features of specific drug overdoses are discussed in more detail in the following subsections.

General Diagnostic Principles

Perform a urine drug screen in all cases of unidentified coma or delirium. If an unidentifiable product is present in the urine, identification may be possible in plasma. The blood drug concentration should be determined. Poison control centers provide valuable assistance, and toxicologists are available by phone.

General Management Principles

The specificities and degree of supportive care needed depend on the drug and the severity of the poisoning. Most children need an intravenous line and careful monitoring of cardiorespiratory status. A continuous electrocardiogram is often required because of concern for arrhythmia. Treat extrapyramidal symptoms with intravenous diphenhydramine 1–2 mg/kg IV given via slow infusion. Specific treatments are discussed here.

Opioid overdose. Although multifactorial, the opioid crisis is one of the major contributing factors to the recent unprecedented decline in life expectancy in the United States. Prescription opioids include fentanyl, hydrocodone, oxycodone, hydromorphone, and others. Illegal opioids include heroin, illegally manufactured fentanyl, and other synthetic opioids.

Clinical features. Opioid overdoses are particularly prevalent in young children under the age of 2, who ingest the substance accidentally, and adolescents in whom opioids may be drugs of abuse. Symptoms of opioid overdose include confusion, delirium, pinpoint pupils, vomiting, and a depressed level of consciousness. Respiratory depression, coma, and death may follow, and mortality is particularly high with fentanyl overdoses since fentanyl is a synthetic opioid many times stronger than other forms.

Management. Naloxone 2 mg intranasal or 0.4–2 mg IV is effective and is the first-line treatment for overdose. Many schools and other public areas have intranasal naloxone available for emergency use; we recommend that all patients with opioids in the home also have naloxone available in case of accidental or intentional overdose.

Tricyclic antidepressant overdose. Tricyclic antidepressants are among the most widely prescribed drugs in the United States and account for a significant percentage of serious overdoses.

Clinical features. The major features of overdose are coma, hypotension, and anticholinergic effects (flushing, dry skin, dilated pupils, tachycardia, decreased gastrointestinal motility, and urinary retention). Seizures and myocardial depression may be present as well.

Management. The main goal of treatment is to provide respiratory and cardiac support until the drug can be metabolized. Cardiac monitoring is required. Correct acidosis and electrolyte abnormalities, and provide respiratory support to avoid hypoxia.

Poisoning

Most accidental poisonings occur in small children ingesting common household products. Usually, the ingestion quickly comes to attention because the child is sick and vomits. Insecticides, herbicides, and products containing hydrocarbons or alcohol are commonly at fault. Clinical features vary depending on the agent ingested. Optimal management requires identification of constituent poisons, estimation of the amount ingested, interval since exposure, cleansing of the gastrointestinal tract, specific antidotes when available, and supportive measures.

Substance Abuse

Alcohol remains the most common substance of abuse in the United States. More than 90% of high school seniors have used alcohol one or more times, and 6% are daily drinkers. Approximately 6% of high school seniors use marijuana daily, but less than 0.1% use hallucinogens or opiates regularly. The use of cocaine, stimulants, and sedatives has been increasing in recent years. Daily use of stimulants occurs in up to 1% of high school seniors.

Clinical features. The American Psychiatric Association defines the diagnostic criteria for substance abuse as: (1) a pattern of pathological use with the inability to stop or reduce use; (2) impairment of social or occupational functioning, which includes school performance in children; and (3) persistence of the problem for 1 month or longer.

The clinical features of acute intoxication vary with the substance used. Almost all disturb judgment, intellectual function, and coordination. Alcohol and sedatives lead to drowsiness, sleep, and obtundation. In contrast, hallucinogens cause bizarre behavior, which includes hallucinations, delusions, and muscle rigidity. Such drugs as phencyclidine (angel dust) and lysergic acid diethylamide produce a clinical picture that simulates schizophrenia.

The usual symptoms of marijuana intoxication are euphoria and a sense of relaxation at low doses, and a dream-like state with slow response time at higher doses. Very high blood concentrations produce depersonalization, disorientation, and sensory disturbances. Hallucinations and delusions are unusual with marijuana and suggest mixed-drug use.

Consider amphetamine abuse when an agitated state couples with peripheral evidence of adrenergic toxicity: mydriasis, flushing, diaphoresis, and reflex bradycardia caused by peripheral vasoconstriction. Cocaine affects the brain and heart. Early symptoms include euphoria, mydriasis, headache, and tachycardia. Higher doses produce emotional lability, nausea and vomiting, flushing, and a syndrome that simulates paranoid schizophrenia. Life-threatening complications are hyperthermia, seizures, cardiac arrhythmia, and stroke. Associated stroke syndromes include transient ischemic attacks in the distribution of the middle cerebral artery, lateral medullary infarction, and anterior spinal artery infarction.

Diagnosis. The major challenge is to differentiate acute substance intoxication from schizophrenia or psychosis. Important clues are a history of substance abuse obtained from family or friends, associated autonomic and cardiac disturbances, and alterations in vital signs. Urinary and plasma screening generally detects the substance or its metabolites.

Management. Management of acute substance abuse depends on the substance used and the amount ingested. Physicians must be alert to the possibility of multiple drug or substance exposure. An attempt should be made to empty the gastrointestinal tract of substances taken orally. Support of cardiorespiratory function and correction of metabolic disturbances are generally required. Intravenous diazepam reduces the hallucinations and seizures produced by stimulants and hallucinogens. Standard cardiac drugs are useful to combat arrhythmias.

Toxicity correlates poorly with drug blood concentrations regarding the following substances: amphetamines, benzodiazepines, cocaine, hallucinogens, and phencyclidine. The basis for management decisions is the patient's condition.

The most vexing problem with substance abuse is generally not the acute management of intoxication, but rather breaking the habit. This requires the patient's motivation and long-term inpatient and outpatient treatment.

TRAUMA

Pediatric neurologists are often involved in the acute care of severe head trauma when seizures occur. Frequently requests for consultation come later when some symptoms persist. Trivial head injuries, without loss of consciousness, are commonplace in children and an almost constant occurrence in toddlers. Suspect migraine whenever transitory neurological disturbances, for example, amnesia, ataxia, blindness, coma, confusion, and hemiplegia, follow trivial head injuries. Important causes of significant head injuries are child abuse in infants, sports and play injuries in children, and motor vehicle accidents in adolescents. Suspect juvenile myoclonic epilepsy in an adolescent driver involved in a single motor vehicle accident, when the driver has no memory of the event but never sustained a head injury. It is likely that an absence seizure caused a loss of control of the vehicle.

Concussion

Concussion is the appearance of neurological symptoms after "shaking of the brain" by a low-velocity injury without obvious structural changes.

Clinical features. Confusion and amnesia are the main features. The confusion and amnesia may occur immediately after the blow to the head or several minutes later. Frequently observed features of concussion include a befuddled facial expression, slowness in answering questions or following instructions, easy distractibility, disorientation, slurred or incoherent speech, incoordination, emotionality, and memory deficits.

In the following days to weeks, the child may have any of these symptoms: low-grade headache, light-headedness, poor attention and concentration, memory dysfunction, easy fatigability, irritability, difficulty with focusing vision, noise intolerance, anxiety, and sleep disturbances.

Among children who have lost consciousness, the child is invariably tired and sleeps long and soundly if left undisturbed after regaining consciousness. Many children complain of headache and dizziness for several days or weeks following concussion (see Posttraumatic Headache in Chapter 3). They may be irritable and have memory disturbances. The severity and duration of these symptoms usually correlate with the severity of injury, but sometimes seem disproportionate.[41]

Focal or generalized seizures, and sometimes status epilepticus, may occur 1 or 2 hours following head injury. Seizures may even occur in children who do not lose consciousness. Such seizures rarely portend later epilepsy.

Diagnosis. Obtain a cranial CT without contrast and with windows adjusted for bone and soft tissue, whenever loss of consciousness, no matter how brief, follows a head injury. This is probably cost-effective because it reduces the number of hospital admissions.

MRI in children with moderate head injury may show foci of hypointensity in the white matter, which indicates axonal injury. Order an EEG for any suspicion that the head injury occurred during a seizure or if neurological disturbances are disproportionate to the severity of the injury.

Management. Mild head injuries do not require immediate treatment, and a child whose neurological examination and CT scan findings are normal does not require hospitalization. Tell the parents to allow the child to sleep.

Severe Head Injuries

The outcome following severe head injuries is usually better for children than for adults, but children less than 1 year have double the mortality of those between 1 and 6 years, and three times the mortality of those between 6 and 12 years. CT evidence of diffuse brain swelling on the day of injury is associated with a higher mortality rate.

Shaking Injuries

Clinical features. Shaking is a common method of child abuse in infants.[42] An unconscious infant arrives at the emergency department with bulging fontanelles. Seizures may have precipitated the hospital visit. The history is fragmentary and inconsistent among informants, and there may be a history of prior social services involvement with the family.

The child often shows no external evidence of head injury, but ophthalmoscopic examination shows retinal and optic nerve sheath hemorrhages. Retinal hemorrhages are more common after inflicted injuries than after accidental injuries and may be due to rotational forces. Many of the hemorrhages may be old, suggesting repeated shaking injuries. On the thorax or back, the examiner notes bruises that conform to the shape of a hand that held the child during the shaking. Healing fractures of the posterior rib cage indicate prior child abuse. Death may result from uncontrollable increased ICP or contusion of the cervicomedullary junction.

Diagnosis. The CT shows a swollen brain but may not show subdural collections of blood if the bleeding is recent. MRI reveals subdural collections of blood or hygromas.

Management. The first step should always be protecting other children in the home or around the possible perpetrator. Notify social work and report the incident to the state's department of child protective services. Neurosurgery consultation for intracranial monitoring, blood evacuation, ventriculoperitoneal shunting, or decompressive procedures is indicated. Overall, the neurological and visual outcomes among victims of shaking are poor. Most have considerable residual deficits.

Closed Head Injuries

Supratentorial subdural hematomas are venous in origin, are frequently bilateral, and usually occur without associated skull fracture. Supratentorial epidural hematomas are usually associated with skull fracture. Epidural and subdural hematomas are almost impossible to distinguish on clinical grounds alone. Progressive loss of consciousness is a feature of both types, and both may be associated with a lucid interval between the time of injury and neurological deterioration. Posterior fossa epidural and subdural hemorrhages occur most often in newborns (see Chapter 1) and older children with posterior skull fractures.

Clinical features. Loss of consciousness is not always immediate; a lucid period of several minutes may intervene between injury and the onset of neurological deterioration. The Glasgow Coma Scale quantifies the degree of responsiveness following head injuries (Table 2.2). Scores of 8 or less correlate well with severe injury.

Acute brain swelling and intracranial hemorrhage cause the clinical features. Increased ICP is always present and may lead to herniation if uncontrolled. Focal neurological deficits suggest intracerebral hemorrhage.

Mortality rates in children with severe head injury are usually between 10% and 15% and have not changed substantially in the past decade. Low mortality rates are sometimes associated with higher percentages of survivors in chronic vegetative states. Duration of coma is the best guide to long-term morbidity. Permanent neurological impairment is an expected outcome when coma persists for 1 month or longer.

Diagnosis. Perform cranial CT as rapidly as possible after closed head injuries. Typical findings are brain swelling and subarachnoid hemorrhage with blood collecting along the falx. Intracranial hemorrhage may be detectable as well. Immediately after injury, some subdural hematomas are briefly isodense and not observed. Later the hematoma appears as a region of increased

TABLE 2.2 Glasgow Coma Scale[a]	
Eye Opening (E)	
Spontaneously	4
To speech	3
To pain	2
None	1
Best Motor Response (M)	
Obeys	6
Localizes	5
Withdraws	4
Abnormal flexion	3
Abnormal extension	2
None	1
Verbal Response (V)	
Oriented	5
Confused conversation	4
Inappropriate words	3
Incomprehensible sounds	2
None	1

[a]Coma score = E + M + V.

density, convex toward the skull and concave toward the brain. With time the density decreases.

Intracerebral hemorrhage is usually superficial but may extend deep into the brain. Frontal or temporal lobe contusion is common. Discrete deep hemorrhages without a superficial extension are not usually the result of trauma. Keep the neck immobilized in children with head injuries until radiographic examination excludes fracture dislocation of the cervical spine. The force of a blow to the skull frequently propagates to the neck. Examine the child for limb and organ injury when a head injury occurs in a motor vehicle accident.

Management. Manage all severe head injuries in an intensive care unit. Essential support includes controlled ventilation, prevention of hypotension, and sufficient reduction in brain swelling to maintain cerebral perfusion. Chapter 4 contains a review of methods to reduce cerebral edema.

Acute expanding intracranial hematomas warrant immediate surgery. Small subdural collections, not producing a mass effect, can remain in place until the patient's condition stabilizes and options are considered. Consult neurosurgery as early as possible for possible

ICP monitoring, shunting, hematoma evacuation, or decompressive procedures.

Open Head Injuries

The clinical features, diagnosis, and management of open head injuries are much the same as described for closed injuries. The major differences are the greater risk of epidural hematoma and infection, and the possibility of damage to the brain surface from depression of the bone.

Supratentorial epidural hematomas are usually temporal or temporoparietal in location. The origin of the blood may be arterial (tearing of the middle meningeal artery), venous, or both. Skull fracture is present in 80% of cases. Increased ICP accounts for the clinical features of vomiting and decreased states of consciousness. Epidural hematoma has a characteristic lens-shaped appearance (Fig. 2.4).

Infratentorial epidural hematoma is venous in origin and associated with an occipital fracture. The clinical features are headache, vomiting, and ataxia. Skull fractures, other than linear fractures, are associated with an increased risk of infection. A depressed fracture is one in which the inner table fragment is displaced by at least the thickness of the skull. A *penetrating* fracture is one in which the dura is torn. Most skull fractures heal spontaneously. Skull fractures that do not heal are usually associated with a dural tear and feel pulsatile. In infants, serial radiographs of the skull may suggest that the fracture is enlarging because the rapid growth of the brain causes the fracture line to spread further in order to accommodate the increasing intracranial volume.

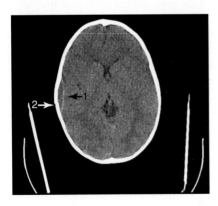

Fig. 2.4 Chronic Epidural Hematoma. Computed tomography scan shows a lens-shaped chronic epidural hematoma *(1)* under a skull fracture *(2)*.

Depressed fractures of the skull vault may injure the underlying brain and tear venous sinuses. The result is hemorrhage into the brain and subdural space. Management includes elevation of depressed fragments, debridement and closure of the scalp laceration, and systemic penicillin.

Basilar skull fractures with dural tears may result in leakage of CSF from the nose or ear and meningitis. Such leaks usually develop within 3 days of injury. The timing and need for dural repair are somewhat controversial, but the need for intravenous antibiotic coverage is established.

Posttraumatic Epilepsy

Posttraumatic epilepsy is one of the most common forms of acquired pediatric epilepsy and a well-recognized complication of traumatic brain injury in children, although specific pediatric studies are limited. Posttraumatic seizures (PTS) are differentiated based on when they occur: seizures occurring at the time of injury are called immediate or impact PTS, while those occurring more than 24 hours after injury are known as "early/delayed" PTS to distinguish them from recurrent later seizures (posttraumatic epilepsy). Immediate/impact seizures are not associated with the later development of epilepsy. Notably, however, mild traumatic brain injury is a clear risk factor for the later development of epilepsy, which may be intractable.[43] History of head injuries should always be taken into account when assessing epilepsy risk factors.

REFERENCES

1. Turkel SB, Tavare CJ. Delirium in children and adolescents. *Journal of Neuropsychiatry and Clinical Neurosciences.* 2003;15:4.
2. Krumholz A, Berg AT. Further evidence that for status epilepticus "one size fits all" does not fit. *Neurology.* 2002;58:515–516.
3. Zamora CA, Nauen D, et al. Delayed posthypoxic leukoencephalopathy: a case series and review of the literature. *Brain and Behavior.* 2015;5(8):e00364.
4. Nakagawa TA, Ashwal S, Mathur M, Mysore M. Society of Critical Care Medicine, Section on Critical Care and Section on Neurology of American Academy of Pediatrics, Child Neurology Society. Clinical report—Guidelines for the determination of brain death in infants and children: an update of the 1987 task force recommendations. *Pediatrics.* 2011;128(3):e720–e740. https://doi.org/10.1542/peds.2011-1511. Epub 2011 Aug 28. PMID: 21873704.

5. Nakagawa TA, Ashwal S, et al. Guidelines for the determination of brain death in infant and children: an update of the 1987 task force recommendations—executive summary. *Annals of Neurology*. 2012;71(4):573–585.

6. Nelson CA, Saha S, Mead PS. Cat-scratch disease in the United States, 2005–2013. *Emerging Infectious Diseases*. 2016;22(10):1741–1746. https://doi.org/10.3201/eid2210.160115. PMID: 27648778; PMCID: PMC5038427.

7. Florin TA, Zaoutis TE, Zaoutis LB. Beyond cat scratch disease: widening spectrum of *Bartonella henselae* infection. *Pediatrics*. 2008;121:e1413–e1425.

8. Saxena R, Gajjar N, Karnath B, Zhou Y. Bartonella neuroretinitis: there is more to cat scratch disease than meets the eye. *American Journal of Case Reports*. 2023;24:e938380. https://doi.org/10.12659/AJCR.938380. PMID: 37118886; PMCID: PMC10158985.

9. Rinka H, Yoshida T, Kubota T, et al. Hemorrhagic shock and encephalopathy syndrome—the markers for an early HSES diagnosis. *BMC Pediatrics*. 2008;8:43. https://doi.org/10.1186/1471-2431-8-43. PMID: 18922188; PMCID: PMC2577649.

10. Halperin JJ. Central nervous system Lyme disease. *Current Neurology and Neuroscience Reports*. 2005;5:446–452.

11. Meissner HC, Steere AC. Management of pediatric Lyme disease: updates from 2020 Lyme guidelines. *Pediatrics*. 2022;149(3): https://doi.org/10.1542/peds.2021-054980. e2021054980.

12. Britton PN, Dale RC, Nissen MD, et al. Parechovirus encephalitis and neurodevelopmental outcomes. *Pediatrics*. 2016;137(2):e20152848. https://doi.org/10.1542/peds.2015-2848. Epub 2016 Jan 20. PMID: 26791970.

13. Jain S, Patel B, Bhatt GC. Enteroviral encephalitis in children: clinical features, pathophysiology, and treatment advances. *Pathogens and Global Health*. 2014;108(5):216–222. https://doi.org/10.1179/2047773214Y.0000000145. PMID: 25175874; PMCID: PMC4153822.

14. Salimi H, Cain MD, Klein RS. Encephalitic arboviruses: emergence, clinical presentation, and neuropathogenesis. *Neurotherapeutics*. 2016;13(3):514–534. https://doi.org/10.1007/s13311-016-0443-5. PMID: 27220616; PMCID: PMC4965410.

15. Stoian A, Stoian M, Bajko Z, et al. Autoimmune encephalitis in COVID-19 infection: our experience and systematic review of the literature. *Biomedicines*. 2022;10(4):774. https://doi.org/10.3390/biomedicines10040774. PMID: 35453524; PMCID: PMC9024859.

16. Siow I, Lee KS, Zhang JJY, Saffari SE, Ng A. Encephalitis as a neurological complication of COVID-19: a systematic review and meta-analysis of incidence, outcomes, and predictors. *European Journal of Neurology*. 2021;28(10):3491–3502. https://doi.org/10.1111/ene.14913. Epub 2021 Jun 2. PMID: 33982853; PMCID: PMC8239820.

17. Garg RK, Paliwal VK, Gupta A. Encephalopathy in patients with COVID-19: a review. *Journal of Medical Virology*. 2021;93(1):206–222. https://doi.org/10.1002/jmv.26207.

18. de Bruijn MAAM, Bruijstens AL, Bastiaansen AEM. CHANCE Study Group. Pediatric autoimmune encephalitis: recognition and diagnosis. *Neurology Neuroimmunology & Neuroinflammation*. 2020;7(3):e682. https://doi.org/10.1212/NXI.0000000000000682. PMID: 32047077; PMCID: PMC7051211.

19. Michev A, Musso P, Foiadelli T, et al. Bickerstaff brainstem encephalitis and overlapping Guillain-Barré syndrome in children: report of two cases and review of the literature. *European Journal of Paediatric Neurology*. 2019;23(1):43–52. https://doi.org/10.1016/j.ejpn.2018.11.008. Epub 2018 Nov 20. PMID: 30502045.

20. Yoshikawa K, Kuwahara M, Morikawa M, Kusunoki S. Bickerstaff brainstem encephalitis with or without anti-GQ1b antibody. *Neurology Neuroimmunology & Neuroinflammation*. 2020;7(6):e889. https://doi.org/10.1212/NXI.0000000000000889.

21. Tenembaum S, Chitnis T, Ness J, et al. Acute disseminated encephalomyelitis. *Neurology*. 2007;68(2):1–17.

22. Banwell B, Ghezzi A, Bar-Or A, et al. Multiple sclerosis in children: clinical diagnosis therapeutic strategies, and future directions. *Lancet Neurology*. 2007;6:887–902.

23. Pohl D, Alper G, Van Haren K, et al. Acute disseminated encephalomyelitis: updates on an inflammatory CNS syndrome. *Neurology*. 2016;87(9 suppl 2):S38–S45. https://doi.org/10.1212/WNL.0000000000002825. PMID: 27572859.

24. Castillo P, Woodruff B, Caselli R, et al. Steroid-responsive encephalopathy associated with autoimmune thyroiditis. *Archives of Neurology*. 2006;63:197–202.

25. Vasconcellos E, Piæa-Garza JE, Fakhoury T, et al. Pediatric manifestations of Hashimoto's encephalopathy. *Pediatric Neurology*. 1999;20:394–398.

26. Sellal F, Berton C, Andriantseheno M, et al. Hashimoto's encephalopathy: exacerbation associated with menstrual cycle. *Neurology*. 2002;59:1633–1635.

27. Ferracci F, Moretto G, Candeago RM, et al. Antithyroid antibodies in the CSF. Their role in the pathogenesis of Hashimoto's encephalopathy. *Neurology*. 2003;60:712–714.

28. Armangue T, Petit-Pedrol M, Dalmau J. Autoimmune encephalitis in children. *Journal of Child Neurology*. 2012;27(11):1460–1469.

29. Florance NR, Davis RL, Lam C, et al. Anti-N-methyl-D-aspartate receptor (NMDAR) encephalitis in children and adolescents. *Annals of Neurology*. 2009;66:11–18.

30. Nabbout R, Mazzuca M, et al. Efficacy of ketogenic diet in severe refractory status epilepticus initiating fever induced refractory epileptic encephalopathy in school age children (FIRES). *Epilepsia.* 2010;51(10):2033–2037.

31. Pardo CA, Nabbout R, et al. Mechanisms of epileptogenesis in pediatric epileptic syndromes: Rasmussen encephalitis, infantile spasms, and febrile infection-related epilepsy syndrome (FIRES). *Neurotherapeutics.* 2014;11:297–310.

32. Huynh W, Cordato DJ, Kehdi E, Masters LT, Dedousis C. Post-vaccination encephalomyelitis: literature review and illustrative case. *Journal of Clinical Neuroscience.* 2008 Dec;15(12):1315–1322. https://doi.org/10.1016/j.jocn.2008.05.002. Epub 2008 Oct 30. PMID: 18976924; PMCID: PMC7125578.

33. Tessier G, Villeneuve E, Villeneuve JP. Etiology and outcome of acute liver failure: experience from a liver transplantation centre in Montreal. *Canadian Journal of Gastroenterology.* 2002;16:672–676.

34. Merritt JL. II, Chang IJ. Medium-chain acyl-coenzyme A dehydrogenase deficiency. 2000 Apr 20 [Updated 2019 Jun 27]. In: Adam MP, Mirzaa GM, Pagon RA, et al., eds. *GeneReviews®* [Internet]. University of Washington, Seattle; 1993–2023. Available from: https://www.ncbi.nlm.nih.gov/books/NBK1424/.

35. Palmer CA. Neurological manifestations of renal disease. *Neurologic Clinics.* 2002;20:23–40.

36. Yasuhara T, Tokunaga K, Hishikawa T, et al. Posterior reversible encephalopathy syndrome. *Journal of Clinical Neuroscience.* 2011;18:406–409.

37. Farooqi AM, Padilla JM, Monteith TS. Acute confusional migraine: distinct clinical entity or spectrum of migraine biology? *Brain Sciences.* 2018;8(2):29. https://doi.org/10.3390/brainsci8020029. PMID: 29414874; PMCID: PMC5836048.

38. Jen JC. Familial hemiplegic migraine. 2001 Jul 17 [Updated 2021 Apr 29]. In: Adam MP, Mirzaa GM, Pagon RA, et al., eds. *GeneReviews®* [Internet]. University of Washington, Seattle; 1993–2023. Available from: https://www.ncbi.nlm.nih.gov/books/NBK1388/.

39. Anghel D, Tanasescu R, Campeanu A, Lupescu I, Podda G, Bajenaru O. Neurotoxicity of immunosuppressive therapies in organ transplantation. *Maedica (Bucur).* 2013;8(2):170–175. PMID: 24371481; PMCID: PMC3865126.

40. Jones CM, Mack KA, Paulozzi LJ. Pharmaceutical overdose deaths, United States, 2010. *JAMA.* 2013;309(7):657–659.

41. American Academy of Neurology. Practice parameters for concussion in sports. *Neurology.* 1997;48:581–585.

42. Duhaime A-C, Christian CW, Rorke LB, et al. Non-accidental head injury in infants—the "shaken baby syndrome." *New England Journal of Medicine.* 1998;338:1822–1829.

43. Keret A, Bennett-Back O, Rosenthal G, et al. Posttraumatic epilepsy: long-term follow-up of children with mild traumatic brain injury. *Journal of Neurosurgery: Pediatrics.* 2017;20(1):64–70. https://doi.org/10.3171/2017.2.PEDS16585. Epub 2017 May 5. PMID: 28474982.

3

Headache

OUTLINE

Approach to Headache, 95
  Sources of Pain, 96
  Taking the History, 96
  Evaluation, 97
Migraine, 97
  Genetics of Migraine, 97
  Triggering Factors, 98
  Clinical Syndromes, 98
  Diagnosis, 99
  Management, 100
Cluster Headache, 103
Indomethacin-Responsive Headache, 104
  Chronic Paroxysmal Hemicrania, 104
  Hemicrania Continua, 104
  Benign Exertional Headache, 104
Chronic Low-Grade Nonprogressive Headaches, 104
  Analgesic Rebound Headache, 105
  Caffeine Headache, 105
  Stress, Depression, and Psychogenic Headaches, 105
  Posttraumatic Headache, 106
  Tension Headache, 106

Headaches Associated with Drugs and Foods, 107
  Food Additives, 107
  Marijuana, 107
  Chronic Progressive Headaches, 108
  Tumor, 108
  Aneurysm, 108
  Increased Intracranial Pressure, 108
Headache and Systemic Disease, 108
  Vasculitis, 108
  Connective Tissue Disorders, 108
  Hypersensitivity Vasculitis, 109
  Hypertension, 109
Pain from other Cranial Structures, 109
  Eyestrain, 109
  Episodic Tension Headache, 109
  Sinusitis, 109
  Temporomandibular Joint Syndrome, 110
  Whiplash and Other Neck Injuries, 110
Seizure Headache, 110
Low-Pressure/Spinal Fluid Leak Headache, 111
References, 111

APPROACH TO HEADACHE

Headache is one of the most common neurological symptoms and the source of frequent referrals to neurology. Proper diagnosis and management of headache has a positive impact on the lives of many children and their parents, and may significantly reduce direct and indirect health care costs. The World Health Organization ranks migraines as one of the top 20 disabilities in the world. Magnetic resonance imaging (MRI) and computed tomography (CT) scans are rarely necessary or justified, and exposing the patient to unnecessary radiation or anesthesia is not a good practice. In most cases a thorough history and neurological examination serve the child better than imaging studies. Migraine is the most common headache diagnosis in children. Some of these children develop more frequent and less disabling headaches due to additional contributing factors (analgesics, caffeine, stress, depression, etc.). The prevalence of migraines increases from 3% in children aged 3–7 years to 4%–11% in children aged 7–11 years and 8%–23% in adolescents. The mean age of onset for boys is 7 years and for girls 11 years.[1] Children with migraine average twice as many days lost from school as those without migraine.

Sources of Pain

Box 3.1 summarizes pain-sensitive structures of the head and neck. The main pain-sensitive structures inside the skull are blood vessels. Mechanisms that stimulate pain from blood vessels are vasodilatation, inflammation, and traction displacement. Increased intracranial pressure causes pain mainly by the traction and displacement of intracranial arteries (see Chapter 4). The brain parenchyma, its ependymal lining, and the meninges, other than the basal dura, are insensitive to pain.

Pain transmission from supratentorial intracranial vessels is by the trigeminal nerve, whereas pain transmission from infratentorial vessels is by the first three cervical nerves. The ophthalmic division of the trigeminal nerve innervates the arteries in the superficial portion of the dura and refers pain to the eye and forehead. The second and third divisions of the trigeminal nerve innervate the middle meningeal artery and refer pain to the temple. In contrast, referred pain from all structures in the posterior fossa is to the occiput and neck.

Several extracranial structures are pain sensitive. Major scalp arteries are present around the eye, forehead, and temple and produce pain when dilated or stretched. Cranial bones are insensitive, but the periosteum, especially in the sinuses and near the teeth, is painful when inflamed. The inflamed periosteum is usually tender to palpation or other forms of physical stimulation. Muscles attached to the skull such as the neck extensors, the masseter muscles, the temporalis, and the frontalis are possible sources of pain. Understanding of the mechanism of muscle pain is incomplete but probably involves prolonged contraction. The extraocular muscles are a source of muscle contraction pain in patients with heterophoria. When an imbalance exists,

especially in convergence, long periods of close work cause difficulty in maintaining conjugate gaze and pain localizes to the orbit and forehead. Decreased visual acuity causes blurred vision, not headaches. Impaired vision is a common delay in the diagnosis and management of migraines.

Pain from the cervical roots and cranial nerves is generally due to mechanical traction from injury or malformation. Pain follows this nerve distribution: the neck and back of the head up to the vertex for the cervical roots and the face for the cranial nerves.

Taking the History

History is the most important tool in diagnosing headaches. The first step is to identify the headache temporal pattern (examples of each type are included; the list is far from exhaustive).

Acute generalized headaches: Systemic or central nervous system (CNS) infections, exertional, cerebrospinal fluid (CSF) leak, postseizure, CNS hemorrhage, hypertension, or metabolic causes (hypoglycemia, hypercapnia, and hypoxia).

Acute localized headaches: Sinusitis, otitis, temporomandibular joint (TMJ), ocular disease, neuralgia (trigeminal, glossopharyngeal, and occipital), trauma, or dental disease.

Acute recurrent headaches: Migraine, cluster, paroxysmal hemicranias, episodic tension headache, icepick, exertional, cough, and intercourse headaches.

Chronic progressive headaches: CNS neoplasm, pseudotumor cerebri, brain abscess, subdural hematoma, and hydrocephalus.

Chronic nonprogressive headaches: Chronic tension, postconcussion, analgesic and caffeine induced, depression, psychogenic, and malingering headaches.

The following four questions are useful in determining the headache pattern:

1. *Is the headache chronic but not disabling, or does it occur occasionally and prevent normal activity?* The number of school days missed because of headache is a good indication of frequency, severity, and disability.
2. *What is the longest period of time that you have been headache free?* This identifies a common headache pattern in which the child has a flurry of headaches over a period of a week or 2 and then, after a prolonged headache-free interval, experiences another flurry of daily headaches.

BOX 3.1   **Sources of Headache Pain**
Intracranial
• Cerebral and dural arteries
• Dura mater at base of brain
• Large veins and venous sinuses
Extracranial
• Cervical roots
• Cranial nerves
• Extracranial arteries
• Muscles attached to skull
• Periosteum/sinuses

3. *How many different kinds of headaches do you have?* A common response is that the child has two kinds of headache: one headache is severe and causes the child to look sick (migraine), and the other is a mild headache that is almost constant but not disabling (analgesic rebound headache/medication overuse headache).

4. *What analgesics have you used and how often?* This helps establish what has worked and what has failed, and may establish the diagnosis of analgesic rebound headache as a contributing factor.

Helpful responses to traditional questions concerning the history of headache can be obtained from children as young as 3 or 4 years old, if they are given time to describe their symptoms. Several typical headache patterns, when present, allow recognition of either the source or the mechanism of pain:

1. A continuous, low-intensity, chronic headache, in the absence of associated symptoms or signs, is unlikely to indicate a serious intracranial disease.

2. Intermittent headaches, especially those that make the child look and feel sick, from which the child recovers completely and is normal between attacks, are likely to be migraine.

3. A severe headache of recent onset, unlike anything previously experienced, from which the child never returns to a normal baseline, is likely due to significant intracranial disease.

4. Brief, intense pain lasting for seconds, in an otherwise normal child, is unusual and suggests an *ice-pick headache.*

5. Periosteal pain, especially inflammation of the sinuses, localizes to the affected sinus and the area is tender to palpation. Sinusitis and allergies as a cause of headache are grossly overstated. Evidence of "sinusitis" is a common feature of MRI studies on children evaluated for other reasons.

6. Cervical root and cranial nerve pain have a radiating or shooting quality.

Evaluation

A routine brain imaging study on every child with chronic headache is not cost effective and is not a substitute for an adequate history and physical examination. A joint committee of the American Academy of Neurology and the Child Neurology Society published a practice parameter for the evaluation of children and adolescents with recurrent headaches. Those with normal neurological examinations require neither electroencephalography (EEG) nor neuroimaging.[2] An MRI of the brain is helpful in most cases of suspected intracranial pathology as the cause of headache. Lumbar puncture (LP), magnetic resonance angiography, and/or CT angiogram are useful when suspecting aneurysm leaks. MRI with magnetic resonance venogram may be useful when suspecting venous thrombosis in cases of increased intracranial pressure (see Chapter 4).

MIGRAINE

Ten percent of children aged 5–15 years old have migraine, and migraine accounts for 75% of headaches in young children referred for neurological consultation. Children with migraine average twice as many days lost from school as those without migraine. Migraine is a hereditary disorder with a multifactorial inheritance pattern. When interviewing both parents, at least one parent gives a history of migraine in most cases. The prevalence of migraine is 1%–3% in children aged 3–7 (both sexes equally affected) and 4%–11% in those aged 7–15 (with an increasing female:male ratio as age increases). The higher incidence of migraine seen in pubertal girls relative to that seen in boys probably relates to the triggering effect of the menstrual cycle on migraine attacks. Approximately one-quarter of children will be migraine free by the age of 25, boys significantly more often than girls, and more than half will still have headaches at age 50 years. Of those who become parents, 50% will have at least one child who suffers from migraine,[3] and there is evidence that children of migraine sufferers tend to experience headache onset at a younger age.[4] When evaluating for a family history of migraine, it is useful to expand your questioning if the parent initially reports a negative family history. Often the family labels their headaches as "normal headaches," "sinus headaches," or "allergy headaches," and when asked about the qualities of these headaches, they describe typical migraines.

Genetics of Migraine

Familial hemiplegic migraine is the only well-established monogenetic migraine syndrome, caused by heterozygous pathogenic mutations in *ATP1A2, CACNA1A,* or *SCN1A*.[5] Other migraine types are more complex, appearing to result from the interaction of genetic susceptibility and environmental factors. Genetic factors are more evident in migraine with aura than in migraine without aura. Migraine and migraine-like headaches are part of several known genetic disorders.

Triggering Factors

Among persons with a predisposition to migraine, the provocation of individual attacks is usually an idiosyncratic triggering factor. Common triggering factors are stress, exercise, head trauma, the premenstrual decline in circulating estrogen, and barometric pressure changes. An allergic basis for migraine is not established. We accept without comment parental statements implicating specific foods and food additives, but we discourage extensive evaluation of food as a trigger or extreme restrictive diets. Triggering foods, when present, are easily recognized by the patient as they consistently trigger a headache after every exposure (red wine, dark chocolate, cured meats, etc.).

Stress and Exercise

Migraine symptoms may first occur during stress or exercise or, more often, during a time of relaxation following a period of stress ("letdown migraines"). When stress is the triggering factor, attacks are most likely to occur in school or just after returning home. Attacks rarely occur upon awakening. Children with migraine do not have a specific personality type. Migraine is just as likely in a relaxed child as in an overachiever. However, the overachiever is more likely to reach the threshold for a migraine, and sometimes the management of anxiety or obsessive-compulsiveness results in decreased migraine frequency in these patients.

Head Trauma

The mechanism by which blows to the head and whiplash head movements provoke migraine attacks is unknown, partially because such injuries usually involve soft tissues with no major abnormalities seen on X-ray or MRI. Trivial blows to the head during competitive sports are significant triggering factors because they occur against a background of vigorous exercise and stress. A severe attack—headache, vomiting, and transitory neurological deficits, following a head injury—suggests the possibility of intracranial hemorrhage rather than migraine. Appreciating the cause-and-effect relationship between head trauma and migraine reduces the number of diagnostic tests requested.

Transient cerebral blindness and other neurological deficits sometimes occur after head trauma in children

with migraine (see Chapter 16). Migraine coma is a rare disorder in which children with familial hemiplegic migraine have depressed consciousness and coma after minor head trauma (see Chapter 2).

Menstrual Cycle

The higher rate of migraine among postpubertal girls, as compared with prepubertal children of both sexes or with postpubertal boys, supports the observation that hormonal changes in the normal female cycle trigger attacks of migraine. The widespread use of oral contraceptives has provided some insight into the relationship between the female hormonal cycle and migraine. Some oral contraceptives increase the frequency and intensity of migraine attacks in females with a history of migraine and may precipitate the initial attack in genetically predisposed females who have previously been migraine free. Conversely, hormonal contraceptives may decrease migraine frequency in pubertal girls with irregular menstrual cycles. Among females taking oral contraceptives, the greatest increase in the frequency of migraine occurs at midcycle. The decline in the concentration of circulating estrogens is probably the critical factor in precipitating an attack.

Clinical Syndromes

Migraine in children is divisible into three groups: (1) migraine with aura, (2) migraine without aura, and (3) migraine equivalent syndromes. Migraine without aura is more than twice as common as migraine with aura in school-age children. Migraine with and without aura are variable expressions of the same genetic defect, and both kinds of attacks may occur in the same individual at different times. The main feature of migraine equivalent syndromes is a transient disturbance in neurological function. Headache is a minor feature or is not present. One percent of migraineurs do not experience headache. Discussion of these syndromes occurs in several other chapters (Box 3.2).

BOX 3.2   Migraine Equivalents

- Acute confusional migraine (see Chapter 2)
- Migraine with brainstem aura (see Chapter 10)
- Benign paroxysmal vertigo (see Chapter 10)
- Cyclic vomiting syndrome
- Hemiplegic migraine (see Chapter 11)
- Retinal migraine (see Chapter 16)
- Paroxysmal torticollis (see Chapter 14)

Ice-pick headache, called *primary stabbing headache* by the International Headache Society, is a peculiar migraine equivalent that occurs mainly during adolescence or later. A severe pain on top of the head drives the patient to the floor. It ends as quickly as it comes. Bouts may repeat over days or months and then remit spontaneously. Ice-pick headaches end so quickly that treatment is often not required, only reassurance; if preventative treatment is desired, the headaches may respond to indomethacin.

Migraine With Aura

Migraine with aura is a biphasic event. In the initial phase a wave of excitation followed by depression of cortical function spreads (cortical spreading depression) over both hemispheres from back to front, and is associated with decreased regional cerebral blood flow and transient neurological dysfunction. The cause of dysfunction is primarily neuronal depression rather than ischemia. The second phase is usually, but not necessarily, associated with increased blood flow in both the internal and external carotid circulations. Headache, nausea, and sometimes vomiting occur in the second phase.

During an attack, the main clinical features (aura) may reflect only the first phase, only the second phase, or both phases. The usual features of the aura are visual aberrations: the perception of sparkling lights or colored lines, blind spots, blurred vision, hemianopia, transient blindness, micropsia, or visual hallucinations. Only a third of children describe visual symptoms. The visual aura tends to be stereotyped and unique to the child. The perception of the imagery may be limited to one eye, one visual field, or without localization.

Visual hallucinations and other visual distortions may disturb time sense and body image. This symptom complex in migraine is called the *Alice-in-Wonderland syndrome*. More extreme disturbances in mental state—amnesia, confusion, and psychosis—are discussed in the sections on confusional migraine (see Chapter 2).

Dysesthesias of the limbs and perioral region are the next most common sensory features. Other possible features of the aura are focal motor deficits, usually hemiplegia (see "Complicated Migraine" section in Chapter 11), ophthalmoplegia (see "Retinal Migraine" section in Chapter 16), or aphasia. Such deficits, although alarming, are transient; normal function usually returns within 24 hours and it is highly unusual for the deficit to last longer than 72 hours.

A migraine attack may terminate at the end of the initial phase without headache. Alternatively, the initial phase may be brief or asymptomatic and headache is the major symptom (see the "Migraine Without Aura" section). The pain is usually dull at first and then becomes throbbing, pulsating, or pounding. A severe headache that is maximal at onset is not suggestive of migraine. Pain is unilateral in approximately two-thirds of patients and bilateral in the rest. It is most intense in the region of the eye, forehead, and temple. Eventually the pain becomes constant and diffuse. Most headaches last for 2–6 hours and are associated with nausea and sometimes vomiting. Anorexia and photophobia are concomitant symptoms. The child looks sick and wants to lie down; always ask the parent, "Does the child look sick?" With migraine, the answer is always "Yes." Vomiting frequently heralds the end of the attack, and the fatigued child falls into a deep sleep. Normal function resumes when the child awakens. Most children average one attack per month but may have long intervals without attacks and other intervals when attacks occur weekly. The intervals with frequent headaches are probably times of stress.

Migraine Without Aura

The attacks of migraine without aura are monophasic. The typical initial symptoms are personality change, malaise, and nausea. Recurrent vomiting may be the only feature of the attack in preschool children.

The headache may be unilateral and pounding, but more often the child has difficulty localizing the pain and describing its quality. When the headache is prolonged, the pain is not of uniform intensity; instead, intermittent severe headaches superimpose on a background of chronic discomfort in the neck and other pericranial muscles. Physical activity aggravates the pain. Migraine without aura may be difficult to separate from other headache syndromes or intercurrent illness. The important clues are that the child appears sick, wants to lie down, and is sensitive to light and sound. Nausea and vomiting may occur repeatedly, need not herald the termination of the attack, and can be more prominent than the headache.

Diagnosis

The clinical features are the basis for migraine diagnosis; migraine is one of the few remaining neurological disorders in which the physician cannot stumble on the diagnosis by imaging the brain. Salient features are a family history of migraine and some combination of recurrent headache, nausea, or neurological disturbances, especially if aggravated by activity and relieved by rest and sleep. Many children will also have an increased perception of all sensory modalities including photophobia (lights), sonophobia (sounds), and osmophobia (smells). The physician should be reluctant to make the diagnosis if questioning both biological parents does not elicit a family history of migraine. When obtaining the history, be certain that you are speaking with the biological parents and that you ask for a family history of *headaches* and not only migraines, as many migraine sufferers are not aware of their diagnosis. Almost half of children with migraine also have a history of motion sickness.

Diagnostic tests are unnecessary when the family history and clinical features clearly establish a migraine diagnosis. Brain imaging is indicated only when uncertainty exists. The main reason is new abnormalities on examination. Lesser reasons are a negative family history or atypical features of the attack. The only reason to request an EEG in children with migraine-like headaches is to exclude the rare possibility of a migraine-associated epilepsy (see Chapter 1).

Management

Some improvement is common after the initial diagnosis of migraine. This is probably due to a reassurance given to the child and the family of not having a tumor or other more serious problem. Once the child's parents are convinced that the headache is due to migraine and not brain tumor, they are less anxious, the child is more relaxed, and headaches either decrease in frequency or become less a topic of discussion and concern. Less commonly, the diagnosis prompts anxiety and fixation on the child's pain, which can worsen attacks. Discourage parents from routinely asking the child if he is in pain; instead, observe and wait for the child to complain of headache or exhibit the usual physical symptoms.

The two approaches to migraine therapy are treatment of the acute attack and prophylaxis. Many children need both. Most boys do not have migraine attacks during adult life, but girls often continue having attacks until menopause.

Good advice for all migraineurs includes (1) healthy eating and sleep habits, (2) avoiding use of caffeine, (3) avoiding overuse of analgesics, (4) avoiding triggers when identified, (5) if possible, undertaking a moderate exercise regimen, and (6) avoiding narcotic use as this may compound the problem. Emotional stress can be a significant trigger in some children, and addressing comorbid anxiety can be an important part of treatment.

Treating the Acute Attack

Acute treatment of migraines is always more effective when given early during the attack. Medication should be available at home, when traveling, and at school if possible. The first line of medications includes ibuprofen or naproxen 10 mg/kg or acetaminophen 15 mg/kg. Nonprescription analgesics and nonsteroidal antiinflammatory drugs, especially ibuprofen, are more effective than a placebo in controlling pain, and ibuprofen is the first-line treatment for most patients.[6]

Nasal sumatriptan (5 or 20 mg) and oral triptans such as sumatriptan (50–100 mg), rizatriptan (5–10 mg), eletriptan (20–40 mg), or zolmitriptan (2.5–5 mg) may be useful. Sumatriptan nasal spray is well tolerated, more effective than placebo, and recommended. Adverse effects include fatigue, tingling of the head and arms, and a sensation of pressure or stiffness in the neck, throat, and chest. The orally dissolved formulations of zolmitriptan and rizatriptan may be useful for children who are unable to swallow pills. The time of absorption is the same as other tablets, as the absorption is not sublingual. For patients requiring faster onset, or when vomiting precludes oral medications, the nasal (5–20 mg) or injectable (3–6 mg) sumatriptan and the nasal or injectable (0.5–1 mg) dihydroergotamine (DHE) are better options, although DHE is increasingly difficult to obtain in the outpatient setting.[7]

Calcitonin gene–related peptide (CGRP) causes blood vessel inflammation and dilation in perivascular trigeminal nerve fibers, leading to pain. CGRP receptor antagonists are newer migraine treatments mainly available for adults, but sometimes used on an off-label basis in adolescents. Rimegepant (Nurtec) can be used both acutely and for migraine prevention. For acute migraine attacks with or without aura, give 75 mg as an oral disintegrating tablet. Nausea, dyspepsia, and abdominal pain are the most common side effects. Ubrogepant (Ubrelvy) 50 mg is approved for the acute treatment of migraine. It provides relief for the majority of patients when used within 2 hours of pain onset and prevents pain in some patients when taken in the premigraine prodromal phase. Potential side effects include nausea and somnolence.

Rectal promethazine (12.5–25 mg) or prochlorperazine injectable (5–10 mg) is also used when vomit interferes with oral administration. Both promethazine and prochlorperazine can be given orally, but sedation from this medication occurs in about 90% of patients and may be as disabling as the illness. These options are helpful and less expensive when the treatment is needed at bedtime. Give prochlorperazine with diphenhydramine (Benadryl) to lessen the risk of extrapyramidal side effects.

In general, we tell patients to avoid coming to the emergency department for their typical migraines unless we have exhausted all possible outpatient management strategies. The emergency department is loud, bright, and chaotic—hardly the ideal environment for a patient to recover from a severe headache. Unfortunately, even excellent outpatient management plans fail at times. Several institutions have protocols for the acute treatment of migraine which serve to decrease unnecessary imaging studies, laboratories, and neurology consults. Such protocols vary among centers, but in general they include hydration (usually via IV fluid bolus), a nonsteroidal anti-inflammatory such as ketorolac IV or ibuprofen orally, and a dopamine antagonist such as metoclopramide or prochlorperazine. The door to the room should be closed and the lights out. Encourage relaxation techniques and rest. Valproic acid may be used adjunctively, and in some cases a dose of IV steroids is helpful.

Intravenous DHE was previously the standard of care but is now used less frequently in the emergency department. DHE administration typically requires admission because several doses may be needed. Pregnancy testing is required for girls over 12 years of age. Use 0.5 mg for children younger than 9 years and 1 mg for children 9 years or older. Doses may be repeated every 6–8 hours.

Migraine Prophylaxis

An extraordinarily large number of agents with diverse pharmacological properties are available for daily use to prevent migraine attacks. Consider prophylactic agents in the following situations:
1. Migraines once a week or more, on average (frequent abortive therapy may lead to medication-induced headaches).
2. Failure to respond to abortive therapy.
3. Migraines are only responsive to abortive medications that also cause sedation (sedation may be as disabling as the migraine in terms of loss of productivity).
4. Disability (loss of school or social activities).

High-quality studies regarding migraine prevention in children are few and far between, and many of the suggestions made below rely on small studies and our personal experiences. In general, daily supplements such as magnesium, riboflavin, and coenzyme Q10 are low risk and may be attractive to families who prefer to avoid prescription medications. However, optimal dosing data for pediatric patients are lacking. Cyproheptadine can be useful in toddlers and very young children with migraine, but side effects including sedation and weight gain become more problematic in older children. Cyproheptadine has proven efficacy in migraine equivalents such as cyclic vomiting syndrome and paroxysmal torticollis.[8] Evidence for other agents is less clear. The Childhood and Adolescent Migraine Prevention (CHAMP) study sought to provide class I evidence for the use of amitriptyline or topiramate in migraine prevention in pediatric patients. The trial concluded early due to a lack of significant between-group differences regarding the primary outcome; amitriptyline and topiramate were found to be no more effective than placebo, and both caused increased side effects as compared to placebo.[9]

The CHAMP study was controversial because it directly contradicted a number of other positive, placebo-controlled, double-blinded studies that led to Food and Drug Administration (FDA) approval of topiramate for use in migraine prophylaxis in patients 12 years of age and older (see FDA product label). The existence of those positive studies, and the absence of other effective treatments, is the reason that amitriptyline and topiramate are still commonly used in pediatric migraine prevention, as are propranolol, zonisamide, and valproic acid. Levetiracetam may be effective in adults, similar but not superior to other anticonvulsants, but there is no evidence of efficacy in children. CGRP receptor antagonists are currently only available for adults and adolescents 18 years of age or older, but clinical trials are underway for pediatric patients. Flunarizine has relatively strong evidence of efficacy in pediatric migraine prevention but is not available in the United States or Japan.

Amitriptyline. Amitriptyline is inexpensive and has an acceptable side-effect profile at low dosages, 0.5–1 mg/kg up to 50 mg at bedtime. The mechanism of action is by inhibiting the membrane pump mechanism responsible for the uptake of norepinephrine and serotonin in adrenergic and serotonergic neurons. Nortriptyline has less sedation and is an acceptable alternative.

Propranolol. Propranolol is a β-adrenergic blocking agent. It decreases headache frequency by at least half in 80% of patients. The mechanism of action is probably central and not by β-adrenergic blockade. Propranolol must have central action, because depression is a common side effect. This and exercise intolerance are the main reasons it is often not used in children and adolescents.

The dosage in children is 2 mg/kg in three divided doses. Because depression is a dose-related adverse reaction and because lower doses may be effective, start treatment at 1 mg/kg/day. Asthma and diabetes are contraindications to usage. The maintenance dose of the sustained-release tablet is one-third greater than that of the short-acting preparation. Plasma levels of propranolol are not useful in determining the effective dose for migraine.

People who respond to propranolol do not develop tolerance to the medication. However, if abruptly stopping the drug after 6–12 months of therapy, some individuals will have rebound headaches of increased frequency. Others will continue to show the benefits achieved during therapy.

Topiramate, zonisamide, and valproate. Topiramate, zonisamide, and valproate are widely used for epilepsy prophylaxis. In children, a dose of topiramate 50–100 mg daily or divided twice a day, zonisamide 50–100 mg nightly, or valproate 250–500 mg twice a day may be useful for migraine prophylaxis. Side effects at low dosages are minimal. Be cautious with the use of valproate in adolescent females because of the significant potential for polycystic ovary syndrome and teratogenicity. We suggest topiramate for children who are overweight and valproate for those who are underweight or have bipolar traits. Zonisamide has fewer cognitive side effects than topiramate; if a patient feels that topiramate was effective but caused unacceptable mental fogginess, zonisamide may be a good alternative. These are also good options for children with epilepsy and migraine as comorbidity.

Levetiracetam. A few small studies have suggested that levetiracetam is safe and effective for migraine prophylaxis in adults.[10] Even in adults, the evidence is scarce, and pediatric studies are virtually nonexistent. We rarely use levetiracetam for migraine prevention in our patients.

Calcitonin gene–related peptide receptor antagonists. Oral CGRP antagonists provide effective migraine prophylaxis, usually with minimal side effects. Rimegepant (Nutrec) is an orally disintegrating tablet given at a dose of 75 mg every other day; common side effects are nausea and abdominal discomfort. Atogepant (Qulipta) is given orally in doses of 10, 30, or 60 mg once daily. Adjust the dose in patients with renal impairment and those who are using CYP3A4 inducers or inhibitors; do not use in patients with severe hepatic impairment. Nausea, constipation, and fatigue are the most commonly reported side effects.

Monoclonal antibodies targeting the calcitonin gene–related peptide receptor. Erenumab-aooe (Aimovig) is a human immunoglobulin G2 (IgG2) monoclonal antibody that has high affinity for binding to the CGRP receptor. It is administered in monthly subcutaneous injections; the usual dose is 70 mg but some patients require 140 mg. Injection site reactions, systemic hypersensitivity reactions, and severe constipation have been reported. As with all such therapies, immunogenicity and the development of neutralizing antibodies may occur.

Monoclonal antibodies targeting the calcitonin gene–related peptide molecule. Eptiezumab (Vyepti) binds the CGRP ligand and is given as a 30-minute infusion every 3 months. Fremanezumab (Ajovy) is administered as a subcutaneous injection monthly (225 mg) or quarterly (675 mg). The recommended dosage of galcanezumab (Emgality) is 240 mg (two consecutive subcutaneous injections of 120 mg each) once as a loading dose, followed by monthly doses of 120 mg injected subcutaneously. All medications in this class may cause hypersensitivity reactions and immunogenicity.

Cyproheptadine. Use cyproheptadine in toddlers or young children with frequent migraines and in those with migraine equivalents such as cyclic vomiting syndrome and paroxysmal torticollis. Give 2–4 mg nightly either as a tablet or in an oral suspension. Sedation and increased appetite are the main side effects and are more pronounced in older children. We never use cyproheptadine for migraine prevention in children over the age of 6 unless the child has a comorbid condition (appetite loss, functional abdominal pain, etc.) that may benefit from administration.

Nerve blocks. Occipital cephalgia is not, in itself, a migraine headache. However, occipital neuralgias and cervicalgias are common triggers for migraines in susceptible patients. The procedure involves injecting a numbing agent, usually lidocaine, into nerves that have been identified as potential pain triggers. The most common nerves treated are the greater occipital nerve, lesser occipital nerve, supraorbital nerve, and auriculotemporal nerve. The procedure can be repeated every 4 months (three times yearly).

Botulinum toxin (Botox). Botulinum toxin is approved for the prevention of chronic migraine in adults; safety and efficacy for episodic migraine and pediatric migraine have not been established. It is administered as a total dose of 155 units divided over 31 separate sites, including the temporalis, frontalis, corrugator, procerus, occipitalis, cervical paraspinals, and trapezius. The mechanism of action is by blocking the release of acetylcholine, although exactly how this leads to migraine reduction remains somewhat unclear. Botulinum toxin can spread distal to the site of injection and may cause serious adverse effects including generalized and focal weakness, dysphagia, and respiratory insufficiency. Some deaths have been reported.

CLUSTER HEADACHE

Cluster headache is rare in children but may have adolescent onset. It occurs mainly in males and rarely affects other family members.[11] Cluster headache is distinct from chronic paroxysmal hemicrania and hemicrania continua (see the "Indomethacin-Responsive Headache" section).

Clinical features. The onset is almost exclusively after age 10. Clusters of headaches recur over periods of weeks or months, separated by intervals of months to years. A cluster of daily attacks lasting for 4–8 weeks may occur once or twice a year, often in the autumn or spring. Headaches do not occur in the interim.

Headache is the initial feature, often beginning during sleep. The pain occurs in bursts lasting for 30–90 minutes and repeats two to six times each day. It is always unilateral and affects the same side of the head in each attack. Pain begins behind and around one eye before spreading to the entire hemicrania. During an attack, the affected individual cannot lie still but typically walks the floor in anguish. This feature distinguishes cluster headache from migraine, in which the child wants to avoid motion and prefers to rest or sleep. Pain is intense and described either as throbbing, sharp, or constant. The scalp may seem edematous and tender. One-third of individuals with cluster headache experience sudden intense jabs of pain suggesting

trigeminal neuralgia/tic douloureux. Nausea and vomiting do not occur, but symptoms of hemicranial autonomic dysfunction—injection of the conjunctiva, tearing of the eye, Horner syndrome, sweating, flushing of the face, and stuffiness of the nose—develop ipsilateral to the headache.

Diagnosis. The clinical features alone establish the diagnosis of cluster headache. Laboratory or imaging studies have no value.

Management. The management of cluster headache consists of suppressing recurrences of a bout that is in progress and relieving acute pain. Prednisone suppresses bouts of cluster headache. An initial dose is 1 mg/kg/day for the first 5 days, followed by a tapering dose over 2 weeks. If headaches reappear during the tapering process, the dose is increased and maintained at a level sufficient to keep the patient headache free. If the bout of cluster headache is prolonged, alternative therapies should be considered to prevent adverse effects from long-term steroid administration.

Injectable sumatriptan or oxygen inhalation both treat the acute attack. The dose of sumatriptan in adults and most adolescents is a 6 mg injection; oral or even nasal administration is typically too slow to be of use. Inhalation of 100% oxygen at a rate of 8–10 L/min relieves an acute attack in most patients, but use is limited by the fact that the patient must carry an oxygen canister and nasal canula with them. Octreotide is a synthetic form of somatostatin available as an injection. It works well for some patients but is both slower and less effective than oxygen and sumatriptan. DHE injection can be considered for patients who have not responded to other standard therapies.

Calcium channel blockers such as verapamil are the first choice for the prevention of cluster headaches. Use doses of 2–6 mg/kg/day. Recently, galcanezumab (Emgality, discussed in the "Migraine Prophylaxis" section) obtained FDA approval for the prevention of cluster headaches in adults; there are no studies in pediatrics at this time. Lithium is useful as a preventative and for patients with a chronic form of cluster headache in which the headache never ceases. Provide increasing doses to achieve a blood concentration of 1.2 mEq/L (1.2 mmol/L). Most patients have at least a partial response to lithium, but only 50% are relieved completely. Occipital nerve blocks and noninvasive vagus nerve stimulation using a hand-held controller prevent attacks in some patients.

INDOMETHACIN-RESPONSIVE HEADACHE

Indomethacin-responsive headache syndromes are a group of seemingly unrelated headache disorders that respond to indomethacin and nothing else. The syndromes include chronic paroxysmal hemicrania, hemicrania continua, ice-pick headache, and benign exertional headache.

Chronic Paroxysmal Hemicrania

Clinical features. As with cluster headache, the main features of chronic paroxysmal hemicrania are unilateral throbbing pain associated with ipsilateral autonomic features. However, the attack duration is briefer but more frequent than in cluster headache.[12] Attacks last for weeks to months followed by remissions that last for months to years. The pain is located in the frontal and retro-orbital regions and is accompanied by conjunctival injection and tearing.

Diagnosis. The clinical features are the basis for diagnosis, and laboratory or imaging studies are normal.

Management. Chronic paroxysmal hemicrania responds to indomethacin. The typical adult dosage is 75 mg/day. Successive attacks often require larger dosages. Acetazolamide may prove successful when indomethacin fails.

Hemicrania Continua

Clinical features. Hemicrania continua is a continuous unilateral headache of moderate severity. Autonomic symptoms may be associated but are not prominent. Some patients have continuous headaches lasting for weeks to months separated by pain-free intervals; others never experience remissions. The episodic form may later become continuous.

Diagnosis. The clinical features establish the diagnosis after excluding other causes of chronic headache, such as increased intracranial pressure and chronic use of analgesics.

Management. The headaches usually respond to indomethacin at dosages of 25–250 mg/day.

Benign Exertional Headache

Exertion, especially during competitive sports, is a known trigger for migraine in predisposed individuals (see the "Migraine" section). Persons who do not have migraine may also experience headaches during exercise. Headache during sexual intercourse may be a form of exertional headache or is at least a comorbid condition.[13] Some adolescents experience this headache type with weight lifting.

Clinical features. Exertional headaches tend to be acute and severe, starting early in the course of exercise, while headaches with sexual activity increase with sexual excitement and may have a dull or throbbing quality. Headache may occur during prolonged sexual arousal as well as during sexual intercourse.

Diagnosis. The association between exertion and headache is easily recognized. Requests for medical consultation are unusual unless the patient is a competitive athlete whose performance is impaired.

Management. Indomethacin use prior to exertion may prevent headache. The prophylactic use of indomethacin, 25 mg three times a day, or propranolol, 1–2 mg/kg/day, also reduces the incidence of attacks.

CHRONIC LOW-GRADE NONPROGRESSIVE HEADACHES

These are almost constant or intermittent daily headaches. Most of the time, the headaches start in a child with a history of migraines and gradually increase in frequency until they occur daily. When presenting to the clinic at this stage, the headaches tend to be multifactorial in origin. The child or adolescent does not appear sick except when having a superimposed migraine attack, but is constantly complaining of headache.

In some cases, the daily headaches precede migraines. Many adolescents with chronic daily headache later convert to migraine.[14] In our experience most patients with daily headaches have a previous history suggestive of migraines.

The most common contributing factors to these multifactorial headaches are (1) frequent analgesic use; (2) frequent caffeine use; (3) stressors, with school being the most frequent; (4) depressed mood or anxiety; and (5) psychogenic etiology. The best way to treat these patients is to address all possible factors from onset to avoid delays in recovery. Do not shy away from discussions about the patient's mood or mental health. Chronic pain itself is associated with depression, and vice versa; many families inherently understand this connection when it is explained in a compassionate way without appearing to trivialize or ignore the child's physical pain.

Analgesic Rebound Headache

Clinical features. Analgesic rebound is one of the more common causes of chronic headache in people of all ages. Individuals with migraine are especially predisposed to analgesic rebound headaches (*extended migraine*). The term refers to a vicious cycle of steadily increasing headaches and analgesic use, ultimately resulting in a state in which the patient uses analgesics daily or even multiple times daily without relief. The pain is generalized, of low intensity, and dull. It interferes with but does not prevent routine activities and activity is not an aggravating factor.[15] This phenomenon has been described in children and adolescents and in infants as young as 17 months.[16–18]

Diagnosis. Any child using nonprescription analgesics every day, or even most days, is likely to suffer from analgesic rebound headache. The risk of chronic daily headache is high if taking two or more doses per week of analgesics, triptans, or narcotics.

Management. Stop all analgesic use and avoid caffeine as well. A short, 5-day course of daily steroids and the initiation of bedtime amitriptyline 0.5–1 mg/kg up to 50 mg often helps the transition to the analgesic-free state. The first few days may be difficult, but a positive effect within weeks reinforces the recommended management. During the first months, the patient should keep a headache calendar to document the decline in headache frequency. Most of the time the migraines or rebound pain may be worse after the initial discontinuation of the offender, and abortive medications for pain such as promethazine, prochlorperazine, and DHE are the only options. Most other medications may have a medication-induced headache effect.

Caffeine Headache

Clinical features. Many children, especially adolescents, drink large volumes of carbonated beverages containing caffeine each day. The amount of caffeine in most popular beverages is equivalent to that in a cup of brewed coffee, and may be much higher in the pervasive "energy drinks." The exact mechanism of the caffeine headache is not established; it could be a withdrawal effect or a direct effect of caffeine. Individuals who regularly drink large amounts of caffeine-containing beverages often notice a dull frontotemporal headache an hour or more after the last use. More caffeine relieves the headache, initiating a caffeine addiction. Withdrawal symptoms may become severe and include throbbing headache, anxiety, and malaise. In our experience the daily use of caffeine alone is rarely the offender leading to daily headaches in a migraineur unless the patient ingests large quantities of energy drinks; however, many patients cannot achieve full remission without cessation of caffeine.

Diagnosis. Most people associate caffeine with coffee and are unaware of the caffeine content of standard soft drinks. Caffeine is also found in iced tea, chocolate milk, and other chocolate products.

Management. Caffeine addiction, like other addictions, is often hard to break. Most patients require abrupt cessation. As in analgesic rebound headache, amitriptyline at bedtime may be useful in breaking the cycle.

Stress, Depression, and Psychogenic Headaches

Most migraine sufferers have an increase in headaches during times of stress. For children and adolescents, school is a common source of stress. The disability imposed by their migraines and the interference with their learning and absences from school further increases the level of stress. Not acknowledging and correcting this cycle may interfere with recovery. Temporary homeschooling or abbreviated days are sometimes necessary to relieve the pressure experienced by the patient.

We also must acknowledge that chronic pain and disability may lead to depression and that mild-to-moderate depression may present as headaches, body aches, gastrointestinal complaints, decreased stamina, or changes in sleeping or eating habits. Some children require management of their depressed mood to regain headache control.

In addition, psychogenic symptoms are common in all ages and headache is likely the most common psychogenic symptom of all. Children or adolescents with limited coping mechanisms for stress may subconsciously use the complaint of headache to protect themselves from overwhelming situations. It is important to examine cases of chronic daily headaches for all of these factors.

Clinical features. The headaches occur without autonomic changes, tachycardia, or hypertension during acute episodes of reportedly severe pain. The neurological examination is normal, and there is a history of depressed mood or psychosocial stressors. Alternatively, incongruity between the level of pain/disability and the reported level of stress (e.g., a child who is unable to attend school or interact with friends, yet insists he is happy and stress free) is suggestive of psychogenic headache.

Diagnosis. There is no confirmatory testing. The diagnosis should be suspected in children or adolescents with chronic headaches unresponsive to medical treatment, with a normal neurological examination, and normal vital signs during a "severe headache."

Management. We often use the help of counselors for children with daily headaches and stressors. In addition, selective serotonin reuptake inhibitors (SSRIs) for children with comorbid anxiety or depression, including citalopram 10–20 mg/day, escitalopram 5–10 mg/day, or sertraline 50–100 mg/day, are often helpful.

Posttraumatic Headache

Prolonged posttraumatic headache represents an important source of morbidity following pediatric traumatic brain injury (TBI) of all severities. The presence of headache does not correlate with the extent of injury and is seen more frequently in patients with mild head injuries. The presence of imaging abnormalities at the time of injury does not predict the severity or persistence of headache. The pathophysiology of chronic posttraumatic headache is not well understood, but animal models suggest that pain is due to a chronic inflammatory response as well as peripheral and central sensitization. Female sex, younger age at the time of injury, preexisting headache disorder, and frequent TBI events seem to be risk factors for the development of prolonged posttraumatic headaches.[19]

Clinical features. Headache is a common symptom immediately after the injury, often characterized by intense, throbbing pain that is holocephalic and involves the neck and shoulders. Nausea and vomiting may occur. The immediate posttraumatic headache resolves within 24–48 hours, although residual muscle soreness may remain for several days, causing dull pain. The initial posttraumatic headache can persist for up to 3 months in 30%–50% of patients.[20]

No consensus exists for the definition of prolonged posttraumatic headache, but it is typically understood to mean a headache that persists for at least 3 months following the initial injury. Migraine-type headache superimposed on chronic daily headache is the most common presentation. Children and adolescents who report persistent posttraumatic headaches perform worse on objective neurocognitive testing and are more likely to report associated symptoms including sleep, mood, and memory disturbances.[21] Preexisting psychiatric disorders such as anxiety and depression are prevalent in patients with prolonged posttraumatic headache. Analgesic rebound headache is a complicating factor, as many of these children use over-the-counter analgesics daily in an attempt to treat the chronic pain.

Diagnosis. Most patients with prolonged posttraumatic headaches have already undergone head CT or brain MRI by the time they see a neurologist. Further imaging is often requested by the family, but is of little clinical utility for patients with previously documented normal imaging studies. The subjective complaint of headache is common, and definitively tying it to a mild TBI is difficult. Diagnosis is based on clinical presentation.

Management. Prolonged headaches are notoriously difficult to treat and are even more difficult in patients with the associated comorbidities mentioned earlier. For the patient with normal neurologic exam and imaging, treatment is limited by several compounding factors. Avoid medication overuse, especially when medications have not proven to be helpful. Neuropsychological testing identifies weaknesses in memory, concentration, and processing and can be used by the school when formulating an educational plan. Identify and treat comorbid psychiatric disorders, that is, depression and anxiety, whether primary or secondary to the injury. Physical therapy is helpful for patients with cervicogenic pain or for those with physical deconditioning. Identify and treat analgesic rebound headache, when present (see the "Analgesic Rebound Headache" section). Daily prophylactic medications such as amitriptyline can be considered, but treatment of comorbidities is perhaps the most important aspect of management. A multidisciplinary approach is often needed.

Tension Headache

The term *tension headache* is time honored.[22] The name suggests that the cause of headache is stress. This etiology is usually true regarding episodic tension headaches (see the "Pain From Other Cranial Structures" section), but the mechanism of chronic tension headache is less well established and is probably multifactorial. One often obtains a family history of chronic tension headache, and about half of adults with chronic tension headache date the onset to childhood. One study found tension headache the most common subtype of chronic daily headache in adolescence.[23] Indeed, adolescence may cause tension headache in all family members. In our opinion, chronic tension headache is a diagnosis that has been overused or incorrectly used without fully evaluating other contributing factors for headaches. Many of these patients suffer from depression and caffeine- and medication-induced headaches. Tension headache seems to be the most appropriate diagnosis for patients who have underlying obsessive-compulsiveness and anxiety traits, which make them prone to respond in this way to stressors.

Clinical features. Individuals with chronic headache of any cause may be depressed and anxious. Pain is usually bilateral and diffuse, and the site of most intense pain may shift during the course of the day. Much of the time, the headache is dull and aching; sometimes it is more intense. Headache is generally present upon awakening and may continue all day but is not aggravated by routine physical activity. Most children describe an undulating course characterized by long periods in which headache occurs almost every day and shorter intervals when they are headache free.

Nausea, vomiting, photophobia, phonophobia, and transitory neurological disturbances are not associated with chronic tension headache. When these features are present, they usually occur only a few times a month and suggest intermittent migraine against a background of chronic tension headache. The neurological examination is normal.

Diagnosis. The diagnosis of chronic tension headache is to some extent a diagnosis of exclusion. Common causes of chronic headache in children that require distinction are migraine and analgesic rebound headache. Both may coexist with chronic tension headache. Brain imaging is sometimes required to exclude the specter of brain tumor. The management of chronic tension headache is often easier after a normal head CT or brain MRI.

Management. Chronic tension headache is by definition difficult to treat, otherwise it would not be a chronic headache. Most children have tried and received no benefit from several nonprescription analgesics before coming to a physician, and analgesic rebound headache often complicates management. The use of more powerful analgesics or analgesic–muscle relaxant combinations has limited value and generally adds upset stomach to the child's distress.

It is not always clear that a child with chronic tension headache is experiencing stress. When a stressful situation is identified (e.g., divorce of the parents, custody battle, unsuitable school placement, physical or sexual abuse), the headache cannot be managed without resolution of the stress. If the child has comorbid anxiety or obsessive-compulsiveness, SSRIs may be helpful.

HEADACHES ASSOCIATED WITH DRUGS AND FOODS

Many psychotropic drugs, analgesics, and cardiovascular agents cause headache. Cocaine use produces a migraine-like headache in individuals who do not have migraine at other times. Drug-induced headache is suspect in a child who has headache following the administration of any drug. These headaches tend to be intermittent rather than daily.

Food Additives

Clinical features. The addition of chemicals to foods preserves shelf life and enhances appearance. Ordinarily, concentrations are low, and adverse effects occur only in genetically sensitive individuals. Nitrites are powerful vasodilators used to enhance the appearance of cured meats such as hot dogs, salami, bacon, and ham. Diffuse, throbbing headaches may occur just after ingestion. Dark chocolate is often implicated as a trigger, but studies are mixed and evidence is insufficient to make firm recommendations. In general, we advise patients that if they have a food trigger, they will know it—migraine onset will occur immediately and consistently after ingestion, and the association is obvious. Obsessive searches for food triggers are not productive and can cause the child to develop a dysfunctional approach to eating.

Diagnosis. The association between ingestion of a specific food and headache is quickly evident to the patient.

Management. Avoiding the offending chemical prevents headache. This avoidance is not easy, as prepared foods often do not contain a list of all additives.

Marijuana

Marijuana is a peripheral vasodilator and causes a sensation of warmth, injection of the conjunctivae, and, sometimes, frontal headache. The headache is mild and ordinarily is experienced only during marijuana use.

However, marijuana metabolites remain in the blood for several days, and chronic headaches may occur in children who are regular users.

Chronic Progressive Headaches

When parents bring a child to the neurologist for evaluation of headaches, ruling out the frightening causes of chronic headache is often their top priority. The potential for space-occupying lesions, increased intracranial pressure, and vascular abnormalities provoke the most concern. In the vast majority of cases the child with headache due to significant underlying intracranial disease will have a clearly abnormal neurological exam or imaging findings, especially if the headache has persisted for more than 3 months. Clearly explaining this to parents is vitally important if the clinician wishes to retain their trust.

We will review chronic progressive headaches only briefly in this chapter. These disorders are discussed in greater detail in Chapter 4.

Tumor

Every parent's greatest fear is that their child has a brain tumor. The term "space-occupying lesion" encompasses benign and malignant tumors. Children with tumors present with seizures (if involving the cortex), focal neurological abnormalities, and symptoms of elevated intracranial pressure.

Aneurysm

Aneurysms are uncommon in children but may occur in patients with certain genetic disorders. Many aneurysms are asymptomatic until they rupture; headache, if present, is an incidental feature. Headache that is sudden, severe, and maximal at onset ("the worst headache of my life"), especially when associated with nausea, vomiting, and meningismus, raises concern for aneurysm rupture.

Increased Intracranial Pressure

Intracranial pressure can be increased via several mechanisms including increased production of CSF, idiopathic intracranial hypertension, and venous sinus thrombosis. The child presents with headache that is consistently worsened by lying flat and is maximal in the morning. Visual disturbances, nausea, and vomiting are common. Cerebral venous sinus thrombosis can cause infarcts that do not correspond to typical arterial territories. Ophthalmologic exam reveals papilledema.

HEADACHE AND SYSTEMIC DISEASE

Vasculitis

Headaches caused by vasculitis, especially temporal arteritis, are important in the differential diagnosis of vascular headaches in adults. Cerebral vasculitis is uncommon in children and usually occurs as part of an autoimmune disease or infection of the nervous system. It is accompanied by focal neurologic symptoms and the patient almost always has an abnormal neurologic exam.

Connective Tissue Disorders

Headache is a feature of systemic lupus erythematosus (SLE) and mixed connective tissue disease. The exact pathophysiology remains unclear.

Clinical features. Severe headache occurs in up to 10% of children with SLE. It may occur in the absence of other neurological manifestations and can be the initial feature of SLE.

Mixed connective tissue disease is a syndrome with features of SLE, scleroderma, and polymyositis. Its course is usually less severe than that of lupus. Thirty-five percent of people with mixed connective tissue disease report headaches. The headaches are moderate and generally do not interfere with activities of daily living. They may be unilateral or bilateral but are generally throbbing. More than half of patients report a visual aura, and some have nausea and vomiting. Some of these children may be experiencing migraine aggravated by the underlying neuroinflammatory disorder; in others, the cause of headache is the neuroinflammation itself.

Diagnosis. The diagnosis of connective tissue disease depends on the combination of a compatible clinical syndrome and the result of specific laboratory tests. The presence of antinuclear antibodies ("positive ANA") is a common and nonspecific finding that does not in itself justify a diagnosis of autoimmunity. Positive ANA in a child with headache, who has no systemic symptoms of connective tissue disease, should suggest the possibility of a genetic susceptibility to autoimmune disease versus an incidental finding.

Management. The ordinary treatment of children with connective tissue disease is corticosteroids and other immune suppressants. In many cases, headaches develop while the child is already taking corticosteroids; this occurrence is not necessarily an indication to increase the dose. Symptomatic treatment may be adequate.

Hypersensitivity Vasculitis

The important causes of hypersensitivity vasculitis in children are serum sickness, Henoch-Schönlein purpura (see Chapter 11), amphetamine abuse, and cocaine abuse. Children with serum sickness or Henoch-Schönlein purpura have systemic symptoms that precede the headache. Persistent headache and behavioral changes are often the only neurological consequences of Henoch-Schönlein purpura. In contrast, substance abuse can cause cerebral vasculitis in the absence of systemic symptoms. The features are headache, encephalopathy, focal neurological deficits, and subarachnoid hemorrhage.

Hypertension

A sudden rise in systemic blood pressure causes the explosive, throbbing hypertensive headache associated with pheochromocytoma. Children with chronic hypertension may have low-grade occipital headache on awakening that diminishes as they get up and begin activity or frontal throbbing headache during the day. However, most children with chronic hypertension are asymptomatic. When a child with renal disease develops headache, hypertension is probably not the cause (see Chapter 2). Instead, pursue alternative causes. Headaches are common in patients undergoing dialysis and may be due to psychological tension, the precipitation of migraine attacks, and dialysis itself. Dialysis headache begins a few hours after terminating the procedure and is characterized by a mild bifrontal throbbing headache, sometimes associated with nausea and vomiting.

PAIN FROM OTHER CRANIAL STRUCTURES

Eyestrain

Clinical features. Prolonged ocular near-fixation in a child with a latent disturbance in convergence may cause dull, aching pain behind the eyes that is quickly relieved when the eyes are closed. The pain is of muscular origin and caused by the continuous effort to maintain conjugate gaze. If work continues despite ocular pain, episodic tension headache may develop.

Diagnosis. Refractive errors are often a first consideration in children with eyestrain. Eyeglasses do not correct the headache. Refractive errors do not cause eyestrain in children, as presbyopia does in adults. Refractive errors cause poor vision and not headaches; when present they delay the diagnosis and management of migraines. These children are often referred to with excellent corrected vision and persistent migraines.

Management. Resting the eyes relieves eyestrain.

Episodic Tension Headache

Clinical features. Episodic tension headache is common in people of all ages and both sexes. Fatigue, exertion, and temporary life stress cause the headache. The mechanism is probably a prolonged contraction of muscles attached to the skull. The pain is constant, aching, and tight. Localization is mainly to the back of the head and neck; the headache sometimes becomes diffuse and is then described as a constricting band around the head. Nausea, vomiting, photophobia, and phonophobia are not present. Headaches usually last for periods ranging from 30 minutes to all day. One episode may last for several days, with some waxing and waning, but not for a week.

Diagnosis. Episodic tension headache differs from chronic tension, which has similar clinical features but persists for weeks, months, or years. Most episodic tension headaches are self-diagnosed, and the individual rarely seeks medical attention.

Management. Rest, relaxation, warm compresses to the neck, massage, and nonprescription analgesics relieve pain.

Sinusitis

When questioned about migraine symptoms, most parents identify their own episodic headache, preceded by scintillating scotomata and followed by nausea and vomiting, as sinusitis. This diagnosis, favored by physicians and patients to describe chronic or episodic headaches, is usually wrong. The vasodilatation that occurs in the trigeminal vasculature of a migraine patient during an attack causes swelling of the turbinates, which may lead to the mistaken impression that the pain has its origin in the sinuses. Use of triptans causes the turbinates to "shrink" and relieves the feeling of pressure.

Clinical features. Children with sinusitis are usually sick. They are febrile and have purulent nasal discharge. Localized tenderness is present over the infected frontal or maxillary sinuses, and inflammation of the ethmoidal or sphenoidal sinuses causes deep midline pain behind the nose and in the upper teeth. Blowing the nose or quick movements of the head, especially bending forward, exaggerate the pain. Concurrent headache caused by fever is common.

Diagnosis. Radiographs reveal clouding of the sinuses and sometimes a fluid level. CT of the skull is exceptionally accurate in identifying sinusitis, but is usually an unnecessary expense. It is impressive how often CT of the head, performed for reasons other than headache, shows radiographic evidence of asymptomatic sinus disease. Clearly, radiographic evidence of sinus disease does not necessarily explain many patients' headache.

Management. The primary objective of treatment is to allow the sinus to drain. Decongestants usually accomplish drainage, but sometimes surgery is required. Antibiotics have limited usefulness if drainage is not established.

Temporomandibular Joint Syndrome

The TMJ syndrome does not cause chronic generalized daily headache, although acute inflammation of the joint can trigger migraine in susceptible patients. The pain is unilateral and centered over and below the TMJ.[24]

Clinical features. TMJ syndrome is an uncommon disease in children, occurring as young as 8 years of age. The duration of symptoms before diagnosis may be as long as 5 years and averages 2 years. The primary disturbance is arthritis of the TMJ causing localized pain in the lower face and crepitus in the joint. Because of pain on one side, chewing occurs on the other, with unwanted overuse of the affected side. The overused masseter muscle becomes tender; a muscle contraction headache ensues. Localization of pain is on the side of the face and the vertex. Bruxism or dental malocclusion is the usual cause of arthritis, but a prior injury of the jaw accounts for one-third of TMJ syndromes in children.

Diagnosis. Radiographs of the TMJ usually show some internal derangement of the joint and may show degenerative arthritis. MRI using surface coils is the most effective technique to show the disturbed joint architecture.

Management. TMJ syndrome treatment based on controlled experiments is not established. Placebos provide considerable benefit, and TMJ syndrome is not an indication for extensive oral surgery. Nonsteroidal antiinflammatory agents, application of heat to the tense muscles, and dental splints may prove useful.

Whiplash and Other Neck Injuries

Whiplash and other neck injuries cause pain by rupturing cervical disks, damaging soft tissue, injuring occipital nerves, and causing excessive muscle contraction. The muscles contract in an effort to splint the area of injury and thereby reduce further tissue damage.

Clinical features. Constant contraction of the neck extensors causes a dull, aching pain not only in the neck but also in the shoulders and upper arms. This pain may persist for up to 3 months after the injury. Holding the head in a fixed position is common. Nausea and vomiting are not associated symptoms.

Diagnosis. Cervical spine radiographs are required after any neck or head injury to determine the presence of fracture or dislocation. Shooting pains, radiating either to the occiput or down the arm and into the fingers, suggest the possibility of disk herniation and require further study with MRI.

Management. Warn the patient and family at the onset that prolonged head and neck pain is an expected outcome after injury and does not indicate a serious condition. Several different interventions achieve pain relief. Lying or sitting with the head supported, superficial application of heat to the painful muscles, muscle relaxants, and nonnarcotic analgesics are potentially effective. When pain persists after 3 months and affects the head as well, the possibility of an analgesic rebound headache is more likely.

SEIZURE HEADACHE

Diffuse headache caused by vasodilatation of cerebral arteries is a frequent occurrence following a generalized tonic-clonic convulsion. In patients who have both epilepsy and migraine, one can trigger the other; frequently, headache and seizure occur concurrently. Approximately 1% of epileptic patients report headache as a seizure manifestation (seizure headache). Most patients with seizure headaches have epilepsy prior to the development of headache. In a small number of children, headache is the only feature of their seizure disorder.

Clinical features. Headache is part of several epilepsy syndromes. The most common syndrome in children is *self-limited occipital epilepsy* (see Chapter 1). The sequence of events suggests migraine. One of the authors evaluated one eloquent adolescent who complained of paroxysmal "head pain unlike other headaches" that was associated with EEG evidence of generalized epileptiform activity. Anticonvulsants relieved head pain.

Headache may also occur as a seizure manifestation in patients known to have epilepsy. Such individuals usually have a long history of partial or generalized seizures before headache becomes part of the syndrome. Associated ictal events depend on the site of the cortical focus and may include auditory hallucinations, visual disturbances, vertigo, déjà vu, and focal motor seizures. Headache may be the initial feature of the seizure or can follow other partial seizure manifestations, such as déjà vu and vertigo. Headache description may be throbbing, sharp, or without an identified quality. Complex partial seizures, simple partial seizures, or generalized tonic-clonic seizures follow the headache phase. Spike foci in patients with seizure headaches are usually temporal in location.

Diagnosis. Chronic headache in children is not an indication for EEG. Interictal discharges, especially rolandic spikes, do not indicate that the headaches are a seizure manifestation, only that the child has a genetic marker for epilepsy. However, children with paroxysmal nonmigrainous headaches may require an EEG study. If interictal spike discharges are seen, an effort should be made to record a headache with an EEG monitor. The observation of continuous epileptiform activity during a headache provides reassurance that headache is a seizure manifestation and anticonvulsant drugs will prove effective.

Management. The response to anticonvulsant therapy is both diagnostic and therapeutic. Because the seizure focus is usually cortical and most often in the temporal lobe, antiepileptic drugs are useful for partial epilepsies (see Chapter 1).

LOW-PRESSURE/SPINAL FLUID LEAK HEADACHE

Low-pressure headache is a common complication of an LP and is rarely the result of a spontaneous CSF leak in children. It occurs in about 1% of spinal surgery patients due to dural tears; 90% require surgical repair.[25]

Clinical features. The most common symptom is a postural headache triggered by standing or by holding an infant in a vertical position. The pain is attenuated or subsides in the supine position. Cognitively normal children and adults will avoid the standing position, but is important to consider this possibility and maintain infants in supine position if they become irritable after an LP.

Diagnosis. The diagnosis is clinical, and laboratory and imaging testing should be normal in the acute and usually self-limited phase. In cases of longer symptom duration, the MRI may show pachymeningeal enhancement.[26]

Management. Supine positioning with IV hydration and caffeine for 48–72 hours is standard care. An epidural blood patch (EBP) is effective in closing the leak. Surgery and epidural fibrin glue are options for refractory cases, but we have never encountered a case refractory to the EBP.

REFERENCES

1. Lewis D, Ashwal S, Hershey A, et al. Practice parameter: pharmacological treatment of migraine headache in children and adolescents. Report of the American Academy of Neurology Quality Standards Subcommittee and the Practice Committee of the Child Neurology Society. *Neurology.* 2004;63:2215-2224.
2. Lewis DW, Ashwal S, Dahl G, et al. Practice parameter: evaluation of children and adolescents with recurrent headaches. Report of the Quality Standards Committee of the American Academy of Neurology and the Practice Committee of the Child Neurology Society. *Neurology.* 2002;59:490-498.
3. Bille B. A 40-year follow-up of school children with migraine. *Cephalalgia.* 1997;17:488-491.
4. Eidlitz-Markus T, Zeharia A. Younger age of migraine onset in children than their parents: a retrospective cohort study. *Journal of Child Neurology.* 2018;33(1):92-97. https://doi.org/10.1177/0883073817739197. PMID: 29246099.
5. Jen JC. Familial hemiplegic migraine (Jul 17, 2001). In: Adam MP, Mirzaa GM, Pagon RA, et al., eds. *GeneReviews® [Internet].* Seattle, WA. University of Washington; 1993–2023. https://www.ncbi.nlm.nih.gov/sites/books/NBK1388/. Updated April 29, 2021.
6. Mather DB. Acute management of migraine. Highlights of the US Headache Consortium. *Neurology.* 2003;60(suppl 2):S21-S23.
7. Silberstein SD, McCory DC. Ergotamine and dihydroergotamine: history, pharmacology, and efficacy. *Headache.* 2003;43:144-166.
8. Madani S, Cortes O, Thomas R. Cyproheptadine use in children with functional gastrointestinal disorders. *Journal of Pediatric Gastroenterology and Nutrition.* 2016 Mar;62(3):409-413. https://doi.org/10.1097/MPG.0000000000000964. PMID: 26308312.
9. Powers SW, Coffey CS, Chamberlin LARD, et al. Trial of amitriptyline, topiramate, and placebo for pediatric

migraine. *New England Journal of Medicine*. 2017;376: 115-124. https://doi.org/10.1056/NEJMoa1610384.

10. Evers S, Frese A, Summ O, Husstedt IW, Marziniak M. Levetiracetam in the prophylactic treatment of episodic migraine: a prospective open label study. *Cephalalgia*. 2022;42(11-12): 1218-1224. https://doi.org/10.1177/03331024221103815. Epub 2022 May 27. PMID: 35633027.

11. Russell MB, Andersson PG, Thomsen LL. Familial occurrence of cluster headache. *Journal of Neurology, Neurosurgery & Psychiatry*. 1995;58:341-343.

12. Goadsby PJ, Lipton RB. A review of paroxysmal hemicranias, SUNCT syndrome and other short lasting headaches with autonomic features, including new cases. *Brain*. 1997;120:193-209.

13. Frese A, Eikermann A, Frese K. Headache associated with sexual activity: demography, clinical features, and comorbidity. *Neurology*. 2003;61:796-800.

14. Wang SJ, Fuh JL, Lu SR, et al. Outcomes and predictors or chronic daily headache in adolescents. A two-year longitudinal study. *Neurology*. 2007;68:591-596.

15. Zwart JA, Dyb G, Hagen K, et al. Analgesic use: a predictor of chronic pain and medication overuse headache. The head-HUNT study. *Neurology*. 2003;61:160-164.

16. Pina-Garza JE, Warner JS. Analgesic rebound headaches in a 17 month old infant. *Journal of Child Neurology*. 2000;15:261.

17. Vasconcellos E, Pina-Garza JE, Millan EJ, Warner JS. Analgesic rebound headaches in children and adolescents. *Journal of Child Neurology*. 1998;13:443-447.

18. Warner JS, Lavin PJ, Pina-Garza JE. Rebound headaches: keys to effective therapy. *Consultant*. 2002:139-142.

19. Blumenfeld A, McVige J, Knievel K. Post-traumatic headache: pathophysiology and management - a review. *Journal of Concussion*. 2022;6. https://doi.org/10.1177/20597002221093478.

20. Schwedt TJ. Post-traumatic headache due to mild traumatic brain injury: current knowledge and future directions. *Cephalalgia*. 2021;41(4):464-471. https://doi.org/10.1177/0333102420970188. Epub 2020 Nov 19. PMID: 33210546.

21. McConnell B, Duffield T, Hall T, Piantino J, Seitz D, Soden D, Williams C. Post-traumatic headache after pediatric traumatic brain injury: prevalence, risk factors, and association with neurocognitive outcomes. *Journal of Child Neurology*. 2020;35(1):63-70. https://doi.org/10.1177/0883073819876473. Epub 2019 Oct 4. PMID: 31581879; PMCID: PMC7308075.

22. Lewis DW, Gozzo YF, Avner MT. The "other" primary headaches in children and adolescents. *Pediatric Neurology*. 2005;33:303-313.

23. Wang S-J, Fuh J-L, Lu S-R, et al. Chronic daily headache in adolescents: prevalence, impact, and medication overuse. *Neurology*. 2006;66:193-197.

24. Rothner AD. Miscellaneous headache syndromes in children and adolescents. *Seminars in Pediatric Neurology*. 1995;21:159-164.

25. Khazim R, Dannawi Z, et al. Incidence and treatment of delayed symptoms of CSF leak following lumbar spinal surgery. *European Spine Journal*. 2015;24(9): 2069-2076.

26. Spears RC. Low pressure/spinal fluid leak headache. *Current Pain and Headache Reports*. 2014;18:425.

4

Increased Intracranial Pressure

OUTLINE

Pathophysiology, 114
Cerebrospinal Fluid, 114
Cerebral Blood Flow, 114
Cerebral Edema, 115
Mass Lesions, 115
Symptoms and Signs, 115
Increased Intracranial Pressure in
    Infancy, 115
Increased Intracranial Pressure in Children, 115
Herniation Syndromes, 117
Medical Treatment, 118
Management of Increased Intracranial Pressure due
    to Severe Traumatic Brain Injury, 118
Head Elevation, 119
Homeostasis, 119
Monitoring Intracranial Pressure, 119
Management of Acutely Increased Intracranial
    Pressure in Severe Traumatic Brain Injury, 119
Hyperventilation, 119
Hyperosmolar Therapy, 120
Pentobarbital Coma, 120
A Note on Hypothermia, 120
Decompressive Craniectomy, 120
Hydrocephalus, 120
Supratentorial Brain Tumors, 120

Choroid Plexus Tumors, 121
Glial, Glianeuronal, and Neuronal Tumors, 122
Astrocytoma, 122
Embryonal Tumors, 124
Ependymoma, 124
Pineal Region Tumors, 125
Other Tumors, 125
Intracranial Arachnoid Cysts, 126
Perinatal Intracranial Hemorrhage, 126
Intraventricular Hemorrhage in the
    Newborn, 126
Intraventricular Hemorrhage at Term, 128
**Increased Intracranial Pressure Related to Vascular
    Abnormalities, 128**
Arterial Aneurysms, 128
Arteriovenous Malformations, 129
Cocaine Abuse, 130
INFECTIOUS DISORDERS, 130
Bacterial Meningitis, 130
Subdural and Epidural Empyema, 135
Fungal Infections, 135
**Idiopathic Intracranial Hypertension (Pseudotumor
    Cerebri), 137**
References, 139

The presenting complaint when dealing with increased intracranial pressure (ICP) (Box 4.1) varies with age. Infants may present with a bulging fontanelle, macrocephaly, or failure to thrive. Older children often present with headache, emesis, diplopia, or change in mentation. The basis of referral for some children is the detection of disk edema during an eye examination. Some conditions causing increased ICP are discussed elsewhere in this book (see Chapters 2, 3, 10, and 15).

This chapter is restricted to conditions in which symptoms of increased ICP are initial and prominent features. The timely management of increased ICP prevents secondary brain insult, regardless of the original cause, which is often a primary central nervous system (CNS) process (infection, abscess, tumor, infarct, etc.). When treating increased ICP the goal is to reduce the pressure while maintaining adequate cerebral perfusion.

113

PATHOPHYSIOLOGY

Normal ICP for children in the resting state has never been definitively established; "normal" ranges are estimates derived from adult data. In general, normal ICP for children is approximately 5–15 cm H_2O, with pressures lower in infants (anywhere from 0–6 cm H_2O). Sustained pressures over 20 cm H_2O are considered abnormal. When the cranial bones fuse during childhood, the skull is a rigid box enveloping its contents. ICP is then the sum of the individual pressures exerted by the brain, blood, and cerebrospinal fluid (CSF). An increase in the volume of any one component requires an equivalent decrease in the size of one or both of the other compartments if ICP is to remain constant. Because the provision of oxygen and nutrients to the brain requires relatively constant cerebral blood flow, the major adaptive mechanisms available to relieve pressure are the compressibility of the brain and the rapid reabsorption of CSF by arachnoid villi. Infants and young children, in whom the cranial bones are still unfused, have the additional adaptive mechanism of spreading the cranial bones apart and bulging of the anterior fontanelle to increase cranial volume.

Cerebrospinal Fluid

The choroid plexus accounts for at least 70% of CSF production, and the transependymal movement of fluid from the brain to the ventricular system accounts for the remainder. The average volumes of CSF are 90 mL in children 4–13 years old and 150 mL in adults. The rate of formation is approximately 0.35 mL/min or 500 mL/day. Approximately 14% of total volume turns over every hour. The rate at which CSF forms remains relatively constant and declines only slightly as CSF pressure increases. In contrast, the rate of absorption increases linearly as CSF pressure exceeds 7 mm Hg. At a pressure of 20 mm Hg, the rate of absorption is three times the rate of formation.

Impaired absorption, not increased formation, is the usual mechanism of progressive hydrocephalus. Choroid plexus papilloma is the only pathological process in which formation sometimes can overwhelm absorption. However, even in cases of choroid plexus papilloma, obstruction of the CSF flow rather than overproduction may be the cause of hydrocephalus. When absorption is impaired, efforts to decrease the formation of CSF are not likely to have a significant effect on volume and ICP.

Cerebral Blood Flow

Systemic arterial pressure is the primary determinant of cerebral blood flow. Normal cerebral blood flow remains remarkably constant from birth to adult life and is generally 50–60 mL/min/100 g brain weight. The autonomic innervation of blood vessels on the surface and at the base of the brain is richer than vessels of any other organ. These nerve fibers allow the autoregulation of cerebral blood flow. Autoregulation refers to a buffering effect by which cerebral blood flow remains constant despite changes in systemic arterial perfusion pressure. Alterations in the arterial blood concentration of carbon dioxide have an important effect on total cerebral blood flow. Hypercarbia dilates cerebral blood vessels and increases blood flow, whereas hypocarbia constricts cerebral blood vessels and decreases flow. Alterations in blood oxygen content have the reverse effect but are less potent stimuli for vasoconstriction or vasodilation than are alterations in the blood carbon dioxide concentration.

Cerebral perfusion pressure (CPP) is the difference between mean systemic arterial pressure and ICP. Reducing systemic arterial pressure or increasing ICP may reduce perfusion pressure to dangerous levels. The autoregulation of the cerebral vessels is lost when CPP decreases to less than 50 cm H_2O, or in the presence of severe acidosis. Arterial vasodilation or obstruction of cerebral veins and venous sinuses increases intracranial blood volume. Increased intracranial blood volume, similar to increased CSF volume, results in increased ICP.

Cerebral Edema

Cerebral edema is an increase in the brain's volume caused by an increase in its water and sodium content. Increased ICP results from either localized or generalized cerebral edema. The categories of cerebral edema are vasogenic, cytotoxic, or interstitial.

Increased capillary permeability causes vasogenic edema; this occurs with brain tumors, abscess, and infection, and to a lesser degree with trauma and hemorrhage. The fluid is located primarily in white matter and responds to treatment with corticosteroids. Osmotic agents have no effect on vasogenic edema, but they reduce total ICP by decreasing normal brain volume. Cytotoxic edema, characterized by swelling of neurons, glia, and endothelial cells, constricts the extracellular space. The usual causes are hypoxia and ischemia. Corticosteroids do not decrease this type of edema, but osmotic agents may relieve ICP by reducing brain volume.

Transependymal movement of fluid causes interstitial edema from the ventricular system to the brain; this occurs when CSF absorption is blocked, and the ventricles enlarge. The fluid collects chiefly in the periventricular white matter. Agents intended to reduce CSF production, such as acetazolamide, topiramate, and furosemide, may be useful. Corticosteroids and osmotic agents are not effective.

Mass Lesions

Mass lesions (e.g., tumor, abscess, hematoma, and arteriovenous malformation [AVM]) increase ICP by occupying space at the expense of other intracranial compartments, provoking cerebral edema, blocking the circulation and absorption of CSF, increasing blood flow, and obstructing venous return.

SYMPTOMS AND SIGNS

The clinical features of increased ICP depend on the child's age and the rate at which pressure increases. Newborns and infants present a special case because the expansion of skull volume allows partial venting of increased pressure; however, the rate of ICP increase is important at all ages. Intracranial structures accommodate slow increases in pressure remarkably well, but sudden changes are intolerable and result in some combination of headache, visual disturbance, personality change, and decreased consciousness.

Increased Intracranial Pressure in Infancy

Measurement of head circumference and palpation of the anterior fontanelle are readily available methods of assessing intracranial volume and pressure rapidly. The measure of head circumference is the greatest anteroposterior circumference. Normal standards are different for premature and full-term newborns. Normal head growth in a term newborn is 2 cm/month for the first 3 months, 1 cm/month for the second 3 months, and 0.5 cm/month for the next 6 months. Excessive head growth is a major feature of increased ICP throughout the first year up to 3 years. Normal head growth does not preclude the presence of increased ICP; for example, in posthemorrhagic hydrocephalus, considerable ventricular dilation precedes any measurable change in head circumference by compressing the brain parenchyma.

The palpable tension of the anterior fontanelle is an excellent measure of ICP. In a quiet infant a fontanelle that bulges above the level of the bone edges and is sufficiently tense to cause difficulty in determining where bone ends and fontanelle begins is abnormal and indicates increased ICP. A full fontanelle, which is clearly distinguishable from the surrounding bone edges, may indicate increased ICP, but alternate causes are crying, edema of the scalp, subgaleal hemorrhage, and extravasation of intravenous fluids. The normal fontanelle clearly demarcates from bone edges, falls below the surface, and pulsates under the examining finger. Although the size of the anterior fontanelle and its rate of closure are variable, increased ICP should be suspected when the separation of the metopic and coronal sutures is sufficient to accommodate a fingertip.

The infant experiences lethargy, vomiting, and failure to thrive when cranial suture separation becomes insufficient to decompress increased ICP. Sixth cranial nerve palsies, impaired upward gaze (setting sun sign), and disturbances of blood pressure and pulse may ensue. Optic disk edema is uncommon in infants.

Increased Intracranial Pressure in Children
Headache

Headache is a common symptom of increased ICP at all ages. Traction and displacement of intracranial arteries are the major causes of headache from increased ICP. As a rule, the trigeminal nerve innervates pain from supratentorial intracranial vessels, and the referral of pain is to the eye, forehead, and temple. In contrast, cervical nerves innervate infratentorial intracranial vessels, and referral of pain is to the occiput and neck.

With generalized increased ICP, as occurs from cerebral edema or obstruction of the ventricular system, headache is generalized and more prominent on awakening and when rising to a standing position. Pain is constant but may vary in intensity. Coughing, sneezing, straining, and other maneuvers, such as Valsalva, that transiently increase ICP exaggerate headache. The quality of the pain is often difficult to describe. Vomiting in the absence of nausea, especially on arising in the morning, is often a concurrent feature. In the absence of generalized increased ICP, localized, or at least unilateral, headache can occur if a mass causes traction on contiguous vessels.

In children younger than 10 years old separation of sutures may relieve symptoms of increased ICP temporarily. Such children may have a symptom-free interval of several weeks after weeks or months of chronic headache and vomiting. The relief of pressure is temporary, and symptoms eventually return with their prior intensity. An intermittent course of symptoms should not direct attention away from the possibility of increased ICP.

An individual who was previously well and then experienced abrupt onset, intense headache, and meningismus probably has suffered a subarachnoid hemorrhage. A small hemorrhage may not cause loss of consciousness, but it still produces sufficient meningeal irritation to cause intense headache and some stiffness of the neck. Fever may be present.

Diplopia and Strabismus

Paralysis or paresis of one or both abducens nerves is a common feature of generalized increased ICP and may be a more prominent feature than headache in children with idiopathic intracranial hypertension (IIH) (pseudotumor cerebri).

Optic Disk Edema

Optic disk edema ("papilledema") is passive swelling of the optic disk caused by increased ICP (Box 4.2). Extension of the arachnoid sheath of the optic nerve to the retina is essential for the development of optic disk edema. This extension does not occur in a small percentage of people, and they can have severe increased ICP without disk edema. The edema is usually bilateral, and when unilateral, it suggests a mass lesion behind the affected eye. Early disk edema is asymptomatic.

BOX 4.2   Differential Diagnosis of a Swollen Optic Disk

- Congenital disk elevation
- Increased intracranial pressure
- Ischemic neuropathy
- Optic glioma
- Optic nerve drusen
- Papillitis
- Retrobulbar mass

Only with advanced disk edema does transitory obscuration of vision occur. Preservation of visual acuity differentiates disk edema from primary optic nerve disturbances, such as optic neuritis, in which visual acuity is always profoundly impaired early in the course (see Chapter 16).

The observation of disk edema in a child with headache or diplopia confirms the diagnosis of increased ICP. The diagnosis of disk edema is not always easy, however, and congenital variations of disk appearance may confuse the issue. The earliest sign of disk edema is the loss of spontaneous venous pulsations in the vessels around the disk margin. Spontaneous venous pulsations occur in approximately 80% of normal adults, but the rate is closer to 100% in children. Spontaneous venous pulsations cease when ICP reaches pathologic levels. Disk edema is not present if spontaneous venous pulsations are present, no matter how obscure the disk margin may appear to be. Conversely, when spontaneous venous pulsations are lacking in children, one should suspect disk edema even though the disk margin is flat and well visualized.

As edema progresses, the disk swells and is raised above the plane of the retina, causing obscuration of the disk margin and tortuosity of the veins (Fig. 4.1). Associated features include small flame-shaped hemorrhages and nerve fiber infarcts known as cotton wool. If the process continues, the retina surrounding the disk becomes edematous so that the disk appears greatly enlarged (Fig. 4.2), and retinal exudates radiate from the fovea. Eventually the hemorrhages and exudates clear, but optic atrophy ensues, and blindness may be permanent. Even if increased ICP is relieved during the early stages of disk edema, 4–6 weeks is required before the retina appears normal again.

Congenitally elevated disks, usually caused by hyaline bodies (drusen) within the nerve head, give the

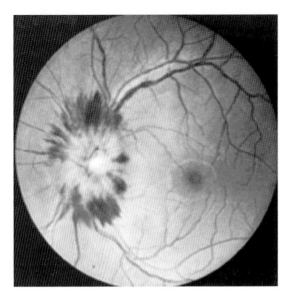

Fig. 4.1 Acute Disk Edema. The optic disk is swollen, and peri-papillary nerve fiber layer hemorrhages are evident.

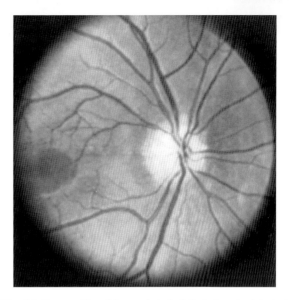

Fig. 4.3 Drusen. The disk margin is indistinct, the physiological cup is absent, and yellowish globular bodies are present on the surface.

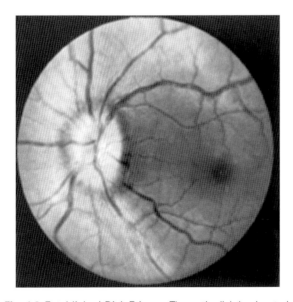

Fig. 4.2 Established Disk Edema. The optic disk is elevated, and opacification of the nerve fiber layer shows around the disk margin and retinal folds (*Paton lines*) temporally.

false impression of disk edema. The actual drusen are not observable before age 10, and only the elevated nerve head is apparent. Drusen continue to grow and can be seen in older children and their parents (Fig. 4.3). Drusen are an autosomal dominant trait and occur more often in Europeans than other ethnic groups.

Spontaneous venous pulsations differentiate disk edema from anomalous nerve head elevations.

Herniation Syndromes

Increased ICP may cause portions of the brain to shift from their normal location into other compartments, compressing structures already occupying that space. These shifts may occur under the falx cerebri, through the tentorial notch, and through the foramen magnum (Box 4.3).

Increased ICP is a relative contraindication for lumbar puncture. The change in fluid dynamics causes herniation in certain circumstances. The hazard is greatest when pressure between cranial compartments is unequal. This prohibition is relative, and early lumbar puncture is the rule in infants and children with suspected infections of the nervous system, despite the presence of increased ICP. In other situations lumbar puncture is rarely essential for diagnosis but is usually accomplished safely in the absence of disk edema. The following imaging criteria define people at increased risk of herniation after lumbar puncture:

- Lateral shift of midline structures
- Loss of the suprachiasmatic and basilar cisterns
- Obliteration of the fourth ventricle
- Obliteration of the superior cerebellar and quadrigeminal plate cisterns

---

BOX 4.3   Herniation Syndromes

Unilateral (Uncal) Transtentorial Herniation
- Declining consciousness
- Increased blood pressure, slow pulse
- Dilated and fixed pupils
- Homonymous hemianopia
- Respiratory irregularity
- Decerebrate rigidity

Bilateral (Central) Transtentorial Herniation
- Decerebrate or decorticate rigidity
- Declining consciousness
- Impaired upward gaze
- Irregular respiration
- Pupillary constriction or dilation

Cerebellar (Downward) Herniation
- Declining consciousness
- Impaired upward gaze
- Irregular respirations
- Lower cranial nerve palsies
- Neck stiffness or head tilt

Falx Herniation

Herniation of one cingulate gyrus under the falx cerebri is more common in the presence of one enlarged hemisphere. The major feature is compression of the internal cerebral vein and the anterior cerebral artery, resulting in still greater increased ICP because of reduced venous outflow and arterial infarction.

Unilateral (Uncal) Transtentorial Herniation

The tentorial notch allows structures to pass from the posterior to the middle fossa. The brainstem, the posterior cerebral artery, and the third cranial nerve are its normal components. Unilateral transtentorial herniation characteristically occurs when enlargement of one temporal lobe causes the uncus or hippocampus to bulge into the tentorial notch. Falx herniation is usually an associated feature. Because considerable ICP is required to cause such a shift, consciousness decreases even before the actual herniation. Direct pressure on the oculomotor nerve causes ipsilateral dilation of the pupil; sometimes dilation of the contralateral pupil occurs because the displaced brainstem compresses the opposite oculomotor nerve against the incisura of the tentorium. Contralateral homonymous hemianopia occurs (but is impossible to test in an unconscious patient)

because of compression of the ipsilateral posterior cerebral artery. With further pressure on the midbrain, both pupils dilate and fix, respirations become irregular, decerebrate posturing is noted, and death results from cardiorespiratory collapse.

Bilateral (Central) Transtentorial Herniation

Central herniation usually is associated with generalized cerebral edema. Both hemispheres displace downward, pushing the diencephalon and midbrain caudad through the tentorial notch. The diencephalon becomes edematous, and the pituitary stalk is avulsed. The clinical features are states of decreasing consciousness, pupillary constriction followed by dilation, impaired upward gaze, irregular respiration, disturbed control of body temperature, decerebrate or decorticate posturing, and death.

Cerebellar Herniation

Increased pressure in the posterior fossa may cause upward herniation of the cerebellum through the tentorial notch or downward displacement of one or both cerebellar tonsils through the foramen magnum. Upward displacement causes compression of the midbrain, resulting in impairment of upward gaze, dilated or fixed pupils, and respiratory irregularity. Downward cerebellar herniation causes compression of the medulla, resulting in states of decreasing consciousness, impaired upward gaze, and lower cranial nerve palsies. One of the earliest features of cerebellar herniation into the foramen magnum is neck stiffness or head tilt in an effort to relieve the pressure by enlarging the surface area of the foramen magnum.

MEDICAL TREATMENT

Several measures to lower increased ICP are available, even in circumstances in which surgical intervention is required (Box 4.4). Management guidelines differ depending on the cause of elevated ICP.

Management of Increased Intracranial Pressure due to Severe Traumatic Brain Injury

Traumatic brain injury (TBI) is unfortunately common in children and adolescents and presents unique treatment challenges, with the goal being the maintenance

BOX 4.4 Medical Measures to Decrease Intracranial Pressure

- Corticosteroids
- Elevation of head
- Hyperosmolality
  - Hypertonic saline
  - Mannitol
- Hyperventilation
- Pentobarbital coma

of adequate CPP. CPP depends on two variables: the mean arterial pressure (MAP) and the ICP. It can be best understood through the following equation:

$$CPP = MAP - ICP.$$

Many hospitals have specific protocols for ICP monitoring and management in the setting of severe TBI. As one can see from the earlier equation, maintenance of appropriate MAPs is equally important for brain survival.

Head Elevation

Elevating the head of the bed 30 degrees above the horizontal improves jugular venous drainage and decreases ICP. Systemic blood pressure remains unchanged, resulting in increased cerebral perfusion. Keep the head midline to avoid compression of the jugular veins.

Homeostasis

Maintain normal glucose. Both hypo- and hyperglycemia may cause further insult. Hyperglycemia may increase oxidative stress. Maintain adequate oxygenation (95%) and CO_2 (35–45 mm Hg). Avoid hypotension and maintain systolic pressure at least above the fifth percentile for age; permissive hypertension is often preferred, but severe hypertension results in the loss of normal adaptive mechanisms and causes further injury. Prevent hyponatremia and maintain osmolality between 300 and 320 mOsmol/L to decrease possible edema with hyponatremia or decreased osmolality. Maintain normal body temperature as every 1°C increases brain metabolism by 5%. Seizures further increase ICP and brain metabolic rate; begin IV levetiracetam and consider continuous electroencephalogram monitoring. Pain and agitation management are important to prevent further elevations in ICP. Paralytics may be needed; use short-acting formulations to allow for intermittent

neurological exams. Sedation should not compromise blood pressure as decrements may result in decreased cerebral perfusion.[1]

Monitoring Intracranial Pressure

ICP monitoring is the standard of care in cases of severe pediatric head trauma. It has limited utility in the treatment of other causes of increased ICP.

Patients requiring ICP monitoring should already be admitted to the ICU. In most institutions ICP is monitored by the placement of an extraventricular drain (EVD) in the nondominant hemisphere via a burr hole. The EVD is then attached to a sensor that allows for accurate ICP measurement. EVDs are a necessary component of treatment but are associated with a wide variety of complications, including infection, hemorrhage, dislodgement, or malfunction. There is no clear consensus regarding whether "true" ICP is more accurate in the injured versus healthy area of the brain. In general, pathologic ICP is defined as pressure over 20 cm H_2O sustained for at least 5 minutes. The presence of an EVD allows for CSF drainage, which is beneficial as increased ICP is unequivocally associated with poorer outcomes. Lumbar drains may be used in some circumstances.

Management of Acutely Increased Intracranial Pressure in Severe Traumatic Brain Injury

Monitor the ICP continuously and use additional management strategies to treat acute increases, defined as pressure greater than or equal to 20 cm H_2O sustained for at least 5 minutes. If an acute increase occurs, the first step is to make sure the patient is adequately ventilated and perfused. Assess for pain, agitation, or active seizures and treat accordingly. If these interventions fail, move on to the following steps.

Severe increased ICP, defined as a measurement of 40 cm H_2O, requires *immediate* intervention to prevent herniation and death. Administer sedatives, osmotic therapies, and hyperosmolar therapies and notify the intensivist and neurosurgeon. Children who experience sustained ICP over 40 cm H_2O refractory to interventions are unlikely to survive.

Hyperventilation

Children with Glasgow Coma Scale scores of less than 8 require intubation to maintain oxygen saturations above 95% and end-tidal carbon dioxide between 35 and 40 mm Hg. ICP decreases within seconds of the initiation of hyperventilation. The mechanism is vasoconstriction resulting from hypocarbia. The goal is to lower the arterial pressure of carbon dioxide to 25–30 mm Hg. Ischemia may result from further or prolonged reductions. The use of hyperventilation is only a transient benefit and should always be followed by immediate neurosurgical consultation.

Hyperosmolar Therapy

Mannitol is the osmotic diuretic most widely used in the United States. A 20% solution of mannitol 0.25–1 g/kg infused intravenously over 15 minutes exerts its beneficial effects as a plasma expander and as an osmotic diuretic. Onset is less rapid than hypertonic saline.

Hypertonic saline is a plasma expander and osmotic diuretic. The typical dosage is 5–10 mL/kg of 3% hypertonic saline solution given over 5–10 minutes.[1] Excretion is by the kidneys, and large doses may cause renal failure, especially when using nephrotoxic drugs concurrently. Maintain serum osmolarity at less than 360 mOsm, serum sodium at less than 160, and adequate intravascular volume.

Pentobarbital Coma

Barbiturates reduce cerebral blood flow, decrease edema formation, and lower the brain's metabolic rate. These effects do not occur at anticonvulsant plasma concentrations but require brain concentrations sufficient to produce a burst-suppression pattern on the electroencephalogram. Barbiturate coma is particularly useful in patients with increased ICP resulting from disorders of mitochondrial function, such as Reye syndrome. Pentobarbital is preferred to phenobarbital (see Chapter 1).

A Note on Hypothermia

There is no conclusive evidence that hypothermia is helpful in cases of severe TBI, and in fact it may be harmful. Children who undergo hypothermia following severe TBI have a greater risk of hypotension, require more vasoactive agents, and have a higher risk of death.[2] Hypothermia does have a role in the treatment of hypoxic-ischemic encephalopathy and anoxic brain injury (see Chapter 1).

Decompressive Craniectomy

Surgical intervention should be considered in cases of increased ICP refractory to medical therapies. It is the only alternative that provides a larger "container" for the increase in intracranial volumes (CSF, blood, and brain parenchyma).

HYDROCEPHALUS

Hydrocephalus is a condition marked by an excessive volume of intracranial CSF. It is termed communicating or noncommunicating, depending on whether the CSF communicates between the ventricular system and the subarachnoid space. Congenital hydrocephalus occurs in approximately 1:1000 births and is generally associated with other congenital malformations. Potential causes include genetic disturbances or intrauterine disorders, such as infection and hemorrhage. Often no cause is determined. Congenital hydrocephalus is discussed in Chapter 18 because its initial feature is usually macrocephaly.

The causes of acquired hydrocephalus are brain tumor, intracranial hemorrhage, or infection. Solid brain tumors generally produce hydrocephalus by obstructing the ventricular system, whereas nonsolid tumors, such as leukemia, impair the reabsorption of CSF in the subarachnoid space.

Intracranial hemorrhage and infection may produce communicating and noncommunicating hydrocephalus and increase ICP through the mechanisms of cerebral edema and impaired venous return. Because several factors contribute to increased ICP, acquired hydrocephalus is discussed by cause in the sections that follow.

Supratentorial Brain Tumors

Primary tumors of the posterior fossa and middle fossa are discussed in Chapters 10, 15, and 16 (Box 4.5). This section discusses tumors of the cerebral hemispheres. Supratentorial tumors comprise approximately half of brain tumors in children. They occur more commonly in children younger than 2 years old, and adolescents.

All children with suspected brain tumors should undergo a contrasted magnetic resonance imaging (MRI) of the brain and total spine. Preferably this is done before surgical intervention, as postoperative blood can complicate radiographic interpretation. Perform lumbar puncture with cytology if feasible and safe; this should not be done in children with acutely elevated ICP. A multidisciplinary team comprising neurologists, neurosurgeons, oncologists, intensivists, nutritionists, and rehabilitative medicine is required in most cases. Aggressive brain tumors in children are rare, and any

BOX 4.5 Brain Tumors in Children

Hemispheric Tumors
- Glial tumors
  - Astrocytoma
  - Ependymoma
  - Oligodendroglioma
  - Primitive neuroectodermal tumors
  - Ganglioglioma
- Pineal region tumors
  - Pineoblastoma
  - Pineocytoma
- Pineal parenchymal tumors
- Germ cell tumors
  - Embryonal cell carcinoma
  - Germinoma
  - Teratoma
- Choroid plexus papilloma
- Other tumors
  - Angiomas
  - Dysplasia
  - Meningioma
  - Metastatic tumors

Middle Fossa Tumors
- Optic glioma (see Chapter 16)
- Sellar and parasellar tumors (see Chapter 16)

Posterior Fossa Tumors
- Astrocytoma (see Chapter 10)
- Brainstem glioma (see Chapter 15)
- Ependymoma (see Chapter 10)
- Hemangioblastoma (see Chapter 10)
- Medulloblastoma (see Chapter 10)

child who has one should be counseled regarding the availability of relevant clinical trials. Often such trials provide the best option for treatment.

General Management of Tumor-Related Increased Intracranial Pressure

The initial management of increased ICP related to tumors is similar to that for severe TBI: head elevation, establishment of a secure airway, and maintenance of homeostasis. Unlike TBI, steroids play an important role, as does surgery. Corticosteroids, such as dexamethasone, are effective in the treatment of vasogenic edema. The intravenous dosage is 0.1–0.2 mg/kg every 6 hours.

The onset of action is 12–24 hours; peak action may be longer. Cerebral blood flow is not affected.

Choroid Plexus Tumors

Choroid plexus tumors arise from the epithelium of the choroid plexus of the cerebral ventricles. They represent only 2%–4% of all pediatric brain tumors, but 10%–20% of tumors that develop in infancy. Two main histological variants exist: choroid plexus papillomas and choroid plexus carcinomas. Choroid plexus papillomas are five times more common than choroid plexus carcinomas. Choroid plexus tumors usually arise from the lateral ventricle, but also may occur in the third ventricle.

Clinical features. Onset is usually during infancy, and the tumor may be present at birth. The main features are those of increased ICP from hydrocephalus. Communicating hydrocephalus may result from excessive production of CSF by the tumor, but noncommunicating hydrocephalus caused by obstruction of the ventricular foramen is the rule. If the tumor is pedunculated, its movement may cause intermittent ventricular obstruction by a ball-valve mechanism. The typical course is one of rapid progression, with only a few weeks from the first symptoms to diagnosis.

Infants with choroid plexus tumors have macrocephaly and often are thought to have congenital hydrocephalus. Older children have nausea, vomiting, diplopia, headaches, and weakness. Disk edema is the rule.

Diagnosis. Multilobular, calcified, contrast-enhancing intraventricular masses are characteristic of choroid plexus tumors. Because affected children show clear evidence of increased ICP, computed tomography (CT) is usually the first test performed. The tumor is located within one ventricle as a mass of increased density with marked contrast enhancement. Hydrocephalus of one or both lateral ventricles is present. Choroid plexus papillomas are vascular and many tumors bleed spontaneously. The spinal fluid may be xanthochromic or grossly bloody. The protein concentration in the CSF is usually elevated.

Management. The choroid plexus receives its blood supply from the anterior and posterior choroidal arteries, branches of the internal carotid artery, and the posterior cerebral artery. This rich vascular network is a major obstacle to complete surgical removal. Yet the extent of surgical resection is the single most important factor that determines the prognosis of a choroid plexus papilloma.[2]

In fact, children with choroid plexus papilloma who undergo complete surgical resection have a survival rate of almost 100%. The success rate is lower for choroid plexus carcinoma, but complete surgical excision still leads to survival rates of 50%–70% on average.

There is no defined optimal therapy. A combination of chemotherapy and radiation may be used for older children with choroid plexus carcinoma. Radiation is not recommended for children under age 3 due to the significant neurological sequelae resulting from irradiation of the young brain.[3]

Glial, Glianeuronal, and Neuronal Tumors

In 2021 the World Health Organization (WHO) released its updated classification for CNS tumors, which placed glial, glianeuronal, and neuronal tumors in their own category.[4] Tumor classification is increasingly reliant on molecular diagnostics in addition to immunohistochemical data, which should in the future allow for more precise and personalized treatment options. However, at present the addition of genetic and molecular information has caused some confusion regarding appropriate therapy, as current treatments were tested in clinical trials utilizing the previous immunohistochemical criteria for enrollment and cohort analysis. The following information is what we felt would be most useful for a clinical pediatric neurologist. More complex diagnostic testing and the development of treatment protocols will rely on pediatric oncologists.

Glial, glianeuronal, and neuronal tumors encompass multiple newly created tumor categories based mainly on molecular characteristics. For the sake of simplicity, we will continue to use the term "tumor of glial origin." This includes both low-grade and high-grade gliomas.

Most of the pediatric low-grade gliomas do not produce an increase in ICP. These tumors are slow-growing and tend to calcify. Common molecular and genetic mutations include alterations in the MAPK signaling pathway (e.g., changes in the tyrosine kinase domain of *FGFR1* or mutations in *BRAF p.V600E*) and the *MYB* or *MYBL1* fusion gene. Overall survival for pediatric diffuse low-grade gliomas is over 90%.

Pediatric high-grade gliomas are more aggressive and may present with increased ICP, although that is rarely the initial symptom. Such gliomas include diffuse midline glioma, anaplastic astrocytoma, glioblastoma multiforme, and diffuse intrinsic pontine glioma (DIPG). Mutations in the histone H3 are associated with particularly poor prognosis. Despite advances in diagnosis, overall survival for high-grade gliomas remains abysmally low, at less than 10%.[5]

There are two autosomal dominant glioma-predisposing syndromes: tuberous sclerosis (subependymal giant cell astrocytoma) and neurofibromatosis type I (pilocytic astrocytoma of the optic pathway and hypothalamus).

Tumors of glial origin constitute approximately 40% of supratentorial tumors in infants and children. The common glial tumors of childhood in order of frequency are astrocytoma, ependymoma, and oligodendroglioma. A mixture of two or more cell types is common. *Oligodendroglioma* occurs exclusively in the cerebral hemispheres, whereas astrocytoma and ependymoma have either a supratentorial or an infratentorial location. Oligodendroglioma is mainly a tumor of adolescence. These tumors grow slowly and tend to calcify. The initial symptom is usually a seizure rather than increased ICP.

Astrocytoma

The traditional grading of hemispheric gliomas by histological appearance into low-grade, anaplastic, and glioblastoma multiforme is gradually incorporating genomic analysis of the tumors. Low-grade gliomas are the most common brain tumors in children.

Pediatric high-grade gliomas and DIPGs are malignant gliomas within the spectrum of anaplastic astrocytoma (WHO grade 3) or glioblastoma multiforme (WHO grade 4). These tumors are associated with mutations in the histones H3.1 and H3.3.

Clinical features. The initial features of glial tumors in children depend on location and may include seizures, hemiparesis, and movement disorders affecting one side of the body. Tumors infiltrating the basal ganglia and internal capsule are less likely to cause seizures than tumors closer to cortical structures. A slow-growing tumor may not cause a mass effect because surrounding neural structures accommodate infiltrating tumors. Epilepsy is a common presenting symptom, particularly in polymorphous low-grade epithelial tumor of the young which involves the temporal lobes in more than 80% of cases.

Headache is a relatively common complaint. Pain localizes if the tumor produces focal displacement of vessels without increasing ICP. A persistent focal headache usually correlates well with tumor location.

The initial features in children with medullary tumors may be progressive dysphagia, hoarseness, ataxia, and hemiparesis. Cervicomedullary tumors cause neck discomfort, weakness or numbness of the hands, and an asymmetric quadriparesis. Midbrain tumors cause features of increased ICP, diplopia, and hemiparesis.

Symptoms of increased ICP, generalized headache, nausea, and vomiting are initial features of hemispheric high-grade glioma in only one-third of children, but are common at the time of diagnosis. ICP is likely to increase when rapidly growing tumors provoke edema of the hemisphere. A mass effect collapses one ventricle, shifts midline structures, and puts pressure on the aqueduct. When herniation occurs or when the lateral ventricles are dilated because of pressure on the aqueduct, the early features of headache, nausea, vomiting, and diplopia are followed by generalized weakness or fatigability, lethargy, and declining consciousness.

Disk edema occurs in children with generalized increased ICP, but macrocephaly occurs in infants. When disk edema is present, abducens palsy is usually an associated symptom. Other neurological findings depend on the site of the tumor and may include hemiparesis, hemisensory loss, or homonymous hemianopia.

Diagnosis. MRI is always preferable to CT when suspecting a tumor. In a CT scan a low-grade glioma appears as low density or cystic areas that enhance with contrast material (Fig. 4.4). A low-density area surrounding the tumor that does not show contrast enhancement indicates edema.

High-grade gliomas have patchy areas of low and high density, sometimes evidence of hemorrhage, and cystic degeneration. Marked contrast enhancement, often in a ring pattern, is noted. When a mass effect is present, imaging studies show a shift of midline structures, deformity of the ipsilateral ventricle, and swelling of the affected hemisphere with obliteration of sulcal markings (Fig. 4.5). A mass effect occurs in half of low-grade astrocytomas and almost all high-grade tumors.

Management.   Treat all children with increased ICP caused by hemispheric gliomas with dexamethasone to reduce vasogenic cerebral edema and with ventriculoperitoneal shunting when hydrocephalus coexists. Headache and nausea frequently are relieved within 24 hours; neurological deficits improve as well.

The recommendation for suspected low-grade gliomas is full surgical resection if possible. There are current clinical trials incorporating the known tumor mutations as targets for the chemotherapeutic or immunologic agents, and mammalian target of rapamycin inhibitors such as sirolimus and verolimus have significant activity against subependymal giant cell astrocytomas.

Children with high-grade gliomas receive surgical resection with radiation therapy and possibly chemotherapy. Patients with DIPGs receive radiation therapy.

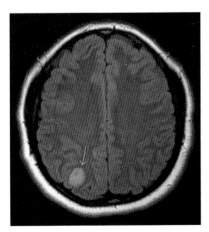

Fig. 4.4 Low-Grade Glioma. Axial T$_2$ flair magnetic resonance imaging shows a well-circumscribed and homogeneous neoplasm (*arrow*).

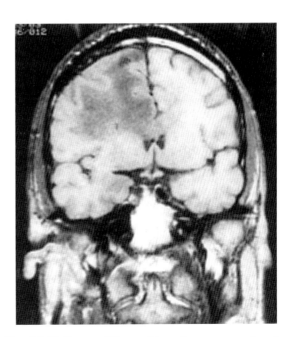

Fig. 4.5 Malignant Glioma. Magnetic resonance imaging shows a malignant astrocytoma invading the corpus callosum.

Children with anaplastic astrocytomas have less than a 30% 5-year survival rate even with radiotherapy, and children with glioblastoma multiforme have less than a 3% 5-year survival. Because the 5-year survival rate of children with high-grade astrocytomas is poor, several chemotherapy and immune therapy protocols are being tried and some enthusiasm exists based on the new genetic targets.

Ependymoma

Ependymomas are tumors derived from cells that line the ventricular system and may be either supratentorial or infratentorial in location (including posterior fossa and spinal cord). They are the second most common malignant brain tumor in children, comprising 9% of childhood brain and spinal cord tumors. Pediatric ependymomas most frequently arise from the lining of the fourth ventricle (see Chapter 10); supratentorial ependymomas are rare but incidence increases in older children and adolescents. Infratentorial ependymoma is discussed in Chapter 10 because the initial symptom is often ataxia. Symptoms of increased ICP are the first feature in 90% of children with posterior fossa ependymoma, and disk edema is present in 75% at the time of initial examination.

The expected location of supratentorial ependymoma is in relation to the third and lateral ventricles. Ependymal tumors may arise within the hemispheres, however, at a site distant from the ventricular system. Such tumors probably derive from ependymal cell rests.

Clinical features. Symptoms of increased ICP are less prominent with supratentorial tumors than with infratentorial tumors. Common manifestations are focal weakness, seizures, and visual disturbances. Disk edema is a common feature in all patients with ependymoma. Hemiparesis, hyperreflexia, and hemianopia are typical features, but some children show only ataxia. The duration of symptoms before diagnosis averages 7 months but can be as little as 1 month for malignant tumors and several years for low-grade tumors.

Diagnosis. A typical MRI appearance of a fourth ventricular ependymoma is that of a homogeneously enhancing solid mass extending out of the foramen of Luschka or the foramen of Magendie with associated obstructive hydrocephalus. Tumor density on CT is usually greater than brain density, and contrast enhancement is present. Small cysts within the tumor are relatively common. Approximately one-third of supratentorial ependymomas contain calcium.

Tumors within the third ventricle cause marked dilation of the lateral ventricles, with edema of the hemispheres and obliteration of sulcal markings. High-grade tumors are likely to seed the subarachnoid space, producing metastases in the spinal cord and throughout the ventricular system. In such cases tumor cells may line the lateral ventricles and produce a "cast" of contrast enhancement around the ventricles.

Management. Complete surgical resection is possible in only 30% of cases. Even after complete resection, the 5-year rate of progression-free survival is 60%–80%.[6] Survival relates directly to the effectiveness of surgical removal followed by either radiation therapy or chemotherapy. The use of radiation in young children with ependymomas was avoided in the past because of the risks of cognitive, endocrine, and developmental side effects. However, the advent of more selective radiation delivery techniques has made postoperative radiation therapy an attractive option for pediatric patients and is offered as part of many clinical trial protocols.[7,8] Several studies suggest that radiation therapy prolongs progression-free survival after subtotal resection of an ependymoma. As such, there is now growing evidence supporting the use of adjuvant radiation for spinal cord and supratentorial ependymomas.[9]

Embryonal Tumors

Atypical teratoid/rhabdoid tumors (ATRTs) and CNS primitive neuroectodermal tumors (PNETs) are biologically distinct entities from other embryonal tumors causing increased ICP such as medulloblastomas (see Chapter 10). Fig. 4.6 shows an example of the imaging characteristics of PNET.

ATRT is an aggressive, fast-growing tumor associated with *SMARCB1* mutations. It typically starts as an intracranial tumor although rarely can begin in other tissues such as the kidney. Because of its rapid progression, it commonly presents with symptoms of increased ICP. On MRI it appears as a large, contrast-enhancing tumor with necrotic and cystic areas. ATRT may spread to other areas of the CNS via CSF. Treatment consists of surgical resection (or at least debulking), chemotherapy, radiation, and clinical trials. Immune therapy and targeted therapies are increasingly available although use in pediatrics remains limited. The overall 5-year survival rate is 32%.

PNETs are in the process of being reclassified based on their molecular characteristics. For the sake of simplicity, we will continue to refer to them as PNETs for the time

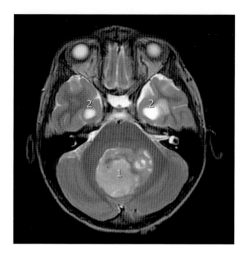

Fig. 4.6 Primitive Neuroectodermal Tumor. T_2 axial magnetic resonance imaging shows *(1)* a 6.5 cm × 3 cm heterogeneous mass with cysts and *(2)* secondary dilation of temporal horns/ hydrocephalus.

being. Subtypes include medulloepithelioma, CNS neuroblastoma, CNS ganglioneuroblastoma, and embryonal tumor with multilayered rosettes and other unspecified embryonal tumors. Like other embryonal tumors, they tend to be aggressive and fast-growing. These are cortical tumors that enhance with contrast and may be associated with cystic fluid collections; multiple tumors are sometimes seen. PNETs are typically supratentorial, although brainstem and spinal PNETs can occur. Metastatic disease is common and about 33% of patients already have metastatic disease at the time of diagnosis. Treatments are similar to those for ATRT: surgery followed by radiation and chemotherapy, possibly with targeted therapies or immune therapies. The 5-year survival rate is not specifically known but is thought to be low.

Pineal Region Tumors

The derivation of tumors in the pineal region comes from several histological types. Grade 1 tumors are slow-growing pineocytomas. Pineal parenchymal or papillary tumors are grade 2 or 3 and have a higher chance of recurrence after resection. Pineoblastomas are categorized as grade 4 and are associated with extension into surrounding brain parenchyma and poorer prognosis. They may metastasize to other areas of the CNS via CSF. Pineoblastomas occur more frequently in patients with a history of bilateral retinoblastoma. Overall, 5-year survival rates are approximately 70%.

The incidence of pineal region tumors is 10 times higher in Japan than in the United States or Western Europe. Pineal region tumors are more common in boys than in girls and generally become symptomatic during adolescence.

Clinical features. Because pineal region tumors are in a midline location, where they can invade or compress the third ventricle or aqueduct, symptoms of increased ICP are common. The first symptoms may be acute and accompanied by midbrain dysfunction. Midbrain dysfunction resulting from pressure by pineal region tumors on the periaqueductal gray is *Parinaud syndrome*: loss of pupillary light reflex, supranuclear palsy of upward gaze with preservation of downward gaze, and retraction-convergence nystagmus when upward gaze is attempted. Eventually paralysis of upward and downward gaze and loss of accommodation may occur.

Tumors growing into or compressing the anterior hypothalamus produce loss of vision, diabetes insipidus, precocious puberty, and emaciation. Precocious puberty occurs almost exclusively in boys. Extension of the tumor into the posterior fossa produces multiple cranial neuropathies and ataxia, and lateral extension causes hemiparesis.

Diagnosis. Pineal tumors typically appear as a solid, contrast-enhancing mass on MRI. Tumors that spread into the ventricular system and have intense contrast enhancement are likely to be malignant pineoblastomas. Tumors that contain abundant amounts of calcium are likely to be benign.

CT or MRI sometimes identifies asymptomatic nonneoplastic pineal cysts in children undergoing imaging for other reasons. These are developmental variants of the pineal gland, which may contain calcium. They only rarely grow to sufficient size to obstruct the aqueduct or cause Parinaud syndrome.

Management. Resection is the first line of treatment and obtains tissue essential to establish the histological type and to plan therapy (typically radiation and chemotherapy). Ventricular drainage relieves hydrocephalus when needed. The common complications of pineal region surgery are ocular dysmotility, ataxia, and altered mental status.

Other Tumors

Cerebral metastatic disease is unusual in childhood. Tumors that produce cerebral metastases most frequently are osteogenic sarcoma and rhabdomyosarcoma in patients younger than 15 years old, and testicular germ cell tumors after age 15. The cerebral hemispheres, more often than posterior fossa structures, are affected. Pulmonary involvement typically precedes cerebral metastasis. Brain metastasis is rarely present at the time of initial cancer diagnosis.

Meningioma is uncommon in children. The initial features may be focal neurological signs, seizures, or increased ICP.

INTRACRANIAL ARACHNOID CYSTS

Primary arachnoid cysts are CSF-filled cavities within the arachnoid. The cause of cyst formation is uncertain. They represent a minor disturbance in arachnoid formation and not a pathological process. Arachnoid cysts are found in 0.5% of postmortem examinations; two-thirds are supratentorial and one-third are infratentorial.

Clinical features. Most cysts are asymptomatic structures identified by CT or MRI. The detection of an arachnoid cyst is often easily perceived as an incidental finding; however, deciding whether the cyst caused the symptom for which the imaging study was required is sometimes problematic. Subarachnoid cysts are usually present from infancy, but may develop, or at least enlarge enough to detect, during adolescence.

Large cysts can produce symptoms by compressing adjacent structures or by increasing ICP. Focal neurological disturbances vary with location but are most often hemiparesis or seizures when the cyst is supratentorial and ataxia when the cyst is infratentorial. Compression of the frontal lobe from early infancy may result in the undergrowth of contralateral limbs.

Increased ICP can result from mass effect or hydrocephalus and is associated with cysts in all locations. Clinical features include macrocephaly, headache, and behavioral change.

Diagnosis. It has become common for children with headache, learning or behavioral disorders, and suspected seizure disorders to undergo imaging studies of the brain. Some of these studies show incidental arachnoid cysts. A cause-and-effect relationship is a consideration only if the cyst is large and clearly explains the symptoms. Positron emission tomography may be useful in deciding whether an arachnoid cyst is having a pressure effect on the brain. Hypometabolism in the surrounding brain indicates brain compression.

Management. Simple drainage of the symptomatic cyst often results in reaccumulation of fluid and recurrence of symptoms. Symptomatic superficial cysts require excision, and deeply located cysts require a shunt into the peritoneal space.

PERINATAL INTRACRANIAL HEMORRHAGE

Intraventricular Hemorrhage in the Newborn

Intraventricular hemorrhage is primarily a disorder of live-born premature neonates with respiratory distress syndrome. The autoregulation of cerebral blood flow, which meets local tissue needs by altering cerebrovascular resistance, is impaired in premature newborns with respiratory distress syndrome. During episodes of systemic hypotension, decreased cerebral blood flow increases the potential for cerebral infarction. Such infarctions usually occur symmetrically in the white matter adjacent to the lateral ventricles. The late finding of these infarcts is termed *periventricular leukomalacia.*

During episodes of systemic hypertension, cerebral blood flow increases. Hemorrhage occurs first in the subependymal germinal matrix, then bursts through the ependymal lining into the lateral ventricle. Such hemorrhages are termed *periventricular-intraventricular hemorrhages* (PIVHs). The predilection of the germinal matrix for hemorrhage during episodes of increased cerebral blood flow is unknown. The likely explanation is a prior ischemic injury that weakens the capillary walls and their supporting structures, making them vulnerable to rupture during episodes of increased cerebral blood flow. Intraventricular hemorrhage also occurs in full-term newborns, but the mechanism of hemorrhage at term is different from that before term.

Periventricular-Intraventricular Hemorrhage in Premature Newborns

The incidence of PIVH in premature newborns with birth weight less than 2000 g has been declining. The reason for the decline is probably attributable to advances in ventilatory care. PIVH occurs in approximately 33% of newborns less than 29 weeks of gestational age. Grade I and II account for 80% of all cases and seem not to have any impact on neurodevelopmental outcomes measured at 1.5–2 years in late premature infants[10]; however, extremely premature infants may suffer long-term neurosensory deficits even with grade I and II hemorrhages.[11] Bleeding occurs within the first 4 days in almost all affected newborns. PIVH originates from the rupture of small vessels in the subependymal germinal matrix. Approximately 80% of germinal matrix hemorrhages extend into the ventricular system. Hemorrhagic lesions into the cerebral parenchyma accompany severe hemorrhages. Parenchymal hemorrhages are usually unilateral and result from hemorrhagic venous infarction in the periventricular region.[12]

The following is a grading system for PIVH:

- Grade I: isolated subependymal hemorrhage.
- Grade II: intraventricular hemorrhage without ventricular dilation.
- Grade III: intraventricular hemorrhage with ventricular dilation.
- Grade IV: intraventricular hemorrhage with ventricular dilation and hemorrhage into the parenchyma of the brain.

Hemorrhage into the parenchyma of the brain (grade IV) is a coexistent process caused by hemorrhagic infarction (periventricular hemorrhagic infarction) and is not an extension of the first three grades of intraventricular hemorrhage.

Clinical features. Routine ultrasound examinations are standard in the care of all newborns whose birth weight is 1800 g or less and often reveal PIVH in newborns in which no clinical suspicion exists. Among this group, some have blood in the CSF, and others have clear CSF. Newborns with grade III and IV hemorrhages have the worst outcomes, but long-term deficits have been reported in premature infants with grade I or II PIVH.

In some premature newborns PIVH produces rapid neurological deterioration characterized by decreasing states of consciousness, severe hypotonia, and respiratory insufficiency. Within minutes to hours, the infant shows obvious evidence of increased ICP: bulging fontanelle, decerebrate posturing, loss of pupillary reflexes, and respiratory arrest. Hypothermia, bradycardia, and hypotension are present, and hematocrit may decrease by as much as 10%.

Often the hemorrhage manifests by stepwise progression of symptoms over hours or days. The initial symptoms are subtle and include change in behavior, diminished spontaneous movement, and either an increase or a decrease in appendicular tone. The fontanelles remain soft, and vital signs are normal. These first symptoms may correspond to grade I hemorrhage.

Some newborns become stable and have no further difficulty. Others undergo clinical deterioration characterized by hypotonia and declining consciousness. This deterioration probably corresponds to the presence of blood in the ventricles. The infant becomes lethargic or obtunded, then may stabilize. If continued bleeding causes acute ventricular dilation, apnea and coma follow. Seizures occur when blood dissects into the cerebral parenchyma.

Newborns with PIVH are at risk for progressive hydrocephalus. The likelihood is much greater among children with grade III or IV hemorrhage. Initial ventricular dilation is probably due to plugging of the arachnoid villi and impaired reabsorption of CSF. The ventricles can enlarge by compressing the brain without causing a measurable change in head circumference. Weekly ultrasound studies are imperative to follow the progression of hydrocephalus.

Diagnosis. Ultrasound is the standard for the diagnosis of intraventricular hemorrhage in the newborn. Ultrasound is preferred over other brain imaging techniques because it is accurate and easily performed at the bedside in the neonatal intensive care unit. MRI during infancy or childhood is useful to show the extent of brain damage (periventricular leukomalacia) from the combination of periventricular strokes and PIVH.

Management. Box 4.6 lists some methods to prevent PIVH. A premature newborn has a significant risk of PIVH and this increases with the amount of intensive care required. Unnecessary manipulation of a premature infant should be avoided, and a quiet environment maintained. The use of paralytics in ventilated

---

BOX 4.6 Prevention of Intra- and Periventricular Hemorrhage

Antenatal
- Delivery in specialized center
- Prevention of prematurity

Postnatal
- Avoidance of rapid volume expansion
- Correction of coagulation abnormalities
- Maintenance of stable systemic blood pressure
- Muscle paralysis of ventilated premature newborns
- Potential pharmacological agents
  - Indomethacin
  - Phenobarbital
- Vitamin K

infants reduces the incidence and severity of PIVH by stabilizing fluctuations of cerebral blood flow velocity. Phenobarbital may dampen fluctuations of systemic blood pressure and cerebral blood flow, and indomethacin inhibits prostaglandin synthesis regulating cerebral blood flow; however, the efficacy of both agents is inconclusive and some concerns about the use of phenobarbital must be considered.

Extension of hemorrhage from grade II or III occurs in 20% of cases. Serial ultrasound scans provide early diagnosis of posthemorrhagic hydrocephalus, which develops in 10%–15% of premature newborns with PIVH. Factors that influence the management of posthemorrhagic hydrocephalus are the rate of progression, ventricular size, and ICP. The hydrocephalus ultimately arrests or regresses in 50% of children and progresses to severe hydrocephalus in the remainder. Rapid ventricular enlargement requires prompt intervention.

When intraventricular hemorrhage has occurred, the direction of treatment is toward the prevention or stabilization of progressive posthemorrhagic hydrocephalus. The efficacy of treatment for posthemorrhagic hydrocephalus is difficult to assess because the role of ventricular dilation in causing chronic neurological impairment is not established. Newborns with progressive posthemorrhagic hydrocephalus also have experienced hypoxic-ischemic encephalopathy, germinal matrix hemorrhage, and periventricular insult. Neurological morbidity correlates better with the degree of parenchymal damage than with ventricular size.

The definitive treatment is the placement of a ventriculoperitoneal shunt. Early shunt placement, while the ventricles still contain blood, has a high incidence of shunt failure and infection. EVDs may be used as a temporizing measure while waiting for ventricular blood to clear.

Intraventricular Hemorrhage at Term

In contrast to intraventricular hemorrhage in a premature newborn, which originates almost exclusively from the germinal matrix, intraventricular hemorrhage at term may originate from the veins of the choroid plexus, from the germinal matrix, or both.

Clinical features. Full-term newborns with intraventricular hemorrhage form two groups. In more than half delivery was difficult, frequently from the breech position and with some degree of sustained intrauterine asphyxia. Usually, these newborns show bruising and require resuscitation. They initially appear to be improving, then multifocal seizures occur on the second day postpartum. The fontanelle is tense, and the CSF is bloody.

The other half of affected infants have experienced neither trauma nor asphyxia and appear normal at birth. During the first hours postpartum, apnea, cyanosis, and a tense fontanelle develop. The mechanism of hemorrhage is unknown. Posthemorrhagic hydrocephalus is common in both groups, and many require shunt placement.

Diagnosis. Ultrasound is as useful for the diagnosis of intraventricular hemorrhage in full-term newborns as in premature newborns.

Management. The treatment of full-term newborns with intraventricular hemorrhage is the same as for premature newborns with intraventricular hemorrhage.

INCREASED INTRACRANIAL PRESSURE RELATED TO VASCULAR ABNORMALITIES

Arterial Aneurysms

Arterial aneurysms are vestiges of the embryonic circulation and are present in a rudimentary form before birth. Only rarely do they rupture during childhood. Symptomatic arterial aneurysms in childhood may be associated with coarctation of the aorta or polycystic kidney disease. Aneurysms tend to be located at the bifurcation of major arteries at the base of the brain.

Clinical features. Subarachnoid hemorrhage is usually the first feature of a ruptured aneurysm. The initial symptoms may be catastrophic: sudden loss of consciousness, tachycardia, hypotension, and evidence of increased ICP, but in most patients the first bleeding is a "warning leak" that may go undiagnosed. Severe headache, stiff neck, and low-grade fever characterize the warning leak. Occasionally aneurysms produce neurological signs by exerting pressure on adjacent cranial nerves. Oculomotor nerve dysfunction is common, resulting in disturbances of gaze and pupillary function.

Physical activity does not relate to the time of rupture. Aneurysmal size is the main predictor of rupture; aneurysms smaller than 1 cm in diameter have a low probability of rupture.

The patient's state of consciousness is the most important predictor of survival. Approximately 50% of patients die during the first hospitalization, some from the initial hemorrhage during the first 14 days. Untreated, another 30% die from recurrent hemorrhage in the next 10 years. Unruptured aneurysms may cause acute severe headache without nuchal rigidity. The mechanism of headache may be aneurysmal thrombosis or localized meningeal inflammation.

Diagnosis. On the day of aneurysmal rupture, CT shows intracranial hemorrhage in all patients, but the blood rapidly reabsorbs, and only two-thirds have visible hemorrhage on the fifth day using standard MRI or magnetic resonance angiography (MRA). Lumbar puncture is common because the stiff neck, headache, and fever suggest bacterial meningitis. The fluid is grossly bloody and thought traumatic unless centrifugation reveals xanthochromic fluid. When a diagnosis of subarachnoid hemorrhage is established, all vessels need to be visualized to determine the aneurysmal site and evaluate for the presence of multiple aneurysms. Four-vessel cerebral arteriography was previously the standard imaging study, but improved MRA technology and CT angiography are often diagnostic and less invasive.

Management. The definitive treatment is surgical clipping and excision of the aneurysm. Early surgery prevents rebleeding in conscious patients.[13] Cerebral vasospasm and ischemia are the leading causes of death and disability among survivors of an initial aneurysm rupture. Pharmacological means to prevent rebleeding are becoming less important with the increasing frequency of early operative intervention. Medical therapy for the prevention and treatment of vasospasm includes a regimen of volume expansion and induced systemic hypertension. Nimodipine is effective for the prevention of delayed ischemia due to vasospasm.

The 6-month survival rate in patients who are conscious at the time of admission is approximately 86%. In contrast, only 20% of patients comatose on admission live 6 months.

Arteriovenous Malformations

Approximately 0.1% of children have an AVM, of which 12%–18% become symptomatic in childhood.[14] The annual hemorrhage rate is difficult to know with certainty but is estimated to be 2%–10%; importantly, the rerupture rate is high, at 2%–4% per year with a mortality rate of up to 25% per event.[15]

All AVMs are congenital anomalies that consist of abnormal arteries and veins without an intervening capillary bed. Two types of malformations occur. One type arises early in gestation from an abnormal communication between primitive choroidal arteries and veins. Such malformations are in the midline and give rise to the vein of Galen malformation, malformations involving the choroid plexus, and shunts between cerebellar arteries and the straight sinus. The other type arises later in gestation or even after birth between superficial arteries and veins. The result is an AVM within the parenchyma of the cerebral hemisphere. Interconnections exist between the vessels of the scalp, skull, and dura, causing anastomotic channels between the extracranial and intracranial circulations to remain patent. Approximately 90% of AVMs are supratentorial, and 10% are infratentorial.

Deep Midline Malformations

Hydrocephalus and high-output cardiac failure during infancy are the presenting features of large deep midline malformations, especially malformations involving the great vein of Galen. They rarely bleed.[16] These malformations are discussed in Chapter 18.

Clinical features. Small, deep midline malformations are rarely symptomatic in childhood. Bleeding into the parenchyma of the brain or the subarachnoid space brings the problem to attention. Secondary venous changes reroute the drainage to the pial veins, which then bleed. Because the bleeding is from the venous rather than the arterial side of the malformation, the initial symptoms are not as catastrophic as with arterial aneurysms. Symptoms may evolve over several hours, and no characteristic clinical syndrome is associated. Most patients describe sudden severe headache, neck stiffness, and vomiting. Fever is frequently an associated symptom. The presence of focal neurological deficits depends on the location of the malformation and may include hemiparesis, sensory disturbances, and oculomotor palsies. Rebleeding risk depends on multiple factors, including prior hemorrhage, size of the malformation, and characteristics of arterial feeding pressures and venous drainage.

Diagnosis. Contrast-enhanced MRI or CT easily reveals most AVMs and shows the degree of ventricular enlargement. Conventional cerebral angiography remains the gold standard for diagnosing and defining AVMs due to the level of detail it provides; however, such details can be obscured if the malformation has already bled and is compressed by a hematoma.

Management. Complete surgical excision is the treatment of choice whenever feasible; the risk of rebleeding remains until the malformation has been completely obliterated. A multidisciplinary approach involving a vascular neurosurgeon, interventional neuroradiologist, and radiation oncologist is recommended. For large AVMs, use conjunctive therapies such as staged endovascular embolization. Stereotactic radiosurgery remains controversial in pediatrics due to the effects of radiation on the developing brain but can be considered for high-grade AVMs or those that lie within the eloquent cortex. Postoperative complications include hemorrhage, thrombosis, stroke, hyperperfusion, seizures, and vasospasm.[17]

Supratentorial Malformations

Clinical features. Among children with AVMs in and around the cerebral hemispheres, the initial feature is intracranial hemorrhage in half and seizures in half. Recurrent vascular headache may precede the onset of hemorrhage, and seizures may develop concurrently. Headaches are usually unilateral but may not occur consistently on the same side. In some patients the headaches have a migraine quality: scintillating scotomata and unilateral throbbing pain. The incidence of these migraine-like headaches in patients with AVMs does not seem to be greater than in the general population; the malformation probably provokes a migraine attack in people who are genetically predisposed. Most patients who have seizures have at least one focal seizure, but among the seizures associated with AVMs, half are focal seizures and half are secondary generalized seizures. No specific location of the malformation is associated with a higher incidence of seizures. Small superficial malformations, especially in the centroparietal region, are associated with the highest incidence of hemorrhage. Hemorrhage may be subarachnoid only or may dissect into the brain parenchyma.

Diagnosis. Contrast-enhanced MRI and CT provide excellent visualization of the malformation in most children. Conventional arteriography provides the necessary level of detail before surgical intervention.

Management. Management is similar to that used for other AVMs.

Cocaine Abuse

Intracranial hemorrhage is associated with cocaine abuse in young adults. The hemorrhages may be subarachnoid or intracerebral in location. A sudden transitory increase in systemic blood pressure is the cause. Cocaine may also lead to ischemic stroke.

INFECTIOUS DISORDERS

Infections of the brain and meninges produce increased ICP by causing cerebral edema, by obstructing the flow and reabsorption of CSF, and by impairing venous outflow. Symptoms of increased ICP are frequently the initial features of bacterial and fungal infections, and occasionally, viral encephalitis. Viral infections are more likely to cause seizures, personality change, or decreased consciousness and are discussed in Chapter 2.

Bacterial Meningitis

The offending organism and the clinical features of bacterial meningitis vary with age. It is useful to discuss the syndromes of bacterial meningitis by age group: newborn, infants and young children (28 days to 5 years), and school-age children.

Meningitis in the Newborn

Meningitis in the newborn has become less common in recent years but remains an important cause of neonatal morbidity and mortality. It is a consequence of septicemia, and organs other than the brain are infected. Maternal infection is the main risk factor for sepsis and meningitis. Group B *Streptococcus* (GBS), *Escherichia coli*, and *Listeria monocytogenes* are the most common causes of meningitis in the first month of life.[14] Intrapartum treatment of maternal GBS infection has greatly reduced the number of associated cases of meningitis; however, GBS remains the most common cause of neonatal meningitis, responsible for approximately 40% of cases. Previously uncommon organisms that are increasing in frequency include multidrug resistant *Acinetobacter baumanii* in Asia, and *Cronobacter* (*Enterobacter*) *sakazakii*, which has been associated with outbreaks of sepsis and meningitis in neonates and infants due to contaminated powdered infant formula. *C. sakazakii* produces brain abscess, subdural empyema, and hydrocephalus, and has a high mortality rate. *Citrobacter diversus* infects neonates even with no known risk factors and may cause a hemorrhagic necrosis of the brain, with liquefaction of the cerebral white matter and abscess formation. Human immunodeficiency virus (HIV) exposure, even if the neonate is not infected, increases meningitis risk.

Early-onset (first 5 days) and late-onset (after 5 days) patterns of meningitis have been identified in newborns. In early-onset meningitis the acquisition of infection is at the time of delivery, and the responsible organisms are usually *E. coli* or GBS. The newborn becomes symptomatic during the first week, and the mortality rate is as high as 50% in developing countries, according to the WHO. In late-onset meningitis the acquisition of infection is postnatal, and symptoms may begin as early as the fourth day postpartum, but usually begin after the first week. Newborns requiring intensive care are specifically at risk for late-onset meningitis because of excessive instrumentation. The responsible organisms are *E. coli*, GBS, enterococci, gram-negative enteric bacilli (*Pseudomonas* and *Klebsiella*), and *L. monocytogenes*. The mortality rate for both forms of meningitis has decreased significantly in the United States.[18] This is mostly the result of antibiotic coverage of all sick newborns until infection is ruled out, and better neonatal intensive care.

Clinical features. Newborns infected in utero or during delivery may experience respiratory distress and shock within 24 hours of birth. Other features that may be associated with septicemia include hyperthermia, hypothermia, jaundice, hepatomegaly, lethargy, anorexia, and vomiting.

In late-onset meningitis the clinical manifestations are variable. Initial symptoms are usually nonspecific and include lethargy, disturbed feeding, and irritability. As meningitis worsens, hyperthermia, respiratory distress or apnea, and seizures are present in about half of newborns, but bulging of the fontanelle occurs in only a quarter, and nuchal rigidity does not occur. Shock is the usual cause of death.

Diagnosis. The diagnosis of septicemia and meningitis in the newborn is often difficult to establish based on symptoms. The first suspicion of septicemia should prompt lumbar puncture. Even in the absence of infection, the CSF of febrile newborns averages 11 leukocytes/mm³ (range 0–20 leukocytes/mm³). Less than 6% are polymorphonuclear leukocytes. The protein concentration has a mean value of 84 mg/dL (0.84 g/L), with a range of 40–130 mg/dL (0.4–1.3 g/L), and the glucose concentration has a mean value of 46 mg/dL (0.46 g/L), with a range of 36–56 mg/dL (0.36–0.56 g/L).

In newborns with meningitis the leukocyte count is usually in the thousands, and the protein concentration may vary from less than 30 mg/dL (<0.3 g/L) to greater than 1000 mg/dL (>10 g/L). A Gram-stained smear of CSF permits the identification of an organism in less than half of cases. Even when the smear is positive, identification may be inaccurate. The use of real-time fluorescence quantitative polymerase chain reaction (PCR) and multiple PCR-based reverse line blot hybridization has a higher sensitivity and similar specificity as cultures. Both techniques are useful in cases already started on antibiotics, as these affect cultures but not PCR results.[19]

Management. Start treatment with the first suspicion of sepsis. Laboratory confirmation is not required. The choice of initial antibiotic coverage varies depending on geographic region and local resistance patterns, but usually includes ampicillin and gentamicin. An alternative regimen is ampicillin and cefotaxime, but cefotaxime-resistant strains are emerging rapidly. Identification of an organism leads to specific therapy. *L. monocytogenes* is particularly resistant to cephalosporins.

Ampicillin and cefotaxime are used to treat *E. coli*, penicillin or ampicillin treats GBS, and cefotaxime and an aminoglycoside treat *Klebsiella pneumoniae*. *Pseudomonas* is difficult to eradicate, and combined intravenous and intrathecal therapy may be required. For late-onset meningitis and concern for nosocomial infections, add vancomycin or a carbapenem.

The duration of treatment for neonatal meningitis is not definitively determined but is at least 14–21 days depending on the organism. Persistently abnormal CSF values should raise suspicion for abscess or empyema.

The type of infecting organism and the gestational age of the infant are the main variables that determine mortality. Mortality has decreased; however, permanent neurological sequelae occur in 30%–50% of survivors, including hydrocephalus, cerebral palsy, epilepsy, cognitive impairment, and deafness. Even when the head circumference is normal, exclusion of hydrocephalus requires ultrasound or MRI evaluation.

Meningitis in Infants and Young Children

For children 6 weeks to 3 months old, GBS remains a leading cause of meningitis, and *E. coli* is less common. The other important organism is *Neisseria meningitidis*. *Haemophilus influenzae*, which had been an important pathogen after 3 months of age, had almost disappeared because of routine immunization, but is now reemerging due to the increasing prevalence of vaccine refusal. *Streptococcus pneumoniae* and *N. meningitidis* are now the principal causes of meningitis in children older than 1 month. For unknown reasons the incidence of *N. meningitidis* started declining after its peak in 1990.

This decline started before the introduction of a vaccine, which is now available for children older than 6 weeks. The vaccine is recommended for all adolescents 11–18 years old and younger children at higher risk of meningococcal disease such as those with asplenia, HIV, and complement deficiency.[20]

Clinical features. The onset of meningitis may be insidious or fulminating. The typical clinical findings include fever, irritability, and neck stiffness. A bulging fontanelle is a feature in young infants. After the fontanelle closes, headache, vomiting, and lethargy are initial features. Seizures occur in about one-third of children with meningitis. They usually occur during the first 24 hours of illness and often bring the child to medical attention. When seizures occur, the state of consciousness declines. Seizures can be focal or secondary generalized, and often difficult to control.

Examination reveals a sick and irritable child who resists being touched or moved. Ophthalmoscopic findings are usually normal or show only minimal disk edema. Focal neurological signs are unusual except in tuberculous meningitis or in cases in which abscess formation has occurred.

The rapidity with which neurological function declines depends on the severity of cerebral edema and cerebral vasculitis. Death may ensue from brainstem compression caused by transtentorial herniation. Peripheral vascular collapse can result from brainstem herniation, endotoxic shock, or adrenal failure. Of children with meningococcemia, 60% have a characteristic petechial or hemorrhagic rash. The rash, although generalized, is most prominent below the waist.

Meningeal irritation causes neck stiffness, characterized by limited mobility and pain on attempted flexion of the head. With the child supine, meningeal irritation is tested. Pain and resistance to extending the knee with the leg flexed at the hip is the Kernig sign. Spontaneous flexion at the hips when passively flexing the neck is the Brudzinski sign. These signs of meningeal irritation occur with subarachnoid hemorrhage and infectious meningitis. The signs of meningeal irritation are rare below the age of 6 months.

Diagnosis. Lumbar puncture and examination of the CSF are essential for the diagnosis of bacterial meningitis. Because bacterial meningitis is often associated with septicemia; the blood, urine, and nasopharynx are also cultured. The peripheral white blood cell count, especially immature granulocytes, is usually increased.

Peripheral leukocytosis is much more common in bacterial than in viral infections but does not rule out viral meningitis. Take note of the platelet count, as some infections are associated with thrombocytopenia. Proper evaluation of the CSF concentration of glucose requires a concurrent measure of the blood glucose concentration. The diagnosis of the syndrome of inappropriate antidiuretic hormone secretion (SIADH) requires measurement of serum electrolytes, especially sodium. SIADH occurs in most patients with acute bacterial meningitis. Every child at risk for tuberculous meningitis requires a tuberculin skin test.

Perform lumbar puncture as quickly as possible when bacterial meningitis is suspected. At times meningitis can present with prominent symptoms of increased ICP, necessitating head imaging before obtaining a lumbar puncture. If the need for head imaging significantly delays lumbar puncture, obtain blood cultures and initiate antimicrobial therapy. Generalized, mild to moderately increased ICP is always part of acute bacterial meningitis and is not a contraindication to lumbar puncture.

Information derived from lumbar puncture includes opening and closing pressures, appearance, white blood cell count with differential count, red blood cell count, concentrations of glucose and protein, identification of microorganisms as shown by Gram stain and culture, and PCRs. The characteristic findings are increased pressure, a cloudy appearance, a cellular response of several thousand polymorphonuclear leukocytes, a reduction in the concentration of glucose to less than half of that in the plasma, and an elevated protein concentration. The expected findings of bacterial meningitis may vary, however, with the organism, the timing of the lumbar puncture, the prior use of antibiotics, and the immunocompetence of the host. The Gram stain and PCR are particularly valuable when tapping a child already on antibiotics, which should be a priority when suspecting bacterial meningitis.

Management. Administer antimicrobials immediately. Do not delay treatment until after obtaining the results of the lumbar puncture. Vancomycin and a third-generation cephalosporin are the initial treatment of meningitis. The final choice awaits the results of culture and antibiotic sensitivity.

The outcome for infants and children with bacterial meningitis depends on the infecting organism and the speed of initiating appropriate antibiotic therapy. Ten percent of children have persistent bilateral or unilateral hearing loss after bacterial meningitis and 4% have neurological deficits. The incidence of hearing loss is 31% after infection with *S. pneumoniae* and 6% after infection with *H. influenzae*. Hearing loss occurs early and probably is not related to the choice of antibiotic. Children with neurological deficits are at risk for epilepsy.

Meningitis in School-Age Children

S. pneumoniae accounts for most cases of bacterial meningitis in previously healthy school-age children in the United States, whereas *Mycobacterium tuberculosis* is a leading cause of meningitis worldwide. Both *H. influenzae* type b and *N. meningitidis* have a much lower incidence. The symptoms of bacterial meningitis in school-age children do not differ substantially from the symptoms encountered in preschool children (see previous section on "Clinical Features" and "Treatment"). In one retrospective study of children treated for bacterial meningitis in the 1980s 8.5% had major neurological deficits (cognitive impairment, seizures, hydrocephalus, cerebral palsy, blindness, or hearing loss) and 18.5% had learning disabilities.[21] Vancomycin and a third-generation cephalosporin are recommended.

Special Circumstances

Pneumococcus. Conditions associated with pneumococcal meningitis are otitis media, cochlear implants, HIV, and sickle cell disease. Children with asplenia and chronic illnesses benefit the most from the pneumococcal conjugate vaccine, which is now part of the recommended vaccination for children older than 2 months in the United States. Penicillin G and ampicillin are equally effective in treating meningitis caused by penicillin-sensitive strains of *S. pneumoniae*. Vancomycin is part of the treatment because of the frequent occurrence of bacteria resistant to penicillin and ceftriaxone.

The incidence of pneumococcal infection before the pneumococcal vaccine in children less than 5 years included 5,000,000 cases of otitis media, 13,000 cases of bacteremia without other known sites of infection, 700 cases of meningitis, and 200 deaths per year in the United States. Based on available clinical trials, the vaccine is expected to have a significant impact similar to the one seen with *Haemophilus* and *Meningococcus* vaccines.[22]

Meningococcus. Children with complement deficiency, HIV, or asplenia require immunization for meningococcus. All household members who may have had saliva exchange contact also require prophylaxis for meningococcal meningitis. A 2-day course of oral rifampin is prescribed, 10 mg/kg every 12 hours for children 1 month to 12 years old, and 5 mg/kg every 12 hours for infants younger than 1 month old. A single 500 mg dose of ciprofloxacin can be used in older adolescents. Intramuscular ceftriaxone (125 mg for children and 250 mg for adults) is another alternative.

Tuberculous Meningitis. Worldwide, tuberculosis remains a leading cause of morbidity and death in children. In the United States tuberculosis accounts for less than 5% of bacterial meningitis cases in children, but it occurs with higher frequency where sanitation is poor and in children who have recently traveled to or emigrated from countries in which infection is endemic. The use of tuberculin skin testing has limited use in children who received vaccinations in their country of origin; a positive purified protein derivative in these cases may reflect immunity rather than active disease. Infection of children follows inhalation of the organism from adults. Tuberculosis occurs first in the lungs and then disseminates to other organs within 6 months.

Clinical features. The peak incidence of tuberculous meningitis is between 6 months and 2 years. The first symptoms tend to be more insidious than with other bacterial meningitides, but they sometimes progress in a fulminating fashion. Tuberculous meningitis, in contrast to fungal meningitis, is not a cause of chronic meningitis. If not treated, a child with tuberculous meningitis dies within 3–5 weeks.

Most often fever develops first, and the child becomes listless and irritable. Headache may cause irritability. Vomiting and abdominal pain are sometimes associated symptoms. Headache and vomiting become increasingly frequent and severe. Signs of meningismus develop during the second week after the onset of fever. Cerebral infarction occurs in 30%–40% of affected children. Seizures may occur early, but more often they occur after meningismus is established. Consciousness declines progressively, and focal neurological deficits are noted. The most common are cranial neuropathies and hemiparesis. Disk edema occurs relatively early in the course.

Diagnosis. Consider the diagnosis of tuberculosis in any child with an affected household contact. The general use of tuberculin skin testing in children is crucial to early detection but is unreliable in children who have received vaccination. In the early stages children with tuberculous meningitis may have only fever. The peripheral white blood cell count generally is elevated (10,000–20,000 cells/mm^3). Hyponatremia and hypochloremia are frequently present because of SIADH. The CSF is usually cloudy and increased in pressure. The leukocyte count in the CSF may range from 10 to 250 cells/mm^3 and rarely exceeds 500 cells/mm^3, with a lymphocytic predominance. The glucose concentration declines throughout the course of the illness and is generally less than 35 mg/dL (<1.8 mmol/L). Conversely, the protein concentration increases steadily and is usually greater than 100 mg/dL (>1 g/L).

Smears of CSF stained by the acid-fast technique generally show the bacillus, if obtained from large CSF samples prepared by centrifuge. Recovery of the organism from the CSF is not always successful even when guinea pig inoculation is used. Newer diagnostic tests include a PCR technique with reported sensitivities of 70%–75% and enzyme-linked immunosorbent assay and radioimmunoassay tests for antimycobacterial antigens in the CSF.

Management. Early treatment enhances the prognosis for survival and for neurological recovery. A positive skin test is a reason to initiate isoniazid therapy in an asymptomatic child. However, immigrants from endemic areas may test positive as they often have been immunized against tuberculosis. Complete neurological recovery is unlikely when the child becomes comatose. Mortality rates of 20% are recorded even when treatment is initiated early.

The standard treatment now consists of a 2-month induction phase with at least isoniazid, rifampin, and pyrazinamide, followed by a 4-month consolidation phase with at least isoniazid and rifampin.[23] The recommended initial drug regimen for treatment of tuberculous meningitis in the first 2 months is isoniazid 20 mg/kg/day orally up to 500 mg/day, rifampin 15 mg/kg/day orally up to 600 mg/day, and pyrazinamide 30 mg/kg/day. Continue isoniazid and rifampin therapy for an additional 4 months. The use of corticosteroids is appropriate to reduce inflammation and cerebral edema.

Communicating hydrocephalus is a common complication of tuberculous meningitis because of impaired reabsorption of CSF. Periodic CT or MRI assessment of ventricular size is routine and specifically indicated when mental function deteriorates. Before the infection is controlled, treatment of communicating hydrocephalus is by repeated lumbar punctures and acetazolamide. In many cases obstructive hydrocephalus develops later; in these cases a surgical shunt is required.

Brain Abscess

The common predisposing factors to pyogenic brain abscess in children are meningitis, chronic otitis media, sinusitis, and congenital heart disease. Brain abscesses in the newborn are usually the result of meningitis caused by *C. diversus*, *C. sakazakii*, and other species of Enterobacteriaceae. Pyogenic abscesses may occur in children younger than 5 months but are rare in older age groups and usually occur in children with hydrocephalus and shunt infection. The organisms most often responsible are *Staphylococcus* species. After 5 months of age, the infecting organisms are diverse, and many abscesses contain a mixed flora. Coagulase-positive *S. aureus* and anaerobic *Streptococcus* are the organisms most frequently recovered.

Clinical features. The clinical features of brain abscess are similar to those of any other space-occupying lesion and depend on the age of the child along with the location and size of the mass. A period of cerebritis, characterized by fever, headache, and lethargy, precedes encapsulation of the abscess. Seizures also may occur, but in the absence of seizures, the initial symptoms may not be severe enough to arouse suspicion of cerebral infection. If the period of cerebritis is not recognized, the initial clinical manifestations are the same as those of other mass lesions. Infants have abnormal head growth, a bulging fontanelle, failure to thrive, and sometimes seizures. Older children show signs of increased ICP and focal neurological dysfunction. Fever is present in only 60% of cases, and meningeal irritation is relatively uncommon. Based on clinical features alone, pyogenic brain abscess is difficult to separate from other mass lesions, such as brain tumor. About 80% of abscesses are in the cerebral hemispheres. Hemiparesis, hemianopia, and seizures are the usual clinical features. Cerebellar abscess most often results from chronic otitis and is manifest as nystagmus and ataxia.

Diagnosis. The combination of headache and disk edema, with or without focal neurological dysfunction, suggests the possibility of a mass lesion and calls for neuroimaging. Most abscesses appear on CT as an area of decreased density surrounded by a rim of intense enhancement referred to as a ring lesion. This lesion, although characteristic, is not diagnostic. Malignant brain tumors may have a similar appearance. Ring enhancement occurs during the late stages of cerebritis, just before capsule formation. After the capsule forms, the diameter of the ring decreases and the center becomes more hypodense. Multiple abscesses may be present.

Management. The development of neuroimaging has altered the management of cerebral abscess. Previously surgical drainage was immediate on diagnosis of abscess formation. Antimicrobials are the initial therapy now even for encapsulated abscesses, with progress assessed by serial scans; however, immediate drainage may be indicated depending on the size of the abscess, mass effect, and the clinical appearance of the patient.

The initial step in treatment is to reduce brain swelling using corticosteroids. Follow the steroids with a broad-spectrum antibiotic regimen, which typically includes a third-generation cephalosporin and metronidazole. Consider vancomycin if the patient has a history of penetrating trauma or recent neurosurgery. Metronidazole covers penicillin-resistant anaerobes and is important if the source of infection is suspected to be the oral cavity or sinuses. Cefepime can treat gram-negative aerobic organisms such as *Pseudomonas*. Patients who are immune compromised may require additional empiric coverage; identification of a specific organism by culture of CSF or blood allows specific antimicrobial therapy. If medical therapy does not resolve the abscess, surgical drainage is necessary. Large abscesses (>2.5 cm diameter) respond poorly to antibiotic treatment alone and typically require surgical drainage and a prolonged antibiotic course.

Subdural and Epidural Empyema

Meningitis in infants and sinusitis in older children are the most common factors causing infection in the subdural space. The subdural space is sterile in children with bacterial meningitis, but contamination may occur when a subdural tap occurs before sterilizing the subarachnoid space with antibiotics. In older children the usual cause of subdural and epidural abscesses is penetrating head injuries or chronic mastoiditis. Infections of the subdural space are difficult to contain and may extend over an entire hemisphere.

Clinical features. Subdural empyema produces increased ICP because of mass effect, cerebral edema, and vasculitis. Vasculitis leads to thrombosis of cortical veins resulting in focal neurological dysfunction and increased ICP. Children with subdural infections have headache, fever, vomiting, seizures, and states of decreasing consciousness. Unilateral and alternating hemiparesis are common.

Diagnosis. Suspect subdural empyema in children with meningitis whose condition declines after an initial period of recovery or in children who continue to have increased ICP of uncertain cause. Examination of the CSF may not be helpful, but the usual abnormality is a mixed cellular response, generally less than 100 cells/mm^3 and with a lymphocytic predominance. The glucose concentration is normal, and the protein concentration is only mildly elevated.

CT is particularly helpful in showing a subdural or epidural abscess. The infected collection appears as a lens-shaped mass of increased lucency just beneath the skull. A shift of midline structures is generally present. In infants subdural puncture provides an abscess specimen for identification of the organism. Subdural puncture also drains much of the abscess.

Management. The treatment of subdural or epidural empyema requires corticosteroids to decrease ICP, antimicrobials to eradicate the organisms, and anticonvulsants for seizures. Medical therapy and CT to monitor progress may replace surgical drainage of subdural empyema in some situations.

Fungal Infections

Fungi exist in two forms: molds and yeasts. Molds are filamentous and divided into segments by hyphae. Yeasts are unicellular organisms surrounded by a thick cell wall and sometimes a capsule. Several fungi exist as yeast in tissue but are filamentous when grown in culture. Such fungi are dimorphic. Box 4.7 lists common

---

BOX 4.7   Common Fungal Pathogens

Yeast Forms
- *Candida*
- *Cryptococcus neoformans*

Dimorphic Forms
- *Blastomyces dermatitidis*
- *Coccidioides immitis*
- *Histoplasma capsulatum*

Mold Forms
- *Aspergillus*

fungal pathogens. Fungal infections of the CNS system may cause an acute, subacute, or chronic meningitis; solitary or multiple abscesses; and granulomas. Fungal infections of the nervous system are most common in children who are immunosuppressed. Fungal infections also occur in immunocompetent children.

Cryptococcus neoformans and *Coccidioides immitis* are the leading causes of fungal meningitis in immunocompetent children. Among clinically recognized fungal CNS disease, *Cryptococcus* and *Candida* infections are the most common, followed by *Coccidioides*, *Aspergillus*, and *Zygomycetes*. Other fungi rarely involve the CNS.

Candidal Meningoencephalitis

Candida is a common inhabitant of the mouth, vagina, and intestinal tract. Ordinarily it causes no symptoms; however, *Candida* can multiply and become an important pathogen in immunosuppressed children taking multiple antibiotics, children with debilitating diseases, transplant recipients, and critically ill neonates undergoing treatment with long-term vascular catheters. The most common sites of infection are the mouth (thrush), skin, and vagina. Candidal meningitis is almost unheard of in healthy, nonhospitalized children.

Clinical features. *Candida* reaches the brain and other organs by vascular dissemination. The brain is involved less often than other organs, and fever, lethargy, and vomiting are the prominent features. Hepatosplenomegaly and arthritis may be present.

Cerebral involvement can be in the form of meningitis, abscess formation, or both. The clinical features of meningoencephalitis are fever, vomiting, meningismus, disk edema, and seizures leading to states of decreased consciousness. In some individuals a single large cerebral abscess forms that causes focal neurological dysfunction and disk edema.

Diagnosis. Suspect cerebral *Candida* infection when unexplained fever develops in children with risk factors for disseminated disease. The organism can be isolated from blood, joint effusion fluid, or CSF. When meningitis is present, a predominantly neutrophilic response is present in the CSF associated with a protein concentration that is generally 100 mg/dL (1 g/L). Reduction of the glucose concentration is small. Children who have a candidal abscess rather than meningitis are likely to have normal or near-normal CSF. CT reveals a mass lesion resembling a pyogenic abscess or tumor.

Management. When a candidal infection develops in a child because of an indwelling vascular catheter, remove the catheter. Treat with amphotericin B and flucytosine, which have a synergistic effect. Dosages are the same as for other fungal infections; administer the drugs for 6–12 weeks, depending on the efficacy of therapy and the presence of adverse reactions.[24]

Coccidioidomycosis

C. immitis is endemic in the San Joaquin Valley of California and all southwestern states. Inhalation is the route of infection, and almost 90% of individuals become infected within 10 years of moving into an endemic area. Only 40% of patients become symptomatic; the other 60% are positive only by skin test.

Clinical features. Malaise, fever, cough, myalgia, and chest pain follow respiratory infection. The pulmonary infection is self-limiting. The incidence of fungal dissemination from the lung to other organs is 1:400. The dissemination rate is considerably higher in infants than in older children and adults.

The usual cause of coccidioidal meningitis is hematogenous spread from the lung to meninges, but sometimes meningitis occurs by direct extension after infection of the skull. Symptoms of meningitis develop 2–4 weeks after respiratory symptoms begin. The main features are headache, apathy, and confusion. These symptoms may persist for weeks or months without concurrent seizures, meningismus, or focal neurological disturbances. If the meningitis becomes chronic, hydrocephalus eventually develops because the basilar meningitis prevents the reabsorption of CSF.

Diagnosis. Suspect coccidioidal meningitis in patients living in endemic areas when headache develops after an acute respiratory infection. Skin hypersensitivity among individuals living in an endemic area is not helpful, because a large percentage of the population is exposed, and they have a skin test positive for the organism. The CSF generally shows increased pressure, and the lymphocytic cellular response is 50–500 cells/mm³. Often, eosinophils also are present. The protein concentration ranges from 100 to 500 mg/dL (1–5 g/L), and the glucose concentration is less than 35 mg/dL (<1.8 mmol/L).

In *C. immitis* meningitis CSF culture is often negative and serological tests may be more useful. Complement-fixing antibody titers above 1:32 or 1:64 are significant. In early infection serology is positive in 70% of patients and increases to 100% in later stages of untreated coccidioidal meningitis.

Management. The introduction of amphotericin B drastically decreased the mortality rate for coccidioidal meningitis, but it is difficult to administer (it must be given both intravenously and intrathecally) and has significant associated morbidity. The introduction of azole therapies such as fluconazole 7 has not improved survival rates but has decreased the side effect burden and is now the recommended treatment.[25]

Cryptococcal Meningitis

Birds, especially pigeons, carry *C. neoformans* and disseminate it widely in soil. Acquisition of human infection is by inhalation. Dissemination is blood borne, but the CNS is a favorite target, causing subacute and chronic meningoencephalitis.

Clinical features. Cryptococcal meningitis is uncommon before age 10, and perhaps only 10% of cases occur before age 20. Male infection rates are greater than female rates. Most children with cryptococcal meningitis are immunosuppressed.

The first symptoms are usually insidious; chronic headache is the major feature. The headache waxes and wanes, but eventually becomes continuous and associated with nausea, vomiting, and lethargy. Body temperature may remain normal, especially in older children and adults, but younger children often have low-grade fever. Personality and behavioral changes are relatively common. The child becomes moody, listless, and sometimes frankly psychotic. Characteristic features of increased ICP are blurred vision, diplopia, and papilledema. Seizures and focal neurological dysfunction are not early features but are signs of vasculitis, hydrocephalus, and granuloma formation.

Diagnosis. Cryptococcal meningitis is difficult to diagnose via culture. The CSF may be normal but more often shows an increased opening pressure and less than 100 cells/mm^3 lymphocytes. The protein concentration is elevated, generally greater than 100 mg/dL (>1 g/L), and the glucose concentration is less than 40 mg/dL (<2 mmol/L). The introduction of cryptococcal antigen via lateral flow assay allowed for rapid and inexpensive diagnosis in resource-poor areas and is both sensitive and specific.[26]

Management. The treatment recommended by the WHO is amphotericin B (0.7–1 mg/kg/day) and flucytosine 100 mg/kg/day. When flucytosine is not available,

fluconazole 800 mg/day may be used. If amphotericin B causes unacceptable side effects due to nephrotoxicity, use it for 5–7 days then transition to fluconazole 800 mg/day for 2 weeks. These doses are for a full-grown adolescent/adult who weighs 70 kg, and dose adjustment is needed for smaller patients.[27,28]

The toxic effects of amphotericin B include chills, fever, nausea, and vomiting. Frequent blood counts and urinalysis monitor for anemia and nephrotoxicity. Manifestations of renal impairment are the appearance of cells or casts in the urine, an elevated blood concentration of urea nitrogen, and decreased creatinine clearance. When renal impairment occurs, discontinue the drug and restart at a lower dose, or transition to fluconazole or flucytosine therapy.

Cytopenia limits the use of flucytosine. Seriously ill patients treated late in the course of the disease also should be given intrathecally administered amphotericin B and miconazole. A decline of the agglutination titer in the CSF indicates therapeutic efficacy. Periodic cranial CT or MRI monitors for the development of hydrocephalus.

Other Fungal Infections

Histoplasmosis is endemic in the central United States and causes pulmonary infection. Miliary spread is unusual. Neurological histoplasmosis may take the form of leptomeningitis, focal abscess, or multiple granulomas. Blastomycosis is primarily a disease of North America. Hematogenous spread from the lungs infects the brain. Multiple abscesses form, which give the CT appearance of metastatic disease. The cellular response in the CSF is markedly increased when fungi produce meningitis and may be normal or only mildly increased with abscess formation. Amphotericin B is the mainstay of therapy for fungal infections; the combination of itraconazole and amphotericin B treats *Histoplasma capsulatum*.

IDIOPATHIC INTRACRANIAL HYPERTENSION (PSEUDOTUMOR CEREBRI)

The term *idiopathic intracranial hypertension* (IIH) characterizes a syndrome of increased ICP, normal CSF content, and a normal brain with normal or small ventricles on brain imaging studies. IIH is a misleading term because at times the syndrome has an identifiable underlying cause as opposed to being truly idiopathic.

BOX 4.8   Causes of Intracranial Hypertension

Drugs
- Corticosteroid withdrawal
- Doxycycline
- Nalidixic acid
- Oral contraceptives
- Tetracycline
- Thyroid replacement
- Vitamin A

Systemic Disorders
- Guillain-Barré syndrome
- Iron deficiency anemia
- Leukemia
- Polycythemia vera
- Protein malnutrition
- Systemic lupus erythematosus
- Vitamin A deficiency
- Vitamin D deficiency

Head Trauma
Infections
- Otitis media (sinus thrombosis)
- Sinusitis (sinus thrombosis)

Metabolic Disorders
- Adrenal insufficiency
- Diabetic ketoacidosis (treatment)
- Galactosemia
- Hyperadrenalism
- Hyperthyroidism
- Hypoparathyroidism
- Pregnancy

Identification of a specific cause is usual in children younger than 6 years old, whereas most idiopathic cases occur after age 11 years. Box 4.8 lists some causes of IIH. An established cause-and-effect relationship is uncertain in many of these conditions. The most frequent causes are obesity and the use of certain drugs including tetracycline, doxycycline, and vitamin A derivatives.

Clinical features. The criteria for diagnosis of pseudotumor cerebri syndrome require the presence of disk edema or sixth nerve palsy as well as ICP over 28 cm of H_2O.[29] The CSF is normal and imaging does not show tumor, inflammation, or infection. Subtle signs of intracranial hypertension, such as an empty sella, cerebellar tonsillar descent, flattening of the posterior sclerae, tortuosity and distention of the subarachnoid perioptic space, protrusion of the optic nerve papillae into the vitreous, and transverse venous sinus stenosis, are frequently seen.

Patients with IIH have headaches that are diffuse, are worse at night, and often wake them from sleep in the early hours of the morning. Sudden movements, such as coughing, aggravate the headache. Headaches may be present for several months before establishing a diagnosis. Some patients complain of dizziness. Transitory loss of vision may occur with the change of position. Vision loss is common and insidious, as central vision is spared until late in the disease. Formal visual field testing may be required to identify patients with early signs of vision impairment. Prolonged disk edema may lead to significant visual loss.

Young children may have only irritability, somnolence, or apathy. Less common symptoms are transitory visual obscurations, neck stiffness, tinnitus, paresthesias, and ataxia. Most children are not acutely ill, and cognitive ability is normal.

Neurological examination is normal except for disk edema and possible abducens nerve palsy. Features of focal neurological dysfunction are lacking. Loss of vision is the main concern. Untreated IIH may lead to progressive disk edema and optic atrophy, with rapid and severe visual loss. Early diagnosis and treatment are essential to preserve vision.

Diagnosis. IIH is a diagnosis of exclusion. Brain imaging including magnetic resonance venography is required in every child with headache and papilledema to exclude a mass lesion, venous sinus thrombosis, or hydrocephalus. The results of imaging studies are usually normal in children with IIH. In some the ventricles are small, and normal sulcal markings are absent. Assess visual fields, with special attention to the size of the blind spot, at baseline and after treatment is initiated. Exclude known underlying causes of IIH by careful history and physical examination. Ordinarily identification of an underlying cause is easily established.

Management. The goals of therapy are to relieve headache and preserve vision. A single lumbar puncture, with the closing pressure reduced to half of the opening pressure, is sufficient to reverse the process in many cases. The mechanism by which lumbar puncture is effective is unknown, but a transitory change in CSF dynamics seems sufficient to readjust the pressure. Remove any possible triggers such as vitamin A, doxycycline, and tetracycline, and address weight reduction when applicable.

The usual treatment for children with IIH is acetazolamide 10 mg/kg/day up to 500 mg three times a day, after the initial lumbar puncture. If therapeutic doses of acetazolamide cannot be tolerated due to metabolic acidosis or other adverse effects, a carbonic anhydrase inhibitor such as topiramate can be substituted, although often less effective. If symptoms return, the lumbar puncture is repeated on subsequent days. Some children require serial lumbar punctures. Severe vision loss may require urgent optic nerve sheath fenestration to preserve vision while other treatments are initiated.

Occasionally, children continue to have increased ICP and evidence of progressive optic neuropathy despite the use of lumbar puncture and acetazolamide. In such patients studies should be repeated to look for a cause other than idiopathic pseudotumor cerebri. If studies are negative, a lumboperitoneal shunt is the usual option to reduce pressure. Optic nerve fenestration relieves papilledema but does not relieve increased ICP.

REFERENCES

1. Pitfield AF, Carroll AB, Kissoon N. Emergency management of increased intracranial pressure. *Pediatric Emergency Care*. 2012;28:200-204.
2. Hutchison JS, Roxanne E, et al. for the Hypothermia Pediatric Head Injury Trial Investigators and the Canadian Critical Care Trials Group. Hypothermia therapy after traumatic brain injury in children. *New England Journal of Medicine*. 2008;358:2447-2456. https://doi.org/10.1056/NEJMoa0706930.
3. Sun MZ, Oh MC, Ivan ME, et al. Current management of choroid plexus carcinomas. *Neurosurgical Review*. 2014;37(2):179-192. https://doi.org/10.1007/s10143-013-0499-1 Epub 2013 Sep 26. PMID: 24068529.
4. Sejda A, Grajkowska W, Trubicka J, et al. WHO CNS5 2021 classification of gliomas: a practical review and road signs for diagnosing pathologists and proper pathoclinical and neuro-oncological cooperation. *Folia Neuropathologica*. 2022;60(2):137-152. https://doi.org/10.5114/fn.2022.118183.
5. Hauser P. Classification and treatment of pediatric gliomas in the molecular era. *Child (Basel)*. 2021;8(9):739. https://doi.org/10.3390/children8090739. PMID: 34572171; PMCID: PMC8464723.
6. Pollack IF, Gerszten PC, Martinez AJ, et al. Intracranial ependymomas of childhood: long-term outcome and prognostic factors. *Neurosurgery*. 1995;37:655-667.
7. Gajjar A, Bowers DC, Karajannis MA, et al. Pediatric brain tumors: innovative genomic information is transforming the diagnostic and clinical landscape. *Journal of Clinical Oncology*. 2015;33(27):2986-2998.
8. Mansur DB, Drzymala RE, Rich KM, et al. The efficacy of stereotactic radiosurgery in the management of intracranial ependymoma. *Journal of Neuro-Oncology*. 2004;66:187-190.
9. Merchant TE, Mulhern RK, Krasin MJ, et al. Preliminary results from a phase II trial of conformation radiation therapy and evaluation of radiation-related CNS effects for pediatric patients with localized ependymoma. *Journal of Clinical Oncology*. 2004;22:3156-3162.
10. Payne AH, Hintz SR, Hibbs AM, et al. Neurodevelopmental outcomes of extremely low gestational age neonates with low grade periventricular-intraventricular hemorrhage. *JAMA Pediatrics*. 2013;167(5):451-459.
11. Bolisetty S, Dhawan A, Abdel-Latif M, et al. on behalf of the New South Wales and Australian Capital Territory Neonatal Intensive Care Units' Data Collection Intraventricular hemorrhage and neurodevelopmental outcomes in extreme preterm infants. *Pediatrics*. 2014;133(1):55-62. https://doi.org/10.1542/peds.2013-0372.
12. Volpe JJ. *Volpe's Neurology of the Newborn*. Philadephia, PA: Elsevier; 2018.
13. Olafsson E, Hauser A, Gudmundsson G. A population-based study of prognosis of ruptured cerebral aneurysm: mortality and recurrence of subarachnoid hemorrhage. *Neurology*. 1997;48:1191-1195.
14. Anand V, Holmen J, Neely M, et al. Closing the brief case: neonatal meningitis caused by *Listeria monocytogenes* diagnosed by multiple molecular panel. *Journal of Clinical Microbiology*. 2016;54(12):3075.
15. El-Ghanem M, Kass-Hout T, Kass-Hout O, et al. Arteriovenous malformations in the pediatric population: review of the existing literature. *Interventional Neurology*. 2016;5(3-4):218-225. https://doi.org/10.1159/000447605. Epub 2016 Sep 1. PMID: 27781052; PMCID: PMC5075815.
16. Meyers PM, Halbach VV, Phatouros CP, et al. Hemorrhagic complications in vein of Galen malformations. *Annals of Neurology*. 2000;47:748-755.
17. El-Ghanem M, Kass-Hout T, Kass-Hout O, et al. Arteriovenous malformations in the pediatric population: review of the existing literature. *Interventional Neurology*. 2016;5(3-4):218-225. https://doi.org/10.1159/000447605. Epub 2016 Sep 1. PMID: 27781052; PMCID: PMC5075815.
18. Nicholson BA. *Genomic Epidemiology and Characterization of Neonatal Meningitis Escherichia coli and Their Virulence Plasmids*. Graduate theses and dissertations. Iowa State University; 2015. http://lib.dr.iastate.edu/etd/14936.
19. Wang Y, Guo G, Yang X, et al. Comparative study of bacteriological culture and real-time fluorescence

quantitative PCR (RT-PCR) and multiplex PCR-based reverse line blot (mPCR/RLB) hybridization assay in the diagnosis of bacterial neonatal meningitis. *BMC Pediatrics.* 2014;14:224.

20. Cohn AC, MacNeil JR, Clark TA, et al. Prevention and control of meningococcal disease. Recommendations of the Advisory Committee on Immunization Practices (ACIP). *Morbidity and Mortality Weekly Report.* 2013;62(2):1-22.

21. Grimwood K, Anderson VA, Bond L, et al. Adverse outcome of bacterial meningitis in school-age survivors. *Pediatrics.* 1995;95:646-656.

22. Centers for Disease Control and Prevention. Epidemiology and Prevention of Vaccine-Preventable Diseases. Hamborsky J, Kroger A, Wolfe S, eds. 13th ed. Public Health Foundation, 2015.

23. Hoshburg CR, Lange CB. Treatment of tuberculosis. *New England Journal of Medicine.* 2015;373:2149-2160.

24. Sanchez JL, Noskin GA. Recent advances in the management of opportunistic fungal infections. *Comprehensive Therapy.* 1996;22:703-712.

25. Johnson R, Ho J, Fowler P, Heidari A. Coccidioidal meningitis: a review on diagnosis, treatment, and management of complications. *Current Neurology and Neuroscience Reports.* 2018;18(4):19. https://doi.org/10.1007/s11910-018-0824-8. PMID: 29536184.

26. Abassi M, Boulware DR, Rhein J. Cryptococcal meningitis: diagnosis and management update. *Current Tropical Medicine Reports.* 2015;2(2):90-99. https://doi.org/10.1007/s40475-015-0046-y. PMID: 26279970; PMCID: PMC4535722.

27. Sanchez JL, Noskin GA. Recent advances in the management of opportunistic fungal infections. *Comprehensive Therapy.* 1996;22:703-712.

28. Loyse A, Thangaraj H, Eastbrook O, et al. Cryptococcal meningitis: improving access to essential antifungal medicines in resource-poor countries. *Lancet Infectious Diseases.* 2013;13(7):629-637.

29. Friedman DI, Jacobson DM. Diagnostic criteria for idiopathic intracranial hypertension. *Neurology.* 2002;59:1492-1495.

5

Psychomotor Delay and Regression

OUTLINE

Developmental Delay, 141
    Language Delay, 141
    Delayed Motor Development, 143
    Global Developmental Delay, 143
Telling Parents Bad News, 143
    Approach to the Child With Developmental Delay of Unknown Cause, 144
Static Encephalopathies, 145
    Perinatal Disorders, 145
    Cerebral Malformations, 145
    Intrauterine Infections, 145
Progressive Encephalopathies with Onset Before Age 2, 152
    Acquired Immunodeficiency Syndrome Encephalopathy, 152
    Disorders of Amino Acid Metabolism, 153

Disorders of Lysosomal Enzymes, 156
Hypothyroidism, 161
Mitochondrial Disorders, 161
Neurocutaneous Syndromes, 163
Other Disorders of Gray Matter, 166
Clinical Features in Males, 168
Other Disorders of White Matter, 169
Progressive Hydrocephalus, 171
Progressive Encephalopathies with Onset After Age 2, 171
    Disorders of Lysosomal Enzymes, 171
    Infectious Diseases, 175
    Other Disorders of Gray Matter, 175
    Other Diseases of White Matter, 178
References, 179

Psychomotor delay or developmental delay refers to the slow progress in the attainment of developmental milestones. This may be caused by either static or progressive encephalopathies. In contrast, psychomotor regression refers to the loss of developmental milestones previously attained. This is usually caused by a progressive disease of the nervous system. In some cases reports of regression may also result from parental misperception of attained milestones, or by the development of new clinical features from an established static disorder as the brain matures (Box 5.1).

DEVELOPMENTAL DELAY

Delayed achievement of developmental milestones is one of the more common problems evaluated by child neurologists. Two important questions require answers: Is developmental delay restricted to specific areas or is it global? and Is development delayed or regressing?

In infants the second question is often difficult to answer. Even in static encephalopathies new symptoms such as involuntary movements and seizures may occur as the child gets older, and delayed acquisition of milestones without other neurological deficits is sometimes the initial feature of progressive disorders. However, once it is clear that milestones previously achieved are lost or that focal neurological deficits are evolving, a progressive disease of the nervous system is a consideration.

The American Academy of Pediatrics recommends that pediatricians perform developmental and behavioral screening evaluations at 9, 18, and 30 months. In addition specific autism screens should be done at 18 and 24 months of age. Multiple formal, validated screening tools are available.

Language Delay

Infants and children have a remarkable facility for acquiring language during the first decade. Those

> **BOX 5.1   Causes of Apparent Regression in Static Encephalopathy**
>
> - Increasing spasticity (usually during the first year)
> - New onset movement disorders (usually during the second year)
> - New onset seizures
> - Parental misperception of attained milestones
> - Progressive hydrocephalus

exposed to two languages concurrently learn both. Vocalization of vowels occurs in the first month, and by 5 months, laughing and squealing are established. At 6 months, infants begin articulating consonants, usually M, D, and B. Parents translate these to mean "mama," "dada," and "bottle" or "baby," although these may not be the infant's intention. These first attempts at vowels and consonants are automatic and sometimes occur even in deaf children. In the months that follow, the infant imitates many speech sounds, babbles and coos, and finally learns the specific use of "mama" and "dada" by the age of 1. Receptive skills are always more highly developed than expressive skills because language must be decoded before it is encoded. By the age of 2, children have learned to combine at least two words, understand more than 250 words, and follow many simple verbal directions.

Developmental disturbances in the language cortex of the dominant hemisphere that occur before the age of 5, and possibly later, displace language to the contralateral hemisphere. This does not occur in older children or adults.

Autistic Spectrum Disorders

Infantile autism is not a single disorder, but rather many different disorders described by a broad behavioral phenotype that has a final common pathway of atypical development.[1] The terms *autistic spectrum disorders* (ASDs) and *pervasive developmental disorders* are used to classify the spectrum of behavioral symptoms. More than 200 autism susceptibility genes have been identified, which make chromosome microarray analysis the recommended first test for the evaluation of ASD.[2] We will discuss autism in more detail in Chapter 19 along with other neurobehavioral disorders.

Clinical features. The major diagnostic criteria are impaired sociability, impaired verbal and nonverbal communication skills, and restricted activities and interests.[3] Failure of language development is the feature most likely to bring autistic children to medical attention and correlates best with the outcome; children who fail to develop language before the age of 5 have the worst outcome. The intelligence quotient (IQ) is less than 70 in most children with autism. However, IQ may be significantly underestimated due to their impaired interactive skills, which make testing difficult and less reliable. Some autistic children show no affection to their parents or other care providers, while others are extremely affectionate on their own terms. Autistic children do not show normal play activity; some have a preoccupation with spinning objects, stereotyped behaviors such as rocking, swinging, and spinning, and relative insensitivity to pain with hypersensitivity to other non-noxious stimuli. An increased incidence of epilepsy in autistic children is probable.

Diagnosis. Infantile autism is a clinical diagnosis and not confirmable by laboratory tests. The autism diagnostic observation schedule is often administered by trained psychologists to confirm the diagnosis; however, it is not required. Infants with profound hearing impairment may display autistic behavior, and hearing tests are a required part of the workup for any child with speech delay. Electroencephalography (EEG) is indicated when seizures are suspected to evaluate for the rare possibility of Landau-Kleffner syndrome. A chromosomal microarray is often performed. The pattern of inheritance for autism is complex and likely multifactorial, which limits the use of genetic testing as a diagnostic tool. However, identifying a genetic susceptibility may be of benefit to the family by providing education and information regarding the diagnosis and prognosis, limiting further diagnostic testing, and providing information regarding the risk for the rest of the family or future pregnancies. In addition a defined diagnosis often makes it easier for the family to obtain developmental therapies and other needed treatments.

Management. Autism is not curable, but several drugs may be useful to control specific behavioral disturbance, including selective serotonin reuptake inhibitors, stimulants, centrally acting alpha-2 receptor agonists, and atypical antipsychotics (see Chapter 19). Behavioral therapy is helpful but can be difficult to obtain.

Hearing Impairment

The major cause of isolated delay in speech development is hearing impairment (see Chapter 17). Hearing loss may occur concomitantly with global developmental delay (GDD), as in rubella embryopathy, cytomegalic inclusion disease, neonatal meningitis, kernicterus, and several genetic disorders. Hearing loss needs not be profound; it can be insidious yet delay speech development. The loss of high-frequency tones, inherent in telephone conversation, prevents the clear distinction of many consonants that we learn to fill in through experience; infants do not have experience in supplying missing sounds.

The hearing of any infant with an isolated delay in speech development requires audiometric testing. Crude testing in the office by slamming objects and ringing bells is inadequate. Hearing loss is suspected in children with global delays caused by disorders ordinarily associated with hearing loss or in cognitively impaired children who fail to imitate sounds. Other clues to hearing loss in children are excessive gesturing and staring at the lips of people who are talking. Brain auditory evoked potentials offer good screening for neonatal hearing deficits. With the implementation of universal hearing screening in the United States, approximately 12,000 children with hearing impairment are identified each year. It is important to identify these children as those with profound or severe sensorineural hearing loss may benefit from cochlear implants. Implants at an early age are associated with better language and social development.[4]

Delayed Motor Development

Infants with delayed gross motor development but normal language and social skills are often hypotonic and may have a neuromuscular disease (see Chapter 6). Isolated delay in motor function is also caused by ataxia (see Chapter 10), mild hemiplegia (see Chapter 11), and mild paraplegia (see Chapter 12). Many such children have a mild form of cerebral palsy, sufficient to delay the achievement of motor milestones, but not severe enough to cause a recognizable disturbance in cognitive function during infancy. The detection of mild disturbances in cognitive function occurs more often when the child enters school. Children with benign macrocephaly may have isolated motor delay in the first 18 months as a result of the difficulty achieving adequate head control with their larger head size.

Global Developmental Delay

GDD is a consideration in children less than 6 years of age, with performance more than two standard deviations below match peers in two or more aspects of development. The incidence of GDD is about 1%–3% and many of these children have intellectual disability (ID). Most infants with GDD have a static encephalopathy caused by an antenatal or perinatal disturbance. However, 1% of infants with developmental delay and no evidence of regression have an inborn error of metabolism and 3.5%–10% have a chromosomal disorder.[5] An exhaustive search for an underlying cause in every infant whose development is slow, but not regressing, is not cost effective. Factors that increase the likelihood of finding a progressive disease include an affected family member, parental consanguinity, organomegaly, and absent tendon reflexes. Unenhanced cranial magnetic resonance imaging (MRI) and chromosome analysis/microarray are a reasonable screening test in all infants with GDD. Consider additional genetic or metabolic testing depending on the presentation.

TELLING PARENTS BAD NEWS

It is not possible to make bad news sound good or even half-bad. The primary goal of telling parents that their child will have neurological or cognitive impairment is that they hear and understand what you are saying. The mind must be prepared to hear bad news. It is a mistake to tell people more than they are ready to accept. Too often parents bring their child for a second opinion because previous doctors "didn't tell us anything." In fact they may have said too much, too fast, and the parents became overwhelmed and tuned out.

Our goal for the first visit is to establish that the child's development is not normal (i.e., not a normal variation), that something is wrong with the brain, and that we share the parents' concerns. When abnormal, review the MRI or genetic testing results with the parents to help their understanding of the problem. Unfortunately, many mothers come alone for this critical visit and must later restate your comments to doubting fathers and grandparents. Most parents cannot handle more information than "the child is not normal" at the first consultation and further discussion awaits a later visit. However, always answer probing questions fully. Parents must never lose confidence in your willingness to be forthright. The timing of the next visit depends on the age of the child and the severity of the cognitive impairment. The more the child falls behind in reaching developmental milestones, the more ready parents will be to accept the diagnosis.

When the time comes to tell a parent that their child has a developmental delay, it is not helpful to describe the deficit as mild, moderate, or severe. Parents want to know what the child will do. Will he walk, need special schools, be able to live alone? The next question is, "What can I do to help my child?" Direct them to programs that provide developmental specialists and other parents who can help them learn how to live with a child with special needs and gain access to community resources.

Providing a prognosis after a brain insult in a neonate or young infant is often difficult. Fortunately, the plasticity of the young brain may offer improved outcomes in some cases, making it difficult to provide a definite prognosis. Prognosis is often better in cases that affect only one hemisphere. In fact complete encephalomalacia of one hemisphere may be associated with better development than having a very injured but still "functional" hemisphere. In all cases we have to make families aware of the spectrum of possibilities and high probability of deficits.

Approach to the Child With Developmental Delay of Unknown Cause

The increasing availability of genetic testing has drastically altered the approach to the child with developmental delay. A search of Orphanet, an online database of rare diseases, yields nearly 2000 results when queried for "intellectual disability–related genes." If one searches the more inclusive Online Mendelian Inheritance of Man (OMIM) website, one will find nearly 3000 identified genes. These are results only for ID; if the search is for nonspecific developmental delay, the results are even more vast.

It is obvious that rote memorization of all potential genetic and metabolic syndromes is a thing of the past. However, the clinical child neurologist must have some awareness of the most common of these disorders. Perhaps more importantly, they must understand how to approach a child with developmental delays.

We begin with the following basic questions, the answers to which will guide the nature of our workup.

Does the delay encompass multiple domains or just one?

Global delays often have a different etiology than isolated delays. ID indicates the involvement of multiple brain regions. Isolated motor delays, on the other hand, may be due to discrete lesions within the central nervous system (CNS) or specific mutations affecting the function of peripheral nerves or muscles. Fine motor delays imply difficulty with coordination, praxis, motor planning, or executive dysfunction. Speech delays may be due to motor problems (apraxia, articulation difficulties), encephalopathy, executive dysfunction (decreased attention), specific neurological deficits (hearing loss, facial nerve palsy), or social deficits (autism, severe anxiety disorders, obsessive-compulsive disorders).

Is the deficit static or progressive? Has clear regression or loss of skills occurred?

A static deficit may appear progressive as the child ages and the extent of the disability becomes clear, but there is no true regression. Regression refers to the loss of previously acquired skills: the toddler who was speaking becomes mute, and the child who was running becomes clumsy and slow. Definable brain injury or malformation leads to static deficits, while progressive deficits or regression is typically due to underlying genetic or metabolic disease.

Does the child have facial dysmorphisms, multiple congenital anomalies, or involvement of other organ systems?

Cardiac, liver, and renal anomalies can be particularly relevant. The presence of epilepsy and cardiac arrhythmia may indicate a channelopathy. Mitochondrial disease can present with liver dysfunction that worsens in a stepwise pattern in conjunction with seizures or developmental regression. Retinal abnormalities can be seen in gangliosidoses, retinitis pigmentosa, and others; optic nerve hypoplasia is part of the septo-optic dysplasia sequence. Renal anomalies are found in multiple genetic disorders. Likewise, facial dysmorphisms are often subtle but, at times, provide important clues. Some disorders have distinctive facies that immediately point the clinician toward the correct diagnosis (e.g., trisomy 21). Hypotelorism can be seen with midline defects; cleft lip and palate are associated with certain trisomies and agenesis of the corpus callosum.

Does the child have social or behavioral abnormalities?

Keep in mind that multiple developmental disabilities can initially present as autism and the diagnosis of autism should not preclude further workup, especially if deficits are global or progressive. Severe anxiety or obsessive-compulsive disorder can present with speech delays. Intelligent and anxious infants sometimes refuse to walk because they realize they might fall and injure themselves.

Does the child have epilepsy?

Dravet syndrome, Lennox-Gastaut syndrome, Aicardi syndrome, and other epileptic encephalopathies are associated with progressive and profound developmental disabilities. Landau-Kleffner causes epileptic aphasia that presents as language regression. Any sufficiently active epilepsy can cause apparent ID; the brain that is constantly seizing cannot learn new skills.

Were there any complications during the pregnancy or delivery?

A traumatic birth requiring extensive resuscitation is an obvious clue as to the potential cause of the delays. Ask about amniotic fluid levels (e.g., oligohydramnios), intrauterine growth restriction, abnormal fetal movements, and any abnormal findings on prenatal ultrasound. Importantly, there are technical limitations to the prenatal head ultrasound and any suspicious findings should be confirmed with fetal MRI or MRI after birth.

What is the family history?

This question requires a certain amount of perseverance and tact. Many genetic abnormalities have incomplete or variable penetrance resulting in a wide variety of phenotypes even within the same family. We ask if anyone in the family has or had developmental delays, learning differences, seizures, speech problems, abnormal movements, or mental health problems. If the child has siblings, obtain their developmental histories as well. Specifically ask if the mother or father received special education services in school (such parents frequently do not self-report as intellectually disabled, but readily admit to needing special classes). Inquire whether the mother has ever suffered a miscarriage, and if so, how many and at what point in the pregnancy. Some X-linked disorders are lethal in a male fetus but result in an intellectually disabled female child.

STATIC ENCEPHALOPATHIES

Static encephalopathies are typically present from birth. Although they are nonprogressive, symptoms continue to evolve as the child ages. Disorders associated with epilepsy may have regression in the setting of poor seizure control; however, regression is not an integral part of the disorder.

Perinatal Disorders

Perinatal infection, asphyxia, maternal drug use, and trauma are the main perinatal events that cause psychomotor delays (see Chapter 1). The important infectious diseases are bacterial meningitis (see Chapter 4) and herpes encephalitis (see Chapter 1). Although the overall mortality rate for bacterial meningitis has improved, many survivors show significant neurological disturbances almost immediately. Cognitive and motor disabilities, hydrocephalus, epilepsy, deafness, and visual loss are the most common sequelae. ID may be the only or the most prominent sequelae. Progressive mental deterioration can occur if meningitis causes secondary hydrocephalus.

Cerebral Malformations

Retrospective reviews have shown the incidence of CNS malformations diagnosed on prenatal ultrasound to be approximately 0.3%.[6] Neural tube defects are the most common malformation, occurring in 1–2 of every 1000 births. Many intrauterine diseases also cause destructive changes that cause malformation of the developing brain. The exposure of an embryo to infectious or toxic agents during the first weeks after conception can disorganize the delicate sequencing of neural development at a time when the brain is incapable of generating a cellular response (see the "Intrauterine Infections" section). Alcohol, lead, prescription drugs, and substances of abuse are factors in the production of cerebral malformations. Various genetic and metabolic disorders can cause malformations such as agenesis of the corpus callosum, heterotopia, or lissencephaly.

Suspect a cerebral malformation in any cognitively impaired child who is dysmorphic, has malformations of other organs, or has an abnormality of head size and shape (see Chapter 18). MRI is the preferred imaging modality due to its greater sensitivity in detecting migration defects and other subtle anomalies.

Intrauterine Infections

The most common intrauterine infections are human immunodeficiency virus (HIV) and cytomegalovirus (CMV). HIV infection can occur in utero, but acquisition of most infections occurs perinatally. Infected infants are asymptomatic in the newborn period and later develop progressive disease of the brain. Rubella embryopathy has almost disappeared because of the mass immunization but reappears when immunization rates decline. Varicella crosses the placenta and can cause fetal demise, microcephaly, or ID. The Zika virus (ZIKV) has emerged as an increasingly prevalent cause of cerebral malformations, microcephaly, and neonatal seizures.

Congenital syphilis. In the United States rates of congenital syphilis decreased from the year 2008 to 2012 but have since risen drastically. In 2019 the rate was 48.5 cases per 100,000 live births, a shocking 477% increase since 2012. Maternal risk factors for syphilis include illicit drug use, incarceration, housing instability, poverty, and transactional sexual activity.

Clinical features. Infection of the fetus is transplacental. Two-thirds of infected newborns are asymptomatic and identified only on screening tests. The more common features in symptomatic newborns and infants are hepatosplenomegaly, periostitis, osteochondritis, pneumonia (pneumonia alba), persistent rhinorrhea (snuffles), and a maculopapular rash that can involve the palms and soles. If left untreated, the classic stigmata of Hutchinson teeth, saddle nose, interstitial keratitis, saber shins, cognitive impairment, hearing loss, and hydrocephalus develop.

The onset of neurological disturbances usually begins after the age of 2 and includes eighth-nerve deafness and cognitive impairment. The combination of nerve deafness, interstitial keratitis, and peg-shaped upper incisors is the *Hutchinson triad.*

Diagnosis. Syphilis screening is typically performed as part of routine prenatal care. All newborns to a mother with reactive nontreponemal (rapid plasma reagin, Venereal Disease Research Laboratory [VDRL]) and treponemal test results should be evaluated with a quantitative nontreponemal serological test performed on the neonate's serum. Cerebrospinal fluid (CSF) should be obtained for VDRL, cell count, and protein to address the question of neurosyphilis. CSF is abnormal in about 10% of asymptomatically infected infants. Suspect concomitant HIV infection in every child with congenital syphilis.

Management. The Centers for Disease Control and Prevention (CDC) recommends one of two regimens for treatment of an infant born to a woman with any stages of syphilis, who has not received appropriate treatment during gestation, or for whom the possibility of congenital syphilis cannot be ruled out: (1) aqueous crystalline penicillin G 100,000–150,000 units/kg/day administered intravenously every 12 hours at a dose of 50,000 units/kg/dose during the first 7 days of life and every 8 hours thereafter for a total of 10 days, or (2) procaine penicillin G 50,000 units/kg/dose intramuscular in a single daily dose for 10 days up to the adult maximum dose of 2.4 million units/dose. Consultation with an infectious disease specialist is advised.

Cytomegalovirus infection. CMV is a member of the herpes virus group and produces a chronic infection characterized by long periods of latency punctuated by intervals of reactivation. CMV is the most common congenital viral infection worldwide (0.2%–2.5% of all live births) and results from primary maternal infection more than from reactivation of the virus in the mother. The seroprevalence of CMV in developing countries is 90%. Congenital CMV is also the most common cause of nonhereditary hearing loss.[7] Pregnancy may cause reactivation of maternal infection. Risks to the fetus are greatest during the first half of gestation. Fortunately, less than 0.05% of newborns with viruria have symptoms of cytomegalic inclusion disease.

Clinical features. Approximately 10%–15% of infected newborns are symptomatic. Clinical manifestations include intrauterine growth retardation, jaundice, petechiae/purpura, hepatosplenomegaly, microcephaly, hydrocephaly, intracerebral calcifications, glaucoma, seizures, and chorioretinitis. Except for the brain, most organ involvement is self-limited.

Migrational defects (lissencephaly, polymicrogyria, and cerebellar agenesis) are the main consequence of fetal infection during the first trimester (Box 5.2). Some infants have microcephaly secondary to intrauterine infection without evidence of systemic infection at birth.

Diagnosis. The virus must be isolated within the first 3 weeks of life to confirm congenital infection. Afterwards virus shedding no longer differentiates congenital from postnatal infection. Although CMV can be isolated from many sites, urine and saliva are preferred samples for congenital CMV infection because

---

BOX 5.2 Examples of Disorders Associated With Cerebral Dysgenesis

- Infectious
  - Cytomegalovirus
  - Chorionic lymphocytic choriomeningitis
  - Toxoplasmosis
- Genetic
  - *GRIN2B* disorders
  - *GRIN1* disorders
  - Coffin-Siris syndrome
  - Disorders of congenital disorders of glycosylation (PMM2-CDG)

of their viral content. For these samples, a technique using monoclonal antibodies to detect CMV is diagnostic. Detection of CMV DNA by polymerase chain reaction (PCR) or in situ hybridization of tissues and fluids is also available. Infected newborns should be isolated from females of childbearing age.

In infants with developmental delay and microcephaly, establishing the diagnosis of cytomegalic inclusion disease is by serological demonstration of prior infection and a consistent pattern of intracranial calcification.

Management. Much of the brain damage from congenital CMV occurs in utero; however, the use of ganciclovir orally at a dose of 16 mg/kg divided twice daily, modestly improved hearing and developmental outcomes when given to affected newborns for 6 months postnatally.[8]

Congenital lymphocytic choriomeningitis.

Clinical features. The lymphocytic choriomeningitis virus (LCMV) causes minor respiratory symptoms when inhaled, and it frequently is entirely asymptomatic. Common house mice are the vector, and an estimated 2%–5% of adults have antibodies to the virus. However, the CDC recognizes fetal infection as a common and likely underreported cause of multiple CNS malformations, particularly hydrocephaly. Other sequelae include migrational abnormalities, microcephaly, periventricular calcifications, pachygyria, and periventricular or porencephalic cysts. Eye findings may include chorioretinal lacunae, panretinal pigment epithelium atrophy, optic nerve hypoplasia, and reduced caliber of retinal vessels.[9]

LCMV is a common cause of hydrocephalus. Up to one-third of newborns with hydrocephalus have positive serology to LCMV, and conversely almost 90% of children with serologically confirmed perinatal infection with LCMV have hydrocephalus. Almost 40% have hydrocephalus at birth; the remainder develop it over the first 3 months of age. Blindness and ID are potential long-term complications. Outcome severity depends on the timing of infection; early infection produces the worse outcomes.

Diagnosis. Imaging of the brain reveals major malformations. Viral culture of blood, CSF, and urine are diagnostic. Immunofluorescent antibody tests or enzyme-linked immunosorbent assays are currently available for serum and CSF. PCR for detection of LCMV RNA in urine, CSF, and serum is possible. Infections in older immunocompetent children are usually asymptomatic or a minor febrile illness, but meningoencephalitis may occur in the immunocompromised.[10]

Management. Much of the brain damage from congenital LCMV occurs in utero and is not influenced by postnatal treatment.

Rubella embryopathy.
The rubella virus is a small, enveloped RNA virus with worldwide distribution. It is responsible for an endemic mild exanthematous disease of childhood (German measles). Major epidemics in which significant numbers of adults are exposed and infected continue to occur with some regularity; however, the incidence of rubella embryopathy in the United States has steadily declined with introduction of the rubella vaccine.

Clinical features. Rubella embryopathy is a multisystem disease characterized by intrauterine growth restriction, cataracts, chorioretinitis, congenital heart disease, sensorineural deafness, hepatosplenomegaly, jaundice, anemia, thrombocytopenia, and rash. Eighty percent of children with congenital rubella syndrome have nervous system involvement. The neurological features are bulging fontanelle, lethargy, hypotonia, and seizures. Seizure onset is from birth to 3 months of age.

Diagnosis. To provide accurate counseling, make every effort to confirm rubella infection in the exposed pregnant woman. The diagnosis is established the best by documenting rubella-specific immunoglobulin M (IgM) antibody in addition to a fourfold or greater rise in rubella-specific immunoglobulin G (IgG).

Management. Prevention is by immunization and avoiding possible exposure during pregnancy. The treatment is not available for active infection in the newborn.

Toxoplasmosis.
Toxoplasma gondii is a protozoan estimated to infect 1 per 1000 live births in the United States each year. The symptoms of toxoplasmosis infection in the mother usually go unnoticed. Transplacental transmission of toxoplasmosis is possible in situations of primary maternal infection during pregnancy or in immunocompromised mothers who have chronic or recurrent infection. The rate of placental transmission is highest during the last trimester, but fetuses infected at that time are least likely to have symptoms. Conversely, the transmission rate is lowest during the first trimester, but fetuses infected at that time have the most serious sequelae.

Clinical features. One-quarter of infected newborns have multisystem involvement (fever, rash, hepatosplenomegaly, jaundice, and thrombocytopenia) at birth. Neurological dysfunction is manifest as seizures, altered states of consciousness, and increased intracranial pressure. The triad of hydrocephalus, chorioretinitis, and intracranial calcification is the hallmark of congenital toxoplasmosis in older children. About 8% of infected newborns who are asymptomatic at birth later show neurological sequelae, especially developmental delay.

Diagnosis. Detection of the organism is diagnostic, as are commercially available serological techniques. Presume any patient with positive IgG and IgM titers to be recently infected. The sensitivity of CSF PCR is only about 50%.[11]

The presence of positive or rising IgM and IgG titers confirms acute *T. gondii* infection in a pregnant woman. Detection of *T. gondii* DNA in amniotic fluid by PCR is less invasive and more sensitive than isolating parasites from fetal blood or amniotic fluid. Serial fetal ultrasonographic examinations monitoring for ventricular enlargement and other signs of fetal infection are recommended.

Management. A combined prenatal and postnatal treatment program for congenital toxoplasmosis can reduce neurological morbidity. When seroconversion indicates acute maternal infection, fetal blood and amniotic fluid are cultured and fetal blood is tested for *Toxoplasma*-specific IgM. Treat with spiramycin monotherapy unless proven fetal infection exists, in which case add pyrimethamine and sulfadoxine. In newborns with clinical evidence of toxoplasmosis, treat with pyrimethamine (Daraprim) and sulfadiazine for 1 year. Because pyrimethamine is a folic acid antagonist, administer folinic acid (leucovorin) during therapy and for 1 week after termination of treatment. Routine monitoring of the peripheral platelet count is required. Newborns with a high protein concentration in the CSF or chorioretinitis also require prednisone 1–2 mg/kg/day. The optimal duration of therapy for congenital toxoplasmosis is unknown, but 1 year is the rule. Because of the high likelihood of fetal damage, termination of pregnancy may be considered if fetal infection is confirmed at less than 16 weeks gestation, or if the fetus shows evidence of hydrocephalus.

Zika virus. The ZIKV was first identified in a rhesus monkey in Uganda in 1947. It is transmitted by the *Aedes aegypti* mosquito and has long caused epidemics in Southeast Asia, sub-Saharan Africa, Micronesia, Polynesia, New Caledonia, and the Cook Islands. In the northern United States, the virus can be transmitted by the *Aedes albopictus* mosquito. Infected males pass the virus to their sexual partners. The virus crosses the placenta in pregnant women and directly infects the fetus, causing microcephaly and other CNS abnormalities.

Zika came to worldwide attention after a large epidemic in Brazil and South-Central America in 2015, which infected an estimated 440,000 to 1.3 million people. Symptoms in immunocompetent individuals are similar to those seen in dengue and chikungunya virus and include fever, malaise, arthralgia, myalgia, and maculopapular rash. Affected adults and children may develop acute inflammatory demyelinating polyradiculoneuropathy, otherwise known as Guillain-Barré syndrome.[12]

There are no effective treatments other than symptomatic management. Pregnant women are advised to avoid areas of high transmission if possible. Local governments have attempted to reduce infection rates by instituting mosquito-control measures.

COVID-19 (SARS-CoV-2). COVID-19 is caused by the severe acute respiratory coronavirus 2 (SARS-CoV-2). Data from the pandemic are still being evaluated and the following comments should be considered preliminary based on data available at the time of publication.

Vertical transmission is relatively rare but can occur. Infection is transplacental and associated with an increased incidence of adverse outcomes for both the mother and neonate. Widespread vaccination has decreased the risk further, and the vaccination of pregnant women is recommended.[13]

Genetic Causes of Static Encephalopathy

There are thousands of genetic mutations associated with ID and developmental delays. Diagnosis has been simplified somewhat by the creating of multigene epilepsy, autism, and ID panels that test for the most common pathogenic variants. Chromosome microarray can identify some of these disorders and is still the first test we recommend whenever genetic abnormalities are suspected.

15q-Related Syndromes

15q11.2–15q13 encompasses the region known as the Prader-Willi Angelman critical region (PWACR). Different abnormalities within this region lead to the distinct disorders as follows.

Prader-Willi syndrome. Affected infants are hypotonic and feed poorly, and most require special feeding strategies to prevent malnutrition. Hypogonadism is universal, and most affected children are infertile and have short stature as well as characteristic facies. As they grow older, they develop an increasingly disruptive obsession with food and quickly become morbidly obese unless access to food is controlled. All have cognitive impairment, which is typically mild. Behavioral difficulties including poor impulse control, obsessive-compulsive tendencies, and manipulative behavior are common.[14]

Diagnosis consists of methylation studies of 15q11.2–15q3 which reveal maternal-only imprinting of the PWACR (paternal imprinting defect), uniparental disomy of the maternal PWACR, or deletion of the paternal PWACR.

Management requires a multidisciplinary approach including nutrition, gastroenterology, endocrinology, and developmental pediatrics. Ensure appropriate therapies and educational support and treat behavioral manifestations symptomatically.

Angelman syndrome. Parents first notice developmental delay around 6 months; however, the typical Angelman phenotype does not become apparent until after the age of 1. The child has a characteristic happy demeanor and appears excitable. Microcephaly, severe developmental delay, tremulousness, and gait ataxia are present, as is epilepsy which may be intractable. Speech delay occurs and most children are nonverbal. Children may have unusual behaviors; in particular, many are fascinated with water, and parents often use pools or splash pads to decrease agitation.

Diagnosis for 80% results from abnormal methylation studies, which reveal uniparental disomy of the paternal PWACR, deletion of the maternal PWACR that includes the *UBE3A* gene, or an imprinting defect of the maternal PWACR. An additional 10% are identified through *UBE3A* sequence analysis demonstrating a pathogenic variant. The final 10% have the Angelman phenotype but the mechanism is unknown.[15]

Management includes epilepsy management with antiseizure medicines; developmental therapy such as physical, occupational, and speech therapies; nutrition monitoring; behavior management; and educational support. Orthopedic surveillance is required for scoliosis and tight Achilles tendons.

Dup15q syndrome. Both maternal and paternal 15q duplication syndromes exist.

Maternal 15q duplication syndrome causes moderate-to-severe hypotonia and delayed motor milestones, speech delay, autism, and ID. Infants may have infantile spasms that develop into intractable epilepsy with an increased risk of sudden unexpected death (SUDEP). The EEG classically demonstrates excessive beta oscillations. Two types exist: a maternal isodicentric 15q11.2–15q13.1 supernumerary chromosome known as idic(15) (comprising 60%–80% of cases) and a maternal interstitial 15q11.12–15q13.1 duplication resulting in 15q11.2–15q13.1 trisomy (comprising 20%–40%). Of the two, idic(15) has the more severe phenotype. Chromosome microarray can identify most cases but cannot reliably differentiate between idic(15) and trisomy. Mosaicism is possible and can complicate the diagnosis.[16]

Paternal 15q duplication syndrome has considerable overlap with the maternal type and is caused by a paternal interstitial duplication of 15q11.2–15q13.1. ID, developmental delays, autism, and seizures are possible. Sleep disorders such as parasomnias may occur. The phenotype is variable and often less severe than the maternal type. Parent-of-origin testing clarifies whether the syndrome is maternal or paternal in origin. Chromosome microarray establishes the diagnosis.

Management consists of symptomatic treatment including antiseizure medications; physical, occupational, and speech therapies; educational supports; and treatment of behavioral and sleep disturbances.

X-Linked Developmental Disorders

There are several X-linked developmental disorders with variable inheritance patterns and phenotypes. As expected, most affect males, but in some cases, females are affected.

Fragile X syndrome. The fragile X syndrome is the most common chromosomal cause of cognitive impairment. Its prevalence in males is approximately 20:100,000. The name derives from a fragile site (constriction) detectable in folate-free culture medium at the Xq27 location. The unstable fragment contains a trinucleotide repeat in the *FMR1* gene that becomes larger in successive generations (genetic anticipation), causing more severe phenotypic expression. A decrease in the repeat size to normal may also occur. Because *FMR1* mutations are complex and may involve several gene-disrupting alterations, abnormal individuals may show atypical presentations with an IQ above 70.[17]

Males with a complete phenotype have a characteristic appearance (large head, long face, prominent forehead and chin, protruding ears), connective tissue findings (joint laxity), and large testes after puberty. Achievement of developmental milestones is delayed; behavioral abnormalities are common and many show signs of autism. The phenotypic features of males with full mutations vary in relation to puberty. Physical features that become more obvious after puberty include long face, prominent forehead, large ears, prominent jaw, and large genitalia.

The phenotype of females depends on both the nature of the *FMR1* mutation and random X-chromosome inactivation. About 50% of females who inherit a full fragile X mutation are cognitively impaired; however, they are usually less severely affected than males with a full mutation. Approximately 20% of males with a fragile X chromosome are normal, while 30% of carrier females are mildly affected. An asymptomatic male can pass the abnormal chromosome to his daughters, who are usually asymptomatic as well. The daughters' children, both male and female, may be symptomatic.

The *FMR1* gene at Xq27.3 normally contains 5–40 consecutive trinucleotide repeats. When 55–200 repeats are present, the gene is prone to further expansion during meiosis. A full expansion of more than 200 repeats is associated with the phenotype of fragile X syndrome.

Treatment consists of pharmacological management for behavior problems and educational intervention.[18]

MECP2 duplication syndrome. The *MECP2* gene lies on the X chromosome and full-scale duplication causes MECP2 duplication syndrome, characterized by hypotonia, motor delays, absent or limited development of speech, severe to profound ID, and a predisposition to infections particularly of the respiratory tract. Epilepsy occurs in 50% of affected children. Spasticity is progressive especially in the lower extremities, but the ID is static. Heterozygous females present with a milder phenotype, but, in rare cases, they can be as severely affected as males.[19] Chromosome microarray reveals the diagnosis. Management is symptomatic.

Alpha-thalassemia X-linked disability syndrome. This syndrome exclusively affects males and is characterized by distinctive facial features, developmental delays, ID that ranges from mild to profound, and genital anomalies ranging from hypospadias and undescended testicles to ambiguous genitalia or even normal female-appearing genitalia. Most affected males have mild alpha-thalassemia that does not require treatment. Diagnosis is made when an affected individual has a 46 XY karyotype and molecular genetic testing reveals a hemizygous pathogenic variant in *ATRX*.[20] Multidisciplinary management includes neurology, urology, and developmental therapies.

Autosomal Dominant Intellectual Disability Syndromes

SYNGAP1-related intellectual disability. All children with *SYNGAP1* disorders have moderate-to-severe ID and developmental delay. Most have generalized epilepsy, occasionally with myoclonic or atonic seizures, as well as autism, behavioral abnormalities, and feeding problems. Brain MRI is usually normal. The disorder is autosomal dominant and almost always occurs via a de novo pathogenic germline mutation; however, in one family, the disorder was inherited from a mildly affected mosaic parent.[21]

There are no established clinical diagnostic criteria. Diagnosis is made when a heterozygous pathogenic variant is discovered in *SYNGAP1* (89%) or a deletion of 6p21.3 (11%). Treatment is symptomatic and includes management of behavioral abnormalities, feeding and nutrition issues, and epilepsy.

GRIN2B-related neurodevelopmental disorder. Numerous *GRIN* mutations exist. *GRIN2B*-related neurodevelopmental disorder is characterized by mild-to-severe ID and developmental delays; epilepsy that may be refractory to treatment; autism; movement disorders including chorea, dyskinesia, and dystonia; and behavioral problems. Many children have abnormal muscle tone, which is variable among patients ranging from hypotonia to spasticity. The movement disorder may cause confusion when attempting to treat epilepsy, as it is not always clear which paroxysmal movements are seizures. Many children require repeated long-term EEG monitoring to help guide treatment. Microcephaly or cortical visual insufficiency may occur. Brain MRI reveals various malformations including extensive polymicrogyria, dysplastic basal ganglia and hippocampi, and hypoplasia of the corpus callosum; the radiographic constellation of findings appears similar to that seen in tubulinopathies (see Box 5.2).[22]

As with other autosomal dominant intellectual disabilities, most pathogenic variants are de novo but parental mosaicism is possible. Molecular genetic testing reveals a pathogenic variant or exon or whole-gene deletion of *GRIN2B*. Treatment comprises symptomatic management of epilepsy, movement disorders, muscle tone, and behavioral problems.

Coffin-Siris syndrome. Multiple different genes are associated with Coffin-Siris syndrome. Affected children have distinctive facies with coarse facial features, bushy eyebrows, thin vermillion of the upper lip, and thick vermilion of the lower lip. Hypertrichosis is present in most individuals. Infants come to medical attention due to multiple congenital anomalies in the CNS, cardiac, and genitourinary systems. The fifth digit demonstrates hypoplasia or aplasia of the fingernail or distal phalanx. Many children have visual problems, hearing impairment, hypotonia, and seizures. ID is typically moderate to severe, and behavioral problems including hyperactivity and aggression may occur. Brain MRI often reveals malformations such as Dandy-Walker variant, simplified gyral pattern, or agenesis of the corpus callosum.

Inheritance is autosomal dominant and usually results from de novo mutations. Multiple genes have been identified, the most common of which is *ARID1B* (37%). Up to 40% of cases have not identified genetic cause.[23]

Management is multidisciplinary and symptomatic. No specific treatment has been identified.

SLC6A1-related neurodevelopmental disabilities. Symptoms include mild-to-severe ID, developmental delays, hypotonia, and epilepsy. Seizures may be intractable, leading to a progressive epileptic encephalopathy with loss of skills. Many children have movement disorders, including tremor, ataxia, tics, and stereotypies. Neuropsychiatric manifestations include autism spectrum disorders, aggression, attention deficit disorder with hyperactivity, and anxiety. Expressive language is frequently affected. Sleep disorders and gastrointestinal symptoms are common.[24]

Inheritance is autosomal dominant, and affected individuals have a 50% chance of passing the disorder on to their offspring. Pathogenic variants are typically de novo but inheritance from a heterozygous parent has been reported. Molecular genetic testing reveals a heterozygous pathogenic variant in *SLC6A1*.

Treatment involves management of seizures, behavioral and psychiatric problems, movement disorders, and gastrointestinal disorders.

Autosomal Recessive Intellectual Disabilities

GRIN1-related disorders. Disorders involving pathogenic variants in the *GRIN1* gene can be inherited in either an autosomal dominant or autosomal recessive pattern. Autosomal dominant pathogenic variants are often de novo, as in the disorders discussed earlier. Autosomal recessive variants are inherited; parents are obligate heterozygotes (carriers).

All affected children have ID, which is usually severe. Microcephaly, hypotonia, spasticity, movement disorders, and cortical visual impairment are common. A subset of children has diffuse bilateral polymicrogyria visualized on brain MRI. Seizures occur in 65%, approximately half of which are refractory to treatment. Feeding difficulties and gastrointestinal disorders require gastrostomy placement in many patients. Neuropsychiatric abnormalities include autism spectrum disorders and behavioral issues; 48% lack expressive language.[25]

In the autosomal dominant form, molecular genetic testing reveals de novo heterozygous pathogenic missense variants in *GRIN1*. Autosomal recessive forms demonstrate biallelic pathogenic missense or truncating variants. Treatment is symptomatic and multidisciplinary.

Creatine deficiency disorders. Creatine deficiency disorders include two subtypes. The first is creatinine biosynthesis disorders: guanidinoacetate methyltransferase (GAMT) deficiency and L arginine:glycine amidinotransferase (AGAT) deficiency. The second subtype consists of creatine transporter (CRTR) deficiency. Creatine biosynthesis disorders (GAMT deficiency and AGAT deficiency) are autosomal recessive. Creatine transporter disorder (CTTR deficiency) is X-linked.

Common symptoms seen in all three disorders include ID, developmental delay, and speech/language disorders. Hypotonia and behavioral problems including autism are often present but are somewhat less consistent. Muscle weakness and myopathy are specific to AGAT deficiency; epilepsy and movement disorders are specific to GAMT and CRTR deficiency. Although affected individuals with AGAT deficiency do not have epilepsy, rare seizures (mainly associated with fever) have been reported in about 10%.

All affected individuals have low cerebral creatine levels. In addition, individuals with GAMT deficiency accumulate neurotoxic levels of guanidinoacetate (GAA).

Low to low-normal plasma, urine, or CSF creatine levels suggest the presence of a creatine deficiency disorder. Elevated GAA levels in plasma, urine, or CSF suggest GAMT deficiency; low GAA levels suggest AGAT deficiency. CRTR deficiency causes elevated creatine-to-creatinine ratio in urine in males; females may have normal or only mildly elevated ratios. Proton magnetic resonance spectroscopy demonstrates an absent or severely depressed creatine peak in all individuals with GAMT and AGAT deficiency, and in males with CRCT deficiency. The creatine peak may be normal in females with heterozygous X-linked CRCT deficiency. Three genes have been associated with creatine deficiency disorders: *GAMT* (33%), *SLC6A8* (64%), and *GATM* (3%). Multigene panels for epilepsy or autism/ID provide the diagnosis in most cases.[26]

Some specific treatment recommendations exist. For creatine biosynthesis disorders (GAMT, AGAT), treat low cerebral creatine with creatine monohydrate, 400–800 mg/kg/day in three to six divided doses. Treat low cerebral creatine caused by deficiency in CRTR with creatine monohydrate 100–200 mg/kg/day in three divided doses, arginine supplementation 400 mg/kg/day in three divided doses, and glycine 150 mg/kg/day in three divided doses. GAMT deficiency causes toxic accumulation of GAA, which is treated by restricting dietary arginine to 15–25 mg/kg/day. Supplement with essential amino acid formula to prevent protein malnutrition.

PROGRESSIVE ENCEPHALOPATHIES WITH ONSET BEFORE AGE 2

The differential diagnosis of progressive diseases of the nervous system that start before the age of 2 is somewhat different from those that begin during childhood, and more often involves metabolic, lysosomal, peroxisomal, or mitochondrial disorders. As with static encephalopathies, genetic testing has drastically changed the approach to the child with progressive disease. The history and physical examination must answer three questions before initiating laboratory diagnosis:

1. Is this multiorgan or only CNS disease? Other organ involvement suggests lysosomal, peroxisomal, and mitochondrial disorders, and/or an underlying genetic defect.
2. Is this a CNS or both central and peripheral nervous systems process? Nerve or muscle involvement

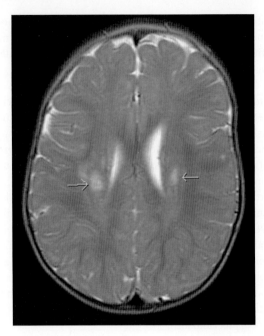

Fig. 5.1 Krabbe Disease. T2 axial magnetic resonance imaging shows an early stage of symmetric demyelination (*arrows*).

suggests mainly lysosomal and mitochondrial disorders.

3. Does the disease affect primarily the gray matter or the white matter? Early features of gray matter disease are personality change, seizures, and dementia. Characteristics of white matter disease are focal neurological deficits, spasticity, and blindness. Whether the process begins in the gray matter or the white matter, eventually clinical features of dysfunction develop in both. The EEG is usually abnormal early in the course of gray matter disease and late in the course of white matter disease. MRI shows cortical atrophy in gray matter disease and cerebral demyelination in white matter disease (Fig. 5.1). Visual evoked responses and motor conduction velocities are useful in documenting demyelination, even subclinical, in the optic and peripheral nerves, respectively.

Acquired Immunodeficiency Syndrome Encephalopathy

Pediatric acquired immunodeficiency syndrome (AIDS) cases result from transplacental, delivery, or breast feeding exposures with subsequent HIV infection. The mother may be asymptomatic when the child becomes infected.

Clinical features. Evidence of infection is apparent during the first year in 30% of children born to untreated AIDS-infected mothers. As a rule, the outcome is worse when the onset of symptoms is early, and the rate of progression in the child relates directly to the severity of disease in the mother.

The spectrum of neurological and nonneurological manifestations in HIV-infected children is somewhat different from adults. Hepatosplenomegaly and bone marrow failure, lymphocytic interstitial pneumonia, chronic diarrhea, failure to thrive, acquired microcephaly, cerebral vasculopathy, and basal ganglia calcification occur more frequently in children. Opportunistic infections that represent recrudescence of previously acquired infections in adults, for example, cerebral toxoplasmosis or progressive multifocal leukoencephalopathy, are rare in infants.

AIDS encephalopathy may be subacute or indolent and is not necessarily associated with failure to thrive or opportunistic infections. The onset of encephalopathy may occur from 2 months to 5 years after exposure to the virus. Ninety percent of affected infants show symptoms by 18 months of age including progressive loss of developmental milestones, microcephaly, dementia, and spasticity. Other features seen in less than 50% of children are ataxia, pseudobulbar palsy, involuntary movement disorders, myoclonus, and seizures. If left untreated, the prognosis is poor.

Diagnosis. Virologic testing should be performed in exposed infants at 14–21 days, 1–2 months, and 4–6 months. It must be performed every 3 months in infants who are breast feeding. Once breast feeding ends, test again in 4 weeks, 3 months, and 6 months. Definitive exclusion of HIV infection requires two negative tests, one at 1 month and the other at 4 months, or two separate negative samples if the infant is above 6 months of age.

Management. The introduction of routine maternal treatment with highly active antiretroviral therapy in 1996 greatly decreased the incidence of pediatric AIDS. Combined treatment with zidovudine (azidothymidine), didanosine, and nevirapine is well tolerated and may have sustained efficacy against HIV-1. Bone marrow suppression is the only important evidence of toxicity. The CDC has published extensive guidelines on the treatment of HIV+ pregnant women, neonates, and infants. These guidelines are available on the CDC website and are frequently updated.

Disorders of Amino Acid Metabolism

Disorders of amino acid metabolism impair neuronal function by causing excessive production of toxic intermediary metabolites and reducing the production of neurotransmitters. The clinical syndromes are either acute neonatal encephalopathy with seizures and cerebral edema (see Chapter 1) or cognitive impairment and dementia. Some disorders of amino acid metabolism cause cerebral malformations, such as agenesis of the corpus callosum. Although the main clinical features of aminoaciduria refer to gray matter dysfunction (cognitive impairment and seizures), myelination is often profoundly delayed or defective. Amino acid disorders are increasingly being recategorized based on the relevant genetic defect.

Homocystinuria

Classic homocystinuria is a disorder of methionine metabolism due to the almost complete deficiency of the enzyme cystathionine β-synthase.[27] Two variants are recognized: B_6-*responsive homocystinuria* and B_6-*nonresponsive homocystinuria*. B_6-responsive homocystinuria is usually milder than the nonresponsive variant. Transmission of all forms is by autosomal recessive inheritance; heterozygotes have partial deficiencies. Cystathionine synthase catalyzes the condensation of serine and homocysteine to form cystathionine (Fig. 5.2). When the enzyme is deficient, the blood and urine concentrations of homocysteine and methionine are increased. Newborn screening programs detect hypermethioninemia.

Clinical features. Affected individuals appear normal at birth. Neurological features include mild-to-moderate cognitive impairment, developmental delay, psychiatric/behavioral symptoms, seizures, and extrapyramidal symptoms. Nonneurological features include ectopia lentis or severe myopia, marfanoid appearance, osteoporosis, pectus excavatum, genu valgum, scoliosis, and cerebral thromboembolism. Intelligence is generally higher in B_6-responsive than in B_6-nonresponsive homocystinuria.

High plasma homocysteine concentrations adversely affect collagen metabolism and are responsible for intimal thickening of blood vessel walls, leading to arterial and venous thromboembolic disease. Cerebral thromboembolism is a life-threatening complication. Emboli may occur in infancy but are seen more frequently in adult life. Young adult heterozygotes are also at risk.

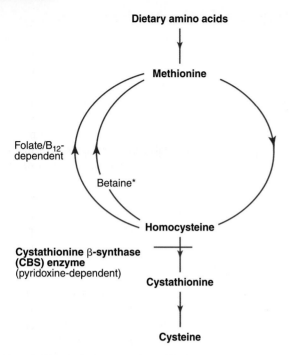

Dietary amino acids

Methionine

Folate/B$_{12}$-
dependent

Betaine*

Homocysteine

**Cystathionine β-synthase
(CBS) enzyme**
(pyridoxine-dependent)

Cystathionine

Cysteine

Fig. 5.2 Metabolic Disturbance in Homocystinuria. Absence of cystathionine β-synthase (cystathionine synthetase) blocks the metabolism of homocysteine, causing the accumulation of homocystine and methionine. Alternate pathway with betaine treatment. (Modified and redrawn from http://www.geneclinics.org.) Sacharow SJ, Picker JD, Levy HL. Homocystinuria caused by cystathionine beta-synthase deficiency. In: Adam MP, Feldman J, Mirzaa GM, et al, eds. GeneReviews®. Seattle, WA. University of Washington; 1993–2024. https://www.ncbi.nlm.nih.gov/books/NBK1524/

Occlusion of the coronary or carotid arteries can lead to sudden death or severe neurological deficits. Thromboembolism is the first clue to the diagnosis in 15% of cases.

Dislocation of the lens, an almost constant feature of homocystinuria, typically occurs between the ages of 2 and 10; dislocation is downward, in contrast to Marfan syndrome in which it is typically upward. Almost all patients have lens dislocation by the age of 40. Older children have osteoporosis, often first affecting the spine resulting in scoliosis. Many children are tall and thin, with blond, sparse, brittle hair, and a Marfanoid habitus. This habitus does not develop until middle or late childhood and serves as a clue to the diagnosis in fewer than 40% of cases.

The diagnosis is suspect in any infant with isolated and unexplained developmental delay, since disease-specific features may not appear until later childhood. The presence of either thromboembolism or lens dislocation strongly suggests homocystinuria.

Diagnosis. The biochemical features of homocystinuria are increased concentrations of plasma homocysteine, total homocysteine, and methionine; increased concentration of urine homocysteine; and reduced cystathionine β-synthase enzyme activity. Molecular testing reveals biallelic pathogenic variants in the *CBS* gene. Family genetic counseling is recommended.

Management. All patients with homocystinuria should receive 10 mg/kg/day of pyridoxine, up to a maximum of 500 mg/day for 6 weeks. Plasma total homocysteine is measured twice before treatment and twice during treatment; the test should not be done if the patient is catabolic. The protein intake should be normal, folate supplements should be given, and vitamin B$_{12}$ deficiency should be corrected before testing. Patients who achieve plasma total homocysteine levels below 50 μmol/L on pyridoxine are clearly B$_6$ responsive and do not need any other treatment, although they will need to remain on pyridoxine for life. Folate and vitamin B$_{12}$ optimize the conversion of homocysteine to methionine and help to decrease homocysteine levels. If the total homocysteine falls more than 20% but remains above 50 μmol/L, additional treatment should be considered (i.e., diet and/or betaine). If total homocysteine falls by less than 20% on B$_6$, the patient is not responsive to B$_6$.[28]

Treatment with betaine, starting at 100 mg/kg/day with increments of 50 mg/g/day weekly up to 200 mg/kg/day or a maximum of 3 g/day in two divided doses, provides an alternate remethylation pathway by donation of a methyl group to convert excess homocysteine to methionine and may help prevent thrombosis.

Maple Syrup Urine Disease

Mutations in three different genes cause maple syrup urine disease (MSUD). These genes encode the catalytic components of the branched-chain alpha-ketoacid dehydrogenase complex, which catalyzes the catabolism of the branched-chain amino acids.

Clinical features. Deficiency is associated with several different phenotypes.[29] Three recognized clinical phenotypes are *classic*, *intermittent*, and *intermediate*. An acute encephalopathy with ketoacidosis characterizes the classic and intermittent forms.

The onset of the intermediate form is late in infancy, often in association with a febrile illness or a large protein intake. In the absence of vigorous early therapeutic intervention, moderate cognitive impairment results. Ataxia, failure to thrive, behavioral problems, and ID occur. Epilepsy, focal neurologic deficits, and acute mental status changes are rare.

A more detailed description of diagnosis and treatment for MSUD can be found in Chapters 1 and 10.

Phenylketonuria

Phenylketonuria (PKU) is a disorder of phenylalanine metabolism caused by partial or total deficiency of the hepatic enzyme phenylalanine hydroxylase (PAH).[30] Genetic transmission is autosomal recessive and occurrence is approximately 1 per 16,000 live births. Failure to hydroxylate phenylalanine to tyrosine leads to further metabolism by transamination to phenylpyruvic acid (Fig. 5.3). Oxidation of phenylpyruvic acid to phenylacetic acid causes a musty odor in the urine.

The completeness of deficiency produces three categories of PAH deficiency as follows: classic PKU, non-PKU hyperphenylalaninemia (HPA), and variant PKU. In *classic PKU*, PAH deficiency is complete or nearly complete. Affected children tolerate less than 250–350 mg of dietary phenylalanine per day to keep plasma phenylalanine concentration below a safe level of 300 μmol/L (5 mg/dL). If untreated, plasma phenylalanine concentrations are greater than 1000 μmol/L and dietary phenylalanine tolerance is less than 500 mg/day. Classic PKU has a high risk of severely impaired cognitive development.

Children with *non-PKU HPA* have plasma phenylalanine concentrations between 120 and 1000 μmol/L on a normal diet and a lower risk of impaired cognitive development without treatment. *Variant PKU* includes individuals who do not fit the description for either PKU or non-PKU HPA.

HPA may also result from the impaired synthesis or recycling of tetrahydrobiopterin (BH4). BH4 is the cofactor in the phenylalanine, tyrosine, and tryptophan hydroxylation reactions. Inheritance of HPA caused by BH4 deficiency is an autosomal recessive trait and accounts for 2% of patients with HPA.

Clinical features. Because affected children are normal at birth, early diagnosis requires compulsory mass screening. The screening test detects HPA, which is not synonymous with PKU. Blood phenylalanine and tyrosine concentrations must be precisely determined in every newborn detected by the screening test to differentiate classic PKU from other conditions. In newborns with classic PKU, HPA develops 48–72 hours after

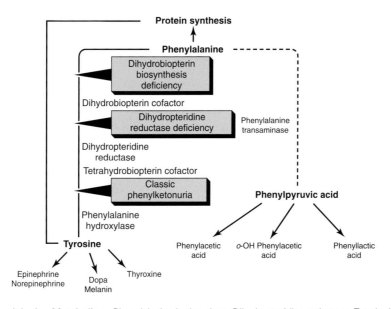

Fig. 5.3 Phenylalanine Metabolism. Phenylalanine hydroxylase. Dihydropteridine reductase. Tetrahydrobiopterin. Phenylalanine transaminase. Tyrosine transaminase. (Reproduced with permission from Swaiman KF. Aminoacidopathies and organic acidemias resulting from deficiency of enzyme activity and transport abnormalities. In: Swaiman KF, Ashwal S, eds. Pediatric Neurology. 3rd ed, Vol 1. Mosby; 1999.)

initiation of milk feeding. Blood phenylalanine concentrations are 20 mg/dL or greater, and serum tyrosine levels are less than 5 mg/dL. When blood phenylalanine concentrations reach 15 mg/dL, phenylalanine spills over into the urine and the addition of ferric chloride solution (5–10 drops of FeCl to 1 mL of urine) produces a green color.

During the first months, the skin may have a musty odor because of phenylacetic acid in the sweat. Developmental delay is sometimes obvious by the third month and always before the end of the first year. By the beginning of the second year, developmental regression is evident. Behavioral disturbances characterized by hyperactivity and aggression are common; focal neurological deficits are unusual. Approximately 25% of affected infants have seizures. Some have infantile spasms and hypsarrhythmia; others have tonic-clonic seizures. Infants with PKU frequently have blond hair, pale skin, and blue eyes owing to diminished pigment production. Eczema is common. These skin changes are the only nonneurological features of PKU.

Diagnosis. Newborn screening detects all cases of PKU. The screening test detects the presence of HPA. Plasma amino acid analysis including phenylalanine concentration, phenylalanine-to-tyrosine ratio, and a complete amino acid profile confirms the diagnosis. Plasma phenylalanine concentrations above 1000 μmol/L in the untreated state are diagnostic. The use of molecular genetic testing is primarily for genetic counseling and prenatal testing. Blood phenylalanine levels less than 25 mg/dL and a normal concentration of tyrosine characterize benign variants of PKU. Disturbances in BH4 underlie the malignant forms of PKU. Seizures are the initial symptom and cognitive impairment and motor deficits come later. Progressive calcification of the basal ganglia occurs in untreated children.

Transitory tyrosinemia occurs in 2% of full-term newborns and in 2% of premature newborns. The cause is a transitory deficiency of the enzyme *p*-hydroxyphenylpyruvic acid. It is a benign condition and can be distinguished from PKU because the blood concentrations of both tyrosine and phenylalanine are elevated.

Management. In classic PKU, initiate a low-protein diet and use of a phenylalanine-free medical formula as soon as possible after birth to achieve plasma phenylalanine concentrations of 120–360 μmol/L (2–6 mg/dL), or 40–240 μmol/L (1–4 mg/dL). Recent studies suggest that the plasma phenylalanine goal should be less than

or equal to 240 μmol/L to expect normal neurocognitive outcomes.[31] Dietary supplementation with 6*R*-BH4 stereoisomer in doses up to 20 mg/kg daily depends on individual needs. Treatment of infants with non-PKU HPA with plasma phenylalanine concentrations consistently less than 600 μmol/L is uncertain.

BH4 is a cofactor for PAH, tyrosine hydroxylase, and tryptophan hydroxylase. Defective recycling or synthesis causes deficiency. In infants with cofactor deficiency, a phenylalanine-restricted diet reduces the blood phenylalanine concentration but does not prevent neurological deterioration. For these children, BH4 administration is the therapy of choice.

Disorders of Lysosomal Enzymes

Lysosomes are cytoplasmic vesicles containing hydrolytic enzymes that degrade the products of cellular catabolism. The causes of lysosomal enzyme disorders are impaired enzyme synthesis, abnormal enzyme targeting, or a defective accessory factor needed for enzymatic processing. When lysosomal enzymes are impaired, abnormal storage of materials occurs causing cell injury and death. One or several organs may be affected, and the clinical features depend on the organ(s) involved. Cognitive impairment and regression are features of many lysosomal enzyme storage diseases. In some diseases, such as acid lipase deficiency (Wolman disease) and ceramide deficiency (Farber lipogranulomatosis), cognitive impairment occurs, but it is neither a prominent nor an initial feature. These disorders are not included for discussion.

Gaucher Disease Type 2 (Glucosylceramide Lipidosis)

Gaucher disease types 2 and 3 were previously distinguished by age at onset; however, there is some overlap between the two disorders. In general children with type 2 develop neurological symptoms before the age of 2, and type 3 presents later in childhood.

All subtypes are caused by mutations in the *GBA* gene encoding the enzyme beta-glucocerebrosidase, leading to toxic lysosomal accumulation of glucocerebrosides. Neurovisceral storage characterizes both types. Type 2 has a more rapid and severe course, and death typically occurs by the ages of 2–4.

Clinical features. Symptom onset in infants with Gaucher disease type 2 is usually before the age of 6 months and frequently before the age of 3 months. The initial features are motor regression and cranial nerve dysfunction. Children are first hypotonic and then spastic. Head retraction, an early and characteristic sign, probably is due to meningeal irritation. Difficulties in sucking and swallowing, trismus, and oculomotor palsies are typical. Mental deterioration is rapid, but seizures are uncommon. Splenomegaly is more prominent than hepatomegaly, and jaundice is not expected. Hypersplenism results in anemia, thrombocytopenia, and leukopenia. Death usually occurs between the ages of 2 and 4.

Diagnosis. Assay of acid β-glucosylceramidase enzyme activity in peripheral blood leukocytes or other nucleated cells is reliable for diagnosis. Glucosylceramidase enzyme activity in peripheral blood leukocytes is 0%–15% of normal. Carrier detection and prenatal diagnosis are available. Inheritance is autosomal recessive. Molecular genetic testing reveals biallelic pathogenic variants of the *GBA* gene.[32]

Management. The International Collaborative Gaucher Group Registry has published surveillance guidelines. Enzyme replacement therapy and substrate reduction therapy are the preferred targeted treatments and are generally well tolerated. They reverse or prevent hematological and visceral abnormalities. If targeted therapies are unavailable, necessary interventions often include partial or total splenectomy for massive splenomegaly and thrombocytopenia, transfusion of blood for severe anemia and bleeding, joint replacement surgery for relief from chronic pain and restoration of function, and supplemental treatment such as oral bisphosphonates for severe osteopenia. Pain is a significant feature and often debilitating. Avoid nonsteroidal anti-inflammatory drugs in patients with thrombocytopenia.

Globoid Cell Leukodystrophy (Krabbe Disease)

Krabbe disease (galactosylceramide lipidosis) is a rapidly progressive demyelinating leukodystrophy caused by deficient activity of the enzyme galactocerebrosidase (GALC).[33] A juvenile and an adult form of the disease also occur. Transmission is by autosomal recessive inheritance, and *GALC* is the gene most often associated with disease. Galactosylceramide is stored within multinucleated macrophages of the white matter of the CNS, forming globoid cells.

Clinical features. The median age of onset is 4 months, with a range of 1–7 months. Initial symptoms are irritability and hyperreactivity to stimuli. Progressive hypertonicity in the skeletal muscles follows. Unexplained low-grade fever is common. Psychomotor

development arrests and then regresses. Within 2–4 months, the infant is in a permanent position of opisthotonos and all previously achieved milestones are lost. Tendon reflexes become hypoactive and disappear. Startle myoclonus and seizures develop. Blindness occurs, and before 1 year 90% of these infants are either dead or in a chronic vegetative state.

Several variant forms of globoid leukodystrophy with different clinical features exist: infantile spasm syndrome (see Chapter 1), focal neurological deficits (see Chapters 10 and 11), and polyneuropathy (see Chapter 7). The juvenile form will be discussed later in this chapter.

Diagnosis. MRI shows diffuse demyelination of the cerebral hemispheres (see Fig. 5.1). Motor nerve conduction velocity of peripheral nerves is usually prolonged, and the protein content of CSF is elevated. Deficient activity of GALC in leukocytes or cultured fibroblasts establishes the diagnosis. Single-gene testing is used for confirmation and reveals pathogenic variants in the *GALC* gene. Several states include Krabbe disease on their standardized newborn screening tests.

Management. Hematopoietic stem cell transplantation performed within the first 7 weeks of life slows the course of disease in children with infantile-onset Krabbe disease. The prognosis for motor function depends largely on the degree of corticospinal tract involvement at birth; some affected infants may have few or no deficits, while others suffer from progressive spasticity or muscular atrophy. There are no specific guidelines regarding monitoring of asymptomatic infants diagnosed on newborn screen, and no helpful biochemical markers have been identified for surveillance purposes.[34]

Glycoprotein Degradation Disorders

Glycoproteins are complex molecules composed of oligosaccharides attached to protein. Disorders of glycoprotein degradation are uncommon and resemble mild forms of mucopolysaccharidosis. The main forms are deficiency of the enzyme α-mannosidase (variety of mutations in the *MAN* gene) and deficiency of the lysosomal enzyme α-fucosidase (*FUCA1* gene).

Clinical features. The clinical features are either a Hurler phenotype (Box 5.3) or a myoclonus-dementia complex. Some patients have macular degeneration (cherry-red spot). Angiokeratoma can be present. These disorders are indistinguishable from other lysosomal storage diseases by clinical features alone.

> **BOX 5.3   The Hurler Phenotype**
> - Abdominal hernia
> - Coarse facial features
> - Corneal opacity
> - Deafness
> - Dysostosis multiplex
> - Cognitive impairment
> - Stiff joints
> - Visceromegaly

> **BOX 5.4   Lysosomal Enzyme Disorders With a Cherry-Red Spot**
> - Cherry-red spot myoclonus (see Chapter 1)
> - Farber lipogranulomatosis
> - GM_1 gangliosidosis
> - GM_2 gangliosidosis
> - Metachromatic leukodystrophy
> - Niemann-Pick disease type A
> - Sialidosis type III

Diagnosis. The urine shows excessive excretion of oligosaccharides or glycoasparagines, but not mucopolysaccharides. Biopsy of the skin and other tissues shows membrane-bound vacuoles containing amorphous material. Tissue concentrations of glycoproteins, and often glycolipids, are increased.

Management. Treatment is supportive.

GM_1 Gangliosidosis

Deficiency of the lysosomal enzyme β-galactosidase causes GM_1 gangliosidosis. The amount and type of residual activity determines whether the phenotype is a generalized gangliosidosis, as in GM_1 gangliosidosis, or visceral storage of mucopolysaccharides with little brain disease, as in Morquio B disease. Mutations in the *GLB1* gene lead to diminished function of the lysosomal enzyme beta-galactosidase and accumulation of toxic GM_1 gangliosides in multiple organs, particularly the brain. Three types exist: type I, the infantile form; type II, presenting in childhood; and type III, representing the chronic or adult form. Inheritance is autosomal recessive.

Clinical features. The onset of type I GM_1 gangliosidosis is between 6 and 18 months. Weakness and incoordination are early features. Spasticity, cognitive impairment, and seizures follow. Psychomotor development is first slow and then regresses. Affected newborns are poorly responsive, hypotonic, and hypoactive. Many elements of the Hurler phenotype are present (see Box 5.3), and a cherry-red spot of the macula is present in 50% of patients (Box 5.4). Death occurs by the age of 2 for patients with the infantile form. Children with type II may live to adolescence or early adulthood.

Diagnosis. The absence of mucopolysacchariduria and the presence of a cherry-red spot distinguish infantile GM_1 gangliosidosis from Hurler syndrome. Showing

enzyme deficiency in leukocytes, cultured fibroblasts, or serum establishes the diagnosis.

Management. Treatment is supportive.

Sandhoff disease. In Sandhoff disease, both hexosaminidase A and B are severely deficient. Disease transmission is by autosomal recessive inheritance. Globosides and GM_2 gangliosides accumulate in brain and viscera.

Clinical features. The clinical features and course of Sandhoff disease are identical to those of Tay-Sachs disease (TSD; discussed later). The only difference is that organs other than the CNS are sometimes involved. Moderate hepatosplenomegaly may be present, and occasionally patients have bony deformities similar to those of infantile GM_1 gangliosidosis.

Diagnosis. Suspect the disease in infants with a Tay-Sachs phenotype who do not have the typical ethnic background. Peripheral lymphocytes are not vacuolated, but foamy histiocytes may be present in the bone marrow. Hexosaminidase deficiency in leukocytes, cultured fibroblasts, or serum establishes the diagnosis in patients and carriers. Prenatal diagnosis is available by the detection of *N*-acetylglucosaminyl oligosaccharides in amniotic fluid.

Management. Treatment is supportive.

Hexa Disorders

Deficiencies of the hexosaminidase A enzyme cause a spectrum of disease encompassing the classic phenotype of TSD, subacute juvenile TSD, and late-onset TSD. Accumulation of the specific glycosphingolipid GM2 ganglioside causes neurotoxicity. Disease severity depends on the amount of residual enzyme activity, with TSD being the most severe type with virtually no functional enzyme. The subacute juvenile and late-onset forms present later in life; we discuss the subacute juvenile form in the "Progressive Encephalopathies with Onset After Age 2" section.

Tay-Sachs disease. Complete deficiency of hexosaminidase A causes TSD (*infantile GM$_2$ gangliosidosis*). The gene frequency is 1:30 in Ashkenazi Jews and 1:300 in other ethnic groups. The CNS is the only affected organ.[35]

Clinical features. The typical initial symptom, onset between the ages of 3 and 6 months, is an abnormal startle reaction (Moro reflex) to noise or light. Motor regression begins between the ages of 4 and 6 months. The infant comes to medical attention because of either delayed achievement of motor milestones or loss of milestones previously attained. A cherry-red spot of the macula is present in almost every patient, but it is not specific for TSD because it is also present in several storage diseases and in central retinal artery occlusion (see Box 5.4). The cherry-red spot develops after retinal ganglion cells in the parafoveal region accumulate stored material, swell, and burst. The red color of the normal fundus is then enhanced. Optic atrophy and blindness follow.

By the age of 1, the infant is severely cognitively impaired, unresponsive, and spastic. During the second year, the head enlarges and seizures develop. Most children die by the age of 5.

Diagnosis. Suspect the diagnosis in any Jewish child with developmental delay and a cherry-red spot of the macula. The diagnosis of HEXA deficiency relies on the demonstration of absent to near-absent β-hexosaminidase A enzymatic activity in the serum or white blood cells of a symptomatic child in the presence of normal or elevated activity of the β-hexosaminidase B isoenzyme. Molecular genetic testing demonstrates biallelic pathogenic variants in the *HEXA* gene. Mutation analysis identifies the carrier state.

Management. Treatment is supportive.

Mucolipidosis Type II (I-Cell Disease)

Deficiency or dysfunction of the enzyme *N*-acetylglucosamine phosphotransferase causes I-cell disease (mucolipidosis II). This enzyme is necessary for the formation of mannose 6-phosphate which is necessary to transport digestive enzymes into lysosomes, resulting in lysosomal accumulation of several mucolipids. The disease is caused by a biallelic pathogenic variant in the *GNPTAB* gene. A milder form, mucolipidosis III, has some retained enzyme activity and produces less severe symptoms that begin later in life. Mucolipidosis II and III are two ends of the spectrum of the same disease.[36]

Clinical features. Mucolipidosis II resembles Hurler syndrome (discussed later) except that symptoms appear earlier, the neurological deterioration is more rapid, and mucopolysacchariduria is not present. Affected newborns are small for gestational age and may have hyperplastic gums and multiple bony abnormalities (*dysostosis multiplex*). Coarsening of facial features and joint contractures occur within the first months, and growth ceases completely after the first year. Profound ID is present, and affected infants suffer from recurrent and prolonged respiratory infections and vocal cord abnormalities. The complete Hurler phenotype is present within the first year, except that corneal opacification is not always present. Gingival hypertrophy is quite striking. Death from congestive heart failure or respiratory insufficiency usually occurs before the age of 5.

Diagnosis. Consider mucolipidosis type II in infants with the Hurler phenotype and negative screening for mucopolysacchariduria. Showing a specific pattern of lysosomal enzyme deficiency in fibroblasts establishes the diagnosis. Molecular genetic testing of the *GNPTAB* coding region identifies causative mutations in more than 95% of affected individuals.[37]

Management. Treatment is supportive.

Mucopolysaccharidoses

Deficiency of the lysosomal enzymes responsible for catalyzing the degradation of glycosaminoglycans (mucopolysaccharides) causes the mucopolysaccharidoses (MPS). Mucopolysaccharides are a normal component of cornea, cartilage, bone, connective tissue, and the reticuloendothelial system. Excessive storage may occur in all these tissues. Transmission of all MPS, except type II, is by autosomal recessive inheritance. Type II is an X-linked trait.

Mucopolysaccharidosis type I (MPS I; Hurler syndrome). The absence of the lysosomal hydrolase α-L-iduronidase causes Hurler syndrome, caused by biallelic pathogenic variants in the *IDUA* gene. Dermatan sulfate and heparan sulfate cannot be fully degraded and appear in the urine. Mucopolysaccharides are stored in the cornea, collagen, and leptomeninges, and gangliosides are stored in cortical neurons.[38]

Clinical features. MPS I is a progressive multisystem disorder with mild-to-severe features. The traditional classification of *Hurler* syndrome, *Hurler-Scheie* syndrome, or *Scheie* syndrome is now discarded in favor of the terms *severe MPS I* or *attenuated MPS I*. Individuals with MPS I appear normal at birth. Coarsening of the facial features occurs within the first 2 years. Progressive skeletal dysplasia (dysostosis multiplex), involving all bones, occurs in all children with severe MPS I. Linear growth stops by the age of 3, hearing loss occurs, and all develop progressive and profound cognitive impairment. Death, caused by cardiorespiratory failure, usually occurs within the first 10 years of life.

The greatest variability occurs in individuals with the attenuated MPS I. Onset is usually between the ages of 3 and 10. Although psychomotor development may be normal in early childhood, individuals with attenuated MPS I may have learning disabilities. The rate of disease progression and severity ranges from death in the second to third decades, to a normal lifespan, with significant disability from progressive, severe restriction in range of motion of all joints. Hearing loss and cardiac valvular disease are common.

Diagnosis. The physical and radiographic appearance suggests the diagnosis. Deficiency of the enzyme α-L-iduronidase in peripheral blood leukocytes or cultured fibroblasts establishes the diagnosis; molecular genetic testing identifies biallelic pathogenic variants in the *IDUA* gene. Mutation analysis is available for prenatal diagnosis.

Management. In addition to symptomatic treatment, hematopoietic stem cell transplantation in selected children with severe MPS I can increase survival, reduce facial coarseness and hepatosplenomegaly, improve hearing, and maintain normal heart function. Enzyme replacement therapy with alpha-L-iduronidase (Aldurazyme) treats the non-CNS manifestations of MPS I and improves liver size, growth, joint mobility, breathing, and sleep apnea in those with attenuated disease.

MPS III (Sanfilippo disease). MPS III is distinct from other MPS types because only heparan sulfate is stored in viscera and appears in the urine. Gangliosides are stored in neurons. Four different, but related, enzyme deficiencies cause similar phenotypes. All are transmitted by autosomal recessive inheritance.

Clinical features. The Hurler phenotype is not prominent, but hepatomegaly is present in two-thirds of cases. Dwarfism does not occur. The major feature is neurological deterioration characterized by delayed motor development beginning toward the end of the second year, followed by an interval of arrested cognitive development, and progressive dementia. Hyperactivity and sleep disorders are relatively common between the ages of 2 and 4. Cognitive impairment in most affected children is severe by the age of 11, and death occurs before the age of 20. However, considerable variability exists, and MPS III is a consideration even when the onset of cognitive regression occurs after the age of 5.

Diagnosis. Suspect the diagnosis in infants and children with progressive psychomotor regression and a screening test positive for mucopolysacchariduria. The presence of heparan sulfate, but not dermatan sulfate, in the urine is presumptive evidence of the disease. Definitive diagnosis requires the demonstration of enzyme deficiency in cultured fibroblasts or molecular genetic testing showing biallelic pathogenic variants in one of the four causative genes: *SGSH, NAGLU, HGSNAT,* or *GNS*.[39]

Management. Treatment is supportive. There are no established therapies, although hematopoietic stem cell transplantation and enzyme replacement therapies are both being evaluated.

Niemann-Pick Disease

Niemann-Pick disease has four distinct subtypes. Niemann-Pick A and B are caused by decreased function of acid sphingomyelinase, with resultant sphingomyelin accumulation and toxicity. Both types A and B result from mutations in the *SMPD1* gene. Niemann-Pick types C1 and C2 are clinically similar but caused by distinct mutations in the *NPC1* and *NPC2* genes, respectively. Type C is most diagnosed in later childhood (see the "Progressive Encephalopathies With Onset After Age 2" section).

Clinical features. Niemann-Pick type A begins in infancy. Affected babies show failure to thrive, hepatosplenomegaly, and a cherry-red spot on ophthalmological examination. Their neurodevelopmental course is normal or only mildly delayed until approximately 1 year of age, when they experience psychomotor regression. With time, emaciation, a tendency toward opisthotonos, exaggerated tendon reflexes, and blindness develop. Seizures are uncommon. Interstitial lung disease is a prominent feature and often leads to death in early childhood, typically by the age of 3. Niemann-Pick type B is similar, but with a milder course. Onset is in mid-childhood, and only one-third of affected children have neurological impairment or a cherry-red spot. Most survive to adulthood.

Diagnosis. Molecular genetic testing is available, but biochemical testing may be needed to confirm the diagnosis.

Management. Treatment for all types is supportive.

Congenital Disorders of Glycosylation

The congenital disorders of glycosylation (CDGs) are a group of genetic, multisystem diseases, with major nervous system involvement.[40] The underlying defect is abnormal glycosylation of *N*-linked oligosaccharides. Multiple different enzymes in the *N*-linked oligosaccharide synthetic pathway may be defective, leading to several subtypes of disease. Deficiency of the carbohydrate moiety of secretory glycoproteins, lysosomal enzymes, and membrane glycoproteins is characteristic of the group. They occur mainly in northern Europeans and transmission is by autosomal recessive inheritance.

Clinical features. PMM2-CDG (formerly CDG-Ia) is the most common subtype of the CDGs. It is caused by deficiency of the phosphomannomutase 2 enzyme, which converts mannose 6-phosphate into mannose 1-phosphate. Affected children have inverted nipples, strabismus, abnormal fat pads, and cerebellar hypoplasia. Failure to thrive, developmental delay, and hypotonia occur early in infancy. Neurological deterioration follows. The main features are ID, ataxia, retinitis pigmentosa, hypotonia, and weakness. Approximately 20% of affected individuals die by their first birthday, usually a result of multiorgan failure; however, the clinical course is highly variable, and some may survive into adulthood. Characteristic features in childhood and adolescence are short stature, failure of sexual maturation, skeletal abnormalities, liver dysfunction, and polyneuropathy.

Children with CDG syndrome type II have a more profound ID, but no cerebellar ataxia or peripheral neuropathy, and those with CDG syndrome types III and IV have severe neurological impairment and seizures from birth.

Diagnosis. The diagnostic test for all types of CDG is analysis of serum transferrin glycoforms. Genetic testing and enzyme assays are available for PMM2-CDG.

Management. Treatment is supportive.

Hypothyroidism

Congenital hypothyroidism secondary to thyroid dysgenesis occurs in 1 per 4000 live births. Mutations in the genes encoding thyrotropin, thyrotropin-releasing hormone, thyroid transcription factor 2, and other factors are causative. Early diagnosis and treatment are imperative to ensure a favorable outcome. Fortunately, newborn screening is universal in the United States and detects virtually all cases.

Clinical features. Affected infants are usually asymptomatic at birth. Clinical features evolve insidiously during the first weeks postpartum, and their significance is not always appreciated. Frequently, gestation lasts for more than 42 weeks, and birth weight is greater than 4 kg. Early clinical features include a wide-open fontanelle, constipation, jaundice, poor temperature control, and umbilical hernia. Macroglossia may interfere with feedings. Edema of the eyes, hands, and feet may be present at birth, but it is often unrecognized in early infancy.

Diagnosis. Radiographs of the long bones show delayed maturation, and radiographs of the skull show excessive numbers of wormian bones. A low serum concentration of thyroxine (T_4) and a high serum concentration of thyroid-stimulating hormone establish the diagnosis.

Management. Initial treatment with levothyroxine at doses of 10–15 μg/kg/day is indicated as soon as detected. Early treatment prevents most, if not all, of the sequelae of congenital hypothyroidism. Each month of delay reduces the ultimate intelligence of the infant.

Mitochondrial Disorders

Mitochondrial disorders involve pyruvate metabolism, the Krebs cycle, and respiratory complexes. Fig. 8.2 depicts the five respiratory complexes, and Box 8.6 lists the disorders assigned to abnormalities in each of these complexes.

Mitochondrial diseases arise from dysfunction of the mitochondrial respiratory chain.[31] Mutations of either nuclear or mitochondrial DNA (mtDNA) are causative. Some mutations affect a single organ, but most involve multiple organ systems and neurological dysfunction is prominent. In general nuclear defects present in childhood, and mtDNA defects present in late childhood or adult life. Many individuals show a cluster of clinical features that fall into a discrete clinical syndrome, but considerable clinical variability exists, and many individuals do not fit into one particular category. Common clinical features of mitochondrial disease include ptosis, retinitis pigmentosa, external ophthalmoplegia, myopathy, exercise intolerance, cardiomyopathy, sensorineural deafness, optic atrophy, seizures, and diabetes mellitus. Serial cranial MRI may show migrating or fluctuating white matter changes. Children tend to decompensate with glucose loads, acute illnesses, or use of valproic acid (contraindicated).

Alexander Disease

Alexander disease is a progressive disorder of cerebral white matter (leukodystrophy; Box 5.5) caused by a heterozygous pathogenic variant in the *GFAP* gene encoding NADH: ubiquinone oxidoreductase flavoprotein-1.[41] Disease transmission is autosomal dominant. Most affected newborns represent new mutations. Rosenthal fibers, the pathological hallmark of the disease, are rod-shaped or round bodies that stain red with hematoxylin and eosin and black with myelin stains. They appear as small granules within the cytoplasm of astrocytes. Rosenthal fibers are scattered diffusely in the cerebral cortex and the white matter, but have a predilection for the subpial, subependymal, and perivascular regions.

Clinical features. In the past, diagnosis depended on autopsy. Expansion of the clinical features expanded with accuracy of antemortem diagnosis. Neonatal, infantile, juvenile, and adult forms are recognized. The neonatal form is the most severe, generally resulting in death by the age of 2. The infantile form is the most common. It accounts for 70% of cases with an identifiable *GFAP* mutation. The onset is any time from birth to early childhood. Affected infants show arrest and regression of psychomotor development, enlargement of the head secondary to megalencephaly, spasticity, and seizures. Megalencephaly may be the initial feature. Optic atrophy does not occur. Death by early childhood is the rule.

Diagnosis. Four of the five following criteria establish an MRI-based diagnosis of Alexander disease: (1) extensive cerebral white matter abnormalities with a frontal preponderance; (2) a periventricular rim of decreased signal intensity on T_2-weighted images and elevated signal intensity on T_1-weighted images; (3) abnormalities of the basal ganglia and thalami; (4) brainstem abnormalities, particularly involving the medulla and midbrain; and (5) contrast enhancement of one or more of the following: ventricular lining, periventricular rim, frontal white matter, optic chiasm, fornix, basal ganglia, thalamus, dentate nucleus, and brainstem.[42] Genetic testing and identification of a heterozygous pathogenic variant of *GFAP*, which encodes glial fibrillary acidic protein, confirms the diagnosis.

Management. Treatment is supportive.

POLG-Related Disorders

The POLG-related disorders encompass a range of clinical phenotypes related to mutations in the *POLG* gene. Common clinical findings include hypotonia, developmental delay, ataxia, extrapyramidal symptoms, psychiatric disorders, epilepsy, ocular symptoms, myopathy, and peripheral neuropathy. There may be considerable clinical overlap between syndromes.[43] We will discuss the most relevant pediatric *POLG* disorders, Alpers-Huttenlocher syndrome (AHS), and childhood myocerebrohepatopathy spectrum (MCHS).

Valproic acid should be avoided in all patients with *POLG*-related disorders as it may accelerate hepatic failure. Monitor liver enzymes frequently when any medication is used that has potential hepatic side effects. As

---

BOX 5.5   Disorders With Specific MRI Findings

- Examples of disorders associated with gray matter abnormalities
  - Mitochondrial disorders
    - Leigh syndrome
    - Alpers-Huttenlocher syndrome
  - Disorders of neurodegeneration with brain iron accumulation
    - Infantile neuroaxonal dystrophy
    - Pantothenate kinase–associated neurodegeneration
- Examples of disorders associated with white matter abnormalities
  - Demyelinating leukodystrophies
    - Alexander disease
    - Globoid cell leukodystrophy (Krabbe disease)
    - X-linked adrenoleukodystrophy
    - Metachromatic leukodystrophy
    - Cerebrotendinous xanthomatosis
  - Hypomyelinating leukodystrophies
    - Pelizaeus-Merzbacher disease
  - Progressive cavitating leukoencephalopathy
  - Canavan disease
  - Vanishing white matter disease

in other mitochondrial disorders, avoid fever, infection, dehydration, and other physical stressors that can precipitate crisis or episodes of regression.

Alpers-Huttenlocher syndrome. AHS is the classic phenotype for POLG disorders and also the most severe. The onset of symptoms is during either infancy or childhood. Seizures usually manifest as progressive myoclonic epilepsy, very refractory to treatment, and some children present with epilepsia partialis continua. A progressive neurological disorder follows with spasticity, myoclonus, and dementia. Neuropathy, headaches (often with visual aura), and cortical visual loss are associated symptoms, and MRI shows atrophy and gliosis, particularly of the occipital lobes. Status epilepticus is often the terminal manifestation. Although clinical signs of liver disease typically appear later in the course, biochemical evidence of liver disease may predate the onset of seizures. Most patients die before the age of 3. Treatment is supportive.

Childhood myocerebrohepatopathy spectrum. MHCS presents between the ages of 3 months and 3 years. Developmental delay, lactic acidosis, failure to thrive, myopathy, hearing loss, pancreatitis, liver failure, and cyclic vomiting syndrome are common symptoms. Unlike AHS, seizures are not present early in the course of the disease. Treatment is supportive.

Leigh Syndrome (Subacute Necrotizing Encephalomyelopathy)

Classic Leigh syndrome, also called subacute necrotizing encephalomyelopathy (SNE), is a progressive disorder primarily affecting neurons of the brainstem, thalamus, basal ganglia, and cerebellum. Over 110 distinct genetic mutations can cause Leigh syndrome spectrum and "Leigh-like" syndrome. Pathogenic variants in nuclear DNA cause the majority, but approximately 20% are related to mtDNA mutations. It is likely that our classification of various disorders within the Leigh syndrome spectrum will continue to evolve over the next several years. Here, we specifically discuss the Leigh syndrome prototype, SNE. Classic Leigh syndrome, also called subacute necrotizing encephalomyelopathy, is a progressive disorder primarily affecting neurons of the brainstem, thalamus, basal ganglia, and cerebellum.

Clinical features. Onset of SNE is typically between the ages of 3 and 12 months. Initial symptoms are vomiting, diarrhea, and dysphagia with resultant failure to thrive. Decompensation, often with lactic acidosis, occurs during an intercurrent illness. Additional symptoms may include psychomotor regression with hypotonia, spasticity, movement disorders, cerebellar ataxia, and peripheral neuropathy. Eye movement abnormalities are common, typically ophthalmoparesis or nystagmus. Optic atrophy may occur. Extraneurological manifestations include hypertrophic cardiomyopathy and progressive respiratory failure.

Most individuals have a progressive course with episodic deterioration interspersed with variable periods of stability during which development may be quite stable or even show some progress. Death typically occurs by the ages of 2–3, most often due to respiratory or cardiac failure. In undiagnosed cases death may appear to be sudden and unexpected. "Leigh-like" syndrome may present later in life (even in adulthood) with slower progression, although this is not universal. ID, neuropathy, ataxia, and pigmentary retinopathy are associated symptoms.

Diagnosis. Lactate concentrations are increased in blood and/or CSF. Lactic acidemia is usually more common in postprandial samples. An oral glucose load causes blood lactate concentrations to double after 60 minutes and is more consistent in CSF samples than in blood samples. Blood concentrations of lactate and pyruvate are usually elevated and rise even higher at the time of clinical exacerbation. MRI greatly increases diagnostic accuracy. MRI features include bilateral symmetrical hyperintense signal abnormality in the brainstem (periaqueductal) and/or basal ganglia on T_2-weighted images. Symmetric MRI changes are a hallmark of the disease (see Box 5.5).

Molecular genetic testing is helpful in some cases, but ultimately SNE remains a diagnosis based on clinical, laboratory, and radiographic findings.

Management. Treatment is supportive and includes the use of sodium bicarbonate or sodium citrate for acidosis and antiepileptic drugs for seizures. Avoid valproic acid and phenobarbital, which adversely affect the mitochondrial respiratory chain. Dystonia can be treated with baclofen, tetrabenazine, or injections of botulinum toxin.

Neurocutaneous Syndromes
Neurofibromatosis Type 1

The neurofibromatoses (NFs) are divisible into a peripheral type (type 1) and a central type (type 2). Transmission of both is by autosomal dominant inheritance with considerable variation in expression. The abnormal gene for neurofibromatosis type 1 (*NF1*) is located on chromosome 17q, and its abnormal protein product is neurofibromin. Approximately 100 mutations of *NF1* have been identified in various regions of the gene. NF1 is the most common of the neurocutaneous syndromes, occurring in approximately 1 in 3000 individuals. Almost 50% of patients with NF1 have new mutations. New mutations are associated with increased paternal age.

Neurofibromatosis type 2 (NF2) is characterized by bilateral acoustic neuromas as well as other intracranial and intraspinal tumors (see Chapter 17).

Clinical features. The clinical manifestations are highly variable. In mild cases café au lait spots and subcutaneous neurofibromas are the only features. Axillary freckles and macrocephaly are common.

Severely affected individuals have developmental and neoplastic disorders of the nervous system. The main CNS abnormalities are optic pathway glioma, intraspinal neurofibroma, dural ectasia, and aqueductal stenosis. Acoustic neuromas are not part of NF1. The usual cognitive defect is a learning disability as opposed to true ID.

Diagnosis. Two or more of the following features are considered diagnostic: (1) six café au lait spots more than 5 mm in diameter in prepubertal individuals or more than 15 mm in postpubertal individuals; (2) two or more neurofibromas, or one plexiform neurofibroma; (3) freckling in the axillary or inguinal region; (4) optic glioma; (5) two or more iris hamartomas (Lisch nodules); (6) a distinctive osseous lesion such as sphenoid dysplasia or thinning of long bones; and (7) a first-degree relative with NF1. Only about half of children with NF1 with no known family history of NF meet the above criteria for diagnosis by the age of 1, but almost all do by the age of 8.

MRI may provide additional diagnostic information (Fig. 5.4). Areas of increased T_2 signal intensity are often present in the basal ganglia, cerebellum, brainstem, and subcortical white matter. The histology of these areas is not established, and they tend to disappear with age. However, the total burden of such areas correlates with intellectual impairment. Molecular genetic testing confirms the clinical diagnosis. MRI surveillance at regular intervals is not recommended as it is unlikely to modify the management. Yearly examinations, on the other hand, provide guidance regarding management and the need for imaging studies.

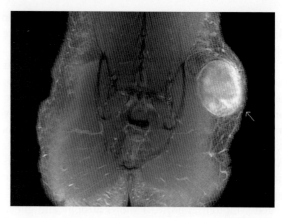

Fig. 5.4 Neurofibromatosis. Pelvic magnetic resonance imaging shows a large single neurofibroma within the subcutaneous tissue of the left superior gluteal region with heterogeneous contrast enhancement. Single large neurofibroma (*arrow*).

Management. Management is primarily supportive: anticonvulsant drugs for seizures, surgery for accessible tumors, and orthopedic procedures for bony deformities. Regular ophthalmological examinations are needed due to the risk of optic pathway gliomas, a type of pilocytic astrocytoma seen in approximately 15% of patients with NF1.[44] Routine MRI studies to screen for optic gliomas in asymptomatic children are unnecessary. Surgical procedures are recommended when gliomas or fibromas are symptomatic, causing mass effect, medically intractable pain, or cosmetic problems. Neuropathic pain associated with spinal neurofibromas may be treated with gabapentin 20–60 mg/kg/day, or pregabalin 2–8 mg/kg/day. Pregabalin is a more effective drug that can be used twice a day as opposed to the three times daily dosing recommended with gabapentin. Both medications may cause increased appetite, edema, and sedation. The sedative effect, when present, may provide hypnotic benefit with larger nighttime doses. Amitriptyline and duloxetine may be helpful as adjunctive therapies for pain management. Selumetinib (Koselugo) was recently approved to treat inoperable plexiform neuromas.

Tuberous Sclerosis

Transmission of the tuberous sclerosis complex (TSC) is by autosomal dominant inheritance with a variable phenotypic expression.[45] Two genes are responsible for TSC. One gene (*TSC1*) is located at chromosome 9q34, and the other (*TSC2*) is near the gene for adult polycystic kidney disease at chromosome 16p13.3. *TSC1*

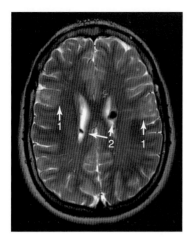

Fig. 5.5 Tuberous Sclerosis. T_2 axial magnetic resonance imaging shows: *(1)* cortical tubers and *(2)* subependymal nodules.

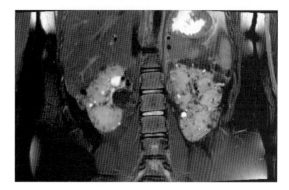

Fig. 5.6 Tuberous Sclerosis. T_2 fat suppression coronal magnetic resonance imaging of abdomen shows kidney cysts and angiomyolipomas (*arrows*).

is more likely than *TSC2* to account for familial cases. As a group, patients with *TSC1* are younger at seizure onset, more cognitively impaired, and have a greater tuber burden.[46]

Clinical features. The most common initial symptom of neurological dysfunction during infancy is seizures, especially infantile spasms (see Chapter 1). Some infants have evidence of developmental delay before the onset of seizures. The delay is often insufficient to prompt medical consultation. Most children with tuberous sclerosis who have cognitive impairment eventually have seizures, and virtually all infants with intractable seizures will later function in the cognitively impaired range. Seizures and ID are due to disturbed histogenesis of the brain, which contains decreased numbers of neurons and bizarrely shaped astrocytes. Subependymal hamartomas are common, tend to calcify with age, and only rarely cause obstructive hydrocephalus. Subependymal giant cell astrocytoma (SEGA) is a possible complication in these children and may obstruct the flow of CSF if left untreated (Fig. 5.5).

Hypomelanotic macules are the most common dermatological manifestation. In late infancy and early childhood, raised plaques of thicker skin may develop (*Shagreen patches*) and are present by 15 years in 50% of affected children. During childhood, adenomata sebaceum (actually angiokeratomas) appear on the face, usually in a butterfly distribution. Other organ involvement includes retinal tumors; rhabdomyoma of the heart;

renal tumors; and cysts of the kidney, bone, and lung (Fig. 5.6). Rhabdomyomas of the heart may manifest as prenatal arrhythmias and are detected by ultrasound. These lesions tend to decrease in size with time.

A shortened life expectancy results from renal disease, cardiovascular disorders, pleural involvement, brain tumors (SEGA), SUDEP, and status epilepticus.

Diagnosis. The clinical diagnosis is established in a child with two major features or one major feature and two or more minor features (Box 5.6). Molecular diagnosis is accomplished when molecular genetic testing reveals heterozygous pathogenic variants in *TSC1* or *TSC2*, regardless of clinical features.[47]

Management. The recommended evaluations in children with TSC are renal ultrasonography every 1–3 years followed by renal computed tomography (CT)/ MRI if large or numerous renal tumors are detected; cranial MRI every 1–3 years (or more frequently if clinically indicated); echocardiography if cardiac symptoms indicate the need; and chest CT if pulmonary symptoms indicate the need.

Anticonvulsant drugs are helpful in reducing seizure frequency, but when compared with other epilepsies a larger percentage of patients remain incompletely controlled. Use vigabatrin for patients with infantile spasms, starting at 50 mg/kg/day divided twice a day, and increasing every 5–7 days up to 250 mg/kg/day or when cessation of spasms and correction of hypsarrhythmia occurs. The concern of possible retinal injury from vigabatrin and associated loss of peripheral vision should not stop its use, since hypsarrhythmia often causes cortical visual impairment and progressive decline in all functions. Transition to a different anticonvulsant after

---

BOX 5.6   Clinical Diagnosis of Tuberous Sclerosis Complex (TSC)

Definite TSC: two major features or one major feature plus two minor features
Probable TSC: one major feature plus one minor feature
Possible TSC: one major feature or two or more minor features

Major Features
- Cardiac rhabdomyoma, single or multiple
- Cortical tuber[a]
- Facial angiofibromas or forehead plaque
- Hypomelanotic macules (three or more)
- Lymphangiomyomatosis[b]
- Multiple retinal nodular hamartomas
- Nontraumatic ungual or periungual fibromas
- Renal angiomyolipoma[b]

- Shagreen patch (connective tissue nevus)
- Subependymal nodule
- Subependymal giant cell astrocytoma

Minor Features
- Bone cysts[c]
- Cerebral white matter radial migration lines[a,c,d]
- "Confetti" skin lesions
- Gingival fibromas
- Hamartomatous rectal polyps[e]
- Multiple randomly distributed pits in dental enamel
- Multiple renal cysts[e]
- Nonrenal hamartoma[e]
- Retinal achromic patch

[a]Cerebral cortical dysplasia and cerebral white matter migration tracts occurring together are counted as one rather than two features of TSC.
[b]When both lymphangiomyomatosis and renal angiomyolipomas are present, other features of tuberous sclerosis must be present before TSC is diagnosed.
[c]Radiographical confirmation is sufficient.
[d]White matter migration lines and focal cortical dysplasia are often seen in individuals with TSC; however, because these lesions can be seen independently and are relatively nonspecific, they are considered a minor diagnostic criterion for TSC.
[e]Histological confirmation is suggested.

---

a few months of correction of hypsarrhythmia and control of infantile spasms to minimize the possibility of retinal or MRI changes.

The hamartin-tuberin complex regulates the activity of the target of rapamycin complex 1, which lies downstream of cellular pathways controlling cell growth and proliferation. Medications such as sirolimus (Rapamune) and everolimus (Afinitor) are known as mTOR (mammalian target of rapamycin) inhibitors and have a positive effect on controlling the growth of affected tissues in patients with tuberous sclerosis. Everolimus received a US Food and Drug Administration (FDA) indication for the treatment of SEGA. Similar medications may be used for the treatment of angiomyolipomas, facial angiofibromas, and lymphangioleiomyomatosis.[48,49] Cognitive impairment is not reversible.

Genetic counseling is an important aspect of patient management. Although disease transmission is autosomal dominant, gene expression is so variable that neither parent may appear affected. One-quarter of parents without a personal or family history of tuberous sclerosis are shown to be affected by a careful history and physical examination, including fundoscopic examination, skin examination with the Wood light, renal ultrasound, and cranial MRI.

Other Disorders of Gray Matter

Infantile Neuronal Ceroid Lipofuscinosis (CLN1 Disease, Batten Disease)

The neuronal ceroid lipofuscinoses (NCLs) are a group of progressive degenerative neurometabolic disorders. These disorders share certain characteristics, such as cognitive and motor regression, seizures, and visual symptoms, but vary in severity and age at onset. The most severe form is CNL1, or infantile neuronal ceroid lipofuscinosis. "Batten disease" is a nonspecific term that is often used interchangeably among various types of infantile and childhood-onset NCLs. Since some NCLs have approved treatments and others do not, a precise diagnosis is required. Here, we discuss CNL1. Classification of these disorders had previously been by age at onset and rapidity of progression, but now are classified by mutation analysis.[50]

The more common NCL types occur after the age of 2 (see the "Progressive Encephalopathies With Onset After Age 2" section) and are caused by mutations at other sites.

Clinical features. Children with CLN1 are normal at birth and usually develop symptoms between the ages of 6 and 24 months. The initial signs include delayed development, then the regression of cognitive and motor skills. Myoclonic jerks, epilepsy, and progressive optic atrophy leading to blindness follow. Head growth slows and microcephaly develops. Most affected individuals are never able to walk or talk and die in early childhood.

Diagnosis. Molecular genetic testing reveals biallelic pathogenic variants in the *PPT* gene which encodes the lysosomal enzyme palmitoyl-protein thioesterase-1. The EEG shows an encephalopathic pattern with myoclonic seizures. Brain MRI demonstrates progressive atrophy.

Management. Seizures and myoclonus are treated with a combination of anticonvulsant drugs (see Chapter 1). No treatment for the underlying metabolic error is available. Zonisamide and levetiracetam are the best choices in the treatment of progressive myoclonic epilepsies. Treatment is supportive, and no specific therapies have been identified.

Infantile Neuroaxonal Dystrophy

Infantile neuroaxonal dystrophy is one of the group of disorders known as neurodegeneration with brain iron accumulations (NBIAs). It is a disorder of axon terminals transmitted by autosomal recessive inheritance, usually via biallelic pathogenic variants in the *PLA2G6* gene. It shares many pathological features with pantothenate kinase–associated neurodegeneration (PKAN) (see Chapter 14) with the exception that symptoms begin in infancy.

Clinical features. Affected children develop normally during the first few months, but most children never walk. Facial dysmorphism includes a prominent forehead, strabismus, small nose, wide mouth, micrognathia, and large, low-set ears.[51] Motor regression occurs at the end of the first year as clumsiness and frequent falling. The infant is first hypotonic and hyporeflexic. Muscle atrophy may be present as well. At this stage, suspect peripheral neuropathy, but the motor nerve conduction velocity and the protein content of the CSF are normal.

After the initial phase of hypotonia, symptoms of cerebral degeneration become prominent. Increasing spastic quadriparesis, optic atrophy, involuntary movements, and cognitive regression are evident. By the age of 2, most children are severely disabled. Deterioration to a vegetative state follows, and death usually occurs by the age of 10.

Diagnosis. The CSF is usually normal. Electromyography shows a denervation pattern consistent with anterior horn cell disease. Motor nerve conduction velocities are normal. MRI shows high iron in the globus pallidus, and the diagnosis is, therefore, a consideration in the differential diagnosis of PKAN.[52]

The majority of affected children have mutations in the *PLA2G6* gene; however, some have no known mutation. A definitive diagnosis requires evidence of neuroaxonal spheroids in peripheral nerve endings, conjunctiva, or brain in the appropriate clinical context. Neuroaxonal spheroids are large eosinophilic spheroids, caused by axonal swelling throughout the gray matter. They are not unique to neuroaxonal dystrophy and are seen in pantothenate kinase deficiency (PKAN), infantile GM_2 gangliosidosis, Niemann-Pick disease type C, and several other neurodegenerative conditions.

Management. Treatment is supportive.

Lesch-Nyhan Disease

Lesch-Nyhan disease is a progressive X-linked neurodegenerative disorder. Mutations in the *HPRT1* gene cause deficiency of the enzyme hypoxanthine-guanine phosphoribosyltransferase (HPRT).[53]

Clinical features. Affected newborns appear normal at birth, except for mild hypotonia. Delayed motor development and poor head control are present during the first 3 months. Progressive limb rigidity and torticollis or retrocollis follow. The progression of neurological disturbance is insidious, and many are misdiagnosed with cerebral palsy. During the second year, facial grimacing, corticospinal tract dysfunction, and involuntary movements (usually chorea but sometimes athetosis) develop. Severe gout with joint swelling and kidney dysfunction occurs. Without adequate HPRT function, the body does not adequately utilize vitamin B_{12}, leading to megaloblastic anemia in some patients.

It is not until after the age of 2, and sometimes considerably later, that affected children begin biting their fingers, lips, and cheeks. Compulsive self-mutilation is characteristic, but not constant, and causes severe disfigurement. Often wrapping the hands or removing teeth is necessary to prevent further harm. In addition to self-directed aggressive behavior, aggressive behavior toward caretakers may be present. Cognitive impairment is constant but of variable severity. Intelligence is difficult to evaluate because of behavioral and motor disturbances.

Diagnosis. Uric acid concentrations in the blood and urine are elevated. Indeed, some parents note a reddish discoloration of diapers caused by uric acid. The demonstration that HPRT activity is less than 1.5% in erythrocytes or cultured fibroblasts establishes the diagnosis, but increasingly the diagnosis is made using molecular genetic testing demonstrating pathogenic variants of the *HPRT1* gene. Such testing also identifies female carriers.

Management. Allopurinol decreases the urinary concentration of uric acid and prevents the development of nephropathy. Levodopa or antipsychotic medications may decrease self-mutilation and aggression. However, no treatment is available to prevent progressive degeneration of the nervous system.

MECP2-Related Disorders

The MECP2-related disorders include classic Rett syndrome and variant Rett syndrome in females and a severe neonatal-onset encephalopathy or severe ID syndrome in males. These disorders are X-linked, caused by heterozygous pathogenic *MECP2* variants in females and hemizygous pathogenic variants in males. Of note, the *MECP2* duplication syndrome is a distinct disorder discussed earlier in this chapter, involving full-scale gene duplication without pathogenic mutations.

Clinical Features in Females. *Classic Rett syndrome.* A period of rapid regression followed by stabilization is the main characteristic of classic Rett syndrome. Affected girls are normal during the first year. Developmental arrest usually begins at 12 months but may appear as early as 5 months, or as late as 18 months. The initial features are deceleration of head growth leading to microcephaly, lack of interest in the environment, and hypotonia. Within a few months, rapid developmental regression occurs characterized by the loss of language skills, gait ataxia or loss of ambulation, seizures, and autistic behavior. A characteristic feature of the syndrome is loss of purposeful hand movements before the age of 3. Stereotyped activity develops that looks like hand wringing or washing. Repetitive blows to the face are another form of stereotyped hand movement.

Continued slower neurological deterioration follows the initial rapid regression. Spastic paraparesis and quadriparesis are frequent endpoints. Dementia is usually severe. Stimulation produces an exaggerated, stereotyped reaction consisting of jerking movements of the trunk and limbs with episodes of disorganized breathing and apnea, followed by tachypnea. Seizures occur in most children before the age of 3. After the period of rapid deterioration, the disease becomes relatively stable, but dystonia may develop later. Females with Rett syndrome usually survive into early adulthood, but have an increased incidence of sudden, unexplained death.

Variant Rett syndrome. Variant Rett syndrome has a broad phenotype which may be milder or more severe than the classic form. In the milder form, ID is less pronounced, and some language may be preserved. Standard clinical findings are similar to those for classic Rett syndrome; sleep disorders are slightly more common.

Mild learning disabilities. Some females with pathogenic *MECP2* mutations do not experience regression and suffer only mild learning disabilities.

Clinical Features in Males. *MECP2-related severe neonatal encephalopathy.* The disorder follows a relentless course, characterized by microcephaly, intractable seizures, movement disorders, and respiratory abnormalities including respiratory insufficiency and central hypoventilation. Death typically occurs by the age of 2.

MECP2 severe ID syndrome. Unlike other *MECP2*-related disorders, microcephaly and seizures usually do not occur. Affected boys have moderate-to-severe ID, ataxia, resting tremor, and psychomotor slowing. The PPM-X syndrome is sometimes seen, which includes pyramidal signs, parkinsonism, and macroorchidism. Progressive spasticity is common.

Syndromic/nonsyndromic ID. Severe ID is the hallmark feature. Speech is absent or impaired in approximately 50%. Behavioral problems may occur, but autism is uncommon. A minority experience regression or progressive spasticity.

Diagnosis. The diagnosis for all *MECP2*-related disorders requires a compatible clinical phenotype in conjunction with a pathogenic variant in the *MECP2* gene. Sequence analysis detects most variants, but 5%–10% require gene-targeted deletion/duplication analysis.[54]

Management. Trofinetide (Daybue) is approved to treat a variety of symptoms in children with classic Rett syndrome. Symptoms studied during phase 3 clinical trials include mood, breathing patterns, stereotypies, nocturnal behaviors, and repetitive behaviors. Trofinetide does not treat seizures. Diarrhea is the most common side effect and can be severe. All laxatives should be stopped before initiation; consider starting a probiotic.

CDKL5 Deficiency Disorder

CDKL5 deficiency disorder was previously thought to be an early-seizure variant of Rett syndrome but has since been classified as its own distinct disorder.

It is X-linked, resulting from pathogenic heterozygous (in females) or hemizygous (in males) variants in the *CDKL5* gene which controls the production of cyclin-dependent kinase 5, an enzyme widely expressed in brain tissue. Females are affected more than males by a 4:1 ratio as affected males lack normal CDKL5, presumably causing in utero fetal demise. When affected males survive to birth, their clinical course is similar to females.

Clinical features. Affected infants have hypotonia, developmental delays, ID, and visual impairment. Severe early-onset seizures characterize the disorder. The median age at seizure onset is 6 weeks, with 90% developing epilepsy by 3 months of age.[55] Infantile spasms are common. The initial epilepsy is explosive and often pharmacoresistant, followed by a "honeymoon" period during which seizures stabilize into a static epileptic encephalopathy before progressing to refractory multifocal and myoclonic epilepsy.

Unlike Rett syndrome, microcephaly does not occur. Severe developmental disabilities are the norm, and only about 25% of affected girls can ambulate or produce spoken words. Repetitive hand movements and stereotypies are present, as well as other movement disorders. Affected children suffer from a variety of sleep disorders, usually poor sleep maintenance with multiple awakenings per night. This also causes strain on caregivers.

Diagnosis. Proposed diagnostic criteria include epilepsy onset within the first year of life, motor and cognitive delays, and a pathogenic variant in the *CDKL5* gene.

Management. Use broad-spectrum anticonvulsants to treat epilepsy, as carbamazepine and oxcarbazepine may cause worsening of seizures. Some children respond well to the ketogenic diet. Ganaxalone, a neurosteroid, was recently approved to treat seizures in children above 2 years of age with CDKL5 deficiency disorders.[56]

ATP7A-Related Copper Transport Disorders: Menkes Syndrome

Menkes syndrome, occipital horn syndrome (OHS), Wilson disease (hepatolenticular degeneration), and *ATP7A*-related distal motor neuropathy comprise the group of disorders caused by defective copper transport due to pathogenic variants in the *ATP7A* gene. Menkes syndrome is the only one that presents in infancy; OHS presents in later childhood with only minor neurological deficits, and *ATP7A*-related distal motor neuropathy presents in adulthood. Wilson disease can present

in adolescence and will be discussed later in this chapter. Tissue copper concentrations are decreased due to impaired intestinal copper absorption, accumulation of copper in other tissues, and reduced activity of copper-dependent enzymes.[57]

Clinical features. Infants with Menkes syndrome are healthy until approximately 2 months of age and then show loss of developmental milestones, hypotonia, and seizures. The appearance of the scalp hair and eyebrows is almost pathognomonic. The hair is sparse, poorly pigmented, and wiry. The shafts break easily, forming short stubble. Radiographs of the long bones suggest osteogenesis imperfecta. Other facial abnormalities include abnormal fullness of the cheeks, a high-arched palate, and micrognathia. Temperature instability and hypoglycemia may be present in the neonatal period. Death usually occurs by the age of 3.

Diagnosis. Low plasma concentrations of ceruloplasmin and copper suggest the diagnosis in older infants but are not useful in infants below 2 months old (in whom serum copper and ceruloplasmin are typically low). The disorder is X-linked and typically affects males, although symptomatic females have been reported. Diagnosis is confirmed when molecular genetic testing reveals a hemizygous (for males) or heterozygous (for females) pathogenic variant of *ATP7A*.[57]

Management. Subcutaneous injections of copper histidinate before the age of 28 days lead to improved neurodevelopmental outcomes and survival, but many infants continue to experience significant symptoms despite treatment, including early death.

Other Disorders of White Matter
Aspartoacylase Deficiency (Canavan Disease)

The inheritance of Canavan disease (also called *spongy degeneration of infancy*) is autosomal recessive. The most common mutation associated with disease is in the *ASPA* gene, which codes for the aspartoacylase enzyme. Enzyme deficiency leads to a buildup of *N*-acetyl-L-aspartic acid in neurons and causes myelin destruction resulting in neurological symptoms.

Clinical features. Psychomotor arrest and regression occur during the first 6 months. Clinical features include decreased awareness of the environment, difficulty in feeding, irritability, and hypotonia. Eventually, spasticity replaces the initial flaccidity. A characteristic posture with leg extension, arm flexion, and head retraction occurs, especially when the child is stimulated. Macrocephaly is evident by the age of 6 months. The head continues to enlarge throughout infancy, and this growth reaches a plateau by the third year. Optic atrophy leading to blindness evolves between 6 and 10 months. Life expectancy varies depending on the severity of the phenotype, but individuals who present in infancy often die during childhood or early adolescence.

Diagnosis. Abnormal excretion of *N*-acetylaspartic acid is detectable in the urine, and aspartoacylase activity in cultured fibroblasts is less than 40% of normal. MRI shows diffuse symmetric leukoencephalopathy even before neurological symptoms are evident. Demyelination of peripheral nerves does not occur, and the CSF is normal. Molecular genetic testing of the *ASPA* gene is available, with several distinct pathogenic variants identified.[58]

Management. Treatment is supportive.

Galactose-1-Phosphate Uridyltransferase Deficiency (Galactosemia)

Three separate inborn errors of galactose metabolism produce galactosemia in the newborn, but only classic galactosemia (type 1) with galactose-1-phosphate uridyltransferase (GALT) deficiency produces significant neurological symptoms. Transmission of the defect is by autosomal recessive inheritance of biallelic pathogenic variants of the *GALT* gene on chromosome 9p13.[59]

Clinical features. Affected newborns appear normal, but cataracts are already developing. The first milk feeding provokes the initial symptoms. These include failure to thrive, vomiting, diarrhea, jaundice, and hepatomegaly. During this time, some newborns have clinical features of increased intracranial pressure, probably resulting from cerebral edema. The combination of a tense fontanelle and vomiting suggests a primary intracranial disturbance and can delay the diagnosis and treatment of the metabolic error.

Diagnosis. Newborn screening detects galactosemia. However, many infants become symptomatic before newborn screen results are available and the disorder should be a consideration in any newborn with vomiting and hepatomegaly, especially when cataracts are present. The best time to test the urine for reducing substances is after feeding. Biallelic pathogenic variants in the *GALT* gene confirm the diagnosis.

Management. Immediate dietary intervention requires replacement of all milk and milk products with a formula that is free of bioavailable galactose. If galactosemia is suspected, these changes should be made immediately rather than awaiting results of confirmatory testing; untreated infants will not survive the newborn period. Most affected females will have primary ovarian insufficiency requiring endocrinology evaluation and management. Even with adequate dietary management, long-term neurologic and hepatic issues may occur.[60] Cataracts, however, appear to be completely reversible.

Pelizaeus-Merzbacher Disease

Pelizaeus-Merzbacher disease (PMD) is a hypomyelinating leukodystrophy transmitted by X-linked recessive inheritance. The gene maps to chromosome Xq22. Defective biosynthesis of a proteolipid protein (*PLP1*) that comprises half of the myelin sheath protein causes the disorder. Mutations in the *PLP1* gene are also responsible for one form of hereditary spastic paraplegia (see Chapter 12). An infantile, a neonatal, and a transitional phenotype of PMD exist.

Pelizaeus-merzbacher-like disease 1 is clinically similar to PMD but is caused by mutations of the *GJC2* gene.[61] Other hypomyelinating leukodystrophies include RNA polymerase-III-related leukodystrophies/4H syndrome (hypomyelination, hypogonadotropic hypogonadism, and hypodontia) and hypomyelination with atrophy of the basal ganglia and cerebellum. We will limit ourselves to PMD in this discussion.

Clinical features. Disorders related to *PLP1* are a continuum of neurological findings from severe CNS involvement to spastic paraplegia. Disease characteristics are usually consistent within families. The first symptoms of the neonatal form suggest spasmus nutans (see Chapter 15). The neonate has an intermittent nodding movement of the head and pendular nystagmus. Chorea or athetosis develops, psychomotor development arrests by the third month, and regression follows. Limb movements become ataxic and tone becomes spastic, first in the legs and then in the arms. Optic atrophy and seizures are late occurrences. Severely affected patients may die in childhood. Children with later disease onset experience slower progression and a milder course. Survival to adult life is relatively common.

Diagnosis. MRI shows diffuse demyelination of the hemispheres with sparing of scattered small areas. Molecular genetic testing is available for diagnosis and carrier detection.

Management. Treatment is supportive.

Progressive Cavitating Leukoencephalopathy

Progressive cavitating leukoencephalopathy describes a progressive degenerative disorder of early childhood characterized by progressive cystic degeneration of the white matter.[62] It may be the result of a mitochondrial depletion syndrome; at least one reported case had an associated *POLG* mutation.[63]

Clinical features. Age at onset is between 2 months and 3.5 years. The initial features are episodes of irritability or focal neurological deficits. Steady clinical deterioration follows often with spasticity and bulbar dysfunction leading to death.

Diagnosis. MRI shows a patchy leukoencephalopathy with cavity formation first affecting the corpus callosum and centrum semiovale. Later, large cystic lesions appear in the brain and spinal cord. Elevated levels of lactate in brain, blood, and CSF suggest a mitochondrial disturbance.

Management. Management is supportive.

Progressive Hydrocephalus

Clinical features. Progressive dilatation of the ventricular system may be a consequence of congenital malformations, infectious diseases, intracranial hemorrhage, or connatal tumors. Whatever the cause, the clinical features of increasing intracranial pressure are much the same. Head circumference enlarges, the anterior fontanelle feels full, and the child becomes lethargic, has difficulty feeding, and vomits. Ataxia and a spastic gait are common.

Diagnosis. Progressive hydrocephalus is often insidious in premature newborns with intraventricular hemorrhage, especially when delayed progression follows initial arrest. Hydrocephalus is always suspected in newborns and infants with excessive head growth. Head ultrasound, CT, or MRI confirm the diagnosis.

Management. Ventriculoperitoneal shunt is the usual procedure to relieve hydrocephalus in newborns and small infants with primary dilatation of the lateral ventricles (see Chapter 18).

PROGRESSIVE ENCEPHALOPATHIES WITH ONSET AFTER AGE 2

Disorders of Lysosomal Enzymes

GM2 Gangliosidosis (Juvenile Tay-Sachs Disease)

Deficiency of *N*-acetyl-β-hexosaminidase (HEXA) underlies both the infantile and juvenile forms of TSD. Unlike in infantile TSD, no ethnic predilection exists.

Clinical features. Affected children develop normally for the first 2 years of life, then develop progressive ataxia and incoordination between the ages of 2 and 10. Children lose language skills and cognition declines. Spasticity and seizures are present by the end of the first decade of life. The loss of vision occurs much later than in the acute infantile form of the disease, and a cherry-red spot is not a consistent finding. Instead, optic atrophy may occur late in the course. A vegetative state with decerebrate rigidity develops by 10–15 years of age, followed within a few years by death, usually due to infection. In some cases, the disease pursues a particularly aggressive course, culminating in death in 2–4 years.

Diagnosis. Serum, leukocytes, and fibroblasts are deficient in HEXA activity. Molecular genetic testing demonstrating biallelic pathogenic variants in the *HEXA* gene confirms the diagnosis. Although involving the same gene, the causative mutations are distinct in the infantile and juvenile forms.

Management. Treatment is supportive.

Gaucher Disease Type 3 (Glucosylceramide Lipidosis)

Gaucher disease encompasses a range of phenotypes from mild to severe and is divided into types 1, 2, and 3. Type 1 presents in infancy with bone and visceral abnormalities, but no neurologic symptoms. Type 2 presents before the age of 2 and was discussed earlier in this chapter. Type 3 presents in childhood. As in other types, the cause of late-onset Gaucher disease is deficiency of the enzyme glucocerebrosidase. Transmission is by autosomal recessive inheritance.

Clinical features. Onset is typically in childhood. As with type 2, hepatosplenomegaly, cardiopulmonary disease, and hematologic abnormalities are common. Hepatosplenomegaly usually precedes neurological deterioration. The most common neurological manifestations are oculomotor apraxia, progressive myoclonic epilepsy, and cognitive regression.[32] Mental regression varies from mild memory loss to severe dementia. Of note, patients with type 3 Gaucher disease have bony abnormalities, while patients with type 2 do not. The presence of vertical oculomotor apraxia is reminiscent of Niemann-Pick disease.

Diagnosis. Gaucher cells are present in the bone marrow and are virtually diagnostic. Confirmation requires the demonstration of deficient glucocerebrosidase activity in hepatocytes or leukocytes, or biallelic pathogenic variants in the *GBA* gene.

Management. Enzyme replacement therapy utilizes imiglucerase (Cerezyme), a recombinant glucosylceramidase enzyme preparation. Regular intravenous infusions of imiglucerase are safe and effective in reversing hematological and visceral involvement, but not neurological disease. Substrate reducing therapy is used where available. Stem cell transplantation has been largely replaced by enzyme replacement therapy.

Globoid Cell Leukodystrophy (Late-Onset Krabbe Disease)

Deficiency of the enzyme galactosylceramide β-galactosidase causes globoid cell leukodystrophy. Transmission is by autosomal recessive inheritance. The onset of symptoms in late infancy and in adolescence can occur in the same family. The severity of the enzyme deficiency is similar in all phenotypes from early infancy to adolescence.

Clinical features. Neurological deterioration usually begins between the ages of 2 and 6 but may start as early as the second year or as late as adolescence. The major features are cognitive regression, cortical blindness, and generalized or unilateral spasticity. The initial feature may be progressive spasticity rather than dementia. Unlike the infantile form, peripheral neuropathy is not a feature of the juvenile form, and the protein content of the CSF is normal. Progressive neurological deterioration results in a vegetative state and death occurs 4–6 years after symptom onset in most cases.

Diagnosis. MRI shows diffuse demyelination of the cerebral hemispheres. Showing the enzyme deficiency in leukocytes or cultured fibroblasts establishes the diagnosis, and molecular genetic testing reveals biallelic pathogenic variants in the *GALC* gene.

Management. Brain MRI with diffusion tensor imaging may show early brainstem atrophy, prompting preparation for increased care needs including apnea and dysfunctional temperature regulation. Evidence for hematopoietic stem cell transplantation is sparse but suggests that transplantation early in the course of late-onset Krabbe (i.e., prior to severe neurological dysfunction) may arrest or slow neurological deterioration.[33] Otherwise, treatment is supportive.

Metachromatic Leukodystrophy (Late-Onset Lipidosis)

Deficiency of the enzyme arylsulfatase A causes the juvenile and infantile forms of sulfatide lipidosis, a demyelinating leukodystrophy and lysosomal storage disease.[64] The late-infantile metachromatic leukodystrophy (MLD) comprises 50%–60% of cases; juvenile MLD comprises about 20%–30%, and the remainder have adult onset. Genetic transmission of both is autosomal recessive inheritance. Two groups of mutations in the gene encoding arylsulfatase A are identified as I and A. Patients with I mutations generate no active enzyme, and those with A mutations generate small amounts. Late-onset disease is associated with I-A genotype, and the adult form with an A-A genotype.

Clinical features. Age of onset within a family is usually similar. All individuals eventually lose motor and intellectual functions. The disease course may be from 3 to 10 or more years in the late-onset infantile form and up to 20 years or more in the juvenile- and adult-onset forms. Death most commonly results from pneumonia or other infection.

Late-onset infantile form. Onset is between 6 months and 4 years of age, but usually less than age 3. Typical presenting symptoms include clumsiness, frequent falls, toe walking, and slurred speech. Weakness and hypotonia are initially observed. Later signs include inability to stand, difficulty speaking, ID, increased muscle tone, pain in the arms and legs, generalized or partial seizures, compromised vision and hearing, and peripheral neuropathy. The final stages include tonic spasms, decerebrate posturing with rigidly extended extremities, feeding by gastrostomy tube, blindness, and general unawareness of surroundings. The expected lifespan is about 5–6 years after symptom onset.

Juvenile form. The onset of symptoms is generally between 5 and 10 years but may be delayed until adolescence or occur as early as late infancy. The early-onset juvenile form is clinically different from the infantile form despite the age overlap. No clinical symptoms of peripheral neuropathy occur, progression is slower, and the protein content of the CSF is normal. Cognitive regression, speech disturbances, and clumsiness of gait are the prominent initial features. Dementia usually progresses slowly over a period of 3–5 years, but sometimes progresses rapidly to a vegetative state. A delay of several years may separate the onset of dementia from the appearance of other neurological disturbances. Ataxia may be an early and prominent manifestation. Spastic quadriplegia eventually develops in all affected children, and most have seizures. Death usually occurs during the second decade.

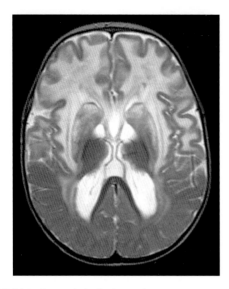

Fig. 5.7 Metachromatic leukodystrophy.

Diagnosis. The juvenile form can overlap in age with a late-onset form, which usually manifests as psychosis or dementia. MRI shows demyelination in the cerebral hemispheres with sparing of the U-fibers (Fig. 5.7). Motor nerve conduction velocities may be normal early in the course. Deficiency of arylsulfatase A in leukocytes or cultured fibroblasts establishes the diagnosis and molecular genetic testing shows biallelic pathogenic variants in the *ARSA* gene.

Management. Treatment is supportive. Targeted gene therapy and hematopoietic stem cell transplantation are both possible future treatments.

ATP7A-Related Copper Transport Disorders: Wilson Disease

Clinical features. Wilson disease can present in childhood, adolescence, or adulthood. Affected children or adolescents often present with hepatic disease or fulminant hepatic failure as the initial symptom. Tremor, dystonia, dysautonomia, and psychiatric disturbance may occur. Slit-lamp examination by an ophthalmologist reveals Keyser-Fleischer rings.

Diagnosis. Consider the diagnosis in adolescents with significant psychiatric disease and unexplained tremor or transaminitis. Demonstration of low serum copper and serum ceruloplasmin, with increased urinary copper excretion, and biallelic pathogenic variants in *ATP7A* establishes the diagnosis.

Management. Initiate treatment with copper chelating agents immediately to prevent further tissue damage from copper accumulation. The American Association for the Study of Liver Diseases has published extensive treatment and management guidelines.[65]

Mucopolysaccharidoses

The MPS are a subset of lyosomal storage diseases resulting from deficiencies of enzymes involved in the catabolism of dermatan sulfate, heparan sulfate, or keratin sulfate. Multiple types of MPS are recognized. Four of these, types I, II, III, and VII, affect the nervous system and cause cognitive impairment/regression. The onset of types I (Hurler syndrome) and III (Sanfilippo syndrome) is in infancy and discussed in the prior section. Types II and VII ordinarily have their onset in childhood following two or more years of normal development.

MPS II (Hunter syndrome). This is the only MPS transmitted by X-linked inheritance.[66] Most affected children are males, but symptomatic heterozygous females have been reported. Most cases are evident by early childhood; in rare cases the disease progresses slowly and may not be apparent until adolescence or later.

Clinical features. Patients with Hunter syndrome have a Hurler phenotype (see Box 5.3) but lack corneal clouding. Iduronate sulfatase is the deficient enzyme; dermatan sulfate and heparan sulfate are stored in the viscera and appear in the urine.

The Hurler phenotype may develop rapidly or evolve slowly during childhood and not be recognized until the second decade or later. A prominent feature is the appearance of a nodular, ivory-colored lesion on the back, usually around the shoulders and upper arms. Affected children have short stature, macrocephaly with or without communicating hydrocephalus, macroglossia, hoarse voice, conductive and sensorineural hearing loss, hepatomegaly and/or splenomegaly, dysostosis multiplex, and joint contractures, which include ankylosis of the temporomandibular joint, spinal stenosis, and carpal tunnel syndrome.

Cognitive regression caused by neuronal storage of gangliosides is slowly progressive, but many patients come to medical attention because of chronic hydrocephalus. Affected children survive into adult life. The accumulation of storage materials in collagen causes the entrapment of peripheral nerves, especially the median and ulnar nerves.

Diagnosis. The presence of mucopolysacchariduria with equal excretion of dermatan sulfate and heparan sulfate suggests the diagnosis. Establishing the diagnosis requires showing iduronate sulfatase deficiency in cultured fibroblasts or serum in the presence of normal activity of at least one other sulfatase. Molecular genetic testing demonstrates hemizygous pathogenic variants in the *IDS* gene.[67]

Management. Treat with idursulfase enzyme replacement therapy (Elaprase) which has been shown to prolong survival. Hematopoietic stem cell transplantation is a potential option but has not been specifically studied in MPS II. Ventriculoperitoneal shunting is often needed to treat obstructive hydrocephalus. Necessary surveillance includes regular cardiac evaluations and pulmonary function testing.

MPS VII (Sly disease). Sly disease is a rare disorder caused by deficiency of the enzyme β-glucuronidase. Transmission is by autosomal recessive inheritance.

Clinical features. Specific to MPS VII is the fact that those with severe disease suffer from nonimmune hydrops fetalis and often are stillborn or die shortly after birth. However, the phenotype varies widely. Macrocephaly, hydrocephalus, and hepatosplenomegaly are common. Heart valve abnormalities occur, as does corneal clouding. As in the other MPS subtypes discussed earlier, dysostosis multiplex, spinal stenosis, and carpal tunnel syndrome are frequently associated symptoms. ID develops after the age of 3 in some but not all cases. Death occurs in infancy for those with severe disease, but many survive to adolescence or adulthood.

Diagnosis. Both dermatan and heparan sulfates are present in the urine, causing a screening test to be positive for mucopolysacchariduria. Specific diagnosis requires the demonstration of β-glucuronidase deficiency in leukocytes or cultured fibroblasts. Molecular genetic testing reveals biallelic pathogenic mutations in the *GUSB* gene.

Management. As in many other lysosomal storage diseases, enzyme replacement therapy is the mainstay of treatment in addition to supportive/symptomatic management. The specific treatment is vestronidase alfa 4 mg/kg given as a slow IV infusion every 2 weeks. Enzyme replacement therapy slows the progression of disease but does not reverse the damage already done. Hematopoietic stem cell therapy has limited data but may be used in some cases. Gene therapy may be a treatment option in the future.[68]

Niemann-Pick Disease Type C (Sphingomyelin Lipidosis)

Niemann-Pick disease type C is another lysosomal storage disease caused by deficient esterification of cholesterol; the nonesterified cholesterol accumulates in the brain and other organs. Types C1 and C2 cannot be distinguished clinically but result from distinct genetic mutations of the *NPC1* and *NPC2* genes, respectively, with *NPC1* mutations being vastly more common. Transmission of the defect is autosomal recessive.[69]

Clinical features. Niemann-Pick C is more common than types A and B and has the most stereotyped clinical features, which tend to be age-dependent although significant overlap exists between types.

Neonatal and infantile forms are uncommon. The phenotype is visceral neurodegenerative, and onset is before the age of 2. Affected infants tend to present with organomegaly; fetal ascites may be evident on late prenatal ultrasound. The lungs contain foam cells causing pulmonary dysfunction. Neurological symptoms follow, including developmental delay and hypotonia. Some infants die quickly as a result of pulmonary and hepatic complications. Those who survive may live for several years.

Late-infantile and childhood forms are the classic neurodegenerative phenotype. Early development is normal. Cerebellar ataxia or dystonia is the initial feature (mean age, 3 years), and apraxia of vertical gaze and cognitive difficulties follow (mean age, 6 years). Oculomotor apraxia, in which the eyes move reflexively but not voluntarily, is unusual in healthy children (see Chapter 15). Vertical gaze apraxia is particularly uncommon and always suggests Niemann-Pick disease type C. Progressive neurological degeneration is relentless. Dementia, seizures, and spasticity cause severe disability during the second decade. Organomegaly is seldom prominent early in the course.

The late-onset form begins in adolescence or adult life and is similar to the delayed-onset form except that the progression is considerably slower. The phenotype is psychiatric/neurodegenerative.

Diagnosis. Biochemical testing that demonstrates impaired cholesterol esterification and positive filipin staining in cultured fibroblasts confirms the diagnosis. Molecular genetic testing demonstrates biallelic pathogenic variants in the *NPC1* or *NPC2* gene.[70]

Management. Published guidelines for the management of NPC exist. Treatment is mainly supportive. Miglustat, a type of substrate reduction therapy used to treat Gaucher disease type 1, is used to treat NPC in many countries but is not approved in the United States.

Infectious Diseases

Infectious diseases are an uncommon cause of progressive dementia in childhood. Several fungal species may cause chronic meningitis characterized by personality change and some decline in higher intellectual function. *Cryptococcus* infection is especially notorious for its indolent course. However, the major features of these infections are fever and headache. Chronic meningitis is not a serious consideration in the differential diagnosis of isolated psychomotor regression.

In contrast, chronic viral infections, especially HIV (see the previous discussion of AIDS encephalopathy), may produce a clinical picture similar to that of many genetic disorders in which dementia is a prominent feature.

Subacute Sclerosing Panencephalitis

Subacute sclerosing panencephalitis (SSPE) is a form of chronic measles encephalitis that was once endemic in several parts of the world but has almost disappeared in countries that require routine measles immunization.[71] In a nonimmunized population, the average age at onset is 8. As a rule, children with SSPE have experienced natural infection with the rubeola virus at an early age, half before the age of 2. A concomitant infection with a second virus at the time of initial exposure to measles and immunosuppression are additional risk factors for SSPE. In the United States, incidence rates are highest in rural areas, especially in the southeastern states and the Ohio River Valley.

Clinical features. The first symptoms of disease are personality change and declining school performance. Personality change may consist of aggressive behavior or withdrawal, and parents may seek psychological rather than medical services. However, retinal examination during this early stage shows pigmentary changes in the macula. Generalized seizures, usually myoclonic, develop next. An EEG at this time shows the characteristic pattern of periodic bursts of spike-wave complexes (approximately every 5–7 seconds) occurring synchronously with the myoclonic jerk. The generalized periodic discharges associated with the myoclonus may contribute to the patient's encephalopathy and are helped by levetiracetam.[72] After the onset of seizures, the child shows rapid neurological deterioration characterized by spasticity, dementia, and involuntary movements.

Within 1–6 years from the onset of symptoms, the child is in a chronic vegetative state.

Diagnosis. Suspect the diagnosis in a child with a compatible clinical course and an EEG characterized by periodic high amplitude sharp and slow-wave bursts associated with myoclonic jerks. Confirmation requires demonstration of an elevated antibody titer against rubeola, usually associated with elevated gamma globulin concentrations in the CSF. The CSF is otherwise normal. The rubeola antibody titer in blood is also markedly elevated.

A similar progressive disorder of the nervous system may occur in children who were born with rubella embryopathy (chronic rubella panencephalitis).

Management. Prevention via vaccination is critical, but unfortunately vaccination rates have been declining in the United States and elsewhere. There is no cure for SSPE. Some patients have improved or stabilized after several 6-week treatments of intraventricular α-interferon, starting at $105\,U/m^2$ body surface area per day combined with oral isoprinosine, 100 mg/kg/day. Repeat courses up to six times at 2- to 6-month intervals. The use of levetiracetam may improve the myoclonus and encephalopathy.

Other Disorders of Gray Matter
Neuronal Ceroid Lipofuscinosis (Batten Disease)

Several neurodegenerative disorders characterized by dementia and blindness are forms of ceroid lipofuscinosis, collectively referred to as Batten disease. When first described, the classification relied on eponyms depending on the age at onset but has since been reorganized according to the causative mutation. There are now 14 different recognized types of neuronal ceroid lipofuscinosis, many of which present in childhood. The common pathological feature is the accumulation of autofluorescent lipopigments, ceroid and lipofuscin within the brain, retina, and some visceral tissues. Genetic transmission of all neuronal lipofuscinoses is by autosomal recessive inheritance except for one adult form which is autosomal dominant. We described CLN1 earlier in this chapter. CLN5, 7, 8, 9, 10, 12, and 14 also present in infants or children, but are less common and less well understood and will not be discussed here.

Late-infantile neuronal ceroid lipofuscinosis (CLN2, Jansky-Bielschowsky disease).

Clinical features. Two forms of CLN2 exist. The most common is the classical type we describe here. Visual failure begins between 2 and 3 years of age and progresses slowly. The onset of seizures and dementia is at 2–4 years. The seizures are myoclonic, akinetic, and tonic-clonic and are usually refractory to anticonvulsant drugs. Severe ataxia develops, owing in part to seizures and in part to motor system deterioration. Myoclonus, involuntary movements, and dementia follow. Dementia sometimes precedes the first seizure.

Ophthalmoscopic findings are abnormal before visual symptoms occur. They include attenuation of vessels, early optic atrophy, and pigmentary degeneration of the macula. The loss of motor, mental, and visual function is relentlessly progressive, and within months the child is in a chronic vegetative state. Death is usually between 10 and 15 years.

CLN6 is a separate disease known as "variant CLN2" because it presents with similar clinical findings. The exact biochemical basis of CLN6 remains unclear, but the disorder is associated with pathogenic variants in the *CLN6* gene.

Diagnosis. Molecular genetic testing reveals biallelic pathogenic variants in the *TPP1/CLN2* gene, which encodes the lysosomal enzyme tripeptidyl peptidase-1. Additional testing shows reduced TPP enzyme activity in leukocytes or cultured fibroblasts.[73]

Management. Cerliponase alfa is a recombinant tripeptidyl peptidase-1 enzyme that has been approved to treat CLN2. It slows the loss of motor function, including motor language regression, in children with CLN2 who are above 3 years of age. CLN2 is the only neuronal ceroid lipofuscinosis with a specific treatment option.

CLN3 (juvenile-onset CLN).

Clinical features. Onset of visual failure is between 4 and 5 years, and the onset of seizures and dementia is between 5 and 9 years. Macular degeneration and pigmentary aggregation are present on ophthalmoscopic examination. Loss of ambulation occurs during the second decade. Myoclonus is prominent. Death occurs between 10 and 20 years.

Diagnosis. Molecular genetic testing is available and demonstrates pathogenic variants in the *CLN3* gene which encodes the protein battenin.

Management. Treatment is supportive and multidisciplinary.

Pantothenate Kinase–Associated Neurodegeneration

PKAN causes progressive motor abnormalities including spasticity, gait abnormalities, and dysarthria as well as dementia and psychiatric disturbance. It is the most common form of the group of disorders known as the NBIAs, caused by pathogenic variants in the *PANK2* gene. There is no cure, and treatment is supportive. PKAN is discussed more fully in Chapter 14.

Juvenile Huntington Disease

Huntington disease (HD) is a chronic degenerative disease of the nervous system transmitted by autosomal dominant inheritance. The HD gene maps to chromosome 4p16.3 and codes a protein known as *huntingtin*. The huntingtin protein is pleiotrophic and interacts with a wide variety of proteins to influence several cell processes.[74] The gene contains an expanded trinucleotide (CAG) repeat sequence. The normal number of repeats is less than 29. Patients with adult-onset HD usually have more than 35 repeats, whereas patients with juvenile-onset HD often have 50 or more repeats.[75]

Clinical features. The age of onset is usually between 35 and 55 years but may be as early as 2 years. Approximately 10% of affected children show symptoms before the age of 20 and 5% before the age of 14. When HD begins in childhood, the father is the affected parent in 83% of cases and may be asymptomatic when the child is born.

The initial features are usually progressive dementia and behavioral disturbances. Declining school performance often brings the child to medical attention. Rigidity, with loss of facial expression and associative movements, is more common than choreoathetosis and hyperkinesia in early-onset cases. Cerebellar dysfunction occurs in approximately 20% of cases and can be a major cause of disability. Ocular motor apraxia may also be present (see Chapter 15). Seizures, which are rare in adult-onset cases, are present in 50% of affected children. The course in childhood is relentlessly progressive, and the average duration from onset to death is 8 years.

Diagnosis. Reliable molecular testing is available to determine the size of the expanded CAG repeat.

Management. Rigidity may be temporarily relieved with levodopa, bromocriptine, and amantadine. Neuroleptics are useful for behavioral control, but treatment is not available for dementia.

Dentatorubral Pallidoluysian Atrophy

Dentatorubral pallidoluysian atrophy is an uncommon disorder in the pediatric population but can present in adolescence with symptoms similar to that of juvenile Huntington disease. Progressive spasticity, dystonia, myoclonic epilepsy, psychiatric disturbances, and dementia define the disease. Like Huntington disease, it is an autosomal dominant trinucleotide repeat disorder, caused by CAG repeats in the *ATN1* gene. Treatment is supportive.[76]

Mitochondrial Encephalomyopathies

The mitochondrial encephalomyopathies are a diverse group of disorders with defects of oxidative metabolism. Descriptions of three such disorders are in the section on progressive encephalopathies of infancy. Progressive external ophthalmoplegia or myopathy is characteristic of later-onset mitochondrial disorders. However, childhood dementia occurs in a syndrome of myoclonic epilepsy associated with ragged-red fibers in skeletal muscle. Genetic transmission is by maternal inheritance.

Myoclonic epilepsy and ragged-red fibers. Point mutations in mtDNA cause the syndrome of myoclonic epilepsy and ragged-red fibers. Ragged-red fibers usually indicate a combined defect of respiratory complexes I and IV.[77] Mutation in more than one mitochondrial gene produces the phenotype. The severity of the clinical phenotype is proportional to the amount of variant mtDNA.[78]

Clinical features. Clinical heterogeneity is common even among members of the same family and ranges from severe CNS dysfunction to myopathy. The four cardinal features are: myoclonus, myoclonic epilepsy, ataxia, and ragged-red fiber in muscle biopsy. Onset may be anytime during childhood or up until the fourth decade. An insidious decline in school performance is often the initial feature, but generalized tonic-clonic seizures or myoclonus may be the symptoms that first prompt medical consultation. Flickering light or watching television may induce seizures. Brief myoclonic twitching develops, often induced by action (action myoclonus), which may interfere with hand movement and posture. Ataxia is a constant feature as the disease progresses, and this may be due to action myoclonus rather than cerebellar dysfunction. Some patients have hearing loss, short stature, and exercise intolerance.

Neurological deterioration is progressive and may include spasticity, sensory loss, and central hypoventilation. Clinical evidence of myopathy is not always present.

Diagnosis. Molecular genetic testing is available. The most common mutation, present in above 80% of individuals with typical findings, is an A-to-G transition at nucleotide 8344 in the mtDNA gene *MT-TK*. Serum concentrations of pyruvate and lactate may be elevated. EEG shows slowing of the background rhythms and a photoconvulsive response. Muscle specimens of weak muscles show ragged-red fibers (see Fig. 8.3) and increased punctuate lipid within myofibers. Unaffected muscles do not contain ragged-red fibers.

Management. Anticonvulsant therapy may provide seizure control early in the course but often fails as the disease progresses. Valproic acid is contraindicated. Avoid glucose loads. Treatment is not available for the underlying defect but coenzyme Q10 (100 mg) and L-carnitine (1000 mg) given three times a day are often used in hopes of improving mitochondrial function.

Xeroderma Pigmentosum

Xeroderma pigmentosum (XP) is a group of uncommon neurocutaneous disorders characterized by susceptibility to sun-induced skin disorders and progressive neurological deterioration. Genetic transmission is autosomal recessive. Several different gene mutations have been associated with these disorders. In the United States, the most common biallelic pathogenic variant is the *XPA* or *XPC* gene. Other implicated genes include *DDB2, ERCC1, ERCC1, ERCC3, ERCC4, ERCC5,* and *POLH*.[79]

Clinical features. Photosensitive dermatitis develops during the first year, and skin cancer may develop as well. Ocular manifestations include severe photophobia, keratitis, and ocular neoplasms. Approximately 25% of affected individuals have neurologic symptoms. After the age of 3, psychomotor regression and poor head growth lead to microcephaly. Sensorineural hearing loss and spinocerebellar ataxia may develop after the age of 7. Approximately one-third of patients are short in stature, and some have a phenotype suggesting Cockayne syndrome, which is a separate genetic error (see Chapter 7) and also involves defective DNA repair. Patients with neurological involvement die earlier than those without neurologic symptoms; the average age of death for those with neurologic impairment is approximately 30.

Diagnosis. The typical skin rash, ocular findings, and neurological deterioration in both the central and peripheral nervous systems suggest the diagnosis. Molecular genetic testing confirms the diagnosis.

Management. Treatment is supportive. Radiation is contraindicated.

Other Diseases of White Matter

X-Linked Adrenoleukodystrophy

X-linked adrenoleukodystrophy is a demyelinating leukodystrophy causing progressive demyelination of the CNS and adrenal cortical failure. Affected children have an impaired ability to oxidize very long-chain fatty acids, especially hexacosanoic acid, because of a deficiency of a peroxisomal acyl coenzyme A (CoA) synthetase. Very long-chain fatty acids accumulate in tissues and plasma.

Distinct phenotypes exist because the cerebral and adrenal systems are involved separately. Cerebral adrenoleukodystrophy (CALD) is the classic presentation that we discuss here. Adrenomyeloneuropathy (see Chapter 12) and primary adrenocortical insufficiency are the other types. Only males develop CALD, but heterozygous females may develop the other subtypes at older ages.

Clinical features. The onset of the cerebral form is between the ages of 4 and 8 but may be as late as adolescence or early adulthood. The first symptoms are usually an alteration in behavior ranging from a withdrawn state to aggressive outbursts. Poor school performance follows and may lead parents to seek psychological services. Neurological deterioration is then relentlessly progressive and includes disturbances of gait and coordination, loss of vision and hearing, and ultimate deterioration to a vegetative state. Seizures are a late manifestation. The average interval from onset to a vegetative state or death is 3 years.

Diagnosis. T_2-weighted MRI shows high signal intensity in the periventricular white matter even in asymptomatic individuals. Adrenal insufficiency, as evidenced by a subnormal response to stimulation by adrenocorticotropic hormone, may be demonstrable even in asymptomatic children.

The level of very long-chain fatty acids in plasma is elevated in males of all ages, even in those who are asymptomatic, and in 85% of female carriers. Molecular genetic testing reveals hemizygous or heterozygous pathogenic variants in the *ABCD1* gene.[80] Newborn screening in the United States includes the disorder.

Management. Assessment of adrenal function and corticosteroid replacement therapy can be lifesaving but have no effect on nervous system involvement. Bone marrow transplantation is an option for boys and adolescents who are in the early clinical stages and have MRI evidence of brain involvement. Dietary therapy has no established benefit. Gene replacement therapy (Skysona) is available in some centers for children with early, active CALD who are between the ages of 4 and 18. Cancer risk is notably increased in recipients of the gene therapy and long-term risks are yet unknown; the FDA approved it under an accelerated approval process that requires ongoing testing to further delineate risks and benefits. The astronomical cost ($3 million) is also a barrier to treatment.

Vanishing White Matter Disease

Vanishing white matter disease is one of the more common childhood leukodystrophies. It is caused by mutations in any of the genes encoding the five subunits of eukaryotic transcription initiation factor 2B (genes *EIF2B1-EIF2B5*). Oligodendrocytes and astrocytes are the most affected cell types.[81]

Clinical features. Progressive cerebellar ataxia characterizes the disease, which typically presents in childhood but may appear at almost any age, from neonates to adults. A unique feature is extreme sensitivity to fever, minor head trauma, and acute fright, which may cause sudden neurological deterioration and coma.[82] Cognition is typically unaffected or only mildly impaired. Death usually occurs a few years after symptom onset.

Diagnosis. Brain MRI reveals the diffuse, symmetric cystic degeneration of white matter tracts. Molecular genetic testing reveals pathogenic variants in one of the *EIF2B* genes.

Management. Treatment is supportive.

Cerebrotendinous Xanthomatosis

Cerebrotendinous xanthomatosis is a rare lipid storage disease.[83]

Clinical features. Affected infants have diarrhea. Dementia begins in early childhood but is insidious in its progression so that affected children seem mildly cognitively impaired rather than actively deteriorating. By the age of 15, cataracts are present and tendinous xanthomas begin to form. They are small at first and may go unnoticed until adult life. Progressive spasticity and ataxia develop during adolescence, and the patient becomes incapacitated in early adult life. A demyelinating neuropathy may be present as well. Speech and swallowing are impaired, and death occurs from brainstem dysfunction or myocardial infarction.

Diagnosis. The symptom complex of diarrhea, cataracts, tendon xanthomas, and progressive neurological deterioration establishes the diagnosis, but complete expression of all features occurs late in the course. The presence of cataracts or Achilles tendon xanthoma is an indication for biochemical screening. Elevated plasma concentrations of cholestanol or xanthomas establish the diagnosis. MRI shows progressive cerebral atrophy and demyelination. Molecular genetic testing is clinically available and shows pathogenic variants in the *CYP27A1* gene.

Management. Long-term treatment with chenodeoxycholic acid normalizes bile acid synthesis, normalizes plasma and CSF concentration of cholestanol, and improves neurophysiological findings. The dose is 15 mg/kg/day in three divided doses for children, or 250 mg three times a day in adults.

REFERENCES

1. Volkmar F, Chawarska K, Klin A. Autism in infancy and early childhood. *Annual Review of Psychology*. 2005;56:315-336.
2. Heil KM, Schaaf CP. The genetics of autism spectrum disorders: a guide for clinicians. *Current Psychiatry Reports*. 2013;15:334.
3. Rapin I. The autistic-spectrum disorders. *New England Journal of Medicine*. 2002;347:302-303.
4. Harris MS, Kronenberger WG, Gao S, et al. Verbal short-term memory development and spoken language outcomes in deaf children with cochlear implants. *Ear and Hearing*. 2013;34(2):179-192.
5. Shevell M, Ashwal S, Donley D, et al. Practice parameter: evaluation of the child with global developmental delay. Report of the Quality Standards Committee of the American Academy of Neurology and the Practice Committee of the Child Neurology Society. *Neurology*. 2003;60:367-380.
6. Onkar D, Onkar P, Mitra K. Evaluation of fetal central nervous system anomalies by ultrasound and its anatomical correlation. *Journal of Clinical and Diagnostic Research*. 2014;8(5):AC05-AC07.
7. Godiers J, Leenher ED, Smets K, et al. Hearing loss and congenital CMV infection a systemic review. *Pediatrics*. 2014;134:972-982.
8. Kimberlin DW, Jester PM, Sanchez PL, et al. Valganciclovir for symptomatic congenital cytomegalovirus disease. *New England Journal of Medicine*. 2015;372: 933-943.
9. Bonthius DJ, Wright R, Tseng B, et al. Congenital lymphocytic choriomeningitis virus infection: spectrum of disease. *Annals of Neurology*. 2007;62:347-355.
10. Aebischer O, Meylan P, Kuns S, et al. Lymphocytic choriomeningitis virus infection induced by percutaneous exposure. *Occupational Medicine*. 2015;66(2):171-173.
11. Olariu TR, Remington JS, Montoya JG. Polymerase chain reaction in cerebrospinal fluid for the diagnosis of congenital toxoplasmosis. *Pediatric Infectious Disease Journal*. 2014;33(6):566-570.
12. Mlakar J, Korva M, Tull N, et al. Zika virus associated microcephaly. *New England Journal of Medicine*. 2016;374: 951-958.
13. Kim YK, Kim EH. Pregnancy and COVID-19: past, present and future. *Obstetrics & Gynecology Science*. 2023;66(3):149-160. https://doi.org/10.5468/ogs.23001. Epub 2023 Mar 20. PMID: 36938588; PMCID: PMC10191757.
14. Driscoll DJ, Miller JL, Cassidy SB. Prader-Willi syndrome. In: Adam MP, Mirzaa GM, Pagon RA, et al., eds. *GeneReviews*. University of Washington; 1993–2023. https://www.ncbi.nlm.nih.gov/sites/books/NBK1330/.
15. Dagli AI, Mathews J, Williams CA. Angelman syndrome. In: Adam MP, Mirzaa GM, Pagon RA, et al., eds. *GeneReviews*. University of Washington; 1993–2023. https://www.ncbi.nlm.nih.gov/books/NBK1144/.
16. Lusk L, Vogel-Farley V, DiStefano C, et al. Maternal 15q duplication syndrome. In: Adam MP, Mirzaa GM, Pagon RA, et al., eds. *GeneReviews*. University of Washington; 1993–2023. https://www.ncbi.nlm.nih.gov/sites/books/NBK367946/.
17. Saul RA, Tarleton JC. FMR-1 related disorders. In: Adam MP, Ardinger HH, Pagon RA, et al., eds. *GeneReviews*. University of Washington; 1993–2019. https://www.ncbi.nlm.nih.gov/books/NBK1384.
18. Michelson DJ, Shevell MI, Sherr EH, et al. Evidence report: genetic and metabolic testing on children with global developmental delay. Report of the Quality Standards Subcommittee of the American Academy of Neurology and the Practice Committee of the Child Neurology Society. *Neurology*. 2011;77:1629-1635.
19. Van Esch H. MECP2 duplication syndrome. In: Adam MP, Mirzaa GM, Pagon RA, et al., eds. *GeneReviews*. University of Washington; 1993–2023. https://www.ncbi.nlm.nih.gov/books/NBK1284/.
20. Stevenson RE. Alpha-thalassemia X-linked intellectual disability syndrome. In: Adam MP, Mirzaa GM, Pagon RA, et al., eds. *GeneReviews*. University of Washington; 1993–2023. https://www.ncbi.nlm.nih.gov/sites/books/NBK1449/.
21. Holder Jr JL, Hamdan FF, Michaud JL. SYNGAP1-related intellectual disability. In: Adam MP, Mirzaa GM, Pagon RA, et al., eds. *GeneReviews*. University of Washington; 1993–2023. https://www.ncbi.nlm.nih.gov/books/NBK537721/.

22. Platzer K, Lemke JR. GRIN2B-related neurodevelopmental disorder. In: Adam MP, Mirzaa GM, Pagon RA, et al., eds. *GeneReviews*. University of Washington; 1993–2023. https://www.ncbi.nlm.nih.gov/books/NBK501979/.

23. Schrier Vergano S, Santen G, Wieczorek D, et al. Coffin-Siris syndrome. In: Adam MP, Mirzaa GM, Pagon RA, et al., eds. *GeneReviews*. University of Washington; 1993–2023. https://www.ncbi.nlm.nih.gov/books/NBK131811/.

24. Goodspeed K, Demarest S, Johannesen K, et al. SLC6A1-related neurodevelopmental disorder. In: Adam MP, Feldman J, Mirzaa GM, et al., eds. *GeneReviews*. University of Washington; 1993–2024. https://www.ncbi.nlm.nih.gov/books/NBK589173/.

25. Platzer K, Lemke JR. GRIN1-related neurodevelopmental disorder. In: Adam MP, Mirzaa GM, Pagon RA, et al., eds. *GeneReviews*: University of Washington; 1993–2023. https://www.ncbi.nlm.nih.gov/books/NBK542807/.

26. Mercimek-Andrews S, Salomons GS. Creatine deficiency disorders. In: Adam MP, Mirzaa GM, Pagon RA, et al., eds. *GeneReviews*. University of Washington; 1993–2023. https://www.ncbi.nlm.nih.gov/books/NBK3794/.

27. Sacharow SJ, Picker JD, Levy HL. Homocystinuria caused by cystathionine beta-synthase deficiency. In: Adam MP, Ardinger HH, Pagon RA, et al., eds. *GeneReviews*. University of Washington; 1993–2019. https://www.ncbi.nlm.nih.gov/books/NBK1524.

28. Morris AAM, Kozich V, Santra S, et al. Guidelines for the diagnosis and management of cystathionine beta-synthase deficiency. *Journal of Inherited Metabolic Disease*. 2017;40:49-74.

29. Strauss KA, Puffenberger EG, Morton DH. Maple syrup urine disease. In: Adam MP, Ardinger HH, Pagon RA, et al., eds. *GeneReviews*. University of Washington; 1993–2019. https://www.ncbi.nlm.nih.gov/books/NBK1319.

30. Regier DS, Greene CL. Phenylalanine hydroxylase deficiency. In: Adam MP, Ardinger HH, Pagon RA, et al., eds. *GeneReviews*. University of Washington; 1993–2019. https://www.ncbi.nlm.nih.gov/books/NBK1384.

31. Jahja R, Huijbregts SCJ, de Soneville LMJ, et al. Neurocognitive evidence for revision of treatment targets and guidelines for phenylketonuria. *Journal of Pediatrics*. 2014;164(4):895-899.

32. Pastores GM, Hughes DA. Gaucher disease. In: Adam MP, Mirzaa GM, Pagon RA, et al., eds. *GeneReviews*. University of Washington; 1993–2023. https://www.ncbi.nlm.nih.gov/books/NBK1269/.

33. Orsini JJ, Escolar ML, Wasserstein MP, et al. Krabbe disease. In: Adam MP, Mirzaa GM, Pagon RA, et al., eds. *GeneReviews*. University of Washington; 1993–2023. https://www.ncbi.nlm.nih.gov/books/NBK1238/.

34. Orsini JJ, Escolar ML, Wasserstein MP, et al. In: Adam MP, Mirzaa GM, Pagon RA, GeneReviews, et al, eds. Krabbe disease. University of Washington; 1993–2023. https://www.ncbi.nlm.nih.gov/books/NBK1238/.

35. Kaback MM, Desnick RJ. Hexosaminidase A deficiency. In: Adam MP, Ardinger HH, Pagon RA, et al., eds. *GeneReviews*. University of Washington; 2011. https://www.ncbi.nlm.nih.gov/books/NBK1218.

36. Dogterom EJ, Wagenmakers MAEM, Wilke M, et al. Mucolipidosis type II and type III: a systematic review of 843 published cases. *Genetics in Medicine*. 2021;23:2047–2056. https://doi.org/10.1038/s41436-021-01244-4.

37. Leroy JG, Cathey S, Friez M. Mucolipidosis II. In: Adam MP, Ardinger HH, Pagon RA, et al., eds. *GeneReviews*. University of Washington; 1993–2019. https://www.ncbi.nlm.nih.gov/books/NBK1828.

38. Clarke LA. Mucopolysaccharidoses type I. In: Adam MP, Ardinger HH, Pagon RA, et al., eds. *GeneReviews*. University of Washington; 1993–2019. https://www.ncbi.nlm.nih.gov/books/NBK1162.

39. Wagner VF, Northrup H. Mucopolysaccharidosis type III. In: Adam MP, Mirzaa GM, Pagon RA, et al., eds. *GeneReviews*. University of Washington; 1993–2023. https://www.ncbi.nlm.nih.gov/books/NBK546574/.

40. Sparks SE, Krasnewich DM. Congenital disorders of N-linked glycosylation and multiple pathway overview. In: Adam MP, Ardinger HH, Pagon RA, et al., eds. *GeneReviews*. University of Washington; 1993–2019. https://www.ncbi.nlm.nih.gov/books/NBK1332.

41. Srivastava S, Naidu S. Alexander disease. In: Adam MP, Ardinger HH, Pagon RA, et al., eds. *GeneReviews*. University of Washington; 1993–2019. https://www.ncbi.nlm.nih.gov/books/NBK1172.

42. van der Knaap MS, Valk J, Barth PG, et al. Leukoencephalopathy with swelling in children and adolescents: MRI patterns and differential diagnosis. *Neuroradiology*. 1995;37:679-686.

43. Cohen BH, Chinnery PF, Copeland WC. POLG-related disorders. In: Adam MP, Mirzaa GM, Pagon RA, et al., eds. *GeneReviews*. University of Washington; 1993–2023. https://www.ncbi.nlm.nih.gov/books/NBK26471/.

44. Listernick R, Louis DN, Packer RJ. Optic pathway gliomas in children with neurofibromatosis type I: consensus statement from the NF-1 optic pathway glioma task force. *Annals of Neurology*. 1997;41(2):143-149.

45. Northrup H, Koenig MK, Pearson DA, et al. Tuberous sclerosis complex. In: Adam MP, Ardinger HH, Pagon RA, et al., eds. *GeneReviews*. University of Washington; 1993–2019. https://www.ncbi.nlm.nih.gov/books/NBK1220.

46. Jansen EE, Braams O, Vincken KL, et al. Overlapping neurologic and cognitive phenotypes in patients

with TSC1 or TSC2 mutations. *Neurology*. 2008;70:908-915.

47. Northrup H, Koenig MK, Pearson DA, et al. Tuberous sclerosis complex. In: Adam MP, Mirzaa GM, Pagon RA, et al., eds. *GeneReviews*. University of Washington; 1993–2023. https://www.ncbi.nlm.nih.gov/books/NBK1220/.

48. Franz DN, Leonard J, Tudor C, et al. Rapamycin causes regression of astrocytomas in tuberous sclerosis complex. *Annals of Neurology*. 2006;59:490-498.

49. Bissler JJ, McCormack FX, Young LR, et al. Sirolimus for angiomyolipoma in tuberous sclerosis complex or lymphangioleiomyomatosis. *New England Journal of Medicine*. 2008;358:140-151.

50. Mole SE, Williams RE. Neuronal ceroid-lipofuscinoses. In: Adam MP, Ardinger HH, Pagon RA, et al., eds. *GeneReviews*. University of Washington; 1993–2019. https://www.ncbi.nlm.nih.gov/books/NBK1428.

51. Seven M, Ozkilic A, Yuksel A. Dysmorphic face in two siblings with infantile neuroaxonal dystrophy. *Genetic Counseling*. 2002;13:465-473.

52. Morgan NV, Westaway SK, Morton JEV, et al. PLA2G6, encoding a phospholipase A2, is mutated in neurodegenerative disorders with high brain iron. *Nature Genetics*. 2006;38:752-754.

53. Nyhan WL, O'Neill JP, Jinnah HA, et al. Lesch-Nyhan syndrome. In: Adam MP, Ardinger HH, Pagon RA, et al., eds. *GeneReviews*. University of Washington; 1993–2019. https://www.nc.

54. Kaur S, Christodoulou J. MECP2 disorders. In: Adam MP, Mirzaa GM, Pagon RA, et al., eds. *GeneReviews*. University of Washington; 1993–2023. https://www.ncbi.nlm.nih.gov/books/NBK1497/.

55. Olson HE, Demarest ST, Pestana-Knight EM, et al. Cyclin-dependent kinase-like 5 deficiency disorder: clinical review. *Pediatric Neurology*. 2019;97:18-25. https://doi.org/10.1016/j.pediatrneurol.2019.02.015. Epub 2019 Feb 23. PMID: 30928302; PMCID: PMC7120929.

56. Knight EMP, Amin S, Bahi-Buisson N, Marigold Trial Group . Safety and efficacy of ganaxolone in patients with CDKL5 deficiency disorder: results from the double-blind phase of a randomised, placebo-controlled, phase 3 trial. *Lancet Neurology*. 2022;21(5):417-427. https://doi.org/10.1016/S1474-4422(22)00077-1. Erratum in: Lancet Neurol. 2022 Jul;21(7):e7. PMID: 35429480.

57. Kaler SG, DiStasio AT. ATP7A-related copper transport disorders. In: Adam MP, Mirzaa GM, Pagon RA, et al., eds. *GeneReviews*. University of Washington; 1993–2023. https://www.ncbi.nlm.nih.gov/books/NBK1413/.

58. Matalon R, Michals-Matalon K. Canavan disease. In: Pagon RA, Bird TD, Dolan CR, et al., eds. *GeneReviews*. University of Washington; 2011. http://www.geneclinics.org. PMID: 20301412. Last updated August 11.

59. Elsas LJ. Galactosemia. In: *Gene Clinics: Medical Genetics Knowledge Base [Database Online]*. University of Washington; 2010. http://www.geneclinics.org. PMID: 20301691. Updated October 26, 2010.

60. Ridel KR, Leslie ND, Gilbert DL. An updated review of the long-term neurological effects of galactosemia. *Pediatric Neurology*. 2005;33:153-161.

61. Nahhas N, Conant A, Orthmann-Murphy J, et al. Pelizaeus-Merzbacher-like disease 1. In: Adam MP, Mirzaa GM, Pagon RA, et al., eds. *GeneReviews*. University of Washington; 1993–2023. https://www.ncbi.nlm.nih.gov/sites/books/NBK470716/.

62. Naidu S, Bibat G, Lin D, et al. Progressive cavitating leukoencephalopathy: a novel childhood disease. *Annals of Neurology*. 2005;58:929-938.

63. Shinagawa A, Hugdal S, Babu J, Rangaswamy R. Progressive cavitating leukoencephalopathy associated with a homozygous *POLG* mutation of 264C>G (p.F88L). *Radiology Case Reports*. 2020;15(7):908-913. https://doi.org/10.1016/j.radcr.2020.04.042. PMID: 32382377; PMCID: PMC7201157.

64. Fluharty AL. Arylsulfatase A deficiency. In: Pagon RA, Bird TD, Dolan CR, et al., eds. *GeneReviews*. University of Washington; 2011. http://www.geneclinics.org. PMID: 20301309.

65. Schilsky ML, Roberts EA, Bronstein JM, et al. A multidisciplinary approach to the diagnosis and management of Wilson disease: 2022 practice guidance on Wilson disease from the American Association for the Study of Liver Diseases. *Hepatology*. 2022;00:1-49. https://doi.org/10.1002/hep.32801.

66. Scarpa M. Mucopolysaccharidosis type II. In: Pagon RA, Bird TD, Dolan CR, et al., eds. *GeneReviews*. University of Washington; 2011. http://www.geneclinics.org.

67. Scarpa M. Mucopolysaccharidosis type II. In: Adam MP, Mirzaa GM, Pagon RA, et al., eds. *GeneReviews*. University of Washington; 1993–2023. https://www.ncbi.nlm.nih.gov/books/NBK1274/.

68. Poswar FO, Henriques Nehm J, Kubaski F, Poletto E, Giugliani R. Diagnosis and emerging treatment strategies for mucopolysaccharidosis VII (Sly syndrome). *Therapeutics and Clinical Risk Management*. 2022;18:1143-1155. https://doi.org/10.2147/TCRM.S351300. PMID: 36578769; PMCID: PMC9791935.

69. Patterson M. Niemann-Pick disease type C. In: Pagon RA, Bird TD, Dolan CR, et al., eds. *GeneReviews*. University of Washington; 2008. http://www.geneclinics.org. PMID: 20301473. Last updated July 22.

70. Patterson M. Niemann-Pick disease type C. In: Adam MP, Mirzaa GM, Pagon RA, et al., eds. *GeneReviews*. University of Washington; 1993–2023. https://www.ncbi.nlm.nih.gov/books/NBK1296/.

71. Honarmand S, Glaser CA, Chow E, et al. Subacute sclerosing panencephalitis in the differential diagnosis of encephalitis. *Neurology*. 2004;63:1489-1493.

72. Becker D, Patel A, Abou-Khalil BW, et al. Successful treatment of encephalopathy and myoclonus with levetiracetam in a case of subacute sclerosing panencephaliti. *Journal of Child Neurology*. 2009;24:763-767.

73. Mole SE, Schulz A, Badoe E, et al. Guidelines on the diagnosis, clinical assessments, treatment and management for CLN2 disease patients. *Orphanet Journal of Rare Diseases*. 2021;16:185. https://doi.org/10.1186/s13023-021-01813-5.

74. Schulte J, Littleton JT. The biological function of huntingtin protein and its relevance to Huntington's disease pathology. *Current Trends in Neurology*. 2011;5:65-78.

75. Warby SC, Graham RK, Hayden MR. Huntington disease. In: Pagon RA, Bird TD, Dolan CR, et al., eds. *GeneReviews*. University of Washington; 2010. http://www.geneclinics.org. PMID: 20301482. Last updated April 22.

76. Rocha Cabrero F, De Jesus O. *Dentatorubral pallidoluysian atrophy*. In: *StatPearls*. StatPearls Publishing; 2023. https://www.ncbi.nlm.nih.gov/books/NBK560862/.

77. Sarnat HB, Marin-Garcia J. Pathology of mitochondrial encephalomyopathies. *Canadian Journal of Neurological Sciences*. 2005;32:152-166.

78. DiMauro S, Hirano M. *MERRF*. In: *GeneClinics: Medical Genetics Knowledge Base [Database Online]*. University of Washington, 2009. http://www.geneclinics.org. PMID: 20301693. Last updated August 18.

79. Kraemer KH, DiGiovanna JJ, Tamura D. Xeroderma pigmentosum. In: Adam MP, Mirzaa GM, Pagon RA, et al., eds. *GeneReviews®*. University of Washington; 1993–2023. https://www.ncbi.nlm.nih.gov/books/NBK1397/.

80. Raymond GV, Moser AB, Fatemi A. X-linked adrenoleukodystrophy. In: Adam MP, Mirzaa GM, Pagon RA, et al., eds. *GeneReviews®*. University of Washington; 1993–2023. https://www.ncbi.nlm.nih.gov/books/NBK1315/.

81. Bugiani Marianna, et al. Leukoencephalopathy with vanishing white matter: a review. *Journal of Neuropathology & Experimental Neurology*. 2010;69(10):987-996. https://doi.org/10.1097/NEN.0b013e3181f2eafa.

82. van der Knaap MS, Pronk JC, Scheper GC. Vanishing white matter disease. *Lancet Neurology*. 2006;5(5):413-423. https://doi.org/10.1016/S1474-4422(06)70440-9. PMID: 16632312.

83. Federico A, Dotti MT, Gallus GN. Cerebrotendinous xanthomatosis. In: Pagon RA, Bird TD, Dolan CR, et al., eds. *GeneReviews*. University of Washington; 2011. http://www.geneclinics.org. PMID: 20301583.

6

The Hypotonic Infant

OUTLINE

The Appearance of Hypotonia, 183
    The Traction Response, 184
    Vertical Suspension, 185
    Horizontal Suspension, 185
Approach to Diagnosis, 185
    Clues to the Diagnosis of Cerebral Hypotonia, 187
    Clues to Motor Unit Disorders, 187
Cerebral Hypotonia, 188
    Benign Congenital Hypotonia, 188
    Chromosomal Disorders, 188
    Chronic Nonprogressive Encephalopathy, 189
    Genetic Disorders, 190

Spinal Cord Disorders, 192
    Hypoxic-Ischemic Myelopathy, 192
    Spinal Cord Injury, 192
Motor Unit Disorders, 193
    Evaluation of Motor Unit Disorders, 193
    Spinal Muscular Atrophies, 194
    Polyneuropathies, 197
    Disorders of Neuromuscular Transmission, 198
    Congenital Myopathies, 199
    Muscular Dystrophies, 202
    Metabolic Myopathies, 204
References, 205

Tone is the resistance of muscle to stretch. Clinicians test two kinds of tones: phasic and postural. *Phasic tone* is a rapid contraction in response to a high-intensity stretch (deep tendon reflexes [DTRs]). Striking the patellar tendon briefly stretches the quadriceps muscle. The spindle apparatus, sensing the stretch, sends an impulse through the sensory nerve to the spinal cord. This information is transmitted to the alpha motor neuron, and the quadriceps muscle contracts (the *monosynaptic reflex*). *Postural tone* is the prolonged contraction of antigravity muscles in response to the low-intensity stretch of gravity. When postural tone is depressed, the trunk and limbs cannot maintain themselves against gravity and the infant appears hypotonic.

The maintenance of normal tone requires intact central and peripheral nervous systems. Not surprisingly, hypotonia is a common symptom of neurological dysfunction and occurs in diseases of the brain, spinal cord, nerves, and muscles (Box 6.1). One anterior horn cell and all the muscle fibers that it innervates make up a *motor unit*. The motor unit is the unit of force. Therefore

weakness is a symptom of all motor unit disorders. A primary disorder of the anterior horn cell body is a *neuronopathy*, a primary disorder of the axon or its myelin covering is a *neuropathy*, and a primary disorder of the muscle fiber is a *myopathy*. In infancy and childhood, cerebral disorders are far more common than motor unit disorders. The term *cerebral hypotonia* encompasses all causes of postural hypotonia caused by cerebral diseases or defects.

THE APPEARANCE OF HYPOTONIA

When lying supine, all hypotonic infants look much the same, regardless of the underlying cause or location of the abnormality within the nervous system. Spontaneous movement may be decreased, full abduction of the legs places the lateral surface of the thighs against the examining table, and the arms lie either extended at the sides of the body or flexed at the elbow with the hands beside the head. Pectus excavatum is present when the infant has long-standing weakness in the chest wall muscles.

BOX 6.1   Differential Diagnosis of Infantile Hypotonia

- Cerebral hypotonia
  - Prader-Willi syndrome
  - Trisomy
  - Benign congenital hypotonia[a]
  - Chromosome disorders
- Chronic nonprogressive encephalopathy
  - Cerebral malformation
  - Perinatal distress[a]
  - Postnatal disorders[a]
- Peroxisomal disorders
  - Cerebrohepatorenal syndrome (Zellweger syndrome)
  - Neonatal adrenoleukodystrophy
- Other genetic defects
  - Familial dysautonomia
  - Oculocerebrorenal syndrome (Lowe syndrome)
- Other metabolic defects
  - Acid maltase deficiency[a] (see the "Metabolic Myopathies" section)
  - Infantile GM$_1$ gangliosidosis (see Chapter 5)
  - Pyruvate carboxylase deficiency
- Spinal cord disorders
- Spinal muscular atrophies[a]
  - Acute infantile
- Chronic infantile
  - Autosomal dominant
  - Autosomal recessive
  - Congenital cervical spinal muscular atrophy
  - Infantile neuronal degeneration
  - Neurogenic arthrogryposis
- Polyneuropathies
  - Congenital hypomyelinating neuropathy
- Giant axonal neuropathy (see Chapter 7)
- Hereditary motor-sensory neuropathies (see Chapter 7)
- Disorders of neuromuscular transmission
  - Familial infantile myasthenia
  - Infantile botulism
  - Transitory myasthenia gravis
- Fiber-type disproportion myopathies
- Congenital fiber-type disproportion myopathy
- Centronuclear myopathy
- Nemaline (rod) myopathy
- Core myopathies
  - Central core disease
  - Multiminicore myopathy
- Metabolic myopathies
  - Acid maltase deficiency/Pompe disease
  - Cytochrome-c oxidase deficiency
- Congenital dystrophinopathy (see Chapter 7)
- Congenital myotonic dystrophy
- Muscular dystrophies
  - Congenital presentation
    - Dystroglycanopathies/tubulinopathies
      - Fukuyama muscular dystrophy
      - Walker-Warburg syndrome
      - Muscle-eye-brain disease
    - LAMA2-related muscular dystrophies
      - Congenital muscular dystrophy type 1A (MCD1A)
  - Collagen VI–related muscular dystrophies
    - Ullrich congenital muscular dystrophy

[a]The most common conditions and the ones with disease-modifying treatments.

Infants who lie motionless eventually develop flattening of the occiput and loss of hair on the portion of the scalp that is in constant contact with the crib sheet. When placed in a sitting posture, the head falls forward, the shoulders droop, and the limbs hang limply.

Newborns who are hypotonic and weak in utero may be born with hip dislocation, multiple joint contractures (*arthrogryposis*), or both due to a lack of mobility. Hip dislocation is a common feature of intrauterine hypotonia. The forceful contraction of muscles pulling the femoral head into the acetabulum is a requirement of normal hip joint formation. Arthrogryposis varies in severity from isolated clubfoot, the most common manifestation, to symmetric flexion deformities of all limb joints. Joint contractures are a nonspecific consequence of intrauterine immobilization. However, among the several disorders that equally decrease fetal movement, some commonly produce arthrogryposis and others never do. Box 6.2 summarizes the differential diagnosis of arthrogryposis. As a rule, newborns with arthrogryposis who require respiratory assistance do not survive extubation unless the underlying disorder is myasthenia. The traction response, vertical suspension, and horizontal suspension further evaluate tone in infants who appear hypotonic at rest.

The Traction Response

The traction response is the most sensitive measure of postural tone and is testable in premature newborns within an incubator. Grasping the hands and pulling the

BOX 6.2 Differential Diagnosis of Arthrogryposis

- Cerebral malformations
- Cerebrohepatorenal syndrome
- Chromosomal disorders
- Motor unit disorders
  - Congenital cervical spinal muscular atrophy
  - Congenital fiber-type disproportion myopathy
  - Congenital hypomyelinating neuropathy
  - Congenital muscular dystrophy
  - Genetic myasthenic syndromes
  - Infantile neuronal degeneration
  - Myotonic dystrophy
  - Neurogenic arthrogryposis
  - Phosphofructokinase deficiency
  - Transitory neonatal myasthenia
- Nonfetal causes

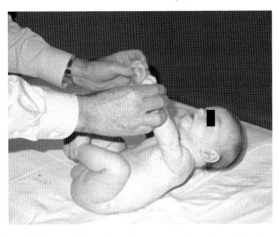

Fig. 6.1 Normal Traction Response. The lift of the head is almost parallel to the body and there is flexion in all limb joints. (Reprinted with permission from Fenichel GM. *Neonatal Neurology.* 4th ed. Elsevier; 2007.)

infant toward a sitting position initiates the response. A normal term infant lifts the head from the surface; the head may lag behind the body, but the neck is not in full extension (Fig. 6.1). During traction, the examiner should feel the infant pulling back against traction and observe flexion at the elbow, knee, and ankle. The traction response is not present in premature newborns of less than 33 weeks' gestation. After 33 weeks, the neck flexors show increasing success in lifting the head. At term, only minimal head lag is present; after attaining the sitting posture, the head may continue to lag or may

erect briefly and then fall forward. The presence of more than minimal head lag and failure to counter traction by flexion of the limbs in the term newborn is abnormal and indicates weakness and hypotonia.

Vertical Suspension

To perform vertical suspension, the examiner places both hands in the infant's axillae, and without grasping the thorax, lifts straight up. The muscles of the shoulders should have sufficient strength to press down against the examiner's hands and allow the infant to suspend vertically without falling through (Fig. 6.2). While in vertical suspension, the head is erect in the midline with flexion at the knee, hip, and ankle joints. When suspending a weak and hypotonic infant vertically, the head falls forward, the legs dangle, and the infant may slip through the examiner's hands because of weakness in the shoulder muscles.

Horizontal Suspension

When suspended horizontally, a normal infant keeps the head erect, maintains the back straight, and flexes the elbow, hip, knee, and ankle joints (Fig. 6.3). A healthy full-term newborn makes intermittent efforts to maintain the head erect, the back straight, and the limbs flexed against gravity. Hypotonic and weak newborns and infants drape over the examiner's hands, with the head and legs hanging limply.

APPROACH TO DIAGNOSIS

Hypotonia is a nonspecific symptom in neonates with critical illnesses. Sepsis, hypothyroidism, genetic disorders, and substance exposures can all cause low tone. For example, females who receive magnesium for preeclampsia often give birth to infants with hypotonia that resolves over hours to days. Assuming that hypotonia is not the result of systemic illness, the first step in diagnosis is to determine whether the disease location is in the brain, spine, or motor unit. More than one site may be involved (Box 6.3). The brain and the peripheral nerves are concomitantly involved in some lysosomal and mitochondrial disorders. Both brain and skeletal muscles are abnormal in infants with acid maltase deficiency and congenital myotonic dystrophy. Newborns with severe hypoxic-ischemic encephalopathy may have hypoxic injury to the spinal cord as well as the brain. Several motor unit disorders produce

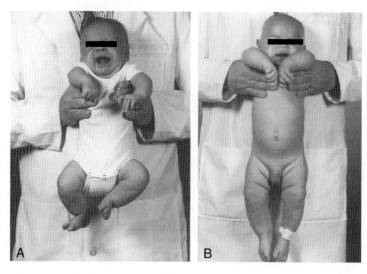

Fig. 6.2 Normal Vertical Suspension. (A) The arms help prop the infant against the examiner's hands, and the legs flex against gravity. (B) The arms and shoulder fail to provide support, and the legs do not resist gravity. The head is in the midline and the legs flex against gravity. (Reprinted with permission from Fenichel GM. *Neonatal Neurology.* 4th ed. Elsevier; 2007.)

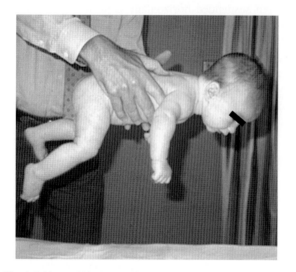

Fig. 6.3 Normal Horizontal Suspension. The head rises intermittently and the head and limbs resist gravity. (Reprinted with permission from Fenichel GM. *Neonatal Neurology.* 4th ed. Elsevier; 2007.)

> ### BOX 6.3   Combined Cerebral and Motor Unit Hypotonia
>
> - Acid maltase deficiency[a]
> - Familial dysautonomia/Riley-Day syndrome
> - Giant axonal neuropathy
> - Hypoxic-ischemic encephalomyopathy
> - Infantile neuronal degeneration
> - Lipid storage diseases
> - Mitochondrial (respiratory chain) disorders
> - Neonatal myotonic dystrophy
> - Perinatal asphyxia secondary to motor unit disease
>
> [a]The most common conditions and the ones with disease-modifying treatments.

> ### BOX 6.4   Motor Unit Disorders With Perinatal Respiratory Distress
>
> - Acute infantile spinal muscular atrophy
> - Congenital hypomyelinating neuropathy
> - Congenital myotonic dystrophy
> - Familial infantile myasthenia
> - Neurogenic arthrogryposis
> - X-linked myotubular myopathy

sufficient hypotonia at birth to impair respiration and cause perinatal asphyxia (Box 6.4). Such infants may then have cerebral hypotonia as well. Spinal cord injuries in newborns are frequently caused by long, difficult deliveries in which brachial plexus injuries and hypoxic-ischemic encephalopathy are concomitant problems.

Central hypotonia (60%–80%) is more common than peripheral hypotonia (15%–30%). Genetic testing reveals a diagnosis in approximately 30% of cases.

The assessment of the hypotonic infant should include the following: three-generation pedigree, history of drug or teratogen exposure (alcohol, solvents, drugs), breech presentation, reduced fetal movements, history of polyhydramnios, family history of recurrent infantile deaths, parental age, consanguinity, history of neuromuscular disease, perinatal asphyxia, Apgar scores, dysmorphism, arthrogryposis, DTRs, and fasciculations.[1]

Testing of the hypotonic infant may include brain imaging, metabolic testing, and chromosomal microarray. Karyotype and targeted genetic testing are useful in infants with clearly syndromic features. Microarray and exome sequencing have the highest yield, but exome sequencing is still difficult to obtain quickly in many institutions. Congenital infections and countless genetic syndromes and chromosomal abnormalities can cause neonatal and infantile hypotonia (see Chapter 5). In this chapter, we will limit ourselves to discussion of a few representative examples.

Clues to the Diagnosis of Cerebral Hypotonia

Cerebral or central hypotonia in newborns usually does not pose diagnostic difficulty. The history and physical examination identify the problem. Many clues to the diagnosis of cerebral hypotonia exist (Box 6.5). Most important is the presence of other abnormal brain functions, such as decreased consciousness and seizures. Cerebral malformation is the likely explanation for hypotonia in an infant with dysmorphic features or with malformations in other organs.

A tightly fisted hand in which the thumb is constantly enclosed by the other fingers and does not open spontaneously (*cortical thumb*), and adduction of the thigh so that the legs are crossed when the infant is suspended vertically (*scissoring*), are early signs of spasticity and indicate cerebral dysfunction; importantly, neonates with hypoxic-ischemic encephalopathy may be hypotonic and hyporreflexic in the acute period. Eliciting postural reflexes in newborns and

infants when spontaneous movement is lacking indicates cerebral hypotonia. In some acute encephalopathies, and especially in metabolic disorders, the Moro reflex may be exaggerated. The tonic neck reflex is an important indicator of cerebral abnormality if the responses are excessive, obligatory, or persist beyond 6 months of age. When hemispheric damage is severe, but the brainstem is intact, turning the head produces full extension of both ipsilateral limbs and tight flexion on the contralateral side. An obligatory reflex is one in which these postures are maintained as long as the head is kept rotated. Tendon reflexes are generally normal or brisk, and clonus may be present.

Clues to Motor Unit Disorders

Disorders of the motor unit are not associated with malformations of other organs except for joint deformities and the maldevelopment of bony structures. The face sometimes looks dysmorphic when facial muscles are weak or when the jaw is underdeveloped.

Tendon reflexes are absent or depressed. Loss of DTRs that is out of proportion to weakness is more likely caused by neuropathy than myopathy, whereas diminished reflexes that are consistent with the degree of weakness are more often caused by myopathy than neuropathy (Box 6.6). Muscle atrophy suggests motor unit disease but does not exclude the possibility of cerebral hypotonia. Failure of growth and even atrophy can be considerable in infants with brain insults. The combination of atrophy and fasciculations is strong evidence of denervation. However, the observation of fasciculations in newborns and infants is often restricted to the tongue, and distinguishing fasciculations from normal random movements of an infant's tongue is difficult unless atrophy is present.

Postural reflexes, such as the tonic neck and Moro reflex, are not imposable on weak muscles. The motor unit is the final common pathway of tone; limbs that will not move voluntarily cannot move reflexively.

BOX 6.5 Clues to Cerebral Hypotonia

- Abnormalities of other brain functions
- Dysmorphic features
- Fisting of the hands
- Malformations of other organs
- Movement through postural reflexes
- Normal or brisk tendon reflexes
- Scissoring on vertical suspension

BOX 6.6 Clues to Motor Unit Disorders

- Absent or depressed tendon reflexes
- Failure of movement on postural reflexes
- Fasciculations
- Muscle atrophy
- No abnormalities of other organs

CEREBRAL HYPOTONIA

Hypotonia is a feature of almost every cerebral disorder in newborns and infants. This section does not deal with conditions in which the major symptoms are states of decreased consciousness, seizures, and progressive psychomotor impairment. Rather, the discussion focuses on conditions in which hypotonia is sufficiently prominent that the examining physician may consider the possibility of motor unit disease.

Benign Congenital Hypotonia

The term *benign congenital hypotonia* is retrospective and refers to infants who are hypotonic at birth or shortly thereafter and later have normal tone. This diagnosis should be reserved for patients that besides recovering normal tone exhibit no other evidence of cerebral dysfunction; however, the majority of children with cerebral hypotonia without clear etiology may later exhibit cognitive impairment, learning disabilities, and other sequelae of cerebral abnormality despite the recovery of normal muscle tone.

Chromosomal Disorders

Despite considerable syndrome diversity, common characteristics of autosomal chromosome aberrations in the newborn are dysmorphic features of the hands and face and profound hypotonia. For this reason, any hypotonic newborn with dysmorphic features of the hands and face, with or without other organ malformation, requires chromosome studies.

MECP2 Duplication Syndrome

The *MECP2* duplication syndrome occurs only in males; inheritance is an X-linked trait. Occasionally, females have been described with a *MECP2* duplication and related clinical findings, often associated with concomitant X-chromosomal abnormalities that prevent inactivation of the duplicated region. The MECP2 duplication syndrome is discussed in more detail in Chapter 5.

Clinical features. Characteristic of the syndrome is infantile hypotonia, severe cognitive impairment with absence of speech, progressive spasticity, recurrent respiratory infections, and seizures. During the first weeks of life, feeding difficulties resulting from hypotonia becomes evident. The child may exhibit difficulty with swallowing and extensive drooling. In some cases, nasogastric tube feeding is required. Dysmorphic features include brachycephaly, midfacial hypoplasia, large ears, and flat nasal bridge.

Generalized tonic-clonic, atonic, and absence seizures are common (50%). Almost 50% die before the age of 25, presumably from complications of recurrent infection. Growth measurements at birth, including head circumference, are usually normal.

Because of hypotonia, delayed motor developmental is the rule. Walking is late, some individuals have an ataxic gait, and one-third never walk independently. Most never develop speech, and some individuals who attain limited speech lose it in adolescence. Hypotonia gives way to spasticity in childhood. The spasticity is greatest in the legs; mild contractures may develop over time. Often, the use of a wheelchair is necessary in adulthood.

Diagnosis. Duplications of *MECP2* ranging from 0.3 to 8 Mb are observable in all affected males and identified by commercially available genetic testing.

Management. Treatment is symptomatic and genetic counseling. The vast majority of affected males inherit the *MECP2* duplication from a carrier mother; however, spontaneous mutations have been reported. If the mother of the proband has an *MECP2* duplication, the chance of transmitting it in each pregnancy is 50%. Males who inherit the *MECP2* duplication will be affected; females who inherit the *MECP2* duplication are usually asymptomatic carriers.

Prader-Willi Syndrome

Hypotonia, hypogonadism, cognitive impairment, short stature, and obesity characterize the Prader-Willi syndrome.[2] Approximately 70% of children with this syndrome have an interstitial deletion of the paternally contributed proximal long arm of chromosome 15(q11-13), known as the Prader-Willi Angelman critical region (PWACR). The basis for the syndrome in most patients who do not have a deletion is *maternal disomy* (both chromosomes 15 are from the mother), but paternal deletion or an imprinting defect are also possible. Paternal disomy of the same region of chromosome 15 causes *Angelman syndrome.*

Clinical features. Decreased fetal movement occurs in 75% of pregnancies, hip dislocation in 10%, and clubfoot in 6%. Hypotonia is profound at birth and tendon reflexes are absent or greatly depressed. Feeding problems are invariable, and prolonged nasogastric tube feeding is common (Box 6.7). Cryptorchidism is present in 84%

and hypogonadism in 100%. However, some newborns lack the associated features and only show hypotonia.[3]

Both hypotonia and feeding difficulty persist until 8–11 months of age and are then replaced by relatively normal muscle tone and insatiable hunger. Delayed developmental milestones and later cognitive impairment are constant features. Minor abnormalities that become more obvious during infancy include a narrow bifrontal diameter of the skull, strabismus, almond-shaped eyes, enamel hypoplasia, and small hands and feet. Obesity is the rule during childhood. The combination of obesity and minor abnormalities of the face and limbs produces a resemblance among children with this syndrome. Major and minor clinical criteria are established (Box 6.8).

Diagnosis. The mainstay of diagnosis is DNA-based testing to detect abnormal parent-specific imprinting within the PWACR on chromosome 15. This testing determines whether the region is maternally inherited only (the paternally contributed region is absent) and detects the majority of individuals.

Management. In infancy, Haberman or slow-flow nipples, or gavage feeding assures adequate nutrition. Physical therapy may improve muscle strength. Strabismus and cryptorchidism require surgical treatment. Growth hormone replacement therapy normalizes height and increases lean body mass. Medication for behavior modification is a consideration. Replacement of sex hormones produces adequate secondary sexual characteristics.

Chronic Nonprogressive Encephalopathy

Cerebral dysgenesis may be due to known or unknown infectious processes, noxious environmental agents, chromosomal disorders, or genetic defects. In the absence of acute encephalopathy, hypotonia may be

---

BOX 6.7 Feeding Difficulty in the Alert Newborn

- Congenital myotonic dystrophy
- Familial dysautonomia
- Genetic myasthenic syndromes
- Hypoplasia of bulbar motor nuclei (see Chapter 17)
- Infantile neuronal degeneration
- Myophosphorylase deficiency
- Neurogenic arthrogryposis
- Prader-Willi syndrome
- Transitory neonatal myasthenia[a]

[a]Denotes treatable conditions.

BOX 6.8 Criteria for the Clinical Diagnosis of Prader-Willi Syndrome

Major Criteria
- Neonatal and infantile central hypotonia with poor suck and improvement with age
- Feeding problems and/or failure to thrive in infancy, with need for gavage or other special feeding techniques
- Onset of rapid weight gain between 12 months and 6 years of age, causing central obesity
- Hyperphagia
- Characteristic facial features: narrow bifrontal diameter, almond-shaped palpebral fissures, downturned mouth
- Hypogonadism
  - Genital hypoplasia: small labia minora and clitoris in females; hypoplastic scrotum and cryptorchidism in males
  - Incomplete and delayed puberty
  - Infertility
- Developmental delay/mild to moderate cognitive impairment/multiple learning disabilities

Minor Criteria
- Decreased fetal movement and infantile lethargy, improving with age

- Typical behavior problems, including temper tantrums, obsessive-compulsive behavior, stubbornness, and rigidity
- Sleep disturbance/sleep apnea
- Short stature for the family by the age of 15
- Hypopigmentation
- Small hands and feet for height age
- Narrow hands with straight ulnar border
- Esotropia, myopia
- Thick, viscous saliva
- Speech articulation defects
- Skin picking

Supportive Findings
- High pain threshold
- Decreased vomiting
- Scoliosis and/or kyphosis
- Early adrenarche
- Osteoporosis
- Unusual skill with jigsaw puzzles
- Normal neuromuscular studies (e.g., muscle biopsy, electromyography, nerve conduction velocity)

the only symptom at birth or during early infancy. Hypotonia is usually worse at birth and improves with time. Suspect cerebral dysgenesis when hypotonia associates with malformations in other organs or abnormalities in head size and shape. Magnetic resonance imaging (MRI) of the brain is advisable when suspecting a cerebral malformation. The identification of a cerebral malformation provides useful information not only for prognosis but also on the feasibility of aggressive therapy to correct malformations in other organs.

Brain injuries occur in the perinatal period, and less commonly throughout infancy secondary to anoxia, hemorrhage, infection, and trauma. The sudden onset of hypotonia in a previously well newborn or infant, with or without signs of encephalopathy, always suggests a cerebral cause. The premature newborn showing a decline in spontaneous movement and tone may have an intraventricular hemorrhage. Hypotonia is an early feature of meningitis in full-term and premature newborns. Tendon reflexes may be diminished or absent during the acute phase.

Genetic Disorders

Familial Dysautonomia (Hereditary Autonomic and Sensory Neuropathy Type III)

Familial dysautonomia, also known as HSAN III or the *Riley-Day syndrome*, is a genetic disorder transmitted by autosomal recessive inheritance in Ashkenazi Jewish people. The abnormality is in the *ELP1* (formerly *IKBKAP*) gene located on chromosome 9q31-q33, which encodes the elongator complex protein 1. Similar clinical syndromes also occur in infants who do not have Ashkenazi Jewish heritage. These syndromes are often sporadic and have an unknown pattern of inheritance.

Clinical features. In the newborn, the important clinical features are meconium aspiration, poor or no sucking reflex, and hypotonia. The causes of hypotonia are disturbances in the brain, the dorsal root ganglia, and the peripheral nerves. Tendon reflexes are hypoactive or absent. Feeding difficulty is common and provides a diagnostic clue. Sucking and swallowing are normal separately but cannot be coordinated for effective feeding. Other noticeable clinical features of the newborn or infants are pallor, temperature instability, the absence of fungiform papillae of the tongue, diarrhea, and abdominal distention. Poor weight gain and lethargy, episodic irritability, absent corneal reflexes, labile blood pressure, and failure to produce overflow tears complete the clinical picture.

Diagnosis. Molecular genetic testing is diagnostic and reveals biallelic pathogenic variants in the *ELP1* gene.[4] Two pathogenic variants account for more than 99% of cases in individuals of Ashkenazi descent. Ophthalmological examination is useful to detect the signs of postganglionic parasympathetic denervation: supersensitivity of the pupil, shown by a positive miotic response to 0.1% pilocarpine or 2.5% methacholine, corneal insensitivity, and absence of tears.

Management. Treatment is symptomatic; improved treatment of symptoms has increased longevity.

Oculocerebrorenal Syndrome (Lowe Syndrome)

Lowe syndrome is caused by markedly reduced activity of the enzyme inositol polyphosphate 5-phosphatase OCRL-1. Transmission is by X-linked recessive inheritance, with affected boys having hemizygous pathogenic variants of the *OCRL* gene.[5] Female carriers show partial expression in the form of minor lenticular opacities.

Clinical features. Lowe syndrome involves the eyes, central nervous system (CNS), and kidneys. All affected boys have dense cataracts and half have glaucoma. Box 6.2 lists the differential diagnosis of cataracts in newborns and infants. Corrected acuity is rarely better than 20/100. Hypotonia is present at birth and the tendon reflexes are usually absent. Hypotonia may improve, but tone never is normal. Motor milestones are achieved slowly, and all boys have some degree of intellectual impairment. Proximal renal tubular dysfunction of the Fanconi type is present, including bicarbonate wasting and renal tubular acidosis, phosphaturia with hypophosphatemia and renal rickets, aminoaciduria, low molecular weight proteinuria, sodium and potassium wasting, and polyuria. Slowly progressive chronic renal failure is the rule, resulting in end-stage renal disease after the ages of 10–20.

Diagnosis. Diagnosis depends on recognition of the clinical constellation and is confirmed with molecular genetic testing. MRI shows diffuse and irregular foci of increased signal consistent with demyelination.

Management. Symptomatic treatment includes early removal of cataracts, nasogastric tube feedings or feeding gastrostomy to achieve appropriate nutrition, occupational or speech therapy to address feeding problems, standard measures for gastroesophageal reflux, and programs to promote optimal psychomotor development.

Peroxisomal Disorders: Zellweger Spectrum Disorder

Peroxisomes are subcellular organelles that participate in the biosynthesis of ether phospholipids and bile acids; the oxidation of very long-chain fatty acids (VLCFAs), prostaglandins, and unsaturated long-chain fatty acids; and the catabolism of phytanate, pipecolate, and glycolate. Hydrogen peroxide is a product of several oxidation reactions catabolized by the enzyme catalase. Mutations in one of the *ZSD-PEX* genes cause the Zellweger spectrum disorders. *PEX* genes encode the proteins required for peroxisomal assembly; pathogenic variants cause peroxisomal biogenesis disorders characterized by an identifiable intrinsic protein membrane but absence of all matrix enzymes.

Zellweger spectrum disorders were previously differentiated into cerebrohepatorenal or Zellweger syndrome, neonatal adrenoleukodystrophy, and infantile Refsum disease, with phenotypes ranging from mild to severe. They are now all considered as a spectrum of a single disease process. Infantile hypotonia is a prominent feature of peroxisomal biogenesis disorders.

Clinical features. Severely affected newborns are poorly responsive and have severe hypotonia, arthrogryposis, and dysmorphic features. Sucking and crying are weak. Tendon reflexes are hypoactive or absent. Characteristic craniofacial abnormalities include a pear-shaped head owing to a high forehead and an unusual fullness of the cheeks, widened sutures, micrognathia, a high-arched palate, flattening of the bridge of the nose, and hypertelorism. Organ abnormalities include biliary cirrhosis, polycystic kidneys, retinal degeneration, and cerebral malformations secondary to abnormalities of neuronal migration.

Limited extension of the fingers and flexion deformities of the knee and ankle characterize the arthrogryposis. Neonatal seizures are common and are often difficult to control. Bony stippling (chondrodysplasia punctata) of the patella and other long bones may occur. Older children have retinal dystrophy, sensorineural hearing loss, developmental delay with hypotonia, and liver dysfunction. Infants with severe Zellweger spectrum disorder are significantly impaired and die during the first year of life, usually having made no developmental progress. The clinical course is variable for those with less severe disease; while some children can be very hypotonic, others learn to walk and talk.

Diagnosis. Measurement of plasma VLCFA levels is often the first step in diagnosis. Elevation of C26:0 and

C26:1 and the ratios C24/C22 and C26/C22 are consistent with a defect in peroxisomal fatty acid metabolism. Molecular genetic testing of the 13 known *ZSD-PEX* genes reveals a biallelic pathogenic variant and confirms the diagnosis. Very rarely, heterozygous variants can cause disease (this has been reported specifically with a variant in *PEX6*).[6]

Management. Treatment is symptomatic and includes anticonvulsants for seizures, hearing aids, cataract removal in infancy. Liver fibrosis is progressive and must be monitored by hepatology. Supplementation of vitamin K and other fat-soluble vitamins is often required. Adrenal insufficiency, dental anomalies, and renal stones are common.

Pyruvate Carboxylase Deficiency

Pyruvate carboxylase deficiency is divided into three types. Type A is the infantile form and causes death in infancy or early childhood. Type B is the severe neonatal form; affected infants usually do not survive beyond 3 months. Type C is a milder intermittent form that will not be discussed here. The initial features of pyruvate carboxylase deficiency types A and B are neonatal hypotonia, tachypnea, and movement disorders.

Clinical features. Types A and B present similarly, but signs and symptoms present earlier and with greater severity in type B. Affected infants are hypotonic with laboratory abnormalities ranging from mild metabolic acidosis (type A) to hypoglycemia, hyperammonemia, and multiple biochemical abnormalities (type B). Episodes of stress precipitate vomiting and tachypnea. High amplitude tremor of the limbs is the rule, and bizarre eye movements are present in some affected infants. Seizures are uncommon but may occur in more severe phenotypes.

Diagnosis. Hypoglycemia, lactic acidosis, and hypercitrullinemia are constant findings. Brain MRI shows cystic periventricular leukomalacia, generalized hypomyelination, and symmetric gliosis or white matter changes. MR spectroscopy shows high levels of lactate and choline and low levels of N-acetylaspartate. Molecular genetic testing reveals biallelic pathogenic variants in the *PC* gene. Inheritance is autosomal recessive, but mosaicism may occur and result in less severe phenotypes.[7]

Treatment. Diet therapy, in the first hours postpartum, with triheptanoin and citrate reverses the biochemical errors. The long-term outcome is not established.

Orthotopic liver transplantation has been successful in correcting biochemical abnormalities in a very small number of cases.

Other Metabolic Defects

Infantile hypotonia is rarely the only manifestation of inborn errors of metabolism. Acid maltase deficiency causes a severe myopathy and is discussed with other metabolic myopathies. Hypotonia may be the only initial feature of generalized GM_1 gangliosidosis (see Chapter 5).

SPINAL CORD DISORDERS

Hypoxic-Ischemic Myelopathy

Hypoxic-ischemic encephalopathy is an expected outcome in severe perinatal asphyxia (see Chapter 1). Affected newborns are hypotonic and areflexic. The main cause of hypotonia is the cerebral injury but spinal cord dysfunction also contributes. Concurrent ischemic necrosis of gray matter occurs in the spinal cord as well as in the brain. The spinal cord component is evident on postmortem examination and by electromyography (EMG) in survivors.

Spinal Cord Injury

Only in the newborn does spinal cord injury enter the differential diagnosis of hypotonia. Injuries to the cervical spinal cord occur almost exclusively during vaginal delivery; approximately 75% are associated with breech presentation and 25% with cephalic presentation. Because the injuries are always associated with a difficult and prolonged delivery, decreased consciousness is common and hypotonia falsely attributed to asphyxia or cerebral trauma. Loss of response to sensory modalities below the mid-chest, absence of reflexes, and absence of the anal wink reflex (can also be seen with peripheral nervous system disorders) should suggest myelopathy.

Injuries in Breech Presentation

Traction injuries to the lower cervical and upper thoracic regions of the cord occur almost exclusively when the angle of extension of the fetal head exceeds 90%. The risk of spinal cord injury to a fetus in breech position whose head is hyperextended is greater than 70%. In such cases, delivery should always be by cesarean section. The tractional forces applied to the extended head are sufficient not only to stretch the cord but also to cause herniation of the brainstem through the foramen magnum. In addition, the hyperextended position compromises the vertebral arteries as they enter the skull.

The spectrum of pathological findings varies from edema of the cord without loss of anatomical continuity to massive hemorrhage (epidural, subdural, and intramedullary). Hemorrhage is greatest in the lower cervical and upper thoracic segments but may extend the entire length of the cord. Concurrent hemorrhage in the posterior fossa and laceration of the cerebellum may be present as well.

Clinical features. Mild tractional injuries, which cause cord edema but not intraparenchymal hemorrhage or loss of anatomical continuity, produce few clinical features. The main feature is hypotonia, often falsely attributed to asphyxia.

Hemorrhage into the posterior fossa accompanies severe tractional injuries. Affected newborns are unconscious and atonic at birth with flaccid quadriplegia and diaphragmatic breathing. Injuries restricted to the low cervical and high thoracic segments produce near-normal strength in the biceps muscles and weakness of the triceps muscles. The result is flexion of the arms at the elbows and flaccid paraplegia. Spontaneous movement and tendon reflexes in the legs are absent, but foot withdrawal from pinprick may occur as a spinal reflex. The infant has a distended bladder and dribbling of urine. The absence of sweating below the injury marks the sensory level, which is difficult to measure directly.

Diagnosis. Radiographs of the vertebrae show no abnormalities because bony displacement does not occur. MRI of the spine shows intraspinal edema and hemorrhage. Unconscious newborns are generally thought to have intracerebral hemorrhage or asphyxia (see Chapter 2), and the diagnosis of spinal cord injury may not be considered until consciousness is regained and the typical motor deficits are observed. Even then, the suspicion of a neuromuscular disorder may exist until disturbed bladder function and the development of progressive spastic paraplegia alerts the physician to the correct diagnosis.

Management. The treatment of spinal cord traction injuries of the newborn is similar to the management of cord injuries in older children (see Chapter 12).

Injuries in Cephalic Presentation

Twisting of the neck during mid-forceps rotation causes high cervical cord injuries in cephalic presentation. The trunk fails to rotate with the head. The risk is greatest when amniotic fluid is absent because of delay from the time of membrane rupture to the application of forceps. The spectrum of injury varies from intraparenchymal hemorrhage to complete transection. Transection usually occurs at the level of a fractured odontoid process, with atlantoaxial dislocation.

Clinical features. Newborns are flaccid and fail to breathe spontaneously. Those with milder injuries may have shallow, labored respirations, but all require assisted ventilation at birth. Most are unconscious at birth owing to edema in the brainstem. When conscious, eye movements, sucking, and the withdrawal reflex are the only movements observed. Tendon reflexes are at first absent but later become exaggerated if the child survives. Bladder distention and overflow incontinence occur. Priapism may be present. Sensation is difficult to assess because the withdrawal reflex is present.

Death from sepsis or respiratory complications is common. Occasionally, children have survived for several years.

Diagnosis. The appearance of children with high cervical cord injuries suggests a neuromuscular disorder, especially infantile spinal muscular atrophy (SMA), because the limbs are flaccid but the eye movements are normal. EMG of the limbs and genetic testing should exclude that possibility. Radiographs of the cervical vertebrae usually do not show abnormalities, but MRI shows marked thinning or disruption of the cord at the site of injury.

Management. Intubation and respiratory assistance commence prior to diagnosis. Chapter 12 discusses management of spinal cord transection.

MOTOR UNIT DISORDERS

Evaluation of Motor Unit Disorders

In the diagnosis of cerebral hypotonia in infants, the choice of laboratory tests varies considerably depending on the disease entity. This is not the case with motor unit hypotonia. The available battery of tests readily defines the anatomy and cause of pathological processes affecting the motor unit (Box 6.9). Molecular genetic testing is now commercially available for many disorders and is preferable to muscle or nerve biopsy.

Serum Creatine Kinase

Increased serum concentrations of creatine kinase (CK) reflect skeletal or cardiac muscle necrosis. Obtain blood before the performance of EMG or muscle biopsy,

---

> **BOX 6.9 Evaluation of Motor Unit Disorders**
>
> - Molecular genetic testing
> - Electrodiagnosis
>   - Electromyography
>   - Nerve conduction studies
>   - Repetitive stimulation
> - Muscle biopsy
> - Nerve biopsy
> - Serum creatine kinase

---

which transiently elevates the serum concentration of CK. Keep in mind that prolonged resuscitation efforts also cause misleadingly high levels. The basis for laboratory reference values for "normal" CK is nonambulatory adults. Normal values tend to be higher in an ambulatory population, especially after exercise. The serum concentration of CK in severely asphyxiated newborns is as high as 1000 IU/L secondary to acidosis. Even normal newborns have a higher-than-normal concentration during the first 24 hours postpartum. A normal CK level in a hypotonic infant is strong evidence against a rapidly progressive myopathy, but it does not exclude fiber-type disproportion myopathies and some metabolic myopathies. Conversely, expect mild elevations in CK concentration in rapidly progressive cases of SMA.

Electrodiagnosis

EMG is extremely useful in the diagnosis of infantile hypotonia when an experienced physician performs the study. It enables the prediction of the final diagnosis in most infants younger than 3 months of age with hypotonia of motor unit origin. Hypotonic infants with normal EMG findings rarely show abnormalities on muscle biopsy. The needle portion of the study helps to distinguish myopathic from neuropathic processes. The appearance of brief, small-amplitude, polyphasic potentials characterizes myopathies, whereas the presence of denervation potentials at rest (fibrillations, fasciculations, sharp waves) and motor unit potentials that are large, prolonged, and polyphasic characterizes denervation. Studies of nerve conduction velocity are useful in distinguishing axonal from demyelinating neuropathies; demyelinating neuropathies cause greater slowing of conduction velocity. Repetitive nerve stimulation studies demonstrate disturbances in neuromuscular transmission.

Muscle Biopsy

Due to the increasing availability of genetic testing, muscle biopsy is rarely required. However, an understanding of the basic concepts remains useful, and many diseases are still classified on the basis of biopsy findings. The muscle selected for biopsy should be weak but still able to contract. Histochemical analysis is essential for the complete evaluation of muscle histology. The demonstration of fiber types, muscle proteins, and storage materials is required. The intensity of the reaction to myosin adenosine triphosphatase (ATPase) at pH 9.4 arbitrarily divides skeletal muscle into two fiber types. Type I fibers react weakly to ATPase, are characterized by oxidative metabolism, and serve a tonic function. Type II fibers react intensely to ATPase, utilize glycolytic metabolism, and serve a phasic function. Type I and II fibers are generally equal in number and randomly distributed in each fascicle. Abnormalities in fiber-type number, fiber-type size, or both characterize some disorders.

Chapter 7 describes and illustrates the structural proteins of muscle. Merosin is the main protein associated with congenital muscular dystrophy (CMD). The important storage materials identified in skeletal muscle are glycogen and lipid. In most storage disorders, vacuoles are present in the fibers that contain the abnormal material. Light microscopy reveals the vacuoles and histochemical reactions identify the specific material.

Nerve Biopsy

Sural nerve biopsy has limited value in the diagnosis of infantile hypotonia, and it is only an option when EMG shows sural neuropathy. Its main utility is in the diagnosis of vasculitis, although abnormalities such as onion bulb formations are present with Dejerine-Sottas syndrome. The latter diagnosis is associated with abnormal nerve conduction studies and may be confirmed by genetic testing.

Historical Note: The Tensilon Test

Edrophonium chloride (*Tensilon*) is a rapidly acting anticholinesterase that temporarily reverses weakness in patients with myasthenia and was previously used to diagnose this disorder at the bedside by demonstrating the reversible nature of the patient's motor deficits. Unfortunately, rare patients are supersensitive to edrophonium chloride and may stop breathing because of depolarization of endplates or an abnormal vagal response, leading to an iatrogenic respiratory crisis.

In addition to presenting a real risk of apnea, the Tensilon test was highly subjective, and for these reasons, it is no longer used. There are multiple safer and more accurate diagnostic options available.

Spinal Muscular Atrophies

The SMAs are genetic disorders in which anterior horn cells in the spinal cord and motor nuclei of the brainstem are progressively lost. The phenotype is variable, and onset ranges from infancy to adulthood. Weakness is typically more evident proximally and is symmetric and progressive in nature. Multiple subtypes were described prior to our current genetic understanding of this disease. Those with onset in infancy usually cause generalized weakness and hypotonia. Infantile SMA is one of the more common motor unit disorders causing infantile hypotonia.

Infantile Spinal Muscular Atrophy

The clinical subtypes of autosomal recessive SMA are a continuum of disease. Discussion of the severe type (SMA I), which always begins before 6 months, follows. Discussion of the intermediate (SMA II) and juvenile (SMA III) types is in Chapter 7, but these should be understood as parts of the same SMA spectrum rather than distinct disease entities. Pathogenic variants in the *SMN1* (survival motor neuron) gene on 5q12.2-q13.3 cause the disease. Normal individuals have both *SMN1* and a variable number of copies of *SMN2*, an almost identical copy of the *SMN1* gene, except for a single substitution that results in a partially functioning protein on the same chromosome. The number of *SMN2* copies affects the observed phenotype and is responsible for differing clinical pictures within the same family.[8]

Clinical features. The age at onset is birth to 6 months. Reduced fetal movement may occur when neuronal degeneration begins in utero. Affected newborns have generalized weakness involving proximal more than distal muscles, hypotonia, and areflexia. Newborns that are hypotonic in utero and weak at birth may have difficulty adapting to extrauterine life and experience postnatal asphyxia and encephalopathy. Most breathe adequately at first and appear alert despite the generalized weakness because facial expression is relatively well preserved and extraocular movement is normal. Some newborns have paradoxical respiration because intercostal paralysis and thoracic collapse occur before diaphragmatic movement is impaired, whereas others have diaphragmatic paralysis as an initial feature. Despite intrauterine hypotonia, arthrogryposis is not present. Neurogenic arthrogryposis may be a distinct entity and is described separately in this chapter.

When weakness begins in infancy, the decline in strength can be sudden or decremental. At times the child seems to improve because of normal cerebral development, but the progression of weakness is relentless. The tongue may show atrophy and fasciculations, but these are difficult to see in newborns. After the gag reflex is lost, feeding becomes difficult and death results from aspiration and pneumonia. When weakness is present at birth, death usually occurs by 6 months of age if untreated, but the course is variable when symptoms develop after 3 months of age. Some infants will attain sitting balance but will not walk. Survival time is not predictable.

Diagnosis. Molecular genetic testing of the *SMN1* gene is available. About 95% of individuals with SMA are homozygous for the absence of exons 7 and 8 of *SMN1*, and about 5% are compound heterozygotes for the absence of exons 7 and 8 of one *SMN1* allele and a point mutation in the other *SMN1* allele. Single gene testing is available; a multiple gene panel can also be done if the differential includes other potential etiologies. The serum concentration of CK is usually normal but may be mildly elevated in infants with rapidly progressive weakness. EMG studies show fibrillations and fasciculations at rest, and the mean amplitude of motor unit potentials is increased. Motor nerve conduction velocities are usually normal.

Muscle biopsy is unnecessary because of the commercial availability of DNA-based testing. The pathological findings in skeletal muscle are characteristic. Routine histological stains show groups of small fibers adjacent to groups of normal-sized or hypertrophied fibers. When the myosin ATPase reaction is applied, all hypertrophied fibers are type I, whereas medium-sized and small fibers are a mixture of types I and II (Fig. 6.4). Type grouping, a sign of reinnervation in which large numbers of fibers of the same type are contiguous, replaces the normal random arrangement of fiber types. Some biopsy specimens show uniform small fibers of both types.

DNA analysis of chorionic villus biopsies provides prenatal diagnosis.

Management. Previously a universally fatal disease, infantile SMA now has several treatment options. All

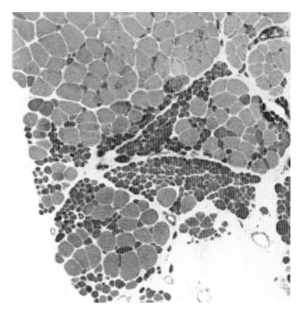

Fig. 6.4 Infantile Spinal Muscular Atrophy (ATPase Reaction). The normal random distribution pattern of fiber types is lost. Groups of large type I fibers (*light shade*) are adjacent to groups of small type II fibers (*dark shade*).

can slow progression of the disease, but none can reverse damage that has already occurred, making early diagnosis and treatment critical. As a result, SMA has been added to many states' newborn screening programs. All the treatment options listed here lead to significantly improved outcomes; primary endpoints in most clinical trials included the ability to sit unsupported for at least 5 seconds and survival at 24 months without the need for permanent ventilation.

The FDA approved the first treatment for SMA in late 2016. Spinraza (nusinersen) is approved for use in a broad range of SMA patients. Results of the ENDEAR clinical trial showed statistically significant improvements in achieving motor milestones (40% versus 0%, $P < .0001$), and decreased mortality in the treatment group (23% versus 43%). Spinraza is delivered intrathecally on a scheduled basis and increases production of full-length SMA protein via the *SMN2* gene. Lifelong treatment is required.[9]

Similar to nusinersen, risdiplam (Evrysdi) is an RNA-splicing modifier directed at *SNM2* to encourage increased production of the full-length SMA protein.[10] It is given as a daily oral medication and is approved for patients 2 months of age and older, making it inappropriate for young symptomatic infants who require immediate initiation of treatment, but useful for presymptomatic infants identified through newborn screening and for those with later-onset SMA disease. The recommended dose is 0.2 mg/kg/day. The most common adverse effects are fever, diarrhea, rash, and respiratory infections.

Zolgensma (onasemnogene abeparvovec) is a one-time gene therapy approved for treatment in children aged 2 years and younger.[11] It uses a viral vector to replace the missing or dysfunctional *SMN1* gene, leading to drastically improved survival rates and acquisition of some motor skills. In clinical trials, approximately 27% of patients experienced transaminitis and one with preexisting liver disease suffered acute liver failure. All patients recovered following treatment with corticosteroids, and a course of steroids before and after dosing is a recommended part of the treatment regimen. Liver enzymes must be checked prior to dosing and for at least 3 months thereafter. Other potential side effects include nausea, vomiting, elevated troponin-I, and thrombocytopenia.

Infantile Spinal Muscular Atrophy With Respiratory Distress Type 1

Originally classified as a variant of SMA I, spinal muscular atrophy with respiratory distress type 1 is a distinct genetic disorder resulting from pathogenic variants in the *IGHMBP2* gene encoding the immunoglobulin μ-binding protein 2.[12]

Clinical features. Clinical features vary somewhat depending on the level of residual enzyme activity; those with more favorable outcomes have greater retained enzymatic activity.[13] Intrauterine growth restriction, weak cry, and foot deformities are the initial features. Most infants come to attention between 1 and 6 months because of respiratory distress secondary to diaphragmatic weakness, weak cry, and progressive distal weakness of the legs. Sensory and autonomic nerve dysfunction accompanies the motor weakness. Sudden infant death occurs without respiratory support, and affected children require permanent mechanical ventilation.

Diagnosis. Consider the diagnosis in infants with an SMA I phenotype lacking the *SMN1* gene abnormality, and those with distal weakness and respiratory failure. Testing for the *IGHMBP2* gene is available.

Management. Treatment is supportive.

Congenital Cervical Spinal Muscular Atrophy

This is a rare sporadic disorder characterized by severe weakness and wasting confined to the arms. Contractures of the shoulder, elbow, and wrist joints are present at birth. The legs are normal. Postnatal progression of weakness does not occur. CNS function is normal. Given that it is nonfamilial and nonprogressive, some authors recommend viewing it as a subtype of neurogenic arthrogryposis.[14]

Neurogenic Arthrogryposis

Neurogenic arthrogryposis is commonly referred to as arthrogryposis multiplex congenita, neurogenic type, and its cause is poorly understood but may be due to poor or absent myelin formation around peripheral nerves. Transmission usually occurs by autosomal recessive inheritance.

Clinical features. In neurogenic arthrogryposis, the most active phase of disease occurs in utero. Severely affected newborns have respiratory and feeding difficulties, and some die of aspiration. The less severely affected ones survive and have little or no progression of their weakness. Indeed, the respiratory and feeding difficulties lessen with time. Contractures are present in both proximal and distal joints. Micrognathia and a high-arched palate may be associated features, and a pattern of facial anomalies suggesting trisomy 18 is present in some newborns. Newborns with respiratory distress at birth may not have a fatal course. Limb weakness may be minimal, and long intervals of stability occur.

Diagnosis. Suspect the diagnosis in newborns with arthrogryposis, normal serum concentrations of CK, and EMG findings compatible with a neuropathic process. Muscle histological examination reveals the typical pattern of denervation and reinnervation. Cranial MRI investigates cerebral malformations in children with microcephaly. Multiple genes have been implicated but genetic testing for the disease remains of limited utility.

Management. Initiate an intensive program of rehabilitation immediately after birth. Surgical release of contractures is often required.

Cytochrome-c Oxidase Deficiency

Cytochrome-c oxidase (COX) deficiency is clinically heterogeneous. Phenotypes range from isolated myopathy to fatal infantile cardioencephalomyopathy.[15] The condition can affect skeletal and cardiac muscle, brain, kidneys, and liver. Phenotypes can vary significantly even within the same family. Although symptoms typically begin before the age of 2, more mildly affected individuals may present later in life. Patients may have symptoms consistent with Leigh syndrome, and it is one of the recognized causes of this disorder (see Chapter 5). Hypertrophic cardiomyopathy, weakness due to myopathy, vomiting, seizures, movement disorders, cognitive impairment, and regression may occur. Mutations in several different genes can cause the COX deficiency phenotype, and may be sporadic, autosomal recessive, or mitochondrial. Diagnosis often requires a multistep workup, with evaluation of lactic acid, genetic panels, or comprehensive genomic testing. Some similar disorders, such as biotinidase deficiency or thiamine transporter-2 deficiency, are potentially treatable and should be ruled out before a final diagnosis is made.

Treatment is supportive.

Polyneuropathies

Polyneuropathies are uncommon in childhood and are even less common during infancy. Box 6.10 lists the polyneuropathies with onset in infancy. They divide into those that primarily affect the myelin

---

BOX 6.10 Polyneuropathies With Possible Onset in Infancy

Axonal
- Familial dysautonomia
- Hereditary motor-sensory neuropathy type II (see Chapter 7)
- Idiopathic with encephalopathy (see Chapter 7)
- Infantile neuronal degeneration
- Subacute necrotizing encephalopathy (see Chapters 5 and 10)

Demyelinating
- Acute inflammatory demyelinating polyneuropathy (Guillain-Barré syndrome) (see Chapter 7)
- Chronic inflammatory demyelinating polyneuropathy (see Chapter 7)
- Congenital hypomyelinating neuropathy
- Globoid cell leukodystrophy (see Chapter 5)
- Hereditary motor-sensory neuropathy type I (see Chapter 7)
- Hereditary motor-sensory neuropathy type III (see Chapter 7)
- Metachromatic leukodystrophy (see Chapter 5)

(demyelinating) or those that affect the axon (axonal). In newborns and infants, the term *demyelinating* also refers to disorders in which myelin has failed to form (hypomyelinating). Only with congenital hypomyelinating neuropathy (CHN) is infantile hypotonia the initial feature. The others are more likely to start as progressive gait disturbance or psychomotor delays. Chapter 7 provides a complete discussion of the clinical approach to neuropathy.

Congenital Hypomyelinating Neuropathy

The term *congenital hypomyelinating neuropathy* (CHN) encompasses several disorders with similar clinical and pathological features. Other terms used to describe this disorder are *severe early onset Charcot-Marie-Tooth* (CMT), CMT3, or *Dejerine-Sottas syndrome*. The disease may be sporadic or inherited in an autosomal recessive fashion. CHN results from a congenital impairment in myelin formation and can be caused by a mutation in the early growth response 2 (*EGR2*) gene[16] or the myelin protein zero (*MPZ*) gene.[17] Mutations in other CMT-causative genes, such as *PMP22, MPZ,* and *GJB*, have also been implicated. Pathogenic variants in the *CNTNAP1* gene are associated with a particularly severe form.[18]

Clinical features. The clinical features are similar to those of acute infantile SMA. Arthrogryposis may be present. Newborns have progressive flaccid weakness and atrophy of the skeletal muscles, a bulbar palsy that spares extraocular motility, and areflexia. Respiratory insufficiency causes death during infancy.

In some children, failure to meet motor milestones is the initial manifestation. Examination shows diffuse weakness, distal atrophy, and areflexia. Weakness progresses slowly and is not life-threatening during childhood. Sensation remains intact.

Diagnosis. The serum concentration of CK is normal, EMG findings are consistent with denervation, and motor nerve conduction velocities are usually less than 10 m/s. The protein concentration of the CSF is markedly elevated in almost every case. Molecular genetic testing is typically performed but may fail to identify a causative mutation.

Management. In general, treatment is supportive. Some infants with hypomyelinating neuropathies respond to treatment with oral prednisone, but reports are anecdotal and evidence-based treatment protocols are lacking.

Disorders of Neuromuscular Transmission

Infantile Botulism

Human botulism ordinarily results from eating food contaminated by preformed exotoxin of the organism *Clostridium botulinum*. The exotoxin prevents the release of acetylcholine, causing a cholinergic blockade of skeletal muscle and end organs innervated by autonomic nerves. Infantile botulism is an age-limited disorder in which ingested *C. botulinum* colonizes the intestinal tract and produces toxin in situ. Dietary contamination with honey or corn syrup accounts for almost 20% of cases, but in most the source is not defined.[19]

Clinical features. The clinical spectrum of infantile botulism includes asymptomatic carriers of organisms; mild hypotonia and failure to thrive; severe, progressive, life-threatening paralysis; and sudden infant death. Infected infants are between 2 and 26 weeks of age and have often been exposed to construction or agricultural soil disruption. The highest incidence is between March and October. A prodromal syndrome of constipation and poor feeding is common. Progressive bulbar and skeletal muscle weakness and loss of tendon reflexes develop 4–5 days later. Typical features on examination include diffuse hypotonia, ptosis, dysphagia, weak cry, and dilated pupils that react sluggishly to light.

Infantile botulism is a self-limited disease generally lasting for 2–6 weeks. Recovery is complete, but relapse occurs in as many as 5% of babies.

Diagnosis. The syndrome suggests acute inflammatory demyelinating polyradiculoneuropathy (Guillain-Barré syndrome), infantile SMA, or generalized myasthenia gravis. Clinical differentiation of infantile botulism from Guillain-Barré syndrome is difficult, and some reported cases of Guillain-Barré syndrome during infancy might have been infantile botulism. Infantile botulism differs from infantile SMA by the early appearance of facial and pharyngeal weakness, the presence of ptosis and dilated pupils, and the occurrence of severe constipation. Infants with generalized myasthenia do not have dilated pupils, absent reflexes, or severe constipation.

Electrophysiological studies provide the first clue to the diagnosis. Repetitive stimulation between 20 and 50 Hz reverses the presynaptic block and produces a gradual increase in the size of the motor unit potentials in 90% of cases. The EMG shows short-duration, low-amplitude, motor unit potentials. The isolation of organisms from the stool is diagnostic.

Management. Intensive care is necessary throughout the period of profound hypotonia, and many infants require ventilator support. Sudden apnea and death are a constant danger. Early use of immune globulin reduces the length of hospitalization and shortens the duration of intensive care, mechanical ventilation, and intravenous or tube feedings.[20,21] Avoid aminoglycoside antibiotics such as gentamicin as they produce presynaptic neuromuscular blockade and may worsen the condition.

Congenital Myasthenic Syndromes

Several genetic defects causing myasthenic syndromes have been identified.[22] All are autosomal recessive traits except for the slow channel syndrome, which is an autosomal dominant trait. All genetic myasthenic syndromes are seronegative for antibodies that bind the acetylcholine receptor (AChR). Both the genetic and clinical features are the basis for classifying congenital myasthenic syndromes.

Clinical Features. Respiratory insufficiency and feeding difficulty may be present at birth. Many affected newborns require mechanical ventilation. Ptosis and generalized weakness are present either at birth or develop during infancy.[23] Arthrogryposis may also be present. Although facial and skeletal muscles are weak, extraocular motility is usually normal. Within weeks many infants become stronger and no longer need mechanical ventilation. However, episodes of weakness and life-threatening apnea occur repeatedly throughout infancy and childhood, sometimes even into adult life.

Diagnosis. The basis for the diagnosis of a congenital myasthenic syndrome is the clinical findings, a decremental EMG response of the compound muscle action potential on low frequency (2–3 Hz) stimulation, negative tests for anti-AChR and anti-MuSK (muscle-specific tyrosine kinase) antibodies in the serum, and lack of improvement in clinical symptoms with immunosuppressive therapy. The intravenous or subcutaneous injection of edrophonium chloride, 0.15 mg/kg, may safely establish the diagnosis in intubated newborns but is rarely used due to its brief effects, which make objective assessment difficult. Several genes encoding proteins expressed at the neuromuscular junction are associated with congenital myasthenic syndrome.

Management. Long-term treatment with neostigmine or pyridostigmine prevents sudden episodes of apnea at the time of intercurrent illness. The weakness in some children responds to a combination of pyridostigmine and diaminopyridine. Diaminopyridine was granted an orphan designation by the FDA in the United States for its use in Lambert-Eaton myasthenic syndrome in 2009. Thymectomy and immunosuppressive therapies are not beneficial.

Transitory Neonatal Myasthenia

A transitory myasthenic syndrome occurs in approximately 15% of newborns of myasthenic mothers.[24] The passive transfer of antibodies directed against fetal AChR from the myasthenic mother to her normal fetus is the presumed cause. Fetal AChR is structurally different from adult AChR. The severity of symptoms in the newborn correlates with the ratio of fetal to adult AChR antibodies in the mother; however, it does not correlate with the severity or duration of maternal symptoms.

Clinical features. Females with myasthenia have a higher rate of complications of delivery. Difficulty feeding and generalized hypotonia are the major clinical features in the infant. Affected children are eager to feed, but the ability to suck fatigues quickly and nutrition is inadequate. Symptoms usually arise within hours of birth but delay until the third day sometimes occurs. Some newborns are hypotonic in utero and born with arthrogryposis. A weak cry and lack of facial expression are present in 50% of affected newborns, but only 15% have limitations in extraocular movement and ptosis. Respiratory insufficiency is uncommon but may occur in severe cases. Weakness becomes progressively worse in the first few days and then improves. The mean duration of symptoms is 18 days, with a range of 5 days to 2 months. Recovery is complete, and transitory neonatal myasthenia does not develop into myasthenia gravis later in life.

Diagnosis. High serum concentrations of the AChR-binding antibody in the newborn and responsiveness to neostigmine or pyridostigmine establish the diagnosis.

Management. Treat newborns with severe generalized weakness and respiratory distress with plasma exchange. For those less impaired, 0.1% neostigmine methylsulfate by intramuscular injection before feeding sufficiently improves sucking and swallowing to allow adequate nutrition. Progressively reduce the dose as symptoms remit. An alternative route for neostigmine is by nasogastric tube at a dose 10 times the parenteral dose. Pyridostigmine is a commonly used alternative.

Congenital Myopathies

Congenital myopathies are developmental disorders of skeletal muscle, and the term currently encompasses seven distinct muscle diseases present from birth or becoming symptomatic during infancy. The main clinical feature is infantile hypotonia and weakness, but symptoms and severity vary considerably from one disorder to the next. Diagnostic testing includes muscle biopsy, CK, EMG, and in some cases molecular genetic testing. The increasing availability of genetic testing is prompting a reassessment of the classification of these disorders, but currently they are still classified based on results of the muscle biopsy.

Nemaline (Rod) Myopathy

Nemaline myopathy (NM) occurs in 1 in 50,000 individuals. Six distinct subtypes have been identified: severe congenital, Amish, intermediate congenital, typical congenital, childhood-onset, and adult-onset. Severe congenital is often fatal, whereas individuals with the adult-onset type tend to be the least affected. The most common type is typical congenital.

Clinical features. NM is characterized by weakness and hypotonia with depressed or absent DTRs. Muscle weakness is usually most pronounced in the face, neck flexors, and proximal limb muscles. Significant differences exist in survival between patients classified as having severe, intermediate, and typical NM. Severe respiratory insufficiency at birth, dilated cardiomyopathy, and the presence of arthrogryposis multiplex congenita are associated with the severe congenital type, and result in death within the first year of life. Mothers of affected infants may report decreased movements in utero. In contrast, infants affected with the typical congenital type appear mildly hypotonic in the neonatal period, often coming to medical attention only when they fail to achieve motor milestones. This form tends to be slowly progressive, with greater weakness in proximal than distal muscles. Weakness of facial muscles causes a dysmorphic appearance in which the face appears long and narrow and the palate is high and arched. Axial weakness leads to scoliosis. Independent ambulation before 18 months of age is a positive predictive feature. Most children with typical NM are eventually able to walk.

Transmission of the childhood-onset form is by autosomal dominant inheritance. Onset of ankle weakness occurs late in the first or early in the second decade. The weakness is slowly progressive, and affected individuals may be wheelchair-dependent as adults.

Diagnosis. The term *NM* refers to a group of genetically distinct disorders linked by common morphological features observed on muscle histology. Muscle fibers show multiple small rod-like or thread-like particles, thought to be derived from lateral expansion of the Z disk. The greatest concentration of particles is under the sarcolemma (Fig. 6.5). Type I fiber predominance is a prominent feature. Electrophysiological studies may suggest a myopathic process but are not specific, and the concentration of serum CK is usually normal or minimally elevated.

At least 12 genes have been implicated in the pathogenesis of NM.[25] *NEB* mutations account for approximately 50% of cases and are autosomal recessive, and *ACTA1* mutations account for 15%–25% and are typically de novo but may be autosomal dominant or autosomal recessive in rare cases. *NEB* mutations are associated with symptom onset in infancy or early childhood. Several different genetic abnormalities cause the same histological features that define the disorder.

Management. Treatment is supportive and aimed at preventing complications. Even patients with mild muscle weakness may experience central hypoventilation during sleep, and this must be closely monitored. Feeding difficulties sometimes necessitate the placement of gastrostomy tubes. Respiratory infections should be treated promptly, and an orthopedist must monitor joint contractures.

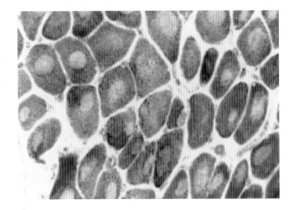

Fig. 6.5 Nemaline (Rod) Myopathy (Trichrome Stain). A spectrum of fiber sizes is present. The small fibers are all type I and contain rod-like bodies in a subsarcolemmal position.

Central Core Disease

Central core disease is one of the two core myopathies and is the most common to occur in infancy. It is a distinct genetic entity transmitted primarily by autosomal dominant inheritance, although recessive and sporadic cases occur. Mutations in the ryanodine receptor–1 gene (*RYR1*) on chromosome 19q13 are responsible for central core disease and malignant hyperthermia.[26] Central core disease was previously thought to be rare, but some literature suggests it is underdiagnosed and may be one of the most common of the congenital myopathies.[27]

Clinical features. Mild hypotonia is present immediately after birth or during infancy. Congenital dislocation of the hips is relatively common. Slowly progressive weakness begins after the age of 5. Weakness is greater in proximal than in distal limb muscles and is greater in the arms than in the legs. Tendon reflexes of weak muscles are depressed or absent. Extraocular motility, facial expression, and swallowing are normal. Some children become progressively weaker, have motor impairment, and develop kyphoscoliosis. In others, weakness remains mild and never causes disability.

Most children with central core disease are assumed to be at risk of malignant hyperthermia and should not be administered anesthetics without appropriate caution (see Chapter 8).

Diagnosis. The serum concentration of CK is normal, and the EMG findings may be normal as well. More frequently, the EMG suggests a myopathic process. The basis for diagnosis is the characteristic histopathological finding of sharply demarcated cores of closely packed myofibrils undergoing varying degrees of degeneration in the center of all type I fibers (Fig. 6.6). Because of the tight packing of myofibrils, the cores are deficient in sarcoplasmic reticulum, glycogen, and mitochondria. Approximately 90% of children with central core disease have mutations in *RYR1*, the gene encoding the ryanodine receptor–1.[28] Sequence analysis identifies about 50% of affected individuals.

Management. Treatment is supportive. Dantrolene is used to abort cases of malignant hyperthermia. Small studies suggest that the beta-agonist salbutamol is helpful with symptom management, although not curative.[29]

Multiminicore Disease

Multiminicore disease comprises the second subtype of the core myopathies. It typically presents in later childhood or adolescence, but infant forms have

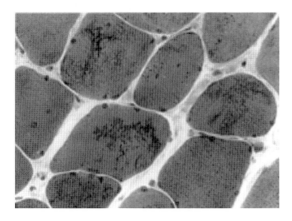

Fig. 6.6 Central Core Disease (DPNH reaction). The center of every fiber has a central core that appears clear when oxidative enzyme reactions are applied.

been described. The presence of multiple small zones ("cores") of sarcomeric disorganization with a lack of oxidative activity defines multiminicore disease.[30] The clinical phenotype is variable, with four main subtypes identified. The classic form comprises 75% of cases and presents congenitally or in early childhood. Affected infants are hypotonic and developmentally delayed, with scoliosis and respiratory involvement, which may lead to heart failure. The antenatal form with arthrogryposis multiplex congenita accounts for less than 10% of cases. Other subtypes include the moderate form, with hand involvement, and the ophthalmoplegic form.[31] Inheritance is autosomal recessive. Some cases are associated with *RYR1* mutations,[32] while others are caused by mutations in the selenoprotein 1 gene (*SEPN1*).[33]

Clinical features. Both sexes are equally affected. Onset is at birth or during infancy. Affected newborns are hypotonic with a high-arched palate and pectus excavatum, or other chest deformities. Delayed achievement of motor milestones characterizes infantile onset. Axial weakness is typical, as evidenced by scoliosis and neck flexor weakness, although the degree of spinal rigidity is variable. Respiratory insufficiency is the norm; however, most individuals are ambulatory despite their symptoms.

Diagnosis. Muscle biopsy specimens show zones of sarcomeric disorganization in both muscle fiber types that do not run the entire length of the fiber. Not every fiber contains a minicore. Type I fibers predominate in number. Genetic testing identifies approximately 50% of cases.

Management. Treatment is supportive. Infants often require respiratory support, and maintenance of good pulmonary toilet is needed. Pulmonary infections or progressive respiratory compromise due to scoliosis may be fatal.

Congenital Fiber-Type Disproportion Myopathy

The congenital fiber-type disproportion myopathies are a heterogeneous group of diseases that have a similar pattern of muscle histology. The initial feature of all these diseases is infantile hypotonia. Both genders are involved equally. Most cases are sporadic; genetic transmission may be autosomal dominant, autosomal recessive, or X-linked.[34] Multiple genes have been implicated, including *TPM2*, *TPM3*, *RYR1*, and *ACTA1*. Despite the label "congenital," an identical pattern of fiber-type disproportion may be present in patients who are asymptomatic at birth and first have weakness during childhood.

Clinical features. The severity of weakness in the newborn varies from mild hypotonia to respiratory insufficiency. Many had intrauterine hypotonia with resultant congenital hip dislocation and joint contractures. Proximal muscles are weaker than distal muscles. Facial weakness, high-arched palate, ptosis, and disturbances of ocular motility may be present. When axial weakness is present in infancy, kyphoscoliosis often develops during childhood. Tendon reflexes are depressed or absent. Intellectual function is normal. Weakness is most severe during the first 2 years and then becomes relatively stable or progresses slowly.

Diagnosis. Type I fiber predominance and hypotrophy are the essential histological features. Type I fibers are 15% smaller than type II fibers. The serum concentration of CK may be slightly elevated or normal, and the EMG may be consistent with a neuropathic process, a myopathic process, or both. Nerve conduction velocities are normal. Genetic testing is available.

Management. Physical therapy should be initiated immediately, not only to relieve existing contractures but also to prevent new contractures from developing. As with other congenital myopathies, respiratory, nutritional, and orthopedic surveillance is necessary to prevent additional complications.

Centronuclear Myopathy

Several clinical syndromes are included in the category of centronuclear (myotubular) myopathy. Transmission of some is by X-linked inheritance, others by autosomal dominant inheritance, and still others by autosomal recessive inheritance. The autosomal dominant form has a later onset and a milder course. The common histological feature of muscle biopsy is the presence of a centrally located nucleus within the muscle fiber, rather than its typical position in the periphery.

X-Linked centronuclear myopathy. X-linked centronuclear myopathy occurs primarily in males. The histological details are the same as for other types of centronuclear myopathies, but the genetic cause is distinct. The abnormal gene maps to the long arm of the X chromosome (Xq28) and is designated *MTM1*. *Myotubularin* is the protein encoded by the *MTM1* gene.[35]

Clinical features. Newborns with X-linked centronuclear myopathy are hypotonic and require respiratory assistance. The face has a myopathic appearance, motor milestones are delayed, and most fail to walk. Death in infancy from complications of respiratory insufficiency is common. Those with forms that are more moderate achieve motor milestones more quickly and about 40% require no ventilator support. In the mildest forms, ventilatory support is only required in the newborn period; delay of motor milestones is mild, walking is achieved, and facial strength is normal. Weakness is not progressive and may improve slowly over time. Female carriers are generally asymptomatic.

Diagnosis. The serum CK is normal. The EMG may suggest a neuropathic process, a myopathic process, or both. Muscle biopsy shows type I fiber predominance and hypotrophy, the presence of many internal nuclei, and a central area of increased oxidative enzyme and decreased myosin ATPase activity. Molecular genetic testing is available.

Management. Treatment is supportive.

Other centronuclear myopathies. Inheritance of milder forms of centronuclear myopathies may be either autosomal dominant or recessive. Multiple genes have been implicated, including *DNM2* (dynamin, autosomal dominant),[36] *BIN1* (usually autosomal recessive, rarely has autosomal dominant forms), and *TTN* (titin, autosomal recessive).

Clinical features. Age at onset varies depending on the causative mutation. Some children with the disease have hypotonia at birth; others come to attention because of delayed motor development. The pattern of limb weakness may be proximal or distal. The axial and neck flexor muscles are weak as well. Ptosis, but

not ophthalmoplegia, is sometimes present at birth. The course is usually slowly progressive. Possible features include ophthalmoplegia, loss of facial expression, and continuing weakness of limb muscles. Some have seizures and cognitive impairment.

Diagnosis. The serum concentration of CK is normal, and EMG findings are abnormal but do not establish the diagnosis. Muscle biopsy is essential for diagnosis, and the histological features are identical to those of the acute form.

Management. Treatment is supportive.

Muscular Dystrophies
Congenital Dystrophinopathy

Dystrophinopathies occasionally cause weakness at birth. In such cases dystrophin is completely absent. Immunofluorescence reactions for all three domains of dystrophin are essential for diagnosis. See Chapter 7 for a complete discussion of dystrophinopathies.

Congenital Muscular Dystrophies

The CMDs are characterized by hypotonia at birth or shortly thereafter, the early formation of multiple joint contractures, and diffuse muscle weakness and atrophy.[37]

Historically, CMDs were classified by the absence or presence of *merosin* (laminin α2) in muscle. Merosin, located in the extracellular matrix, is the linking protein for the dystroglycan complex (see Fig. 7.2). CMDs have since been reclassified according to the genetic defect.

LAMA2 Muscular Dystrophy

The spectrum of *LAMA2* muscular dystrophies includes CMD type 1A (MDC1A) and late-onset *LAMA2* muscular dystrophy.[38]

Clinical features. MDC1A presents from birth through age 6 months, and it is characterized by severe hypotonia, delayed motor milestones, joint contractures, and feeding difficulties. Neck weakness, scoliosis, and myopathic facies are present; macroglossia results in tongue protrusion. Most infants have some level of respiratory insufficiency and may require ventilatory support. Cognition is typically normal. Affected children may sit independently, but rarely achieve independent ambulation. Seizures and progressive sensorimotor neuropathy are less common but may occur. Cardiomyopathy is rare.

Diagnosis. Serum CK is several times higher than normal during the first 2 years of life. Brain MRI demonstrates white matter abnormalities, and migrational defects such as lissencephaly and polymicrogyria are present in almost all affected individuals. Extensive migrational defects are more likely to cause refractory symptomatic epilepsy. Muscle biopsy demonstrates deficiency of laminin α2. Molecular genetic testing reveals biallelic pathogenic variants in the *LAMA2* gene.

Management. Treatment is supportive. Respiratory, dietary, and orthopedic surveillance are required. Epilepsy may be refractory.

Ullrich Congenital Muscular Dystrophy (Collagen Type VI–Related Dystrophy)

Ullrich congenital muscular dystrophy (UCMD) is the most severe form of the collagen VI–related dystrophies (COLD6-RDs).

Clinical features. UCMD causes severe hypotonia and weakness present from birth with proximal joint contractures and noticeable laxity of the distal joints. Respiratory insufficiency is universally present and affected children typically require noninvasive nocturnal ventilatory support by their second decade. Some children ambulate independently, but this milestone is lost by age 10. Intelligence is normal.[39]

Diagnosis. Serum CK is normal or mildly elevated. Muscle MRI demonstrates characteristic abnormalities, particularly in the vastus lateralis and rectus femoris. Molecular genetic testing demonstrates biallelic pathogenic variants in the *COL6A1*, *COL6A2*, or *COL6A3* genes.

Management. Patients usually require nocturnal ventilatory support such as BiPAP by the age of 10 or 11.

Fukuyama Congenital Muscular Dystrophy

Fukuyama muscular dystrophy is characterized by weakness, hypotonia, and migrational CNS defects. It is one of the dystroglycanopathies causing CMD. Dystroglycanopathy is a general term for disorders in which normal glycosylation of the dystroglycan molecule is impaired.

Clinical features. Affected infants are born with hypotonia, symmetric muscle weakness, and contractures of the hips, knees, and interphalangeal joints. Brain MRI shows extensive malformations, including cobblestone lissencephaly, cerebellar polymicrogyria and cerebellar cysts, dilation of the lateral ventricles and white matter abnormalities. Epilepsy is common and may be difficult to control. All affected individuals have

intellectual disability, usually with retained social skills; autism is not present. The early course is static, but rapid diffuse muscle atrophy begins in mid-childhood, followed by progressive joint contractures. Cardiac involvement progresses slowly and is milder than that seen in Duchenne muscular dystrophy.[40]

Diagnosis. As with the other CMDs, inheritance is autosomal recessive. CK in young children is 10–60× above normal. Molecular genetic testing reveals biallelic pathogenic variants in the *FKTN* gene.

Management. Physical therapy may delay contractures to some extent. All patients require cardiac, respiratory, and dietary surveillance. Epilepsy is treated with anticonvulsants but is often refractory.

Other Dystroglycanopathies

Multiple genes cause the various subtypes of the dystroglycanopathies, three of which are associated with CMD. The first is Fukuyama muscular dystrophy, discussed earlier. The other two types are Walker-Warburg syndrome and muscle-eye-brain disease. As noted earlier, extensive cerebral dysgenesis is characteristic; thus, these disorders can also be classified as *tubulinopathies* (disorders involving tubulin, which is critical for proper cortical development). The serum concentration of CK is generally elevated, and the EMG indicates a myopathy. Muscle biopsy specimens show excessive proliferation of adipose tissue and collagen out of proportion to the degree of fiber degeneration. Molecular genetic testing confirms the diagnosis. Treatment for all types is supportive.

Walker-Warburg syndrome. At least a dozen genes have been implicated in the development of Walker-Warburg syndrome. A subset of patients have pathogenic variants in the *FKTN* gene, similar to Fukuyama muscular dystrophy. Brain MRI shows cobblestone lissencephaly, hydrocephalus, and cerebellar dysplasia. Some infants are born with encephalocele. Multiple eye anomalies are present such as microphthalmos, chorioretinal dysplasia, cataracts, and abnormalities of the optic nerve. Hypotonia and muscle weakness are present.

Muscle-eye-brain disease. Pathogenic variants in *POMT1, POMT2, POMGNT1*, and others cause muscle-eye-brain disease. Infants are hypotonic and weak. Eye anomalies include glaucoma, cataracts, severe myopia, buphthalmos, and megalocornea. Erratic, uncontrollable eye movements may occur. Cerebral malformations may include brainstem hypoplasia, hydrocephalus, and lissencephaly. Seizures occur in some patients.

Congenital Myotonic Dystrophy

Myotonic dystrophy is a multisystem disorder transmitted by autosomal dominant inheritance.[41] Symptoms usually begin in the second decade (see Chapter 7). An unstable DNA triplet in the *DMPK* gene (chromosome 19q13.2-13.3) causes the disease. Repeats may increase 50 to several thousand times in successive generations. The number of repeats correlates with the severity of disease, but repeat size alone does not predict phenotype. Repeat size changes from mother to child are greater than from father to child, and for this reason, the mother is usually the affected parent when a child has CMD. A mother with repeats of 100 units has a 90% chance that her child will have repeats of 400 units or more.

The main features during pregnancy are reduced fetal movement and polyhydramnios. Fifty percent of babies are born prematurely. Inadequate uterine contraction may prolong labor and vacuum or forceps assistance is common. Severely affected newborns have inadequate diaphragmatic and intercostal muscle function and are incapable of spontaneous respiration. In the absence of prompt intubation and mechanical ventilation, many will die immediately after birth.

Prominent clinical features in the newborn include facial diplegia, in which the mouth is oddly shaped so that the upper lip forms an inverted V (Fig. 6.7); generalized muscular hypotonia; joint deformities ranging from bilateral clubfoot to generalized arthrogryposis; and gastrointestinal dysfunction, including choking, regurgitation, aspiration, swallowing difficulties, and gastroparesis. Limb weakness in the newborn is more often proximal than distal. Tendon reflexes are usually absent in weak muscles. Percussion does not elicit myotonia in newborns, nor is EMG a reliable test.

Mortality in the first year of life is estimated at 30%, frequently due to cardiomyopathy. Survivors usually gain strength and become ambulatory; however, a progressive myopathy similar to the late-onset form occurs eventually. Severe cognitive impairment is the rule, and may result from a combination of early respiratory failure and a direct effect of the mutation on the brain.

Diagnosis. Suspicion of the diagnosis of CMD in the newborn requires examination of the mother. She is likely to have many clinical features of the disease and

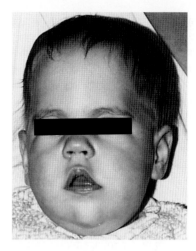

Fig. 6.7 Infantile Myotonic Dystrophy. The mouth has an inverted V position. (Reprinted with permission from Amato AA, Brook MH. Disorders of skeletal muscle. In: Bradley WG, Daroff RB, Fenichel GM, Jankovic J, eds. *Neurology in Clinical Practice.* 5th ed. Elsevier; 2008.)

show myotonia on EMG. Showing DNA amplification on chromosome 19 in both mother and child confirms the diagnosis. Carrier testing is available for at-risk, nonsymptomatic family members.

Management. The immediate treatment is intubation and mechanical ventilation. Joint contractures respond to physical therapy and casting. Metoclopramide alleviates gastroparesis.

Metabolic Myopathies
Acid Maltase Deficiency (Pompe Disease, Glycogen Storage Disease Type II)

Acid maltase is a lysosomal enzyme, present in all tissues, that hydrolyzes maltose and other branches of glycogen to yield glucose.[42] It has no function in maintaining blood glucose concentrations. Two distinct clinical forms are recognized: infantile and late-onset (see Chapter 7). Transmission of all forms is by autosomal recessive inheritance. Biallelic pathogenic variants of the *GAA* gene cause disease.

Clinical features. The infantile form may begin immediately after birth but usually appears during the second month. Profound generalized hypotonia and congestive heart failure are the initial symptoms. Muscle atrophy is typically not present. Hypotonia is the result of glycogen storage in the brain, spinal cord, and skeletal muscles, causing mixed signs of cerebral and motor unit dysfunction, decreased awareness, and depressed tendon reflexes. The mixed signs may be confusing, but the presence of cardiomegaly is almost diagnostic. The electrocardiogram shows abnormalities, including short PR intervals and high QRS complexes on all leads. Without enzyme replacement therapy, most patients die of cardiac failure by the age of 1.

Characteristics of a second, milder subtype of the infantile form are less severe cardiomyopathy, absence of left ventricular outflow obstruction, and less than 5% of residual acid maltase activity. Such patients can survive without enzyme replacement therapy but require long-term invasive ventilation.

Diagnosis. Measurement of acid α-glucosidase enzyme activity is diagnostic; confirm the diagnosis with molecular genetic testing. Muscle biopsy reveals muscle fibers with large vacuoles packed with glycogen. Acid maltase activity is deficient in fibroblasts and other tissues.

Management. Individualized care of cardiomyopathy is required. Begin enzyme replacement therapy with Lumizyme (alglucosidase alfa) as soon as possible. Most infants treated before the age of 6 months and before requiring ventilatory assistance showed improved survival, ventilator-independent survival, acquisition of motor skills, and reduced cardiac mass compared to untreated controls. Improvements of skeletal muscle functions also occurred.

REFERENCES

1. Prasad AN, Prasad C. Genetic evaluation of the floppy infant. *Seminars in Fetal & Neonatal Medicine.* 2011;16: 99-108.
2. Driscoll DJ, Miller JL, Schwartz S, et al. Prader Willi syndrome. In: Adam MP, Ardinger HH, Pagon RA, et al., eds. *GeneReviews.* University of Washington; 1993–2019. https://www.ncbi.nlm.nih.gov/books/NBK1330.
3. Miller SP, Riley P, Shevell MI. The neonatal presentation of Prader-Willi syndrome revisited. *Journal of Pediatrics.* 1999;134:226-228.
4. Bar-Aluma BE. Familial dysautonomia. In: Adam MP, Mirzaa GM, Pagon RA, et al., eds. *GeneReviews®.* University of Washington; 1993–2023. https://www.ncbi.nlm.nih.gov/books/NBK1180/. Updated November 4, 2021.
5. Lewis RA, Nussbaum RL, Brewer ED. Lowe syndrome. 2001 Jul 24 [Updated 2019 Apr 18]. In: Adam MP, Mirzaa GM, Pagon RA, et al., eds. *GeneReviews®.* University of Washington; 1993–2023. https://www.ncbi.nlm.nih.gov/books/NBK1480/.
6. Steinberg SJ, Raymond GV, Braverman NE, et al. Zellweger spectrum disorder. 2003 Dec 12 [Updated 2020 Oct 29]. In: Adam MP, Mirzaa GM, Pagon RA, et al., eds. *GeneReviews®.* University of Washington; 1993–2023. https://www.ncbi.nlm.nih.gov/books/NBK1448/.
7. Wang D, De Vivo D. Pyruvate carboxylase deficiency. 2009 Jun 2 [Updated 2018 Mar 1]. In: Adam MP, Mirzaa GM, Pagon RA, et al., eds. *GeneReviews®.* University of Washington; 1993–2023. https://www.ncbi.nlm.nih.gov/sites/books/NBK6852/.
8. Prior TW, Leach ME, Finanger E. Spinal muscular atrophy. 2000 Feb 24 [Updated 2020 Dec 3]. In: Adam MP, Mirzaa GM, Pagon RA, et al., eds. *GeneReviews®.* University of Washington; 1993–2023. https://www.ncbi.nlm.nih.gov/books/NBK1352/.
9. Finkel RS. Primary efficacy and safety results from the Phase 3 ENDEAR study of nusinersen in infants diagnosed with spinal muscular atrophy (SMA). *Paper presented at: 43rd Annual Congress of the British Paediatric Neurology Association;* January 11-13, 2017; Cambridge, UK.
10. Dhillon S. Risdiplam: first approval. *Drugs.* 2020;80(17): 1853-1858. https://doi.org/10.1007/s40265-020-01410-z. PMID: 33044711.
11. Day JW, Finkel RS, Chiriboga CA, et al. Onasemnogene abeparvovec gene therapy for symptomatic infantile-onset spinal muscular atrophy in patients with two copies of SMN2 (STR1VE): an open-label, single-arm, multicentre, phase 3 trial. *Lancet Neurology.* 2021;20(4):284-293. https://doi.org/10.1016/S1474-4422(21)00001-6. Epub 2021 Mar 17. PMID: 33743238.
12. Grohmann K, Varon R, Stolz P, et al. Infantile spinal muscular atrophy with respiratory distress type 1 (SMARD). *Annals of Neurology.* 2003;54: 719-724.
13. Eckart M, Guenther U-P, Idkowiak J, et al. The natural course of infantile spinal muscular atrophy with respiratory distress type I (SMARD-1). *Pediatrics.* 2012;129(1).
14. Hageman G, Ramaekers VT, Hilhorst BG, Rozeboom AR. Congenital cervical spinal muscular atrophy: a non-familial, non-progressive condition of the upper limbs. *Journal of Neurology, Neurosurgery, and Psychiatry.* 1993;56(4):365-368.
15. Rubio-Gozalbo MD, Smeitink JAM, Ruitenbeek W, et al. Spinal muscular atrophy-like picture, cardiomyopathy, and cytochrome-c-oxidase deficiency. *Neurology.* 1999; 52:383-386.

16. Warner LE, Mancians P, Butler IJ, et al. Mutations in the early growth response 2 (EGR2) gene are associated with hereditary myelinopathies. *Nature Genetics.* 1998;18:382-384.

17. Kochanski A, Drac H, Kabzinska D, et al. A novel MPZ gene mutation in congenital neuropathy with hypomyelination. *Neurology.* 2004;8:2122-2123.

18. Lesmana H, Vawter Lee M, Hosseini SA, et al. CNTNAP1-related congenital hypomyelinating neuropathy. *Pediatric Neurology.* 2019;93:43-49. https://doi.org/10.1016/j.pediatrneurol.2018.12.014. Epub 2018 Dec 28. PMID: 30686628.

19. Cherington M. Clinical spectrum of botulism. *Muscle & Nerve.* 1998;21:701-710.

20. Arnon SS, Shechter R, Maslanka SE, et al. Human botulism immune globulin for the treatment of infant botulism. *The New England Journal of Medicine.* 2006;354:462-471.

21. Underwood K, Rubin S, Deakers T, et al. Infant botulism: a 30-year experience spanning the introduction of botulism immune globulin intravenous in the intensive care unit at Children's Hospital Los Angeles. *Pediatrics.* 2007;120:e1380-e1385.

22. Abicht A, Muller J, Lochmuller H. Congenital myasthenic syndromes. In: Adam MP, Ardinger HH, Pagon RA, et al., eds. *GeneReviews.* University of Washington; 1993–2019. https://www.ncbi.nlm.nih.gov/books/NBK1168.

23. Mullaney P, Vajsar J, Smith R, et al. The natural history and ophthalmic involvement in childhood myasthenia gravis at The Hospital for Sick Children. *Ophthalmology.* 2000;107:504-510.

24. Hoff JM, Daltveit AK, Gilhus NE. Myasthenia gravis. Consequences for pregnancy, delivery, and the newborn. *Neurology.* 2003;61:1362-1366.

25. Sewry CA, Laitila JM, Wallgren-Pettersson C. Nemaline myopathies: a current view. *Journal of Muscle Research and Cell Motility.* 2019;40(2):111-126. https://doi.org/10.1007/s10974-019-09519-9. Epub 2019 Jun 21. PMID: 31228046; PMCID: PMC6726674.

26. Malicdan MCV, Nishino I. Central core disease. In: Adam MP, Ardinger HH, Pagon RA, et al., eds. *GeneReviews.* University of Washington; 1993–2019. https://www.ncbi.nlm.nih.gov/books/NBK1391.

27. Jungbluth H. Central core disease. *Orphanet Journal of Rare Diseases.* 2007;2:25.

28. Wu S, Ibarra CA, Malicdan MCV, et al. Central core disease is due to RYR1 mutations in more than 90% of patients. *Brain.* 2006;129:1470-1480.

29. Messina S, Hartley L, Main M, et al. Pilot trial of salbutamol in central core and multi-minicore diseases. *Neuropediatrics.* 2004;35(5):262-266.

30. Ferreiro A, Estounet B, Chateau D, et al. Multi-minicore disease – searching for boundaries: phenotype analysis of 38 cases. *Annals of Neurology.* 2000;48:745-757.

31. Beggs AH, Agrawal PB. Multiminicore disease. *GeneReviews.* University of Washington; 2013. http://www.geneclinics.org.

32. Ferreiro A, Monnier N, Romero NB, et al. A recessive form of central core disease, transiently presenting as multi-minicore disease, is associated with a homozygous recessive mutation in the ryanodine receptor type 1 gene. *Annals of Neurology.* 2002;51:750-759.

33. Ferreiro A, Quijano-Roy S, Pichereau C, et al. Mutations of the selenoprotein N gene, which is implicated in rigid spine muscular dystrophy, cause the classical phenotype of multiminicore disease: reassessing the nosology of early-onset myopathies. *American Journal of Human Genetics.* 2002;71:739-749.

34. Clarke NF, Smith RLL, Bahlo M, et al. A novel X-linked form of congenital fiber-type disproportion. *Annals of Neurology.* 2005;58:767-772.

35. Dowling JJ, Lawlor MW, Das S. X-linked myotubular myopathy. In: Adam MP, Ardinger HH, Pagon RA, et al., eds. *GeneReviews.* University of Washington; 1993–2019. https://www.ncbi.nlm.nih.gov/books/NBK1432.

36. Bitoun M, Maugenre S, Jeannet PY, et al. Mutations in dynamin 2 cause dominant centronuclear myopathy. *Nature Genetics.* 2005;37:1207-1209.

37. Sparks S, Quijano-Roy S, Harper A, et al. Congenital muscular dystrophy overview. In: Adam MP, Ardinger HH, Pagon RA, et al., eds. *GeneReviews.* University of Washington; 1993–2019. https://www.ncbi.nlm.nih.gov/books/NBK1291.

38. Oliveira J, Parente Freixo J, Santos M, et al. LAMA2 muscular dystrophy 2012 Jun 7 [Updated 2020 Sep 17]. In: Adam MP, Mirzaa GM, Pagon RA, et al., eds. *GeneReviews®.* University of Washington; 1993–2023. https://www.ncbi.nlm.nih.gov/books/NBK97333/.

39. Foley AR, Mohassel P, Donkervoort S, et al. Collagen VI-related dystrophies 2004 Jun 25 [Updated 2021 Mar 11]. In: Adam MP, Mirzaa GM, Pagon RA, et al., eds. *GeneReviews®.* University of Washington; 1993–2023. https://www.ncbi.nlm.nih.gov/books/NBK1503/.

40. Saito K. Fukuyama congenital muscular dystrophy. 2006 Jan 26 [Updated 2019 Jul 3]. In: Adam MP, Mirzaa GM, Pagon RA, et al., eds. *GeneReviews®.* University of Washington, Seattle; 1993–2023. https://www.ncbi.nlm.nih.gov/books/NBK1206/.

41. Bird TD. Myotonic dystrophy type I. In: Adam MP, Ardinger HH, Pagon RA, et al., eds. *GeneReviews*. University of Washington; 1993–2019. https://www.ncbi.nlm.nih.gov/books/NBK1165.

42. Leslie N, Bailey L. Pompe disease. In: Adam MP, Ardinger HH, Pagon RA, et al., eds. *GeneReviews*. University of Washington; 1993–2019. https://www.ncbi.nlm.nih.gov/books/NBK1261.

7

Flaccid Limb Weakness in Childhood

OUTLINE

Clinical Features of Neuromuscular Disease, 208
   The Initial Complaint, 208
   Physical Findings, 209
Progressive Proximal Weakness, 210
   Spinal Muscular Atrophies, 211
   GM$_2$ Gangliosidosis, 212
   Myasthenic Syndromes, 212
   Muscular Dystrophies, 213
   Inflammatory Myopathies, 217
   Metabolic Myopathies, 219
   Endocrine Myopathies, 220
Progressive Distal Weakness, 220
   Diagnosis in Neuropathy and Neuronopathy, 220

   Neuronopathy, 222
   Neuropathy, 222
   Myopathies, 225
Acute Generalized Weakness, 227
   Infectious Disease, 227
   Neuromuscular Blockade, 230
Periodic Paralyses, 231
   Familial Hypokalemic Periodic Paralysis, 231
   Familial Hyperkalemic Periodic Paralysis
      Type 1, 232
   Familial Normokalemic Periodic Paralysis, 232
   Andersen-Tawil Syndrome, 232
References, 233

The majority of children with flaccid limb weakness have a motor unit disorder. Flaccid leg weakness may be the initial feature of disturbances in the lumbosacral region, but other symptoms of spinal cord dysfunction are usually present. Consult Box 12.1 when considering the differential diagnosis of flaccid leg weakness without arm impairment. Cerebral disorders may cause flaccid weakness, but dementia (see Chapter 5) or seizures (see Chapter 1) are usually concomitant features.

CLINICAL FEATURES OF NEUROMUSCULAR DISEASE

Weakness is decreased strength, as measured by the force of a maximal contraction. Fatigue is an inability to maintain a less-than-maximal contraction, as measured by exercise tolerance. Weak muscles are always more easily fatigued than normal muscles, but fatigue may occur in the absence of weakness. Chapter 8 discusses conditions in which strength is normal at rest but muscles fatigue or cramp on exercise.

The Initial Complaint

Limb weakness in children is usually noted first in the legs and then in the arms (Box 7.1). The reason for this is that the legs are required to bear weight and are subject to continuous testing while standing or walking. Delayed development of motor skills is often an initial or prominent feature in the history of children with neuromuscular disorders. Marginal motor delay in children with otherwise normal development rarely raises concern and is often considered part of the spectrum of normal development. Prompts for neurological consultation in older children with neuromuscular disorders are failure to keep up with peers, frequent falls, or easy fatigability.

An abnormal gait can be the initial symptom of either proximal or distal leg weakness. With proximal weakness, the pelvis fails to stabilize and waddles from side to side as the child walks. Running is especially difficult and accentuates the hip waddle. Descending stairs is particularly difficult in children with quadriceps weakness; the knee cannot lock and stiffen. Difficulty with

- Abnormal gait
  - Steppage
  - Toe walking
  - Waddling
- Easy fatigability
- Frequent falls
- Slow motor development
- Specific disability
- Arm elevation
  - Climbing stairs
  - Hand grip
  - Rising from floor

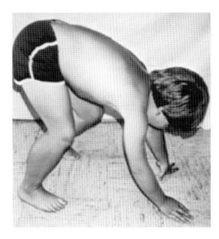

Fig. 7.1 Gower Sign. The child rises from the floor by pushing off with the hands to overcome proximal pelvic weakness.

ascending stairs suggests hip extensor weakness. Rising from the floor or a deep chair is difficult, and the hands help to push off.

Stumbling is an early complaint when there is distal leg weakness, especially weakness of the evertors and dorsiflexors of the foot. Falling is first noted when the child walks on uneven surfaces. The child is thought to be clumsy, but after a while parents realize that the child is "tripping on nothing at all." Repeated ankle spraining occurs because of lateral instability. Children with foot drop tend to lift their knees high in the air so that the foot will clear the ground. The weak foot then comes down with a slapping motion (*steppage gait*).

Toe walking is commonplace in Duchenne muscular dystrophy (DMD) because the pelvis thrusts forward to shift the center of gravity and the gastrocnemius muscle is stronger than the peroneal muscles. Toe walking occurs also in upper motor neuron disorders that cause spasticity and in children who have tight heel cords but no identifiable neurological disease. Toe walking with progressive foot deformity suggests hereditary spastic paraplegia. Compulsive tiptoe walking should be suspected in children with a normal examination and obsessive-compulsive traits. Muscular dystrophy is usually associated with hyporeflexia and spasticity with hyperreflexia. However, the ankle tendon reflex may be difficult to elicit when the tendon is tight for any reason.

Adolescents, but usually not children, with weakness complain of specific disabilities. A young person with proximal weakness may have difficulty keeping their arms elevated to brush their hair or rotating the shoulder to get into and out of garments. Weakness of hand muscles often comes to attention because of difficulty

with handwriting. Adolescents may notice difficulty in unscrewing jar tops or working with tools. Teachers report to parents when children are slower than classmates in climbing stairs, getting up from the floor, and skipping and jumping. Parents may report a specific complaint to the physician, but more often they define the problem as inability to keep up with peers.

A child whose limbs are weak also may have weakness in the muscles of the head and neck. Specific questions should be asked about double vision, drooping eyelids, difficulty chewing and swallowing, change of facial expression and strength (whistling, sucking, chewing, blowing), and the clarity and tone of speech. Weakness of neck muscles is frequently noticed when the child is a passenger in a vehicle that suddenly accelerates or decelerates, as it is normal in the first couple of months of life. The neck muscles are unable to stabilize the head, which snaps backward or forward.

Physical Findings

The examination begins by watching the child sit, stand, and walk. A normal child sitting cross-legged on the floor can rise to a standing position in a single movement without using the hands. This remarkable feat is lost sometime after the age of 15 years in most children, in which case rising from a low stool is a better test of proximal leg strength. The child with weak pelvic muscles uses the hands for assistance (Fig. 7.1), and with progressive weakness the hands are used to climb up the legs (*Gower sign*).

BOX 7.2   Signs of Neuromuscular Disease

Observation
- Atrophy and hypertrophy
- Fasciculations
- Functional ability

Palpation
- Muscle texture
- Tenderness

Examination
- Joint contractures
- Myotonia
- Strength
- Tendon reflexes

BOX 7.3   Progressive Proximal Weakness

- Spinal cord disorders (see Chapter 12)
- Juvenile spinal muscular atrophies
  - Autosomal dominant
  - Autosomal recessive
- GM_2 gangliosidosis (hexosaminidase A deficiency)
- Myasthenic syndromes
  - Acquired limb-girdle myasthenia
  - Slow-channel syndrome
- Muscular dystrophies
  - Bethlem myopathy
  - Dystrophinopathies
  - Facioscapulohumeral syndrome
  - Severe childhood autosomal recessive muscular dystrophy
- Inflammatory myopathies
  - Dermatomyositis[a]
  - Polymyositis[a]
- Metabolic myopathies
  - Acid maltase deficiency[a]
  - Carnitine deficiency[a]
  - Debrancher enzyme deficiency[a] (see Chapter 8)
  - Lipid storage myopathies
  - Mitochondrial myopathies (see Chapter 8)
  - Myophosphorylase deficiency (see Chapter 8)
- Endocrine myopathies
  - Adrenal cortex[a]
  - Parathyroid[a]
  - Thyroid[a]

[a]The most common conditions and the ones with disease modifying treatments.

After normal gait is observed, the child is asked to walk first on the toes and then on the heels (Box 7.2). Inability to walk on the toes indicates gastrocnemius muscle weakness and inability to walk on the heels indicates weakness of the anterior compartment muscles. Push-ups are a quick test of strength in almost all arm muscles. Most normal children can do at least one push-up. Then ask the child to touch the tip of the shoulder blade with the ipsilateral thumb. This is an impossible task when the rhomboids are weak.

Finally, face and eye movements are tested. The best test of facial strength is to blow out the cheeks and hold air against compression. Normally the lips are smooth. Wrinkling of the perioral tissues and failure to hold air indicate facial weakness. During this period of observation and again during muscle strength testing, the physician should look for atrophy or hypertrophy. Muscle wasting in the shoulder causes bony prominences to stand out even further. Wasting of hand muscles flattens the thenar and hypothenar eminences. Wasting of the quadriceps muscles causes a tapering appearance of the thigh that exaggerates when the patient tenses the thigh by straightening the knee. Atrophy of the anterior tibial and peroneal muscles gives the anterior border of the tibia a sharp appearance, and atrophy of the gastrocnemius muscle diminishes the normal contour of the calf.

Loss of tendon reflexes occurs early in denervation, especially when sensory nerves are involved, but parallels the degree of weakness in myopathy. Tendon reflexes are usually normal even during times of weakness in patients with myasthenia gravis and may be normal between episodes of recurrent weakness in those with metabolic myopathies. The description of myotonia, a disturbance in muscle relaxation following contraction, is in the section on "Myotonic Dystrophy."

PROGRESSIVE PROXIMAL WEAKNESS

Progressive proximal weakness in childhood is most often due to myopathy, usually a muscular dystrophy (Box 7.3). Juvenile spinal muscular atrophy (SMA) and the limb-girdle muscular dystrophies (LGMDs) cause proximal greater than distal weakness with onset in late childhood or adolescence. Electromyography (EMG) and muscle biopsy readily distinguish it from myopathic disorders. Limb-girdle myasthenia is rare but is an important consideration because specific treatment is available (Table 7.1).

TABLE 7.1 Distinguishing Features in Proximal Weakness

	Neuronopathy	Myopathy	Myasthenia
Tendon reflexes	Absent	Depressed or absent	Normal
Electromyography	Fasciculations; denervation potentials; high-amplitude polyphasic motor potentials	Brief, small-amplitude polyphasic motor units	Normal
Nerve conduction	Normal or mildly slow	Normal	Abnormal repetitive stimulation
Creatine kinase concentration	Normal or mildly elevated	Elevated	Normal
Muscle biopsy	Group atrophy; group typing	Fiber necrosis; fatty replacement; excessive collagen	Normal

Spinal Muscular Atrophies

SMA is the most common inherited disorder of the spinal cord resulting in hypotonia and weakness in infants with an incidence of approximately 1 in 6000 to 1 in 11,000 live births in the United States. It is an autosomal recessive disorder with a molecular defect leading to increased apoptosis in anterior horn cells and in motor nuclei of lower cranial nerves. In approximately 95% of cases the genetic defect is homozygous deletion of the survival motor neuron 1 gene (*SMN1*), which is located on the telomeric region of chromosome 5q13.[1,2] A virtually identical centromeric gene on 5q13, referred to as *SMN2*, encodes a similar but less active product.[3] The protein product of *SMN2* partially appears to rescue the SMA phenotype such that a larger *SMN2* copy number generally results in a milder disease. Although age at onset distinguishes three subtypes of SMA, the subtypes are actually a continuum. The infantile type (SMA I) always begins before 6 months of age (see Chapter 6), the intermediate type (SMA II) begins between 6 and 18 months, and the juvenile type (SMA III) begins after 18 months.

Clinical features. In intermediate SMA (SMA II) fetal movements are normal and the child is normal at birth. The initial feature of SMA II is delayed motor development. As a rule, affected children achieve sitting balance but are unable to stand unsupported and are wheelchair confined. A fine hand tremor is often present. Contractures of the hips and knees and scoliosis eventually develop. Some of those affected die in childhood because of respiratory failure, but most survive into adult life. Muscle weakness is a constant feature of the disease but tends to be diffuse rather than proximal.

In contrast, the initial feature of juvenile SMA (SMA III) is gait instability caused by proximal weakness. Similar to SMA II, a fine-action tremor is common. Disease progression is very slow, sometimes in a stepwise fashion, and often seems arrested. Weakness may progress either to the distal muscles of the legs or to the proximal muscles of the arms. The hands are the last parts affected. Facial muscles may be weak, but extraocular motility is always normal. Tendon reflexes are hypoactive or absent. The sensory examination is normal. Cases with ophthalmoplegia are probably genetically distinct.

Some children have more profound weakness in the arms than in the legs and are likely to have facial weakness as well. Within a family, some children may have predominant leg weakness, whereas their siblings may have predominant arm weakness.

Diagnosis. The discovery of biallelic pathogenic variants of the *SMN1* gene establishes the diagnosis. EMG and muscle biopsy are unnecessary if genetic analysis shows the appropriate mutation. The findings on both tests are similar to those described for SMA I in Chapter 6. The serum concentration of creatine kinase (CK) may be two to four times the upper limit of normal, and the increase in concentration correlates directly with the duration of illness.

Management. The treatment for intermediate and juvenile SMAs is focused on modified RNA splicing of the *SMN2* gene, encouraging increased production of the full-length SMA protein. Nusinersen (Spinraza) is delivered intrathecally on a scheduled basis. Risdiplan (Evrysdi) is a daily oral medication given at a dose of 0.2 mg/kg/day. Lifetime treatment is required.

Zolgensma, a one-time gene therapy treatment, is only approved for those patients who are 2 years of age or younger and therefore is not useful for most of the later-onset SMAs.

GM$_2$ Gangliosidosis

The typical clinical expression of hexosaminidase A deficiency is *Tay-Sachs disease* (see Chapter 5). Several phenotypic variants of the enzyme deficiency exist, with onset throughout childhood and adult life. Transmission of all variants is by autosomal recessive inheritance. The initial features of the juvenile-onset type mimic those of juvenile SMA.[4]

Clinical features. Weakness, wasting, and cramps of the proximal leg muscles begin after infancy and frequently not until adolescence. Distal leg weakness, proximal and distal arm weakness, and tremor follow. Symptoms of cerebral degeneration (personality change, intermittent psychosis, and dementia) become evident after motor neuron dysfunction is established.

Examination shows a mixture of upper and lower motor neuron signs. The macula is usually normal and the cranial nerves are intact, with the exception of atrophy and fasciculations in the tongue. Fasciculations also may be present in the limbs. Tendon reflexes are absent or exaggerated, depending on the relative severity of upper and lower motor neuron dysfunction. Plantar responses are sometimes extensor and sometimes flexor. Tremor, but not dysmetria, is present in the outstretched arms, and sensation is intact.

Some children never develop cerebral symptoms and have only motor neuron disease; some adults have only dementia and psychosis. The course is variable and compatible with prolonged survival.

Diagnosis. The serum concentration of CK is normal or only mildly elevated. Motor and sensory nerve conduction velocities are normal, but needle EMG shows neuropathic motor units. Showing a severe deficiency or absence of hexosaminidase A activity in leukocytes or cultured fibroblasts establishes the diagnosis.

Management. No treatment is available. Heterozygote detection is possible because enzyme activity is partially deficient. Prenatal diagnosis is available. Gene therapy or enzyme replacement therapy research may eventually lead to a treatment to slow progression or cure Tay-Sachs.

Myasthenic Syndromes

Proximal weakness and sometimes wasting may occur in acquired immune-mediated myasthenia and in genetic myasthenic syndromes.

Limb-Girdle Myasthenia

Limb-girdle myasthenia makes up 10%–15% of congenital myasthenic syndromes. A pathogenic variant in the *DOK7* gene causes the disorder in most cases.

Clinical features. Onset is often in mid-childhood, with symptoms characterized by a waddling gait due to weakness of the pelvic musculature. Some patients have ptosis, but extraocular ophthalmoplegia is not seen. The vast majority of limb-girdle myasthenias are caused by pathogenic variants in the *DOK7* gene which adversely affect the AChR clustering pathway. Approximately 1%–2% have limb-girdle myasthenia with glycosylation deficiencies caused by mutations in *DPAG1*, *GFPT1*, or *GMPPB* genes. In these cases there is no ptosis or ophthalmoplegia, but intellectual disability and increased CK concentration may be present.[5] Tendon reflexes are usually present but may be hypoactive. The clinical features suggest limb-girdle dystrophy or polymyositis.

Diagnosis. Multigene panels, exome sequencing, or genomic sequencing provide the diagnosis. In children with glycosylation deficiency muscle biopsy sometimes demonstrates tubular aggregates.

Management. Limb-girdle myasthenia caused by *DOK7* mutations is unresponsive to acetylcholinesterase inhibitors and such drugs may actually worsen the symptoms. Ephedrine or beta-2-agonists such as albuterol are the preferred therapies. Limb-girdle myasthenia associated with *DPAG1*, *GFPT1*, or *GMPPB* responds to AChE inhibitors similarly to other forms of antibody-positive myasthenia (see Chapter 15).

Slow-Channel Congenital Myasthenic Syndrome

Slow-channel syndrome comprises 50% of the congenital myasthenic syndromes. It can be inherited in an autosomal dominant or autosomal recessive fashion and is caused by pathogenic variants in the *CHRNA1*, *CHRNB1*, *CHRND*, or *CHRNE* genes.[5]

Clinical features. No symptoms are present at birth. The phenotype is highly variable, with onset from childhood through adulthood with mild to severe impairment. Selective severe weakness in the neck, wrist, and finger extensors characterizes the disorder. Progressive respiratory insufficiency occurs, and assisted ventilation may be required in some patients.

Diagnosis. Weakness does not respond either to injection or oral administration of anticholinesterase medication. Molecular genetic testing either with a multigene panel or exome sequencing provides the diagnosis.

Management. Cholinesterase inhibitors, thymectomy, and immunosuppression are not effective. Quinidine sulfate improves strength and fluoxetine is equally beneficial in patients who do not tolerate quinidine.[6] Fluoxetine, which is known to have potential anticholinergic side effects, works by blocking mutant acetylcholine receptors and normalizing prolonged synaptic currents; most patients require high doses, but some have been reported to respond well to low-dose treatments. Albuterol has been reported to be beneficial in some patients.[7]

Muscular Dystrophies

No agreed-upon definition of muscular dystrophy exists. We prefer to use the term to embrace *all genetic myopathies caused by a defect in a structural protein of the muscle* (Fig. 7.2). Enzyme deficiencies, such as acid maltase deficiency, are not dystrophies but rather *metabolic myopathies*. For most dystrophies the abnormal gene and gene product are established.

X-linked muscular dystrophies include Duchenne and Becker muscular dystrophy (BMD) (*dystrophinopathies*). Not discussed is *Danon disease*, an X-linked cardiomyopathy and skeletal myopathy, with onset in late adolescence.[8]

The term *limb-girdle muscular dystrophy* (LGMD) encompasses several muscular dystrophies characterized by progressive proximal muscle weakness. While LGMDs are clinically similar to the dystrophinopathies, they occur in both sexes and are caused by mutations affecting the functioning of dysferlin, calpain, sarcoglycans, and other muscle cell membrane proteins that interact with dystrophin.

The more common forms of muscular dystrophy transmitted by autosomal dominant inheritance are facioscapulohumeral dystrophy (FSHD; see Chapter 17), the dominant form of Emery-Dreifuss dystrophy, and Bethlem myopathy. LGMD transmitted by autosomal recessive inheritance includes LGMDR1, LGMDR2, and the sarcoglycanopathies (discussed later in this chapter).

Autosomal recessive types may begin in childhood or adult life. These are distinguishable by the location of the abnormal gene and in some cases by the abnormal gene product (Table 7.2).

Bethlem Myopathy

Bethlem myopathy is the milder form of the collagen VI–related myopathies (the severe form, Ullrich congenital muscular dystrophy, was discussed in Chapter 6). It is a slowly progressive LGMD transmitted by autosomal dominant or autosomal recessive inheritance due to pathogenic variants in the *COL6A1*, *COL6A2*, or *COL6A3* genes.

Clinical features. The onset of contractures or weakness always occurs in the first 2 years. Diminished fetal movements and congenital hypotonia may be present. The usual initial features are congenital flexion

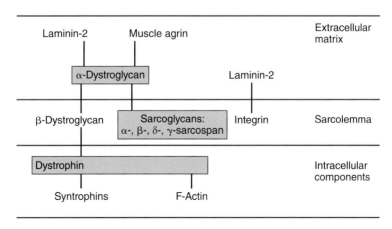

Fig. 7.2 The Structural Proteins of Muscle Fibers.

TABLE 7.2   Autosomal Recessive Limb-Girdle Muscular Dystrophies

LGMD Type	Location	Gene Product	Clinical Features
LGMDR1	15q	Calpain-3	Onset at 8–15 years, progression variable
LGMDR2	2p13-16	Dysferlin	Onset at adolescence, mild weakness; gene site is the same as for Miyoshi myopathy
LGMDR3	13q12	Sarcoglycan	Duchenne-like, severe childhood autosomal recessive muscular dystrophy (SCARMD1)
LGMDR4	17q21	A-Sarcoglycan (adhalin)	Duchenne-like, severe childhood autosomal recessive muscular dystrophy (SCARMD2)
LGMDR5	4q12	B-Sarcoglycan	Phenotype between Duchenne and Becker muscular dystrophies
LGMDR6	5q33-34	Sarcoglycan	Slowly progressive, growth retardation

LGMDs, Limb-girdle muscular dystrophies.

contractures of the elbows, ankles, and interphalangeal joints of the last four fingers, but sparing the spine. The contractures are at first mild and unrecognized by parents. Mild proximal weakness and delayed motor development are common. Both the contractures and the weakness progress slowly and produce disability in middle life but do not shorten the life span. Tendon reflexes are normal or depressed. Cardiomyopathy does not occur.

Diagnosis. Molecular genetic testing is available. The serum concentration of CK is normal or slightly elevated, EMG usually shows myopathy, and muscle biopsy shows a nonspecific myopathy.

Management. Physical therapy for contractures is the main treatment.

Dystrophinopathies: Duchenne and Becker Muscular Dystrophy

DMD and BMD are variable phenotypic expressions of pathogenic mutations of the *DMD* gene located at Xp21 (Box 7.4). The abnormal gene product in both DMD and BMD is a reduced muscle content of the structural protein dystrophin, hence the term *dystrophinopathy*. Dystrophinopathies are clinically similar to the LGMDs but comprise a separate class of disorders. Other phenotypes include *DMD*-associated dilated cardiomyopathy, asymptomatic increased serum CK levels, and exercise intolerance with cramping and myoglobinuria, which we will not discuss here. Males with hemizygous pathogenic mutations are affected; heterozygotic female carriers can experience a range of clinical symptoms.

BOX 7.4   Phenotypes Associated With the Xp21 Gene Site

- Becker muscular dystrophy
- Dilated cardiomyopathy without skeletal muscle weakness
- Duchenne muscular dystrophy
- Familial X-linked myalgia and cramps (see Chapter 8)
- McLeod syndrome (elevated serum creatine kinase concentration, acanthocytosis, and absence of Kell antigen)
- Intellectual disability and elevated serum creatine kinase
- Quadriceps myopathy

In DMD the dystrophin content is 0%–5% of normal, and in BMD the dystrophin content is 5%–20% of normal. DMD has a worldwide distribution with a mean incidence of 1 per 3500 male births. The traditional phenotypic difference between the two dystrophies is that BMD has a later age of onset (after age 5 years), unassisted ambulation after age 15 years, and survival into adult life. However, a spectrum of intermediate phenotypes exists depending on dystrophin content. Survival into the 30s and beyond is not uncommon for DMD.[9]

Clinical features. The initial feature in most boys with DMD is a gait disturbance; onset is always before age 5 years and is often before age 3 years. Toe walking and frequent falling are typical complaints. Often one obtains a retrospective history of delayed achievement of motor milestones. Early symptoms are insidious and likely dismissed by both parents and physicians. Only when proximal weakness causes difficulty in rising from the floor with an obvious waddling gait is medical attention sought. At this stage, mild proximal weakness is present in the pelvic muscles and the Gower sign is present (see Fig. 7.1). The calf muscles are often large (Fig. 7.3). The ankle tendon is tight, and the heels do not quite touch the floor. Tendon reflexes may still be present at the ankle and knee but are difficult to obtain.

The decline in motor strength is linear throughout childhood. Motor function usually appears static between the ages of 3 and 6 years because of cerebral maturation. Most children maintain their ability to walk and climb stairs until 8 years of age. Between ages 3 and 8, the child shows progressive contractures of the ankle tendons and the iliotibial bands, increased lordosis, a more pronounced waddling gait, and increased toe walking. Gait is more precarious, and the child falls more often. Tendon reflexes at the knees and ankles are lost, and proximal weakness develops in the arms. Considerable variability of expression occurs even within the DMD phenotype. On average, functional ability declines rapidly after 8 years of age because of increasing muscle weakness and contractures. By 9 years

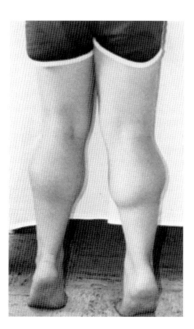

Fig. 7.3 Enlarged Calf Muscles in Duchenne Muscular Dystrophy. Enlarged calves also occur in other neuromuscular disorders.

of age, some children require a wheelchair, but most can remain ambulatory until age 12 and may continue to stand in braces until age 16.

The range of intelligence scores in boys with DMD shifts downward. While most affected boys function in the normal range, the percentage of those with learning disabilities and cognitive impairment is increased.

Scoliosis occurs in some boys and can exacerbate progressive respiratory insufficiency. Deterioration of vital capacity to less than 20% of normal leads to symptoms of nocturnal hypoventilation. The child awakens frequently and is afraid to sleep. The immediate cause of death is usually a combination of respiratory insufficiency and cardiomyopathy. In some patients with chronic hypoxia, intercurrent infection or aspiration causes respiratory arrest.

Diagnosis. Before 5 years of age, the serum concentration of CK is 10 times the upper limit of normal. The concentration then declines with age at an approximate rate of 20% per year. BMD tends to have lower concentrations of serum CK than DMD.

Mutation analysis is the standard for diagnosis, carrier detection, and fetal diagnosis. Intragenic deletions account for the majority of pathogenic mutations and single-gene testing (deletion/duplication analysis, followed by gene sequencing if needed) is the first-line diagnostic test. Multigene panels are also available.[10] Dystrophin analysis of muscle is useful to distinguish DMD from BMD. However, muscle biopsy is not essential when the molecular diagnosis is positive.

Management. Although DMD is not curable, it is treatable. Cardiology must be involved as soon as the diagnosis is made in order to monitor and treat cardiomyopathy. Prednisone 0.75 mg/kg/day or deflazacort 0.9 mg/kg/day increases strength and function. The mechanism of action is not clearly understood. Steroid therapy should be started as soon as motor skills start to decline, as evidence suggests that earlier treatment may delay loss of function. Scoliosis can be treated with bracing, but spinal fusion is usually required.

Certain mutations are amenable to dystrophin restoration therapies using antisense oligonucleotide treatments. These target dystrophin premessenger RNA to skip out-of-frame variants. Drisapersen, eteplirsen, golodirsen, and casimersen are examples of such treatments. Gene transfer and gene editing therapies are potential future treatment options.

Facioscapulohumeral Dystrophy

Although the classification of progressive facioscapulo-humeral (FSHD) weakness is as a muscular dystrophy, patients with genetic FSH weakness may have histological evidence of myopathy, neuropathy, and inflammation. FSHD is autosomal dominant and associated with a deletion within a repeat motif named *D4Z4* at chromosome 4q35.[11] Most cases are inherited but a minority result from de novo mutations. The size of the deletion correlates with the severity of disease. Considerable interfamily and intrafamily heterogeneity exists. A negative family history may result because affected family members are unaware that they have a problem.

Clinical features. Weakness usually begins in the second decade. Initial involvement is often in the shoulder girdle (Fig. 7.4), with subsequent spread to the humeral muscles. The deltoid is never affected. Facial weakness is present but often overlooked until late in the course. The progression of weakness is insidious and delays the diagnosis. Late in the course, leg muscles may be involved. Anterior tibial weakness is most prominent, but proximal weakness may occur as well.

The course of FSHD is variable. Many patients do not become disabled, and their life expectancy is normal. About 20% of patients eventually become wheelchair dependent. In the infantile form progression is usually rapid and disability is always severe[12] (see Chapter 17). Deafness and retinal vascular abnormalities are part of the phenotype. The most severe manifestations are retinal telangiectasia, exudation, and detachment (*Coats-like disease*).

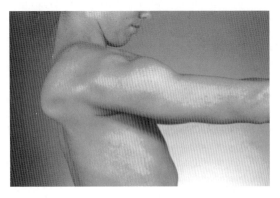

Fig. 7.4 Asymmetrical Scapular Winging in Facioscapulohumeral Dystrophy. (Reproduced with permission from Preston DC, Shapiro BA, Robinson JA. Proximal, distal, and generalized weakness. In: Bradley WG, Daroff R, Fenichel G, Jankovic J, eds. *Neurology in Clinical Practice.* 5th ed. Elsevier; 2008.)

Diagnosis. Molecular genetic testing is the standard for diagnosis. The serum concentration of CK can be normal or increased to five times normal. The EMG may show denervation potentials, myopathic motor units, or both. Histological changes are minimal in many limb muscles and are never diagnostic. Occasional fibers are myopathic, some appear denervated, and inflammatory cells may be present.

Management. No treatment for the weakness is available. Low-intensity aerobic exercise, management of chronic pain by physical therapy and medications, ventilatory support for hypoventilation, lubricants or eyelid taping for incomplete eye closure to decrease conjunctival dryness and keratitis, and ankle/foot orthotics to prevent falls may be helpful. Retinal examination for Coats-like disease is required. Coagulation of retinal telangiectasia prevents blindness.

Limb-Girdle Muscular Dystrophies

There are multiple types of LGMDs, many of which do not become symptomatic until adulthood. We will discuss some of the childhood-onset forms, but this should not be considered an exhaustive discussion, as many uncommon subtypes exist and will not be covered in this brief review.

The classification system has been updated multiple times. Currently, LGMD is classified based on whether it is autosomal dominant (LGMDD) or autosomal recessive (LGMDR). Groups are further subdivided based on the order of discovery and the specific genetic mutation. Many gene products have been implicated, but the three most common are dysferlinopathies, sarcoglycanopathies, and calpainopathies.

Limb-Girdle Muscular Dystrophy R1

LGMDR1 begins in mid-childhood, but onset may be later in some cases. It is a *calpainopathy*, caused by pathogenic variants in the *CPAN3* gene.[13]

Clinical features. As with all LGMDs, weakness begins in the pelvic or shoulder girdle muscles. Affected children have a waddling gait and a tendency to walk on tiptoe. Scoliosis and scapular winging may occur. Intelligence is normal, and there are usually no cardiac manifestations.

Diagnosis. Molecular genetic testing reveals biallelic (or, less frequently, heterozygous pathogenic) variants in the *CAPN3* gene. Muscle biopsy shows absent or reduced calpain-3. As with all of the LGMDs, serum CK is elevated.

Management. Physical therapy, orthotics, release of tendon contractures, and good pulmonary toilet are essential. Avoid excessive exercise; use caution with volatile anesthetics.

Limb-Girdle Muscular Dystrophy R2

LGMDR2 is one of the milder phenotypes and typically begins in late childhood, adolescence, or early adulthood. It is caused by biallelic pathogenic variants in the dysferlin gene (*DYSF*).[14]

Clinical features. Average age at onset is the late teens or early 20s, with symptoms characterized by weakness and atrophy of the pelvic and shoulder girdle muscles or proximal lower extremity muscles. Patients may note a waddling gait and difficulty raising or maintaining their arms above their heads. The disease progresses slowly. Some adolescents present with scapuloperoneal manifestations, with weakness of the shoulder girdle muscles and distal leg musculature.

Diagnosis. LGMDR2 is one of the *dysferlinopathies*, caused by mutations of the *DYSF* gene. Single-gene testing is first line, but more specific gene-targeted duplication/deletion analysis or RNA analysis of *DYSF* in myogenic cells may be required. If the clinical picture is unclear, a less specific muscular dystrophy multigene panel may be more helpful. CK is massively elevated. Distal muscle involvement is often clinically asymptomatic but can be detected on muscle magnetic resonance imaging (MRI).

Management. No specific treatment exists. Management is supportive with the focus on activities of daily living and surveillance of respiratory and cardiac functioning.

Sarcoglycanopathies

A deficiency of any of the four subunits of the sarcoglycan complex of proteins associated with dystrophin causes a severe form of autosomal recessive LGMDR. These disorders were previously referred to as severe childhood autosomal recessive muscular dystrophy (SCARMD) (see Table 7.2).

Clinical features. The sarcoglycanopathies are the most severe forms of LGMD and affect both genders equally. The clinical features are identical to those described for the dystrophinopathies.

Diagnosis. Consider the diagnosis of sarcoglycanopathy in all girls with a Duchenne phenotype and in boys who appear to have DMD but show normal dystrophin content in muscle and/or negative genetic testing. Homozygous mutations of *SGC* gene isoforms (*SGCG*, *SGCA*, *SGCB*, and *SGCD*) have been implicated.

Management. Management is as for DMD including the use of steroids, which has been reported to be beneficial for some patients, although the mechanism of action remains unclear. Genetic therapies are being explored but are not yet available.

Myotonic Dystrophy 2 (Proximal Myotonic Dystrophy)

Myotonic dystrophy 2 (DM2), previously called proximal myotonic dystrophy, is genetically distinct from the more common distal form (DM1). A CCTG repeat expansion is present in the *CNBP* gene at locus 3q21. Unlike DM1, a congenital form does not exist, and there is no anticipation. The size of the repeat expansion does not correlate with disease severity. Onset of symptoms is usually between the third and fourth decade of life, although myotonia may be present in childhood. Therefore the discussion of the disorder is outside the spectrum of this book, except that molecular genetic testing is available for children at risk and may provide an answer for the cases of early-onset myotonia.[15]

Inflammatory Myopathies

The inflammatory myopathies are a heterogeneous group of disorders whose causes are infectious, immune mediated, or both. A progressive proximal myopathy occurs in adults, but not in children, with acquired immunodeficiency syndrome (AIDS). However, the concentration of serum CK is elevated in children with AIDS treated with zidovudine. The description of *acute infectious myositis* is in the section on "Acute Generalized Weakness." The conditions discussed in this section are immune mediated.

Dermatomyositis

Dermatomyositis is a systemic angiopathy in which vascular occlusion and infarction account for all pathological changes observed in muscle, connective tissue, skin, gastrointestinal tract, and small nerves. More than 30% of adults with dermatomyositis have an underlying malignancy, but cancer is not a factor before the age of 16. The childhood form of dermatomyositis is a relatively homogeneous disease. The female-to-male ratio is about 2:1 with a reported incidence between 1.2 and 17 per 1,000,000 and prevalence between 5 and 11 per 100,000.

An increase in both incidence and prevalence during the last century is likely due to awareness and better diagnostic tools.[16]

Clinical features. Peak incidence is generally between the ages of 5 and 10 years, but onset may be as early as 4 months. The initial features may be insidious or fulminating. Characteristic of the insidious onset is fever, fatigue, and anorexia in the absence of rash or weakness. These symptoms may persist for weeks or months and suggest an underlying infection. Dermatitis precedes myositis in most children. An erythematous discoloration and edema of the upper eyelids that spread to involve the entire periorbital and malar regions is characteristic. Erythema and edema of the extensor surfaces overlying the joints of the knuckles, elbows, and knees develop later. With time, the skin appears atrophic and scaly. In chronic, long-standing dermatomyositis of childhood, the skin changes may be more disabling than the muscle weakness.

Proximal weakness, stiffness, and pain characterize the myopathy. Weakness generalizes, and flexion contractures develop rapidly and cause joint deformities. Tendon reflexes become increasingly difficult to obtain and finally disappear.

Calcinosis of subcutaneous tissue, especially under discolored areas of skin, occurs in 60% of children and is extraordinarily painful. When severe, it produces an armor-like appearance, termed *calcinosis universalis*, on radiographs. In some children stiffness is the main initial feature, and skin and muscle symptoms are only minor. In the past gastrointestinal tract infarction was a leading cause of death. The mortality rate is less than 5% with modern treatment.

Diagnosis. The combination of fever, rash, myalgia, and weakness is compelling evidence for the diagnosis of dermatomyositis. The serum concentration of CK is usually elevated early in the course. During the time of active myositis, the resting EMG shows increased insertional activity, fibrillations, and positive sharp waves; muscle contraction produces brief, small-amplitude polyphasic potentials. The diagnostic feature on muscle biopsy is perifascicular atrophy (Fig. 7.5). Capillary necrosis usually starts at the periphery of the muscle fascicle and causes ischemia in the adjacent muscle fibers. The most profound atrophy occurs in fascicular borders that face large connective tissue septae.

Management. Corticosteroids are the mainstay of treatment. Initiate prednisone at 0.5–1.5 mg/kg/day, not

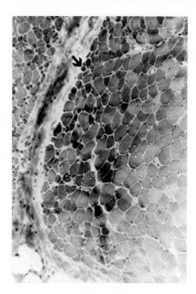

Fig. 7.5 Perifascicular Atrophy in Childhood Dermatomyositis (Trichrome Stain). The muscle fibers at the edge of each fascicle are atrophied (*arrow*).

to exceed 100 mg/day. The response follows a predictable pattern. Temperature returns to normal within 48 hours. The serum CK concentration returns to normal by the second week, and muscle strength increases simultaneously. When these events occur, reduce the prednisone dosage to alternate-day therapy to reduce the frequency and severity of corticosteroid-induced side effects. The prednisone can then be slowly tapered at a rate of 5% per month. When the response is inadequate or high-dose steroids are not tolerated, use a steroid-sparing agent such as methotrexate, azathioprine, or cyclophosphamide. Intravenous immunoglobulin (IVIG) is a useful adjunct.

Dermatomyositis is primarily a skin disease, and it is vital to use protective clothing and sunscreen to prevent symptom exacerbation. The response of the skin rash to prednisone is variable; in some children the rash heals completely, but most will have some permanent scarring from the disease. Calcinosis can be managed with calcium channel blockers such as diltiazem, and especially painful focal lesions can be surgically removed.

Although most children show a dramatic improvement and seem normal within 3 months, long-term treatment is typically required.

Polymyositis

Polymyositis without evidence of other target organ involvement is uncommon before puberty. It is similar to dermatomyositis except the characteristic skin rash is absent. Children with systemic lupus erythematosus may have myalgia and arthralgia as early symptoms but rarely have muscle weakness at onset. Skin, joint, and systemic manifestations usually precede the onset of myopathy. Polymyositis in children is similar to the disorder in adult life except that malignancy is not a causative factor.

Clinical features. Polymyositis begins as a symmetric proximal weakness that develops insidiously and progresses to a moderate disability within weeks to months. The patient may have prolonged periods of stability or even remission that suggest the diagnosis of LGMD because of the slow progress. Tendon reflexes are present early in the course but are less active as muscle bulk is lost. Cardiorespiratory complications are less common in childhood than in adult polymyositis.

Diagnosis. The serum CK concentration is not always increased, but EMG usually shows both myopathic and neuropathic features. Muscle biopsy may show several different patterns of abnormality, and perivascular inflammation may not be present. Instead, one observes features of myopathy, denervation, or both.

Management. The same treatment schedule suggested for childhood dermatomyositis is useful for children with polymyositis. Unfortunately, the response to corticosteroids is far less predictable in polymyositis than in dermatomyositis. Treat those who fail to respond to corticosteroids with methotrexate or other steroid-sparing agents. Plasmapheresis and IVIG are reasonable alternatives when other therapies fail.

Metabolic Myopathies
Late-Onset Pompe Disease

Pompe disease (also known as acid maltase deficiency or glycogen storage disease type II) is an autosomal recessive deficiency of the lysosomal enzyme acid α-1,4-glucosidase (acid maltase) characterized by skeletal myopathy. Prominent cardiomyopathy characterizes the infantile-onset form, whereas the late-onset form is defined by proximal muscle weakness and progressive respiratory insufficiency. The enzyme defect is the same regardless of the age of onset, and different ages of onset may occur within the same family. The speed of progression is variable, but the severity of cardiorespiratory involvement correlates with the amount of residual enzyme activity.

Clinical features. Infants with acid maltase deficiency have glycogen storage in both skeletal and cardiac muscles. Death occurs from cardiac failure during infancy (see Chapter 6). The childhood form involves only skeletal muscle, and the main clinical feature is slowly progressive proximal limb weakness. Tendon reflexes are hypoactive or unobtainable. Some children have mild hypertrophy of the calves simulating DMD. The weakness is steadily progressive and leads to disability and respiratory insufficiency by 20 years of age. Onset at a later age predicts a more benign course.

Diagnosis. Molecular genetic testing reveals biallelic pathogenic variants in the GAA gene.[17] Routine histochemical stains show accumulation of glycogen in lysosomal vacuoles and within the sarcoplasm. The diagnosis is confirmed with biochemical assay of enzyme (acid maltase) activity in muscle or cultured skin fibroblasts. Complete deficiency is associated with classic infantile-onset, whereas residual activity produces later-onset disease.

Management. Begin enzyme replacement therapy with Myozyme (alglucosidase alfa) as soon as the diagnosis is established. Myozyme initiated before age 6 months and before the need for ventilatory assistance improves ventilator-independent survival and acquisition of motor skills. Genetic counseling is needed for the families of affected children.

Other Carbohydrate Myopathies

Slowly progressive proximal weakness is sometimes the initial feature of McArdle disease and debrancher enzyme deficiency. Consider both disorders in the differential diagnosis of proximal weakness. The initial symptom of these disorders is usually exercise intolerance which is discussed in Chapter 8.

Carnitine Deficiency

Carnitine is an essential cofactor in the transfer of long-chain fatty acids across the inner mitochondrial membrane and modulates the ratio of acyl to acyl-coenzyme A. For this reason, carnitine is one of the supplements often given in cases of suspected mitochondrial disease. Its deficiency causes a failure in the production of energy for metabolism and the storage of triglycerides. It occurs as follows: (1) in newborns receiving total parenteral alimentation, (2) in several systemic disorders, (3) as the result of several genetic disorders of organic acid metabolism, (4) in children treated with valproate,

(5) as primary genetic defects that cause deficiency of the cellular carnitine transporter, and (6) may occur if not supplemented while receiving ketogenic diet therapy. The myopathic and systemic forms are caused by different genetic loci.

Transmission of the primary genetic defect on chromosome 5q33.1 is by autosomal recessive inheritance. Primary carnitine deficiency is rare (1:40,000–1:140,000 newborns) except in the Faroe Islands (1:300). The clinical features include hypoketotic hypoglycemia, hepatic encephalopathy, skeletal and cardiac myopathy, and arrhythmia.[18]

Clinical features. The main clinical feature of muscle carnitine deficiency is the childhood onset of slowly progressive proximal weakness affecting the legs before, and more severely, than the arms. Sudden exacerbations or fluctuations are superimposed. Cardiac manifestations are prominent, and death from dilated cardiomyopathy can occur prior to diagnosis.

Diagnosis. Molecular genetic testing reveals biallelic pathogenic variants in the *SLC22A5* gene.[19] The serum concentration of CK is elevated. EMG findings are nonspecific. Muscle biopsy specimens show a vacuolar myopathy with lipid storage mainly in type I fibers. The biochemical measurement of carnitine, both free and total, establishes the diagnosis.

Management. Dietary therapy with L-carnitine is usually effective. Diarrhea and a fishy odor are the most common side effects. The usual dosage is 100 mg/kg/day in three or four divided doses.

Other Lipid Myopathies

Children with progressive proximal weakness associated with lipid storage in muscle and normal carnitine content usually have a disturbance of mitochondrial fatty acid oxidation. These disorders are genetically heterogeneous and difficult to distinguish from other mitochondrial myopathies.

Clinical features. Progressive proximal weakness begins any time from early childhood to adolescence. The legs are affected first and then the arms. Exercise intolerance is noted, and in some cases, the ingestion of fatty foods leads to nausea and vomiting. The pattern and progression of weakness may simulate those of DMD even to the presence of calf hypertrophy. Limb weakness is steadily progressive, and cardiomyopathy may develop.

Diagnosis. The serum concentration of CK is markedly elevated. EMG findings are abnormal and are consistent with a myopathic process. Muscle biopsy is critical to diagnosis. Type I muscle fibers contain fatty droplets. Carnitine and carnitine palmitoyltransferase concentrations are normal.

Management. Patients with fat intolerance may show improvement on a diet free of long-chain fatty acids. Avoid stressors including excessive aerobic exercise, infection, cold exposure, and prolonged fasting. Episodes of rhabdomyolysis should be managed with standard treatments.

Endocrine Myopathies

Progressive proximal limb weakness may occur in children with hyperthyroidism, hypothyroidism, hyperparathyroidism, hypoparathyroidism, hyperadrenalism, and hypoadrenalism.

Clinical features. Systemic features of endocrine disease usually predate the onset of weakness. However, weakness may be the initial feature in primary or secondary hypoparathyroidism and in thyroid disorders. Weakness is much more prominent in the legs than in the arms. Tendon reflexes, even in weak muscles, are normal or diminished but generally are not absent.

Diagnosis. The serum concentration of CK is typically normal. EMG is not useful for diagnosis. Many endocrinopathies produce both neuropathy and myopathy. In Cushing disease and in hyperparathyroidism muscle histological studies show type II fiber atrophy. Other endocrinopathies show nonspecific myopathic changes that vary with the severity of disease.

Management. These disorders should be evaluated in cases of weakness of unknown etiology as they are correctable causes of weakness. Treating the underlying endocrinopathy corrects the weakness.

PROGRESSIVE DISTAL WEAKNESS

Neuropathy is the most common cause of progressive distal weakness (Box 7.5). Among the slowly progressive neuropathies of childhood, hereditary disorders are far more common than acquired disorders. The only common acquired neuropathy is acute inflammatory demyelinating polyradiculoneuropathy (AIDP) (Guillain-Barré syndrome [GBS]), in which weakness evolves rapidly.

Diagnosis in Neuropathy and Neuronopathy

The initial feature of neuropathy in children is progressive symmetric distal weakness affecting the legs

BOX 7.5 Progressive Distal Weakness

- Spinal cord disorders (see Chapter 12)
- Motor neuron diseases
  - Autosomal dominant forms
  - Autosomal recessive forms
  - Juvenile amyotrophic lateral sclerosis
  - Monomelic (see Chapter 13)
  - Spinal muscular atrophies
- Neuropathies
- Hereditary motor sensory neuropathies
  - Charcot-Marie-Tooth disease
  - Familial amyloid neuropathy (see Chapter 9)
  - Giant axonal neuropathy (16q24)
  - Other genetic neuropathies
  - Other lipid neuropathies
  - Pyruvate dehydrogenase deficiency (see Chapter 10)
  - Refsum disease
  - Sulfatide lipidosis: metachromatic leukodystrophy
- Neuropathies with systemic diseases
- Drug induced[a]
- Systemic vasculitis[a]
- Toxins[a]
- Uremia[a]
- Idiopathic neuropathy
  - Chronic axonal neuropathy[a]
  - Chronic demyelinating neuropathy[a]
- Myopathies
  - Autosomal dominant childhood myopathy
  - Autosomal dominant infantile myopathy
  - Autosomal recessive distal (Miyoshi) myopathy
  - Inclusion body myopathies
  - Myotonic dystrophy
- Scapulo (humeral) peroneal syndrome
  - Emery-Dreifuss muscular dystrophy type 1
  - Emery-Dreifuss muscular dystrophy type 2
  - Scapuloperoneal myopathy
  - Scapuloperoneal neuronopathy

[a]The most common conditions and the ones with disease modifying treatments.

TABLE 7.3 Electrodiagnosis in Neuropathy

	Neuronopathy	Axonal	Demyelinating
Fasciculations	+++	+++	+
Denervation potentials	+++	+++	+
Reduced number of motor units	+++	+++	0
High-amplitude potentials	+++	+++	0
Slow motor velocity	0	+	+++
Reduced sensory potentials	0	+	+++

0, Absent; +, rare; +++, common.

and then the arms. When sensation is disturbed, dysesthesias are experienced. These consist of tingling, "pins and needles," or a burning sensation in the feet. Dysesthesias usually occur in acquired but not in hereditary neuropathies. The progression of weakness and sensory loss is in a distal to proximal direction (glove-and-stocking distribution). Tendon reflexes are lost early, especially when sensory fibers are affected.

An important first step in diagnosis is to determine the primary site of the disorder: cell body (anterior horn cell), nerve axon, or myelin. Electrodiagnosis accomplishes localization (Table 7.3). In primary disorders of the cell body (neuronopathy) resting muscle shows fibrillations and fasciculations, which is a sign of

denervation. Voluntary contraction activates reduced numbers of motor unit potentials whose amplitude is normal or increased because of collateral reinnervation. Motor conduction nerve velocity is normal or only slightly diminished, and the amplitude of sensory action potentials is normal. In axonopathies the EMG shows fibrillations at rest and a reduced number of motor unit potentials that are normal or increased in amplitude. High-amplitude potentials may be polyphasic. Motor nerve conduction velocity slows and sensory action potentials have reduced amplitude. Marked slowing of motor conduction velocity and reduced amplitude of sensory evoked potentials characterize demyelinating neuropathies. EMG findings may be normal early in the course.

Neuronopathy

Juvenile Amyotrophic Lateral Sclerosis

Juvenile amyotrophic lateral sclerosis (JALS) is distinct from adult ALS in that more cases are associated with defined genetic defects (40% versus approximately 10%). Multiple causative genes have been identified and there are several different clinical phenotypes. Weakness and atrophy combined with spasticity and hyperreflexia (combined upper and lower motor neuron signs) are common to all presentations.

Clinical features. Pathogenic variants in the *FUS* gene represent the most common genetic cause of JALS. Although *FUS* mutations also cause some forms of adult-onset ALS, the specific mutation implicated in JALS is distinct. Affected patients present with combined upper and lower motor neuron symptoms. Onset is typically in adolescence or early adulthood. Some patients experience executive dysfunction, frontal lobe deficits, and a decline in cognition. The course is rapid and relentless. Death occurs within 1–2 years, usually due to respiratory failure.

Pathogenic variants in sentaxin (*SETX*) are associated with an autosomal dominant form of JALS known as ALS4. Onset is in mid-adolescence. Lower extremity weakness and gait disturbance are the initial features, followed by hand weakness and involvement of the proximal musculature. Bulbar and respiratory muscles are typically spared. Many patients have ataxia on examination, in addition to the expected upper and lower motor neuron signs.

Other genetic causes include variants in the *ALS2*, *SOD1*, *SPTLC1*, *SPG11*, *UBQNL2*, *SIGMAR1*, *GNE*, *ERLIN1*, *TARDBP*, and *VRK1*.[20]

Diagnosis. Multigene panels and whole exome sequencing identify pathogenic variants. Keep in mind that a significant percentage of JALS cases have no known genetic cause. In such cases the diagnosis remains based on clinical presentation and electrodiagnostic findings.

Management. Only supportive therapy is available.

Neuropathy

Charcot-Marie-Tooth Inherited Neuropathies

An exhaustive description of Charcot-Marie-Tooth (CMT) is beyond the scope of this book. Instead, we will focus on the most common forms of CMT and the symptoms that should alert the clinician to consider CMT in the differential diagnosis. CMT represents a large number of genetically distinct disorders with a common overarching phenotype. It was historically classified as demyelinating, axonal, or dominant-intermediate, based on the results of nerve conduction velocity testing. Further understanding of the genetic causes of CMT rendered this classification system increasingly unwieldy; most authors now classify CMT based on the underlying genetic defect. As a result, there are over 70 forms of CMT currently identified and more are likely to come to light in the future. Inheritance can be autosomal dominant, autosomal recessive, or X-linked.

Clinical features. Patients begin experiencing distal weakness between the first and third decades of life, typically in the peroneal muscles. Affected individuals may note repeated episodes of "rolling" or spraining their ankles. With time the anterior tibial as well as the peroneal muscles become weak, producing foot drop. Calf muscles may atrophy or hypertrophy depending on the causative mutation. Eventually, usually after 20 years of age, weakness spreads to the proximal muscles of the legs and hands. Scoliosis is unusual. Cramps with exercise are present in weak muscles. Mild-to-moderate sensory neuropathy results in impaired position sense in the fingers and toes. Dysesthesias are uncommon but can occur. Physical examination reveals depressed or absent tendon reflexes and characteristic *pes cavus* foot deformity (high-arched feet). Intellectual disability, cognitive regression, epilepsy, and blindness do not occur. If such features are present, the diagnosis of CMT should be reconsidered.

Diagnosis. Eight genetic defects account for the majority of CMT phenotypes: *GDAP1*, *GJB1*, *HINT1*, *MFN2*, *MPZ*, *PMP22*, *SH3CT2*, and *SORD*. Of these, *PMP22* is by far the most common, comprising approximately 50% of CMT cases.[21] Single-gene *PMP22* deletion/duplication analysis is a reasonable initial diagnostic test; multigene panels are also available, but one must be sure that they specifically perform *PMP22* deletion/duplication analysis (not all do).

Multiple other disorders mimic the symptoms of CMT, including a variety of distal myopathies, other hereditary motor neuropathies, hereditary sensory neuropathies, hereditary sensory and autonomic neuropathies, and acquired causes of neuropathy. Many of these entities are discussed later in this chapter. Specific symptoms, family history, and examination findings help distinguish CMT from these other entities. If the clinical picture is unclear, consider broad-spectrum genetic testing such as exome sequencing.

Management. Treatment of CMT is supportive. Gene therapy treatment is a potential future treatment option, and clinical trials are ongoing.[22]

Other Genetic Neuropathies

Giant axonal neuropathy. Giant axonal neuropathy (GAN) is a rare disorder transmitted by autosomal recessive inheritance. Biallelic pathogenic variants of the *GAN* gene encoding gigaxonin cause the disorder. The underlying defect is one of generalized intermediate filament organization, with neurofilaments predominantly affected. Central and peripheral axons are both affected.

Clinical features. Patients with GAN have severe early-onset peripheral motor and sensory neuropathy and characteristic tightly curled hair that differs markedly from that of the parents. Patients often show signs of central nervous system involvement including cognitive impairment, seizures, cerebellar signs (ataxia, nystagmus, dysarthria), and pyramidal tract signs.

Both genders are at equal risk, and many are from consanguineous marriages. Affected children are pale and thin and have chronic polyneuropathy accompanied by curly pale hair. Gait impairment usually begins by 3 years of age but can appear later. Most patients become wheelchair dependent during the second decade of life. Symmetric distal atrophy of leg muscles is a constant early feature. Impairment of vibratory and proprioceptive sensations in the legs is profound and diminished or absent tendon reflex response is the rule. Central involvement may result in cerebellar dysfunction, dementia, optic atrophy, and cranial neuropathies.

Diagnosis. Diagnosis is suspected based on the clinical findings, slow nerve conduction velocity, and T_2 abnormalities on MRI. It is confirmed by the detection of a biallelic pathogenic variant in the *GAN* gene or a decreased quantity of gigaxonin on immunogenic testing. Sural nerve biopsy shows enlarged axons filled with disrupted neurofilaments surrounded by thin or fragmented myelin sheaths, but biopsy is rarely required now that genetic testing is available.[23]

Management. Treatment is symptomatic and includes occupational and physical therapy, special education, speech therapy, orthopedics for foot deformities, and ophthalmological treatment of diplopia.

Sulfatide lipidosis: metachromatic leukodystrophy. Metachromatic leukodystrophy (MLD) is an autosomal recessive inherited disorder of myelin metabolism caused by deficient activity of the enzyme arylsulfatase A (ASA), with the inability to degrade galactosylceramide 3-*O*-sulfate (sulfatide) and galactosylsphingosine 3-*O*-sulfate (lysosulfatide). The accumulation of these sulfatides within oligodendrocytes results in myelin and axonal injury both centrally and peripherally. Sulfatide levels correlate with the severity of injury.[24] Infantile, juvenile, and adult forms are recognized. This section only discusses the late infantile form.

Clinical features. After a period of normal development, gait disturbances develop, usually before 2 years of age, but sometimes not until age 4. Initial features may be spasticity, ataxia, or distal weakness of the feet with loss of the ankle tendon reflex. Progressive weakness of all limbs results in generalized hypotonia and hyporeflexia. Weakness, dementia, and optic atrophy are progressive. Death occurs within several years of onset.

Diagnosis. At the time of initial leg weakness, the protein content of the cerebrospinal fluid is elevated and motor nerve conduction velocities are reduced. Brain MRI shows subcortical demyelination with a posterior predominance of white matter abnormalities and sparing of the subcortical U-fibers. MLD is suggested by ASA enzyme activity in leukocytes that are less than 10% of normal controls using the Baum-type assay or by elevated urine sulfatides. The presence of the biallelic *ASA* pathogenic variant on genetic testing confirms the diagnosis.[24]

Management. Hematopoietic stem cell transplantation early in the course of the juvenile and adult-onset forms of the disease may slow its progress; however, it is ineffective in late infantile MLD.[25] Enzyme replacement therapy and gene therapy, both systemic and intrathecally, are being explored as potential therapies.

Other lipid disorders. Peripheral neuropathy occurs in globoid cell leukodystrophy (Krabbe disease) but is not as prominent a feature as in MLD. The usual initial features are psychomotor retardation and irritability rather than flaccid weakness (see Chapter 5). Tendon reflexes may be absent or hyperactive, and half of cases show slowing of motor nerve conduction velocity. The cerebrospinal fluid protein concentration is always elevated. Krabbe disease is autosomal recessive due to deficiency in galactocerebrosidase (GALC) activity, which results in the production of abnormal myelin. Many states in the United States now include GALC in neonatal screens. The diagnosis is confirmed by detecting with genetic testing.[26]

Progeria, small stature, ataxia, retinitis pigmentosa, deafness, and cognitive decline are characteristics of *Cockayne syndrome* (see Chapter 16). A primary segmental demyelinating neuropathy is present in 10%–20% of cases but is not an initial symptom. The main features are hyporeflexia and reduced motor nerve conduction velocity. Other disorders of lipid metabolism in which demyelinating neuropathy is present, but not an important feature, include Niemann-Pick disease (see Chapter 5), Gaucher disease, and Farber disease.

Neuropathies With Systemic Disease

Drug-induced neuropathy. Several medications can cause neuropathy. Such neuropathies are often subclinical and detected only by electrodiagnosis, or because of loss of the ankle tendon reflex. Drugs that commonly produce clinical evidence of motor and sensory neuropathy are isoniazid, nitrofurantoin, vincristine, and zidovudine. Vitamin B_6 (pyridoxine) has been implicated as a potential cause of neuropathy in several case reports; however, it was often being used in patients with tuberculosis on isoniazid therapy, or with other emaciating conditions, which may have been the true underlying cause of the neuropathy. We have not seen the development of neuropathy in cases of pyridoxine-dependent epilepsy (which requires high doses of pyridoxine for treatment), or when pyridoxine is used empirically to treat irritability.

Isoniazid

Clinical features. The initial symptoms are numbness and paresthesias of the fingers and toes. If treatment is continued, superficial sensation diminishes in a glove-and-stocking pattern. Distal limb weakness follows and is associated with tenderness of the muscles and burning dysesthesias. Reduced or absent ankle tendon reflexes are expected.

Diagnosis. Suspect isoniazid neuropathy whenever neuropathy develops in children taking the drug.

Management. Isoniazid interferes with pyridoxine metabolism and produces neuropathy by causing a pyridoxine deficiency state. The administration of pyridoxine along with isoniazid prevents neuropathy without interfering with antituberculous activity. The longer the symptoms progress, the longer the time until recovery. Although pyridoxine can prevent the development of neuropathy, it has little effect on the speed of recovery once neuropathy is established.

Nitrofurantoin

Clinical features. Nitrofurantoin neuropathy most often occurs in patients with impaired renal function. A high blood concentration of nitrofurantoin causes an axonal neuropathy. The initial features are usually paresthesias, followed within a few days or weeks by glove-and-stocking sensory loss, and weakness of distal muscles. Pure motor neuropathy is occasionally present.

Diagnosis. Suspect nitrofurantoin neuropathy in any child with neuropathy taking the drug. It may be difficult to distinguish from uremic neuropathy.

Management. Complete recovery usually follows complete cessation of the drug. Occasional patients have developed complete paralysis and death despite discontinuation of nitrofurantoin.

Vincristine

Clinical features. Neuropathy is an expected complication of vincristine therapy. The ankle tendon reflex is lost first; later, other tendon reflexes become less reactive and may be lost. The first symptoms are paresthesias, often starting in the fingers rather than the feet and progressing to mild loss of superficial sensation but not position sense. Weakness follows sensory loss as evidenced by clumsiness in the hands and cramps in the feet. Distal muscles are affected more than proximal muscles and extensors more than flexors. Weakness may progress rapidly, with loss of ambulation in a few weeks. The initial weakness may be asymmetric and suggests mononeuropathy multiplex.

Diagnosis. Electrodiagnostic features are consistent with axonal neuropathy, fibrillations, and fasciculations on needle EMG but with normal motor nerve conduction velocity.

Management. The neuropathy is dose related, and usually the patient recovers 1–3 months after discontinuing the drug although the loss of tendon reflexes is often permanent. Gabapentin, pregabalin, duloxetine, amitriptyline, and carbamazepine all show some efficacy in treating chemotherapy-induced neuropathy.

Toxins. Several heavy metals, inorganic chemicals, and insecticides produce polyneuropathies in children. In adults industrial exposure, agricultural exposure, or attempted homicide are the usual causes of heavy metal poisoning. Small children who have a single accidental ingestion are more likely to have acute symptoms of systemic disease or central nervous system dysfunction than a slowly progressive neuropathy. Sometimes progressive distal weakness is an early sign in older children who have an addiction to inhalants. Even in these cases symptoms of central nervous system dysfunction are usually present.

Uremia. Some degree of neuropathy occurs at some time in many children undergoing long-term periodic hemodialysis. Uremic neuropathy is more common in males than in females, but the reason for the gender bias is unknown.

Clinical features. The earliest symptoms may be muscle cramps in the hands and feet, burning feet or restless legs, and loss of the ankle tendon reflex. After the initial sensory symptoms, the disorder progresses to a severe distal, symmetric, mixed motor and sensory polyneuropathy affecting the legs more than the arms. The rate of progression is variable and may be fulminating or may evolve over several months.

Pure motor neuropathy develops in some children with uremia. Symptoms begin after starting hemodialysis. The rapid progression of distal weakness in all limbs does not respond to dialysis but may reverse after renal transplantation.

Diagnosis. Uremia causes an axonal neuropathy, but chronic renal failure causes segmental demyelination that is out of proportion to axonal changes. Therefore repeated measures of motor nerve conduction velocity are a useful way to monitor neuropathy progression. Slow conduction velocities are present even before clinical symptoms occur. Reduced creatine clearance correlates with slowing of the conduction velocity.

Management. Early neuropathy resolves with correction of the underlying uremia. Patients with severe neuropathy rarely recover fully despite adequate treatment.

Vasculitis and vasculopathy. Polyneuropathy and mononeuropathy multiplex are relatively common neurological complications of vasculitis in adults but not in children. Children with lupus erythematosus are generally sicker than adults, but peripheral neuropathy is neither an initial nor a prominent feature of their disease. Motor and sensory neuropathies occur in children with chronic juvenile rheumatoid arthritis.

Myopathies
Hereditary Distal Myopathies

The hereditary distal myopathies, as a group, are uncommon except for myotonic dystrophy.[27] Forms that usually have an adult onset are not discussed here.

Laing early-onset distal myopathy. Laing distal myopathy is one of four known childhood-onset distal myopathies and is typically inherited in an autosomal dominant manner, although rare autosomal recessive cases have been reported. The disorder is caused by a mutation in *MYH7*, which encodes the beta-heavy chain of myosin expressed in type 1 skeletal muscle and cardiac muscle.[28]

Clinical features. Age at onset is after 4 years and may delay to the third decade. The initial weakness is in the toe and ankle extensors and the neck flexors. Weakness of the finger extensors develops years later, with relative sparing of the finger flexors and intrinsic hand muscles. Some proximal limb muscles become weak late in life without impairing walking.

Diagnosis. EMG findings are consistent with a myopathic process. CK is mildly elevated, and muscle biopsy shows hypertrophy of type 1 fibers with core/minocore lesions. Muscle MRI shows involvement of the anterior compartment muscles of the lower leg. The diagnosis may be confirmed by genetic testing and sequencing of *MHT7* gene.

Management. Treatment is symptomatic.

Autosomal Recessive Distal Myopathies

Dysferlinopathies. Dysferlin mutations cause four different phenotypes. LGMD type R2 causes proximal weakness (discussed earlier in this chapter in the section on "Limb Girdle Muscular Dystrophies"). *Miyoshi myopathy* and *distal myopathy with anterior tibial onset (DMAT)* cause distal weakness. A fourth phenotype causes asymptomatic elevation of CK levels.

Clinical features. Miyoshi myopathy becomes symptomatic in late adolescence. Weakness begins in the distal parts of the legs, especially the gastrocnemius and soleus muscles. Over a period of years, the weakness and atrophy spread to the thighs and gluteal muscles. The forearms may become mildly atrophic with a decrease in grip strength, but the small muscles of the hands are spared. Most patients lose the ability to ambulate independently approximately 20 years after symptom onset.

DMAT becomes symptomatic earlier and, in contrast to Myoshi myopathy, predominantly involves the anterior muscles of the lower leg. Foot drop is the most common manifestation.

Diagnosis. The peculiar pattern of calf atrophy is almost pathognomonic for Myoshi myopathy. CK is elevated in both disorders, but more significantly in Myoshi myopathy. Molecular genetic testing demonstrates biallelic pathogenic variants in *DYSF*.[15]

Management. Treatment is supportive. Although disease progression is slow, most patients will eventually require assistive devices and mobility aids.

Nebulin myopathy. Nebulin myopathy is one of the nemaline rod myopathies, characterized by the presence of nemaline rods on muscle biopsy. Nebulin myopathy is the only subtype that can cause predominantly distal myopathy. Inheritance is usually autosomal recessive, but rare autosomal dominant cases have occurred.

Clinical features. Onset is in childhood with extensor weakness of the feet and later the hands. Weakness is slowly progressive and most adults do not experience severe disability.

Diagnosis. MRI shows fatty degeneration of the anterior compartment muscles of the lower leg. CK is normal to mildly elevated. Molecular genetic testing reveals biallelic, usually missense variants of the *NEB* gene.

Management. Treatment is supportive.

Myotonic dystrophy. Myotonic dystrophy type 1 is a multisystem disorder transmitted by autosomal dominant inheritance with variable penetrance. It is caused by a larger number of CTG trinucleotide repeats (>34) in the *DMPK* gene.[29] Amplification (increasing size of trinucleotide repeats) occurs in successive generations and correlates with more severe disease with earlier onset (anticipation). A neonatal form occurs in children born to mothers with myotonic dystrophy (see Chapter 6).

A proximal form of myotonic dystrophy (myotonic dystrophy type 2) is a distinct genetic disorder and considered in the section on "Progressive Proximal Weakness."

Clinical features. The onset of symptoms is usually during adolescence or later. The major features are myotonia (a disturbance characterized by decreased muscle relaxation after contraction), weakness in the face and distal portion of the limbs, cataracts, frontal baldness, and multiple endocrinopathies. The pattern of muscle atrophy in the face is so stereotypical that all patients with the disease have similar facies. The face is long and thin because of wasting of the temporal and masseter muscles, and the neck is thin because of atrophy of the sternocleidomastoid muscles. The eyelids and corners of the mouth droop and the lower part of the face sags, producing the appearance of sadness.

Although seeking medical treatment is rare before adolescence, myotonia is usually present in childhood

and is detectable by EMG, or by clinical examination. Percussion of muscle demonstrates myotonia. When percussed, the thenar eminence dimples and remains dimpled at the site of percussion. In addition, the thumb adducts and remains in that position for several seconds. The physician can also detect myotonia by shaking hands with the patient, who has difficulty letting go and releases the grip in part by flexing the wrist to force the finger flexors to open.

Some patients have little or no evidence of muscle weakness, only cataracts, frontal baldness, or endocrine disturbances. However, the presence of muscle weakness before the age of 20 years is likely to be relentlessly progressive, causing severe distal weakness in the hands and feet by adult life. Smooth and cardiac muscle involvement may be present. Disturbed gastrointestinal motility is characteristic. Endocrine disturbances include testicular atrophy, infertility in females, hyperinsulinism, diabetes, hypothyroidism, adrenal atrophy, and disturbances in growth hormone secretion. Many patients have an intellectual disability and an "avoidant" or apathetic personality.

Diagnosis. The basis for the diagnosis of myotonic dystrophy is usually the clinical features, the family history, and genetic analysis. EMG and muscle biopsy are unnecessary. Studies to show the presence and number of trinucleotide repeats are commercially available and are the best method to detect asymptomatic individuals and the best for prenatal diagnosis.

Management. Myotonia frequently responds to drugs that stabilize membranes; mexiletine is probably the most effective. Patients should undergo cardiac evaluation prior to taking mexiletine as it can rarely exert proarrhythmic effects on cardiac muscle. However, weakness and not myotonia disables the patient. Braces for foot drop are usually required as the disease progresses. Avoid statins, as they may increase weakness and pain, and use caution with paralytics and anesthetics which may cause malignant hyperthermia. Screen for hypothyroidism, diabetes, cataracts, and cardiac arrhythmias.

Emery-Dreifuss muscular dystrophy. Emery-Dreifuss muscular dystrophy is defined by the clinical triad of joint contractures, slowly progressive muscle weakness and atrophy, and cardiac involvement. Autosomal dominant and X-linked forms exist which have slightly different clinical characteristics. Autosomal recessive forms have been reported but are extremely rare. Mutations in emerin (*EMD*), lamins A/C (*LMNA*), and FHL isoforms (*FHL1*) cause the disease.

Clinical features. The onset of symptoms is between 5 and 15 years of age, although age of onset and severity of disease demonstrate significant variability even within families. Joint contractures develop early and involve the elbows, ankles, and posterior cervical muscles. This is followed by muscle weakness and wasting in the biceps and triceps muscles, and then in the deltoid and other shoulder muscles. The peroneal muscles are severely affected. Calf hypertrophy does not occur. The progression of symptoms is slow. Loss of ambulation is common in individuals with the autosomal dominant form, but rare with X-linked disease.

Cardiac involvement may be extensive and comprises arrhythmias, conduction defects, dilated cardiomyopathy, and congestive heart failure. Pacemakers are often required, and there are reports of some patients experiencing sudden death despite pacemaker placement.

Diagnosis. Molecular genetic testing demonstrates hemizygous pathogenic variants in *EMD* or *FHL1*; heterozygous pathogenic variants in *LMNA*, or (rarely) biallelic pathogenic variants in *LMNA*.[30]

Management. Treatment for skeletal muscle weakness is symptomatic; surgery may help release joint contractures and improve range of motion. Early implantation of a permanent pacemaker is lifesaving. Antithrombotic agents prevent stroke in patients with left ventricular dysfunction or arrhythmias. Avoid depolarizing muscle relaxants and volatile anesthetics, which increase the risk of malignant hyperthermia.

ACUTE GENERALIZED WEAKNESS

The sudden onset or rapid evolution of generalized flaccid weakness in the absence of symptoms of encephalopathy is always due to disorders of the motor unit (Box 7.6). Among these disorders, AIDP (GBS) is by far the most common.

The combination of acute weakness and rhabdomyolysis, as evidenced by myoglobinuria, indicates that muscle is degenerating rapidly. This may occur in some disorders of carbohydrate and fatty acid metabolism (see Chapter 8), after intense and unusual exercise, in some cases of infectious and idiopathic polymyositis, and in intoxication with alcohol and cocaine. Death from renal failure is a possible outcome in patients with

---

BOX 7.6 Acute Generalized Weakness

Infectious Disorders
- Acute infectious myositis
- Acute inflammatory polyradiculoneuropathy[a] (Guillain-Barré syndrome)
- Acute axonal neuropathies
- Chronic inflammatory polyradiculoneuropathy[a] (CIDP)
- Enterovirus infections

Metabolic Disorders
- Acute intermittent porphyria (see Chapter 9)
- Hereditary tyrosinemia (see Chapter 9)

Neuromuscular Blockade
- Botulism[a]
- Corticosteroid-induced quadriplegia[a]
- Intensive care unit weakness
- Tick paralysis[a]

Periodic Paralysis
- Andersen-Tawil syndrome
- Familial hypokalemic[a] (FPPI)
- Familial hyperkalemic[a] (FPPII)
- Familial normokalemic (FPPIII)

[a]The most common conditions and the ones with disease modifying treatments.

---

rhabdomyolysis. Intravenous fluids are needed to prevent this outcome.

Infectious Disease
Acute Infectious Myositis

Acute myositis in children most often follows influenza or enterovirus infections.[31] Boys are affected more often than girls.

Clinical features. Ordinarily prodromal respiratory symptoms persist for 3–8 days before the onset of severe symmetric muscle pain and weakness, which may cause severe disability within 24 hours. Pain and tenderness are most severe in the calf muscles. Tendon reflexes are present.

Diagnosis. The serum concentration of CK is elevated, usually more than 10 times the upper limit of normal.

Management. Spontaneous resolution of myositis occurs quickly. Bed rest is required for 2–7 days until pain subsides, after which the patient recovers completely. Intravenous fluids at rates higher than maintenance are needed to prevent renal failure when rhabdomyolysis with high CK levels is detected.

Acute Inflammatory Demyelinating Polyradiculoneuropathy

AIDP, more commonly called Guillain-Barré syndrome or GBS, is an acute monophasic demyelinating neuropathy. Peripheral nerves are the target of an abnormal immune response. More than half of patients describe an antecedent viral infection. Respiratory tract infections are more common than gastrointestinal infections.[32] Enteritis caused by specific strains of *Campylobacter jejuni* 19 is more often the inciting disease in the acute axonal form of GBS than in the demyelinating form. Approximately 85%–90% of cases are demyelinating and 10%–15% are axonal in nature.

Clinical features. The natural history of AIDP in children is substantially the same as in adults. The clinical features are sufficiently stereotypical that establishing the diagnosis usually does not require laboratory confirmation. This is especially important because the characteristic laboratory features may not be present at the onset of clinical symptoms. The two essential features are progressive motor weakness involving more than one limb, and areflexia. Frequently insidious sensory symptoms precede the onset of weakness; in some cases pain is a significant complaint, and affected children may display a degree of irritability that appears out of proportion to their objective physical symptoms. Weakness progresses rapidly, and approximately 50% of patients will reach a nadir by 2 weeks, 80% by 3 weeks, and the rest by 4 weeks. The weakness is usually ascending and relatively symmetric qualitatively, if not quantitatively. Tendon reflexes are absent in all weak muscles and are absent even before the muscle is weak. Bilateral facial weakness occurs in as many as half. Autonomic dysfunction (arrhythmia, labile blood pressure, and gastrointestinal dysfunction) is commonly associated, and a syndrome of acute autonomic dysfunction without paralysis may be a variant.

Recovery of function usually begins 2–4 weeks after progression stops. In children recovery is usually complete. The prognosis is best when recovery begins early. Respiratory paralysis is unusual, but by supporting respiratory function during the critical time of profound paralysis, complete or near-complete recovery is expected.

Diagnosis. Examination of the cerebrospinal fluid was once critical in distinguishing GBS from acute poliomyelitis. In the absence of poliomyelitis this examination is less important. A physician first sees most children during the second week of symptoms. At that time the concentration of protein may be normal or elevated, and the number of mononuclear leukocytes per cubic millimeter may be 10 or fewer.

Electrophysiological studies are more important than cerebrospinal fluid analysis for diagnosis, especially to distinguish AIDP from acute axonal neuropathy, which has a worse prognosis. However, EMG and nerve conduction studies may be normal during the initial portion of the illness.

Management. Careful monitoring of respiratory function is critical. Intubation is essential if vital capacity falls rapidly to less than 50% of normal. Adequate control of respiration prevents death from the disorder. Corticosteroids are not helpful, because although they may produce some initial improvement, they tend to prolong the course. Plasma exchange or the use of intravenous immune globulin hastens recovery from GBS.[33] We prefer the use of IVIG 2 g/kg over 2 days.

Acute Motor Axonal Neuropathy

The axonal form of GBS occurs more often in rural and economically deprived populations than does AIDP and often follows *C. jejuni* enteritis.

Clinical features. The clinical features are indistinguishable from AIDP except that sensation is not usually affected. Maximal weakness, symmetric quadriparesis, and respiratory failure occur rapidly, often over a few days. Tendon reflexes are absent early in the course. Distal atrophy occurs. Recovery is slow, and the mean time to ambulation is 5 months.

Diagnosis. The cerebrospinal fluid cell count is normal, but the protein concentration increases after 1 or 2 weeks. Electrophysiological studies are consistent with an axonopathy rather than a demyelinating neuropathy, and sensory nerve action potentials are normal.

Management. Respiratory support is often required. Treatment is the same as for the demyelinating forms.

Chronic Inflammatory Demyelinating Polyradiculoneuropathy

Acquired demyelinating polyradiculoneuropathies occur in both an acute and a chronic form. The acute form is the GBS described in the section earlier. The chronic form is *chronic inflammatory demyelinating polyradiculoneuropathy* (CIDP). The acute and chronic forms may be difficult to distinguish from each other at the onset of symptoms, but their distinguishing feature is the monophasic or recurrent course.[34]

CIDP, like GBS, is immune mediated. The preceding infection is more often a respiratory illness than a gastrointestinal illness. However, both are so common in all school-age children that the cause-and-effect relationship is difficult to establish.

Clinical features. CIDP is more common in adults than in children. The usual initial features are weakness and paresthesias in the distal portions of the limbs causing a gait disturbance. Cranial neuropathies are unusual. Mandatory criteria for diagnosis are: (1) progressive or relapsing motor and sensory dysfunction of more than one limb, of a peripheral nerve nature, developing over at least 2 months; and (2) areflexia or hyporeflexia, usually affecting all four limbs. The course is monophasic in one-quarter of children and has a relapsing course in the remainder. Three-quarters have residual weakness.

Diagnosis. Exclusionary criteria in establishing the diagnosis of CIDP are a family history of a similar disorder, pure sensory neuropathy, other organ involvement, or abnormal storage of material in nerves. The protein content of the cerebrospinal fluid is always greater than 0.45 g/L, and a small number of mononuclear cells may be present. Motor nerve conduction velocity is less than 70% of the lower limit of normal in at least two nerves. Sural nerve biopsy is not mandatory but shows features of demyelination, cellular infiltration of the nerve, and no evidence of vasculitis.

Electrodiagnosis differentiates acquired demyelinating neuropathies from familial demyelinating neuropathies. Acquired neuropathies show a multifocal disturbance of conduction velocity, whereas slowing of conduction velocity is uniform throughout the length of the nerve in hereditary disorders.

Management. Steroids and IVIG are first-line treatments. Proceed quickly with plasma exchange if steroids and IVIG are ineffective. As a rule, long-term therapy is essential, and relapse may follow discontinuation of therapy. The outcome is more favorable in children than in adults. Steroids, IVIG, and subcutaneous immunoglobulins may be used for maintenance; if these required doses are high, consider escalating to immunosuppressant or immunomodulatory drugs. Neuropathic pain requires symptomatic treatment with gabapentin, pregabalin, or other agents.[35]

Viral Infections

Enterovirus infections. Poliovirus, coxsackievirus, and the echovirus group are RNA viruses that inhabit the intestinal tract of humans. They are neurotropic and produce paralytic disease by destroying the motor neurons of the brainstem and spinal cord. Of this group, poliovirus causes the most severe and devastating disease. Coxsackievirus and echoviruses are more likely to cause aseptic meningitis, although they can cause an acute paralytic syndrome similar to that of poliomyelitis.

Enterovirus D68 is associated with outbreaks of respiratory illness and acute flaccid myelitis in the United States. Acute flaccid myelitis, a polio-like illness, was first recognized in 2012 in California and has occurred seasonally since that time.

Clinical features. Enterovirus infections occur in epidemics during the spring and summer. Acute flaccid myelitis and poliovirus infection present similarly. There is an initial brief illness characterized by fever, malaise, and gastrointestinal symptoms. Aseptic meningitis occurs in more severe cases. The extreme situation is acute flaccid myelitis or paralytic poliomyelitis. After a brief period of apparent well-being, fever recurs in association with headache, vomiting, and signs of meningeal irritation. Pain in the limbs or over the spine is an antecedent symptom of limb paralysis. Flaccid muscle weakness develops rapidly thereafter. The pattern of muscle weakness varies but is generally asymmetric and may be ascending or descending. One arm or leg is often weaker than the other limbs. Reflexes in the weak limbs are hypoactive or absent. Bulbar symptoms may occur, but extraocular muscles are usually spared. Muscles of respiration become weak and intubation with mechanical ventilation may be necessary. Long-term disability is common, and most patients require extensive rehabilitation with only incomplete recovery.[36]

Diagnosis. Suspect the diagnosis from the clinical findings. Isolation and viral typing from stool and nasopharyngeal specimens provide confirmation. The cerebrospinal fluid initially shows a polymorphonuclear reaction, with the cell count ranging from 50 to 200/mm^3. After 1 week, lymphocytes predominate; after 2–3 weeks, the total cell count decreases. The protein content is elevated early and remains elevated for several months.

Management. Treatment is supportive and includes ventilatory support during the acute phase and rehabilitation with physical, occupational, and speech/feeding therapies once symptoms have stabilized.

The introduction of inactivated poliomyelitis vaccine in 1954, followed by the use of live-attenuated vaccine in 1960, abolished the disease in the Western hemisphere and Europe. Vaccine-associated poliomyelitis is rare since inactivated polio vaccine replaced the live-attenuated vaccine. No vaccine is available for the strains of enterovirus associated with acute flaccid myelitis.

West Nile virus. West Nile virus (WNV) has spread across the United States since arriving in New York in 1999.[37] It is now the most important cause of arboviral meningitis, encephalitis, and acute flaccid paralysis in the continental United States.[38] Almost all transmission occurs from the bite of an infected mosquito. Rare person-to-person transmission occurs through organ transplantation, blood and blood product transfusion, and intrauterine spread. Only 20% of humans infected with WNV become symptomatic, and neurological disease occurs in 1% of all infected.[39] The saliva of the *Culex tarsalis* mosquito is a potent enhancer for the virus to cause viremia.[40]

Clinical features. Within 3–14 days of a mosquito bite, a flu-like illness occurs. Three neurological syndromes may occur: meningitis, encephalitis, or anterior myelitis (acute flaccid paralysis). Myelitis occurs in about 17.5% of neurological cases and is caused by direct invasion of anterior horn cells. The encephalitic form may present with focal neurological deficits, tremors, ataxia, confusion, or seizures, and may evolve into coma and death.

Diagnosis. EMG indicates severe denervation in affected muscles. Both EMG and MRI studies localize the abnormality to the motor neuron or ventral horn. The detection of WNV RNA in blood is possible 4 days before the appearance of IgM antibodies.

Management. Treatment is supportive. Ribavirin, interferon, and WNV-specific IVIG lack evidence in humans and are currently not recommended treatments according to the Centers for Disease Control and Prevention.

Neuromuscular Blockade

Children treated for prolonged periods with neuromuscular blocking agents for assisted ventilation may remain in a flaccid state for days or weeks after discontinuing the drug. This is especially true in newborns receiving several drugs that block the neuromuscular junction.

Botulism

Clostridium botulinum produces a toxin that interferes with the release of acetylcholine at the neuromuscular junction. Chapter 6 describes the infantile form, but most cases occur after infancy in people who eat food, usually preserved at home, contaminated with the organism.

Clinical features. The first symptoms are blurred vision, diplopia, dizziness, dysarthria, and dysphagia, which have their onset 12–36 hours after the ingestion of toxin. Some patients have only bulbar signs; in others flaccid paralysis develops in all limbs. Patients with generalized weakness always have ophthalmoplegia with sparing of the pupillary response. Tendon reflexes may be present or absent.

Diagnosis. Repetitive supermaximal nerve stimulation at a rate of 20–50 stimuli per second produces an incremental response characteristic of a presynaptic defect. The electrical abnormality evolves with time and may not be demonstrable in all limbs on any given day.

Management. Botulism can be fatal because of respiratory depression. Treatment relies primarily on supportive care, which is similar to the management of GBS. Antitoxin is recommended in confirmed cases. Equine-derived heptavalent botulism antitoxin causes anaphylaxis in 1%–2% of recipients. Antihistamine, epinephrine, and possibly intensive care may be required.[41]

Corticosteroid-Induced Quadriplegia

The administration of high-dose intravenous corticosteroids, especially in combination with a neuromuscular blocking agent, may cause acute generalized weakness.

Clinical features. Most patients with this syndrome receive corticosteroids to treat asthma. The onset of weakness is 4–14 days after starting treatment. The weakness is usually diffuse at onset but may be limited to proximal or distal muscles. Tendon reflexes are usually preserved. Complete recovery is the rule.

Diagnosis. The serum CK concentration may be normal or elevated. EMG shows brief, small-amplitude polyphasic potentials, and the muscle is electrically unresponsive to direct stimulation.

Management. Respiratory assistance may be required. Cessation of the offending drugs usually ends the disorder and allows the patient to recover spontaneously.

Tick Paralysis

Tick paralysis is caused by a neurotoxin that female ticks secrete through their salivary glands, rather than by an infectious organism. The disease is most common in North America and Australia, and over 40 species of ticks have been implicated in the disease. The mechanism of paralysis is unknown.[42]

Clinical features. Affected children are usually less than 5 years of age. The clinical syndrome is similar to GBS, except that ocular motor palsies and pupillary abnormalities are more common. A severe generalized flaccid weakness, usually first affecting the legs, develops rapidly and is sometimes associated with bifacial palsy. Respiratory paralysis requiring assisted ventilation is common. Tendon reflexes are usually absent or greatly depressed. Dysesthesias and irritability may be present at the onset of weakness, but examination fails to show loss of sensation.

Diagnosis. Consider the diagnosis in all children who present with acute ataxia. The cerebrospinal fluid protein concentration is normal. Nerve conduction studies may be normal or may show mild slowing of motor nerve conduction velocities. Decreased amplitude of the compound muscle action potentials is common. High rates of repetitive stimulation may show a normal result or an abnormal incremental response. Unfortunately, no specific testing exists, and a clinically compatible syndrome with discovery of an engorged tick is usually needed to make a definitive diagnosis.

Management. In most cases strength returns quickly on removing the causative tick. However, the tick may be hard to find because it hides in body hair. Certain tick species produce more severe paralysis which worsens over 1–2 days after removal of the tick before improvement begins.

Intensive Care Unit Weakness

Almost 2% of children admitted to critical care units develop muscle weakness.[43] Most were organ transplant recipients treated with neuromuscular blocking agents, corticosteroids, and aminoglycoside antibiotics. The usual clinical feature is failure to wean from a respirator. Some exemplify "corticosteroid-induced quadriplegia" described earlier. Corticosteroid myopathy accounts for some. These show increased blood concentrations of CK and histological evidence of myofiber necrosis. Another possible cause is the depletion of myosin from muscle. Muscle biopsy distinguishes the several types of prolonged weakness that may occur in people with severe illness requiring intensive care.

PERIODIC PARALYSES

The usual classification of periodic paralyses is in relation to serum potassium: hyperkalemic, hypokalemic, or normokalemic. In addition, periodic paralysis may be primary (genetic) or secondary. The cause of secondary hypokalemic periodic paralysis is urinary or gastrointestinal loss of potassium. Urinary loss accompanies primary hyperaldosteronism, licorice intoxication, amphotericin B therapy, and several renal tubular defects. Gastrointestinal loss most often occurs with severe chronic diarrhea, prolonged gastrointestinal intubation, vomiting, and a draining gastrointestinal fistula. Either urinary or gastrointestinal loss, or both, may occur in children with anorexia nervosa who overuse diuretics or induce vomiting. Thyrotoxicosis is an important cause of hypokalemic periodic paralysis, especially in Asians. Secondary hyperkalemic periodic paralysis is associated with renal or adrenal insufficiency.

Familial Hypokalemic Periodic Paralysis

Genetic transmission of familial hypokalemic periodic paralysis (FHPP) is by autosomal dominant inheritance with decreased penetrance in females. FHPP is caused by a mutation in either calcium or sodium sarcolemmal ion channels: *CACNA1S* (the majority of cases) and *SCN4A*.

Clinical features. The onset of symptoms occurs before 16 years of age in 60% of cases and by 20 years of age in the remainder. Attacks are not truly periodic as their frequency is variable. Factors that trigger an attack include rest after exercise (therefore many attacks occur early in the morning), a large meal with high carbohydrate content (pizza is the trigger of choice in adolescents), emotional or physical stress, alcohol ingestion, and exposure to cold. Before and during the attack the patient may have excessive thirst and oliguria. The weakness begins with a sensation of aching in the proximal muscles. Sometimes only the proximal muscles are affected; at other times there is complete paralysis so that the patient cannot even raise the head. Facial muscles are rarely affected, and extraocular motility is always normal. Respiratory distress does not occur. When the weakness reaches extreme, the muscles feel swollen, and the tendon reflexes are absent. Most attacks last for 6–12 hours and some for the whole day. Strength recovers rapidly, but after several attacks residual weakness may be present.

Diagnosis. Molecular genetic testing is available, but the clinical features usually establish the diagnosis. During the attack, the serum concentration of potassium ranges from 0.9 to 3.0 mL (normal range 3.5–5 mL), and electrocardiographic (ECG) changes occur, including bradycardia, flattening of T waves, and prolongation of the PR and Q-T intervals. The muscle is electrically silent and not excitable. The oral administration of glucose 2 g/kg, with 10–20 units of crystalline insulin given subcutaneously, provokes attacks but is not recommended.

Management. Acute attacks are associated with respiratory difficulty in some patients, and respiratory status should be closely monitored as should cardiac function. Treatment of attacks in patients with good renal function is with repeated oral doses of potassium and avoidance of glucose. Give intravenous infusions for severe hypokalemia, with continuous ECG monitoring and serial serum potassium measurements. Hyperthyroidism may provoke attacks; monitor thyroid function. Preventative medications include daily potassium supplementation, acetazolamide, and potassium-sparing diuretics.[44]

Familial Hyperkalemic Periodic Paralysis Type 1

Genetic transmission of familial hyperkalemic periodic paralysis type 1 is by autosomal dominant inheritance. The frequency is the same in both genders. The cause is a defect of the gene encoding the sodium channel, *SCN4A*.

Clinical features. The onset of weakness is in early childhood and sometimes in infancy. Attacks are initially rare but increase in frequency over time. As in hypokalemic periodic paralysis, resting after exercise may provoke attacks. However, only moderate exercise is required. Weakness begins with a sensation of heaviness in the back and leg muscles. Sometimes the patient can delay the paralysis by walking or moving about. In infants and small children characteristic attacks are episodes of floppiness in which the child lies around and cannot move. In older children and adults both mild and severe attacks may occur. Factors causing attacks are potassium-rich foods, rest after exercise, a cold environment, emotional stress, glucocorticoids, and pregnancy. Mild attacks last for less than an hour and do not produce complete paralysis. More than one mild attack may occur in a day. Severe attacks are similar to the complete flaccid paralysis seen in hypokalemic periodic paralysis and may last for several hours. Residual weakness may persist after several severe attacks. Mild myotonia of the eyelids, face, and hands may be present between attacks. Older patients may develop a progressive myopathy.

Diagnosis. Between attacks, the serum concentration of potassium is normal but increases at least 1.5 mmol/L during attacks. When the potassium concentration is high, ECG changes are consistent with hyperkalemia. Oral administration of potassium chloride just after exercise in the fasting state provokes an attack, but such dangerous maneuvers are not recommended since molecular genetic testing is readily available. During the attack, the muscles are electrically silent. Myotonia in patients with hyperkalemic periodic paralysis is mild and may occur only on exposure to cold.

Management. Acute attacks seldom require treatment because they are brief. Prophylactic measures include avoidance of meals rich in potassium (grapefruit juice) and cold exposure. Should an attack occur, it can sometimes be shorted or aborted by continuing mild exercise or carbohydrate ingestion, use of albuterol, or IV administration of calcium gluconate. Use caution with anesthetics.[45]

Familial Normokalemic Periodic Paralysis

This is the rarest form of periodic paralysis and is also due to mutations of the skeletal muscle sodium channel alpha subunit (*SCN4A*). The clinical picture is so similar to the hyperkalemic form that many feel familial normokalemic periodic paralysis (FNKPP) represents a variant of hyperkalemic paralysis.[46,47]

Andersen-Tawil Syndrome

Andersen-Tawil syndrome is a distinct channelopathy affecting both skeletal and cardiac muscles.[48] The genetic defect involves the α-subunit of the skeletal muscle sodium channel and the cardiac muscle potassium channel responsible for most long Q-T intervals.

Clinical features. The main features are short stature, dysmorphic features, periodic paralysis, cardiac arrhythmias, and a prolonged Q-T interval. Dysmorphic features include hypertelorism, low-set ears, a small mandible, scoliosis, clinodactyly, and syndactyly. Periodic paralysis may be associated with hyperkalemia, hypokalemia, or normokalemia. The prolonged Q-T interval may be the only feature in some individuals. The initial feature may be an arrhythmia, especially ventricular tachycardia, or attacks of paralysis.

Diagnosis. Suspect the diagnosis in any dysmorphic child with a prolonged Q-T interval and periodic paralysis. This can be confirmed by a pathogenic variant in *KCNJ2*.

Management. The arrhythmias associated with prolonged Q-T interval are life threatening and must be treated. Cardiology evaluation for a cardioverter-defibrillator is recommended for patients with tachycardia-induced syncope. Affected members with periodic paralysis are responsive to oral potassium when potassium is lower than 3 mmol/L.

REFERENCES

1. Ogino S, Wilson RB. Genetic testing and risk assessment for spinal muscular atrophy. *Human Genetics.* 2002;111:477-500.
2. Prior TW, Finanger E. Spinal muscular atrophy. In: Adam MP, Ardinger HH, Pagon RA, et al., eds. *GeneReviews®.* University of Washington; 1993–2023. https://www.ncbi.nlm.nih.gov/books/NBK1352.
3. Swoboda KJ, Prior TW, Scott CB, et al. Natural history of denervation in SMA: relation to age, SMN2 copy number, and function. *Annals of Neurology.* 2005;57:704-712.
4. Navon R, Khosravi R, Melki J, et al. Juvenile-onset spinal muscular atrophy caused by compound heterozygosity for mutations in the HEXA gene. *Annals of Neurology.* 1997;41:631-638.
5. Abicht A, Müller JS, Lochmüller H. Congenital Myasthenic Syndromes Overview. In: Adam MP, Mirzaa GM, Pagon RA, et al., eds. *GeneReviews®.* University of Washington; 1993–2023. https://www.ncbi.nlm.nih.gov/books/NBK1168/. Updated December 23, 2021.
6. Harper CM, Fukodome T, Engel AG. Treatment of slow-channel congenital myasthenic syndrome with fluoxetine. *Neurology.* 2003:1710-1713.
7. Finlayason E, Spillane J, et al. Slow channel congenital myasthenic syndrome responsive to a combination of fluoxetine and salbutamol. *Muscle Nerve.* 2013;47(2):279-282.
8. Sugie K, Yamamoto A, Murayama K, et al. Clinicopathological features of genetically confirmed Danon disease. *Neurology.* 2002;58:1773-1778.
9. Birnkrant DJ, Bushby K, Bann CM, et al. Diagnosis and management of Duchenne muscular dystrophy, part 1: diagnosis, and neuromuscular, rehabilitation, endocrine, and gastrointestinal and nutritional management. *Lancet Neurology.* 2018;17(3):251-267.
10. Darras BT, Urion DK, Ghosh PS. Dystrophinopathies. 2000 Sep 5 [Updated 2022 Jan 20]. In: Adam MP, Mirzaa GM, Pagon RA, et al., eds. *GeneReviews®.* University of Washington; 1993–2023. https://www.ncbi.nlm.nih.gov/sites/books/NBK1119/.
11. Lemmers R, Miller DG, van der Maarel SM. Facioscapulohumeral muscular dystrophy. In: Adam MP, Ardinger HH, Pagon RA, et al., eds. *GeneReviews®.* University of Washington; 1993–2019. https://www.ncbi.nlm.nih.gov/books/NBK1443.
12. Chen TH, Wu YZ, Tseng YH. Early-onset infantile facioscapulohumeral muscular dystrophy: a timely review. *International Journal of Molecular Sciences.* 2020;21(20):7783. https://doi.org/10.3390/ijms21207783. PMID: 33096728; PMCID: PMC7589635.
13. Angelini C. Calpainopathy. 2005 May 10 [Updated 2022 Dec 1]. In: Adam MP, Mirzaa GM, Pagon RA, et al., eds. *GeneReviews®.* University of Washington; 1993–2023. https://www.ncbi.nlm.nih.gov/books/NBK1313/.
14. Aoki M, Takahashi T. Dysferlinopathy. 2004 Feb 5 [Updated 2021 May 27]. In: Adam MP, Mirzaa GM, Pagon RA, et al., eds. *GeneReviews®.* University of Washington; 1993–2023. https://www.ncbi.nlm.nih.gov/books/NBK1303/.
15. Soltanzadeh P. Myotonic dystrophies: a genetic overview. *Genes (Basel).* 2022;13(2):367. https://doi.org/10.3390/genes13020367. PMID: 35205411; PMCID: PMC8872148.
16. Iaccarino L, Ghiradello A, Bettio S, et al. The clinical features, diagnosis and classification of dermatomyositis. *Journal of Autoimmunity.* 2014;48-49:122-127.
17. Leslie N, Bailey L. Pompe disease. 2007 Aug 31 [Updated 2017 May 11]. In: Adam MP, Mirzaa GM, Pagon RA, et al., eds. *GeneReviews®.* University of Washington; 1993–2023. https://www.ncbi.nlm.nih.gov/books/NBK1261/.
18. El-Hattab AW. Systemic primary carnitine deficiency. In: Adam MP, Ardinger HH, Pagon RA, et al., eds. *GeneReviews®.* University of Washington; 1993–2019. https://www.ncbi.nlm.nih.gov/books/NBK84551.
19. El-Hattab AW. Systemic primary carnitine deficiency. 2012 Mar 15 [Updated 2016 Nov 3]. In: Adam MP, Mirzaa GM, Pagon RA, et al., eds. *GeneReviews®.* University of Washington; 1993–2023. https://www.ncbi.nlm.nih.gov/books/NBK84551/.
20. Lehky T, Grunseich C. Juvenile amyotrophic lateral sclerosis: a review. *Genes (Basel).* 2021;12(12):1935. https://doi.org/10.3390/genes12121935. PMID: 34946884; PMCID: PMC8701111.
21. Bird TD. Charcot-Marie-Tooth hereditary neuropathy overview. 1998 Sep 28 [Updated 2023 Feb 23]. In: Adam MP, Mirzaa GM, Pagon RA, et al., eds. *GeneReviews®.* University of Washington; 1993–2023. https://www.ncbi.nlm.nih.gov/books/NBK1358/.
22. Stavrou M, Sargiannidou I, Georgiou E, Kagiava A, Kleopa KA. Emerging therapies for Charcot-Marie-Tooth inherited neuropathies. *International Journal of Molecular Sciences.* 2021;22(11):6048. https://doi.org/10.3390/ijms22116048. PMID: 34205075; PMCID: PMC8199910.

23. Kuhlenbaumer G, Timmerman V, Bomont P. Giant axonal neuropathy. In: Adam MP, Ardinger HH, Pagon RA, et al., eds. *GeneReviews*®. University of Washington; 1993–2019. https://www.ncbi.nlm.nih.gov/books/NBK1136.

24. Gomez-Ospina N. Arylsulfatase A deficiency. In: Adam MP, Ardinger HH, Pagon RA, et al., eds. *GeneReviews*®. University of Washington; 1993–2019. https://www.ncbi.nlm.nih.gov/books/NBK1130.

25. Van Rappard DF, Boelens JJ, Wolf NI. Metachromatic leukodystrophy: disease spectrum and approaches for treatment. *Best Practice & Research Clinical Endocrinology & Metabolism*. 2015;29(2):261-273.

26. Saavedra-Matiz CA, Luzi P, Nichols M, et al. Expression of individual mutations and haplotypes in the galactocerebrosidase gene identified by the newborn screening program in New York State and in confirmed cases of Krabbe's disease. *Journal of Neuroscience Research*. 2016;94(11):1076-1083.

27. Saperstein DS, Amato AA, Barohn RJ. Clinical and genetic aspects of distal myopathies. *Muscle & Nerve*. 2001;24:1440-1450.

28. Savarese M, Sarparanta J, Vihola A, et al. Panorama of the distal myopathies. *Acta Myologica*. 2020;39(4):245-265. https://doi.org/10.36185/2532-1900-028. PMID: 33458580; PMCID: PMC7783427.

29. Bird TD. Myotonic dystrophy type I. In: Adam MP, Ardinger HH, Pagon RA, et al., eds. *GeneReviews*®. University of Washington; 1993–2019. https://www.ncbi.nlm.nih.gov/books/NBK1165.

30. Bonne G, Leturcq F, Ben Yaou R. Emery-Dreifuss muscular dystrophy. 2004 Sep 29 [Updated 2019 Aug 15]. In: Adam MP, Mirzaa GM, Pagon RA, et al., eds. *GeneReviews*®. University of Washington; 1993–2023. https://www.ncbi.nlm.nih.gov/books/NBK1436/.

31. Torricelli R. Acute muscular weakness in children. *Arquivos de Neuro-Psiquiatria*. 2017;75(4):248-254.

32. Paradiso G, Tripoli J, Galicchio S, et al. Epidemiological, clinical, and electrodiagnostic findings in childhood Guillain-Barre syndrome: a reappraisal. *Annals of Neurology*. 1999;46:701–707.

33. Hughes RAC, Wijdicks EFM, Barohn R, et al. Practice parameter: immunotherapy for Guillain-Barre syndrome. Report of the Quality Standards Committee of the American Academy of Neurology. *Neurology*. 2003;61:736-740.

34. Ryan MM, Grattan-Smith PJ, Procopis PG, et al. Childhood chronic inflammatory demyelinating polyneuropathy: clinical course and long-term outcome. *Neuromuscular Disorders*. 2000;10:398-406.

35. Van den Bergh PYK, van Doorn PA, Hadden RDM, et al. European Academy of Neurology/Peripheral Nerve Society guideline on diagnosis and treatment of chronic inflammatory demyelinating polyradiculoneuropathy: report of a joint Task Force-Second revision. *Journal of the Peripheral Nervous System*. 2021;26(3):242-268. https://doi.org/10.1111/jns.12455. Epub 2021 Jul 30. Erratum in: *Journal of the Peripheral Nervous System*. 2022;27(1):94. Erratum in: *European Journal of Neurology*. 2022;29(4):1288. PMID: 34085743.

36. Murphy OC, Messacar K, Benson L, AFM Working Group Acute flaccid myelitis: cause, diagnosis, and management. *Lancet*. 2021;397(10271):334-346. https://doi.org/10.1016/S0140-6736(20)32723-9. Epub 2020 Dec 23. PMID: 33357469; PMCID: PMC7909727.

37. Li J, Loeb JA, Shy ME, et al. Asymmetric flaccid paralysis: a neuromuscular presentation of West Nile virus infection. *Annals of Neurology*. 2003;53:703-710.

38. Davis LE, DeBiasi R, Goade DE, et al. West Nile virus neuroinvasive disease. *Annals of Neurology*. 2006;60:286-300.

39. Gray TJ, Webb CE. A review of the epidemiological and clinical aspects of West Nile virus. *International Journal of General Medicine*. 2014;7:193.

40. Moser LA, Lim PY, StyerL M, et al. Parameters of mosquito-enhanced West Nile virus infection. *Journal of Virology*. 2016;90(1):292-299.

41. Schussler E, Sobel J, Hsu J, et al. Workgroup report by the joint task force involving American Academy of Allergy, Asthma & Immunology (AAAAI); Food Allergy, Anaphylaxis, Dermatology and Drug Allergy (FADDA) (Adverse Reactions to Foods Committee and Adverse Reactions to Drugs, Biologicals, and Latex Committee); and the Centers for Disease Control and Prevention Botulism Clinical Treatment Guidelines Workgroup—allergic reactions to botulinum antitoxin: a systematic review. *Clinical Infectious Diseases*. 2017;66(suppl 1):S65-S72.

42. Vednarayanan VV, Evans OB, Subramony SH. Tick paralysis in children. Electrophysiology and possibility of misdiagnosis. *Neurology*. 2002;59:1088-1090.

43. Banwell BL, Mildner RJ, Hassall AC, et al. Muscle weakness in critically ill children. *Neurology*. 2003;61:1779-1782.

44. Weber F, Lehmann-Horn F. Hypokalemic periodic paralysis. 2002 Apr 30 [Updated 2018 Jul 26]. In: Adam MP, Mirzaa GM, Pagon RA, et al., eds. *GeneReviews*®. University of Washington; 1993–2023. https://www.ncbi.nlm.nih.gov/books/NBK1338/.

45. Weber F. Hyperkalemic periodic paralysis. 2003 Jul 18 [Updated 2021 Jul 1]. In: Adam MP, Mirzaa GM, Pagon RA, et al., eds. *GeneReviews*®. University of Washington; 1993–2023. https://www.ncbi.nlm.nih.gov/sites/books/NBK1496/.

46. Chinnery PF, Walls TJ, Hanna MG, et al. Normokalemic periodic paralysis revisited: does it really exist? *Annals of Neurology*. 2002;52:251-252.

47. Fu C, Wang Z, Chen J, Liu X. Familial normokalemic periodic paralysis associated with mutation in the SCN4A p. M1592V. *Frontiers in Neurology*. 2018;9:430.

48. Veerapandiyan A, Statland JM, Tawil R. Andersen-Tawil syndrome. In: Adam MP, Ardinger HH, Pagon RA, et al., eds. *GeneReviews*®. University of Washington; 2004. 1993–2018. www.geneclinics.org. Last updated 2018 Jun 7.

8

Cramps, Muscle Stiffness, and Exercise Intolerance

OUTLINE

Abnormal Muscle Activity, 237
  Continuous Motor Unit Activity, 237
  Myotonic Disorders, 238
  Systemic Disorders, 239
Decreased Muscle Energy, 240
  Clinical Features of Decreased Muscle
    Energy, 241
  Defects of Carbohydrate Utilization, 241
  Defects of Long-Chain Fatty Acid Metabolism, 242
  Mitochondrial (Respiratory Chain)
    Myopathies, 243

Adenosine Monophosphate Deaminase Deficiency
  (Myoadenylate Deaminase Deficiency), 244
Myopathic Stiffness and Cramps, 244
  Brody Myopathy, 245
  Tubular Aggregate Myopathies, 245
  Familial X-Linked Myalgia and Cramps, 245
  Malignant Hyperthermia, 246
  Neuroleptic Malignant Syndrome, 246
  Rigid Spine Syndrome, 246
  Rippling Muscle Disease (Caveolinopathies), 247
References, 247

A cramp is an involuntary painful contraction of a muscle or part of a muscle. Cramps can occur in normal children during or after vigorous exercise, and after excessive loss of fluid or electrolytes. The characteristic electromyography (EMG) finding for such cramps is the repetitive firing of normal motor unit potentials. Stretching the muscle relieves the cramp. Partially denervated muscle is particularly susceptible to cramping not only during exercise but also during sleep. Night cramps may awaken patients with neuronopathies, neuropathies, or root compressions. Cramps during exercise occur also in patients with several different disorders of muscle energy metabolism. The EMG characteristic of these cramps is electrical silence.

Muscle stiffness and spasms are not cramps but are actually prolonged contractions of several muscles that are able to impose postures. Such contractions may or may not be painful. When painful, they lack the explosive character of cramps. Prolonged contractions occur when muscles fail to relax (myotonia) or when motor unit activity is continuous (Box 8.1). Prolonged, painless muscle contractions occur also in dystonia and other movement disorders (see Chapter 14).

Many normal children, especially preadolescent boys, complain of pain in their legs at night and sometimes during the day, especially after a period of increased activity. These pains are not true cramps. The muscle is not in spasm, the pain is diffuse, and aching in quality, and the discomfort lasts for an hour or longer. Stretching the muscle does not relieve the pain. This is not a symptom of neuromuscular disease and is called *growing pains*, for want of better understanding. One-third of the cases are associated with abdominal pain or headaches, which suggests a common ground with migraines.[1] Mild analgesics or heat relieve symptoms.

Exercise intolerance is a relative term for an inability to maintain exercise at an expected level. The causes of exercise intolerance considered in this chapter are fatigue and muscle pain. Fatigue is a normal consequence of exercise and occurs in everyone at some level of activity. In general, weak children become fatigued more quickly than children who have normal strength. Many children with exercise intolerance and cramps, but no permanent weakness, have a defect in an enzyme needed to produce energy for muscular contraction (Box 8.2). A known mechanism underlies several such

BOX 8.1 Diseases With Abnormal Muscle Activity

- Continuous motor unit activity
  - Neuromyotonia
  - Paroxysmal ataxia and myokymia (see Chapter 10)
  - Schwartz-Jampel syndrome
  - Stiff person syndrome
  - Thyrotoxicosis[a]
- Cramps-fasciculation syndrome
- Myotonia
  - Myotonia congenita
  - Myotonia fluctuans
- Systemic disorders
  - Hypoadrenalism[a]
  - Hypocalcemia[a] (tetany)
  - Hypothyroidism[a]
  - Strychnine poisoning[a]
  - Uremia[a]

[a]Denotes the most common conditions and the ones with disease-modifying treatments.

BOX 8.2 Diseases With Decreased Muscle Energy

- Defects of carbohydrate utilization
  - Lactate dehydrogenase deficiency
  - Myophosphorylase deficiency
  - Phosphofructokinase deficiency
  - Phosphoglycerate kinase deficiency
  - Phosphoglycerate mutase deficiency
- Defects of fatty acid oxidation
  - Carnitine palmitoyltransferase 2 deficiency
  - Very-long-chain acyl-coenzyme A dehydrogenase deficiency
- Mitochondrial (respiratory chain) myopathies
- Myoadenylate deaminase deficiency

BOX 8.3 Electromyography in Muscle Stiffness

Normal Between Cramps[a]
- Brody myopathy
- Defects of carbohydrate metabolism
- Defects of lipid metabolism
- Mitochondrial myopathies
- Myoadenylate deaminase deficiency
- Rippling muscle disease
- Tubular aggregates

Silent Cramps
- Brody disease
- Defects of carbohydrate metabolism
- Rippling muscle disease
- Tubular aggregates

Continuous Motor Activity
- Neuromyotonia
- Myotonia
- Myotonia congenita
- Myotonic dystrophy
- Schwartz-Jampel syndrome
- Stiff person syndrome

Myopathy
- Emery-Dreifuss muscular dystrophy
- Rigid spine syndrome
- X-linked myalgia

[a]Or may be myopathic.

with decreased energy for muscle contraction, and myopathies. As a rule, the first and third groups are symptomatic at all times, whereas the second group is symptomatic only with exercise. The first group usually requires EMG for diagnosis. EMG is the initial diagnostic test in children with muscle stiffness that is not due to spasticity or rigidity and often leads to the correct diagnosis (Box 8.3).

ABNORMAL MUSCLE ACTIVITY

Continuous Motor Unit Activity

The cause of continuous motor unit activity (CMUA) is the uncontrolled release of acetylcholine (ACh) packets at the neuromuscular junction. The EMG features of CMUA are repetitive muscle action potentials in response to a single nerve stimulus; high-frequency bursts of motor unit potentials of normal morphology abruptly start and

inborn errors of metabolism. However, even when the full spectrum of biochemical and genetic tests is available, identification of a metabolic defect is not possible in some children with cramps during exercise.

Myasthenia gravis is a disorder characterized by fatigability and exercise intolerance but is not covered in this chapter because the usual initial symptoms are either isolated cranial nerve disturbances (see Chapter 15) or limb weakness (see Chapters 6 and 7).

Conditions that produce some combination of cramps and exercise intolerance are divided into three groups: diseases with abnormal muscle activity, diseases

---

---

stop. Rhythmic firing of doublets, triplets, and multiplets occurs. During long bursts the potentials decline in amplitude. This activity is difficult to distinguish from normal voluntary activity. CMUA occurs in a heterogeneous group of disorders characterized clinically by some combination of muscle pain, fasciculations, myokymia, contractures, and cramps (Box 8.4).

The primary defect in CMUA disorder may reside within the spinal cord (stiff person syndrome) or the peripheral nerve (neuromyotonia). The original name for neuromyotonia is *Isaac syndrome*. These disorders may be sporadic or familial in occurrence. When familial, the usual mode of transmission is autosomal dominant inheritance.

Neuromyotonia

The primary abnormality in neuromyotonia (or *nondystrophic myotonia*) is the decreased outward potassium current of voltage-gated potassium channel function. Most childhood cases are sporadic in occurrence, but some show a pattern of autosomal dominant inheritance. An autoimmune process directed against the potassium channel may account for some sporadic cases. Some cases may be paraneoplastic, but this is rarely the case in children.

Clinical features. Unlike myotonic dystrophy, progressive weakness does not occur. The clinical triad for neuromyotonia includes involuntary muscle twitching (fasciculations or myokymia), muscle cramps or stiffness, and myotonia. Excessive sweating is frequently associated with muscle stiffness. The age at onset is any time from birth to adult life.

The initial features are muscle twitching and cramps brought on by exercise. Later these symptoms occur also at rest and even during sleep. The cramps may affect only distal muscles, causing painful posturing of the hands and feet. As a rule, leg weakness is greater than arm weakness. These disorders are not progressive and do not lead to permanent disability, although they may cause transient difficulty with walking and coordination of motor tasks. Rarely, myotonia may be associated with excessive salivation, hallucinations, chorea, or personality changes. In such cases the disorder is termed *Morvan syndrome*.

In some children cramps and fasciculations are not as prominent as stiffness, which causes abnormal limb posturing associated frequently with excessive sweating. Leg involvement is more common than arm involvement, and the symptoms suggest dystonia (see Chapter 14). Limb posturing may begin in one foot and remain asymmetric for months. Most cases are sporadic.

Muscle mass, muscle strength, and tendon reflexes are normal. Fasciculations are sporadic and seen only after prolonged observation.

Diagnosis. Some adult-onset cases are associated with malignancy, but this is virtually never the case in children. Muscle fibers fire repetitively at a rate of 100–300 Hz, either continuously or in recurring bursts, producing a pinging sound. The discharge continues during sleep and persists after procaine nerve block.

A significant portion of patients have antibodies to voltage-gated potassium channels. There is a known association with thymoma; perform testing for ACh receptor antibodies if thymoma is suspected. Hereditary cases exist, but causative genes are not yet known.

Management. Carbamazepine and phenytoin, at usual anticonvulsant doses, are both effective in reducing or abolishing symptoms. Intravenous immunoglobulin and plasmapheresis may be an option for patients with known autoimmune causes.[2]

Myotonic Disorders
Myotonia Congenita

Myotonia congenita is a genetic disorder characterized by episodic muscle stiffness and hypertrophy. Weakness does not typically occur, but stiffness may impair muscle function. The disease can be transmitted as either an autosomal dominant (*Thomsen disease*) or autosomal recessive (*Becker disease*) trait with considerable overlap of clinical features. Pathogenic heterozygous or biallelic pathogenic variants in the *CLCN1* chloride channel gene underlie all cases. It is often not possible to tell the mode of inheritance based solely on the child's genetic testing.[3]

Clinical features. Age of onset is variable. In the dominant form age at onset is usually in infancy or early childhood; in the recessive form the age of onset is slightly older, but both may begin in adult life. The autosomal recessive form of myotonia congenita is often more severe than the dominant form. Individuals with the recessive form may have mild, progressive, distal weakness, and transitory attacks of weakness induced by movement after rest.

Clinical features of the dominant form are stereotyped. After resting, muscles are stiff and difficult to move. With activity, the stiffness disappears, and movement may be normal (the "warm-up" effect). One of our patients played Little League baseball and could not sit while he was waiting to bat for fear that he would be unable to get up. Myotonia may cause generalized muscle hypertrophy, giving the infant a Herculean appearance. The tongue, face, and jaw muscles are sometimes involved. Cold exposure exacerbates stiffness, which is painless. Percussion myotonia is present. Strength and tendon reflexes are normal.

Diagnosis. EMG and molecular genetic testing establish the diagnosis. Repetitive discharges at rates of 20–80 cycles/s are recorded when the needle is first inserted into the muscle and again on voluntary contraction. Two types of discharges occur: a biphasic spike potential of less than 5 ms and a positive wave of less than 50 ms. The waxing and waning of the amplitude and frequency of potentials produces a characteristic sound (dive-bomber). Dystrophy is not present. The serum concentration of creatine kinase (CK) may be normal to moderately elevated, and muscle biopsy specimens do not contain necrotic fibers. Genetic testing reveals pathogenic variants in *CLCN1*.

Management. Myotonia does not always require treatment, but if it is needed, mexiletine is the most effective drug.

Myotonia Fluctuans

Myotonia fluctuans is a distinct disorder caused by mutations of the muscle sodium channel gene *SCN4A*.[4] Transmission is by autosomal dominant inheritance. Allelic disorders with overlapping clinical phenotypes include hyperkalemic periodic paralysis and paramyotonia congenita.

Clinical features. The onset of stiffness is usually in the second decade and worsens with exercise or potassium ingestion. Cramps in the toes, fingers, and eyelids, especially when tired or cold, begin in childhood.

Physical examination reveals mild myotonia affecting the trunk, limbs, and extraocular muscles but normal strength. The severity of myotonia fluctuates on a day-by-day basis. "Warming up" usually relieves symptoms, but exercise may also worsen symptoms. A bad day may follow a day of exercise or potassium ingestion, but neither precipitant causes immediate worsening of myotonia. Cooling does not trigger or worsen myotonia.

Diagnosis. EMG shows myotonia and a mild reduction in the amplitude of compound muscle action potential on cooling and administration of potassium. Molecular genetic testing reveals heterozygous pathogenic variants in *SCN4A*.

Management. Daily use of mexiletine or acetazolamide may relieve the stiffness.[5]

Systemic Disorders

Hypoadrenalism

A small percentage of patients with Addison disease complain of cramps and pain in their truncal muscles. At times, paroxysmal cramps occur in the lower torso and legs and cause the patient to double up in pain. Hormone replacement relieves the symptoms.

Hypocalcemia and Hypomagnesemia

Tetany caused by a dietary deficiency of calcium is rare in modern times, except in newborns fed cows' milk. Hypocalcemic tetany is more likely to result from hypoparathyroidism or hyperventilation-induced alkalosis.

The initial symptom of tetany is tingling around the mouth and in the hands and feet. With time the tingling increases in intensity and becomes generalized. Spasms in the muscles of the face, hands, and feet follow. The hands assume a typical posture in which the fingers extend, the wrists flex, and the thumb abducts. Fasciculations and laryngeal spasms may be present. Percussion of the facial nerve, either just anterior to the ear or over the cheek, produces contraction of the muscles innervated by that branch of the nerve (*Chvostek sign*).

A similar syndrome occurs with magnesium deficiency. In addition to tetany encephalopathy occurs. Restoring the proper concentration of serum electrolytes relieves the cramps associated with hypocalcemia and hypomagnesemia.

Thyroid Disease

Myalgia, cramps, and stiffness are the initial features in up to half of patients with hypothyroidism. Stiffness is worse in the morning, especially on cold days, and the probable cause is the slowing of muscular contraction and relaxation. This is different from myotonia, in which only relaxation is affected. Indeed, activity worsens the stiffness of hypothyroidism, which may be painful, whereas activity relieves myotonia and is painless. The slowing of muscular contraction and relaxation is sometimes demonstrated when tendon reflexes are tested. The response tends to "hang up."

Percussion of a muscle produces a localized knot of contraction called myoedema. This localized contraction lasts for up to 1 minute before slowly relaxing.

Myokymia, CMUA of the face, tongue, and limbs, and muscle cramps develop occasionally in patients with thyrotoxicosis. Restoring the euthyroid state reverses all the neuromuscular symptoms of hypothyroidism and hyperthyroidism.

Uremia

Uremia is a known cause of polyneuropathy (see Chapter 7). However, 50% of patients complain of nocturnal leg cramps and flexion cramps of the hands even before clinical evidence of polyneuropathy is present. Excessive use of diuretics may be the triggering factor. Muscle cramps occur also in approximately one-third of patients undergoing hemodialysis. Monitoring with EMG during dialysis documents a buildup of spontaneous discharges. After several hours, usually toward the end of dialysis treatment, repetitive high-voltage discharges occur associated with clinical cramps. Because standard dialysis fluid is slightly hypotonic, many nephrologists have attempted to treat the cramps by administering hypertonic solutions. Either sodium chloride or glucose solutions relieve cramps in most patients. The cramps apparently result from either extracellular volume contraction or hypoosmolarity. Similar cramps occur in children with severe diarrhea or vomiting.

DECREASED MUSCLE ENERGY

Three sources for replenishing adenosine triphosphate (ATP) during exercise are available: the phosphorylation of adenosine diphosphate (ADP) to ATP by phosphocreatine (PCr) within the exercising muscles; glycogen and lipids within the exercising muscles; and glucose and triglycerides brought to the exercising muscles by the blood. A fourth and less efficient source

derives from ADP via an alternate pathway using adenylate kinase and deaminase. PCr stores are the main source that replenishes ATP during intense activity of short duration. During the first 30 seconds of intense endurance exercise, PCr decreases by 35% and muscle glycogen stores reduce by 25%. Exercise lasting longer than 30 seconds is associated with the mobilization of substantial amounts of carbohydrates and lipids.

The breakdown of muscle glycogen (glycogenolysis) and the anaerobic metabolism of glucose to pyruvate (glycolysis) provide the energy to sustain a prolonged contraction (Fig. 8.1). Anaerobic glycolysis is an inefficient mechanism for producing energy and is not satisfactory for endurance exercise. Endurance requires further aerobic metabolism in the mitochondria of pyruvate generated in muscle by glycolysis. Oxidative metabolism provides high levels of energy for every molecule of glucose metabolized (see Fig. 8.1).

The central compound of oxidative metabolism in mitochondria is acetyl-coenzyme A (acetyl-CoA). Acetyl-CoA derives from pyruvate, fatty acids, and amino acids. When exercise is prolonged, fatty acids become an important substrate to maintain muscular contraction. Oxidation of acetyl-CoA is through the

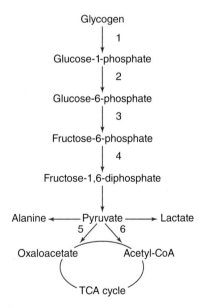

Fig. 8.1 Glycogen Metabolism. *(1)* Myophosphorylase initiates glycogen breakdown; *(2)* phosphoglucomutase; *(3)* phosphoglucose isomerase; *(4)* phosphofructokinase; *(5)* pyruvate carboxylase; and *(6)* pyruvate dehydrogenase complex.

Krebs cycle. Hydrogen-ion release reduces nicotinamide adenine dinucleotide. These reduced compounds then enter a sequence of oxidation-reduction steps in the respiratory chain, which liberates energy. Energy is stored as ATP. This process of releasing and storing energy is *oxidation-phosphorylation coupling*. Disorders that prevent the delivery of glucose or fatty acids, prevent the oxidation process in the mitochondria, or prevent the creation of ATP can all impair the production of energy for muscular contraction.

Clinical Features of Decreased Muscle Energy

Exercise intolerance is the invariable result of any disturbance in the biochemical pathways that support muscle contraction. The common symptom is fatigue. Other symptoms are myalgia and cramps. Muscle pain is the expected outcome of unaccustomed exercise. Muscle pain develops during exercise when the mechanisms to supply energy for contraction are impaired.

The ischemic exercise test was historically the first step in the diagnosis of muscle energy disorders, but it is rarely used now due to the ease of genetic testing, tissue diagnosis by muscle biopsy, and the commercial availability of methods for measuring enzyme activity in fibroblasts.

Defects of Carbohydrate Utilization
Myophosphorylase Deficiency (McArdle Disease, Glycogen Storage Disease Type V)

Myophosphorylase deficiency exists in two forms: phosphorylase-a is the active form and phosphorylase-b is the inactive form. Phosphorylase-b kinase is the enzyme that converts the inactive form to the active form and is itself activated by a protein kinase. Deficiencies of either enzyme result in exercise intolerance.

Genetic transmission of myophosphorylase deficiency is the result of a mutation in the *PYGM* gene. The defective myophosphorylase enzyme fails to break down glycogen into glucose-1-phosphate, which is the first step in transforming glycogen into glucose. The muscle then has insufficient energy, at least until additional sources of glucose can be mobilized (the "second wind" effect). Myophosphorylase is found only in muscle. Liver phosphorylase concentrations are normal, and hypoglycemia does not occur.

Clinical features. The severity of symptoms varies with the percentage of enzyme activity. Children with only mild deficiency have few or no symptoms until adolescence. Aching becomes increasingly prominent and then, after an episode of vigorous exercise, severe cramps occur in the exercised muscles. Myoglobinuria is sometimes present. The pain can last for hours. Thereafter, exercise leads to repeated bouts of cramps that cause a decline in the overall level of activity. Pain begins soon after initiating vigorous exercise, and myoglobinuria is present several hours later. Some patients exercise through the pain by slowing down just before the time of fatigue. Once passing that point, exercise may continue unimpeded. This "second wind" phenomenon is probably due to an increase in cardiac output, the use of blood glucose and free fatty acids as a substrate for muscle metabolism, and the recruitment of more motor units.

Muscle mass, muscle strength, and tendon reflexes are usually normal. Only adult patients develop weakness, and even then, the tendon reflexes are normal.

An alternate presentation of myophosphorylase deficiency is a slowly progressive proximal weakness beginning during childhood or adult life. Affected individuals may never complain of cramps during exercise or of myoglobinuria. Tendon reflexes are present until late in the course of disease.

Diagnosis. EMG examination is usually normal. The serum concentration of CK is elevated, and myoglobin may appear in the urine coincidentally with the cramps.

Salient features of muscle biopsy specimens are histochemical evidence of subsarcolemmal vacuoles containing glycogen and the absence of phosphorylase. Muscle fiber degeneration and regeneration are present immediately after an episode of cramps and myoglobinuria. Definitive diagnosis requires the biochemical demonstration of decreased myophosphorylase activity or confirmatory genetic testing.

Management. Creatine supplementation may increase muscle function.[6] Moderate aerobic conditioning improves exercise capacity.[7] Ingestion of oral sucrose 30–40 minutes before aerobic exercise may also improve exercise tolerance.[8] Patients usually learn to live with their disorder by controlling their level of exercise.

Other Disorders of Glucose Utilization

Four other enzyme deficiencies associated with the anaerobic glycolysis of carbohydrates produce a syndrome identical to myophosphorylase deficiency, that is, cramps on exercise and myoglobinuria (see Fig. 8.1).

They are muscle phosphofructokinase (PFK) deficiency (glycogen storage disease type VII, Tarui disease), muscle phosphoglycerate kinase (PGK) deficiency (glycogen storage disease type IX), muscle phosphoglycerate mutase deficiency (glycogen storage disease type X), and lactate dehydrogenase deficiency (glycogen storage disease type XI). All are autosomal recessive traits except phosphoglycerate kinase deficiency, which is an X-linked trait. PFK deficiency is the most common member of this group and also causes infantile hypotonia (see Chapter 6). Attacks may be associated with nausea, vomiting, and muscle pain. The mutase deficiency occurs mainly in people with African ancestry.

Muscle biopsy results show subsarcolemmal collections of glycogen, but the histochemical reaction for phosphorylase is normal. Biochemical analysis correctly identifies the disorders.

Defects of Long-Chain Fatty Acid Metabolism

Long-chain fatty acids are the principal lipids oxidized to produce acetyl-CoA.

Carnitine Palmitoyltransferase 2 Deficiency

The mitochondrial oxidation of fatty acids is the main source of energy for muscles during prolonged exercise and fasting. The carnitine palmitoyltransferase (CPT) enzyme system is essential for the transfer of fatty acids across the mitochondrial membrane. This system includes CPT-1 in the outer mitochondrial membrane and CPT-2 and carnitine-acylcarnitine translocase in the inner mitochondrial membrane.

CPT-2 deficiency is an autosomal recessive trait with three main phenotypes: the lethal neonatal form, the severe infantile hepatocardiomuscular form, and the myopathic form, which we discuss here. Exercise intolerance with myoglobinuria characterizes the myopathic form, which is the least severe phenotype of CPT-2 deficiency of muscle. CPT-2 deficiency is the most common disorder of lipid metabolism affecting skeletal muscle.[9]

Clinical features. Age at onset of symptoms ranges from 1 year to adult life. In 70% the disease starts by age 12 years, and in most of the rest between 13 and 22 years. Performing heavy exercise for a short duration poses no difficulty. However, pain, tenderness, and swelling of muscles develop after sustained aerobic exercise. Severe muscle cramps, as in myophosphorylase

deficiency, do not occur. Associated with the pain may be actual muscle injury characterized by an increased serum concentration of CK and myoglobinuria. Muscle injury may also accompany periods of prolonged fasting, especially in patients on low-carbohydrate, high-fat diets.

In the interval between attacks results of muscle examination, serum concentration of CK, and EMG are usually normal. People with CPT-2 deficiency are at risk for malignant hyperthermia (MH).

Diagnosis. The clinical features suggest the diagnosis. Molecular genetic testing reveals biallelic pathogenic variants in the *CPT2* gene, and measuring the concentration of CPT-2 in muscle provides confirmation. Muscle histology is usually normal between attacks.

Management. Frequent carbohydrate feedings and the avoidance of prolonged aerobic activity minimize muscle destruction.

Very-Long-Chain Acyl-Coenzyme A Dehydrogenase Deficiency

The chain length of their preferred substrates describes four mitochondrial acyl-CoA dehydrogenases: short, medium, long, and very long (very-long-chain acyl-CoA dehydrogenase [VLCAD]). The first three are located in the mitochondrial matrix, and deficiency causes recurrent coma (see Chapter 2). VLCAD is bound to the inner mitochondrial membrane, and deficiency causes exercise-induced myoglobinuria in the later-onset myopathic form.[10] There is also a severe, early-onset form associated with cardiomyopathy and a hypoglycemic form of VLCAD deficiency, which are not discussed here.

Clinical features. Onset is usually in the second decade but can be as early as 4 years. Pain and myoglobinuria occur during or following prolonged exercise or fasting. Weakness may be profound. Carbohydrate ingestion before or during exercise reduces the intensity of pain. Examination between attacks is normal.

Diagnosis. The serum CK concentration is slightly elevated between attacks and increases further at the time of myoglobinuria. EMG is consistent with myopathy, and muscle biopsy shows lipid storage in type I fibers. Plasma-free fatty acids, but not ketones, increase during a 24-hour fast, suggesting impaired ketogenesis.

Management. Frequent small carbohydrate feeds, dietary fat restriction, and carnitine supplementation reduce the frequency of attacks.

Mitochondrial (Respiratory Chain) Myopathies

The respiratory chain, located in the inner mitochondrial membrane, consists of five protein complexes: complex I (NADH-coenzyme Q reductase); complex II (succinate-coenzyme Q reductase); complex III (reduced coenzyme Q-cytochrome c reductase); complex IV (cytochrome c oxidase); and complex V (ATP synthase) (Fig. 8.2).

Coenzyme Q is a shuttle between complexes I and II and complex III. The clinical syndromes associated with mitochondrial disorders are continually expanding and revised. The organs affected are those highly dependent on aerobic metabolism: nervous system, skeletal muscle, heart, and kidney (Box 8.5). Exercise intolerance, either alone or in combination with symptoms of other organ failure, is a common feature of mitochondrial disorders. Some of the more common mitochondrial myopathies include Kearns-Sayre syndrome, myoclonic epilepsy with ragged-red fibers, and mitochondrial encephalomyopathy with lactic acidosis and stroke. The several clinical syndromes defined do not correspond exactly with any one of the respiratory complexes (Box 8.6).

Clinical features. The age at which mitochondrial myopathies begin ranges from birth to adult life but occurs before 20 years in most patients. The symptomatology varies, but most patients will have exercise intolerance, ptosis, or ophthalmoplegia. Weakness, cardiac disturbances, vomiting, seizures, and encephalopathy may be present.

Exercise intolerance usually develops by 10 years of age. With ordinary activity, active muscles become tight, weak, and painful. Cramps and myoglobinuria are unusual but may occur. Nausea, headache, and breathlessness are sometimes associated features. During these

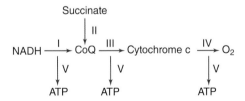

Fig. 8.2 Respiratory complexes: complex I (NADH: coenzyme Q reductase); complex II (succinate-coenzyme Q reductase); complex III (reduced coenzyme Q: cytochrome c reductase); complex IV (cytochrome c oxidase); and complex V (ATP synthase). *ATP*, Adenosine triphosphate; *NADH*, nicotinamide adenine dinucleotide (hydrogen).

BOX 8.5   Clinical Features of Mitochondrial Disease

Nervous System
- Ataxia
- Central apnea
- Cognitive impairment
- Deafness-sensorineural[a]
- Dementia
- Dystonia
- Hypotonia[a]
- Migraine-like headaches
- Neuropathy-sensorimotor
- Ophthalmoplegia[a]
- Optic atrophy
- Polyneuropathy
- Retinitis pigmentosa
- Seizures
- Spinal muscular atrophy

Heart
- Cardiomyopathy
- Conduction defects

Kidney
- Aminoaciduria
- Hyperphosphaturia

Skeletal Muscle
- Exercise intolerance
- Myopathy[a]

[a]Denotes the most common conditions and the ones with disease-modifying treatments.

---

episodes, the serum concentration of lactate and CK may increase. Generalized weakness with ptosis and ophthalmoplegia may follow prolonged periods of activity or fasting. Such symptoms may last for several days, but recovery is usually complete.

Diagnosis. Mitochondrial myopathy is a consideration in all children with exercise intolerance and ptosis or ophthalmoplegia. This combination of symptoms may also suggest myasthenia gravis. However, in myasthenia the ocular motor features fluctuate, whereas in mitochondrial myopathies they are constant.

Some children with mitochondrial myopathies have an increased concentration of serum lactate after exercise. Previously clinicians utilized the glucose-lactate tolerance test. During an ordinary oral glucose tolerance test, lactate and glucose concentrations are measured simultaneously. In some children with mitochondrial

BOX 8.6 Mitochondrial Disorders

Complex I (NADH: Coenzyme Q Reductase)
- Congenital lactic acidosis, hypotonia, seizures, and apnea
- Exercise intolerance and myalgia
- Kearns-Sayre syndrome (see Chapter 15)
- Metabolic encephalopathy, lactic acidosis, and stroke (see Chapter 11)
- Progressive infantile poliodystrophy (see Chapter 5)
- Subacute necrotizing encephalomyelopathy (see Chapter 5)

Complex II (Succinate: Coenzyme Q Reductase)
- Encephalomyopathy

Complex III (Coenzyme Q: Cytochrome c Reductase)
- Cardiomyopathy
- Kearns-Sayre syndrome (see Chapter 15)
- Myopathy and exercise intolerance with or without progressive external ophthalmoplegia

Complex IV (Cytochrome c Oxidase)
- Menkes syndrome (see Chapter 5)
- Myoclonus epilepsy and ragged-red fibers
- Progressive infantile poliodystrophy (see Chapter 5)
- Subacute necrotizing encephalomyelopathy (see Chapter 5)
- Transitory neonatal hypotonia (see Chapter 6)

Complex V (Adenosine Triphosphate Synthase)
- Congenital myopathy
- Neuropathy, retinopathy, ataxia, and dementia
- Retinitis pigmentosa, ataxia, neuropathy, and dementia

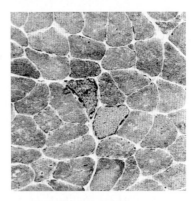

Fig. 8.3 Ragged-Red Fibers (Trichrome Stain). The mitochondria are enlarged and stain intensely with hematoxylin.

Adenosine Monophosphate Deaminase Deficiency (Myoadenylate Deaminase Deficiency)

Adenosine monophosphate (AMP) deaminase deficiency is caused by mutations in the *AMPD1* gene. Deficiency of AMP deaminase is clearly a familial trait, and the mode of inheritance is autosomal recessive. The deficiency state occurs in infants with hypotonia, in children with progressive myopathies and recurrent rhabdomyolysis, in children and adults with exercise intolerance, and asymptomatic individuals. Establishing a cause-and-effect relationship between AMP deaminase deficiency and exercise intolerance in any particular individual is often difficult because most people in the deficiency state are asymptomatic.

Clinical features. The typical history is one of intermittent muscle pain and weakness with exercise. The pain varies from a diffuse aching to a severe cramping type associated with muscle tenderness and swelling. Between attacks, the children are normal. Symptoms last for 1–20 years, with a mean duration of less than 9 years.

Diagnosis. During attacks, the serum concentration of CK may be normal or markedly elevated. EMG and muscle histological studies are usually normal. There is a genetic testing registry for the disease.

Management. Treatment is not available and often is not needed.

disorders lactic acidosis develops and glucose is slow to clear. We no longer use this test as it may precipitate a crisis in children with severe mitochondrial disease.

Muscle biopsy specimens, taken from a weak muscle, show a clumping of the mitochondria, which become red when the Gomori trichrome stain is applied (Fig. 8.3). These muscle cells are *ragged-red fibers*. Commercial laboratories can identify several specific respiratory complex disturbances.

Management. The following supplements are worth trying but often fail to provide benefits: coenzyme Q 10–20 mg/kg/day, riboflavin 100 mg/day, pyridoxine 30 mg/kg/day, biotin 5–20 mg/kg/day, and carnitine 50–100 mg/kg/day.

MYOPATHIC STIFFNESS AND CRAMPS

This section deals with several conditions that cause muscle stiffness or cramps, or both, in which the primary abnormality is thought to be in skeletal muscle.

Brody Myopathy

Brody myopathy is a rare, likely underdiagnosed muscle disease caused by a mutation in the *ATP2A1* gene that encodes the fast-twitch skeletal muscle calcium-activated ATPase in the sarcoplasmic reticulum.[11]

Clinical features. The main clinical feature is difficult relaxation after contraction. EMG supports the diagnosis. Symptoms of exercise-induced stiffness and cramping begin in the first decade, but weakness does not occur, and many patients are actually quite athletic. Muscles of the legs, arms, and face (particularly eyelids) are most often involved, and myoglobinuria may be present. Muscle strength and tendon reflexes are normal. As with many other neuromuscular disorders, patients are at risk of malignant hyperthermia (see the "Malignant Hyperthermia" section).[12]

Diagnosis. Muscle histology reveals type II atrophy. Establishing the diagnosis requires showing the biochemical defect.

Management. Dantrolene, which reduces the myofibrillar Ca^{2+} concentration by blocking Ca^{2+} release from the sarcoplasmic reticulum, provides symptomatic relief for some patients. Verapamil may also be useful.

Tubular Aggregate Myopathies

Tubular aggregates are abnormal double-walled structures that originate from the sarcoplasmic reticulum and are located in a subsarcolemmal position (Fig. 8.4). Aggregates appear in the muscle biopsy specimens of patients with several neuromuscular disorders. In some families patients have a progressive myopathy, while others only experience cramps or myalgia.

Clinical features. Because tubular aggregate myopathies are heterogeneous, the presentation varies widely. The most prevalent symptoms include myalgias and limb weakness, followed by cramps, fatiguability, and muscle stiffness. Cold weather exacerbates cramps, which are often worse at night and may interfere with sleep. Pupillary changes, dysphagia, and dysarthria are less common, occurring in approximately 5% of patients.[13]

Diagnosis. Several causative genetic changes have been identified, which may be autosomal dominant or autosomal recessive. In a significant portion of cases a genetic cause is never identified. CK may be normal but is often elevated. Myoglobinuria is rare but has been reported in some cases. EMG may be normal or show myopathic changes. Muscle histology results are the basis for a diagnosis. Light and electron microscopic

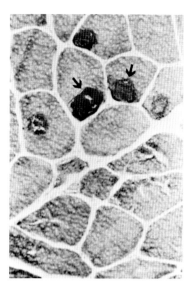

Fig. 8.4 Tubular Aggregates (ATPase Reaction). Dark material is present beneath the sarcolemma in type I and type II fibers (*arrows*). *ATPase*, Adenosine triphosphatase.

examinations show tubular aggregates in type II fibers. Evidence of glycogen or lipid storage is not present.

Management. The cramps typically do not respond to medication.

Familial X-Linked Myalgia and Cramps

Familial X-linked myalgia and cramps are another phenotype associated with a decreased amount of skeletal muscle dystrophin, which is usually associated with Becker muscular dystrophy (see Chapter 7). Almost all cases are male,[14] except for one female who also had hypertrophy of the calves.[15] Half of the males and one female showed a deletion in the dystrophin gene.

Clinical features. Symptoms begin in early childhood, frequently between 4 and 6 years. The boys first have cramps with exercise and then cramps at rest. Usually the limb muscles are affected, but chest pain may occur as well. The cramping continues throughout life but is not associated with atrophy or weakness. Tendon reflexes are normal.

Diagnosis. Affected family members have elevated concentrations of serum CK, especially after exercise. The EMG and muscle biopsy are usually normal or show only mild, nonspecific changes. This disorder and the McLeod phenotype (acanthocytosis, elevated serum concentration of CK, and absence of the Kell antigen) are allelic conditions. EMG and muscle specimens show nonspecific myopathic changes. DNA analysis may be normal or may show a deletion in the first third of the dystrophin gene or exons 45–52.

Management. Pharmaceutical agents do not relieve the cramps. Exercise avoidance is the only way to avoid cramping.

Malignant Hyperthermia

MH is a disorder of calcium regulation in skeletal muscle that causes uncontrolled muscle hypermetabolism. Transmission is autosomal dominant; however, many families are unaware they carry the trait until one family member experiences a crisis in response to anesthesia. Mutations in the skeletal muscle ryanodine receptor are the main cause, leading to the release of calcium from the sarcoplasmic reticulum, glycogenolysis, and increased cellular metabolism when exposed to a triggering substance. Pathogenic heterozygous variants in *RYR1*, *CACNA1S*, and *STAC3* cause the disorder.[16] Several neuromuscular disorders, such as CPT-2, muscular dystrophy, and central core disease, predispose to the syndrome. The administration of several inhalation anesthetics or succinylcholine triggers attacks of muscular rigidity and necrosis associated with a rapid rise in body temperature. Nonanesthetic triggers of rhabdomyolysis in susceptible persons include strenuous exercise in hot conditions, neuroleptic drugs, alcohol, and infections.

Clinical features. The first symptoms are tachycardia, tachypnea, muscle fasciculations, and increasing muscle tone. Body temperature rises dramatically, as much as 2°C per hour. All muscles become rigid, a progressive and severe metabolic acidosis develops, and seizures and death follow. *Prompt recognition and treatment are vital.*

Diagnosis. MH is typically diagnosed after it occurs as an adverse event in the operating room or during the immediate postoperative period. The basis for diagnosis is the response to anesthesia or succinylcholine. The serum concentration of CK rises to 10 times the upper limit of normal. Molecular diagnosis is available; some institutions are also able to perform a muscle contraction test in which biopsied muscle fibers are exposed to halothane or caffeine and the amount of muscle contraction is measured.

Management. Treatment includes termination of anesthesia, body cooling, treatment of metabolic acidosis, and intravenous injection of dantrolene, 1–2 mg/kg repeated every 5–10 minutes up to a total dose of 10 mg/kg. Avoid causative agents including volatile anesthetics and succinylcholine; exercise is permissible, but patients should avoid extreme heat.

Neuroleptic Malignant Syndrome

Neuroleptic malignant syndrome, like MH, is a disorder of the skeletal muscle calcium channels.

Clinical features. Several neuroleptic agents may induce an idiosyncratic response characterized by muscle rigidity, hyperthermia, altered states of consciousness, and autonomic dysfunction in susceptible individuals. Implicated agents include phenothiazines, butyrophenones, and thioxanthenes. Persons of all ages are affected, but young males predominate. Symptoms develop over 1–3 days. The first symptoms are rigidity and akinesia, followed by fever, excessive sweating, urinary incontinence, and hypertension. Consciousness fluctuates, and the 20% mortality rate is due to respiratory failure.

Diagnosis. The clinical findings are the basis of diagnosis. The only helpful laboratory test results are an increased serum concentration of CK and leukocytosis.

Management. The offending neuroleptic agent must be promptly withdrawn, and general supportive care provided. Bromocriptine reverses the syndrome completely.

Rigid Spine Syndrome

Rigid spine syndrome is now recognized as the severe classic form of multiminicore myopathy,[17] and has been linked to mutations in the *SEPN1* gene.[18] Multiminicore myopathy is divisible into four groups: the classic form comprises 75% of the total, and the other three (moderate form with hand involvement, antenatal form with arthrogyposis, and the ophthalmoplegic form) each comprise less than 10%. The classic form is usually perinatal and characterized by neonatal hypotonia, delayed motor development, axial muscle weakness, scoliosis, and significant respiratory depression. Spinal rigidity of varying severity is present.

Clinical features. Marked limitations in flexion of the dorsolumbar and cervical spine begin in infancy or early childhood secondary to contractures in the spinal extensors. Movement of the spine and the thoracic cage is lost. Extension of the elbow and ankles may be limited. The condition is not progressive, but scoliosis often leads to respiratory failure.

Diagnosis. The presence of multiple "minicores" visible on a muscle biopsy using oxidative stains is the traditional basis for diagnosis. Genetic testing for *SEPN1* mutations is available.

Management. Management is symptomatic.

Rippling Muscle Disease (Caveolinopathies)

Caveolin is a muscle-specific membrane protein.[19] Disorders of caveolin produce several different phenotypes within the same family. One is *rippling muscle disease* in which mechanical stimulation of muscle produces electrically silent contractions. Transmission of the disorder is by autosomal dominant inheritance. Autosomal dominant limb-girdle muscular dystrophy type 1C, as well as some cases of isolated hyperCKemia and isolated hypertrophic cardiomyopathy, are allelic disorders.[20]

Clinical features. Frequent falls are the initial feature in children with the caveolin-3 gene mutation. Other features include muscle pain and cramps following exercise that persists for several hours. Stiffness occurs during rest after the child exercises or maintains posture for long periods. Percussion of muscles causes local swelling and a peculiar rippling movement that lasts for 10–20 seconds. Muscle hypertrophy develops. Muscle strength, tone, and coordination, as well as tendon reflexes, are normal.

Diagnosis. The serum CK concentration is mildly elevated, and muscle biopsy findings are normal. EMG of the muscle swelling after percussion shows no electrical activity. Molecular genetic diagnosis confirms the diagnosis.

Management. Management is symptomatic.

REFERENCES

1. Abu-Arafeh I, Russell G. Recurrent limb pain in schoolchildren. *Archives of Disease in Childhood.* 1996;74:336-339.
2. Van den Berg JSP, et al. Acquired neuromyotonia: superiority of plasma exchange over high-dose intravenous human immunoglobulin. *Journal of Neurology.* 1999;246(7):623-625.
3. Dunø M, Vissing J. Myotonia Congenita. (August 3, 2005). In: Adam MP, Mirzaa GM, Pagon RA, et al., eds. *GeneReviews®.* University of Washington; 1993–2023. https://www.ncbi.nlm.nih.gov/books/NBK1355/. Updated February 25, 2021.
4. Colding-Jorgensen E, Dunø M, Vissing J. Autosomal dominant monosymptomatic myotonia permanens. *Neurology.* 2006;67:153-155.
5. Meola G, Hanna MG, Fontaine B. Diagnosis and new treatment in muscle channelopathies. *Journal of Neurology, Neurosurgery, and Psychiatry.* 2009;80:360-365.
6. Vorgerd M, Zange J, Kley R, et al. Effect of high-dose creatine therapy on symptoms of exercise intolerance in McArdle disease. *Archives of Neurology.* 2002;59:97-101.
7. Haller RG, Wyrick P, Taivassalo T, et al. Aerobic conditioning: an effective therapy in McArdle's disease. *Annals of Neurology.* 2006;59:922-928.
8. Vissing J, Haller R. The effect of oral sucrose on exercise tolerance in patients with McArdle's disease. *New England Journal of Medicine.* 2003;349:2503-2509.
9. Wieser T. Carnitine palmitoyltransferase II deficiency. (August 27, 2004). In: Adam MP, Mirzaa GM, Pagon RA, et al., eds. *GeneReviews®.* University of Washington; 1993–2023. https://www.ncbi.nlm.nih.gov/books/NBK1253/. Updated January 3, 2019.
10. Gregersen N, Andresen BS, Corydon MJ, et al. Mutation analysis in mitochondrial fatty acid oxidation defects: exemplified by acyl-CoA dehydrogenase deficiencies, with special focus on genotype-phenotype relationship. *Human Mutatation.* 2001;18:169-189.
11. Odermatt A, Taschner PEM, Scherer SW, et al. Characterization of the gene encoding human sarcolipin (SLN), a proteolipid associated with SERCA1: absence of structural mutations in five patients with Brody disease. *Genomics.* 1997;45:541-553.
12. Molenaar JP, Verhoeven JI, Rodenburg RJ, et al. Clinical, morphological and genetic characterization of Brody disease: an international study of 40 patients. *Brain.* 2020;143(2):452-466. https://doi.org/10.1093/brain/awz410. PMID: 32040565; PMCID: PMC7009512.
13. Gang Q, Bettencourt C, Brady S, et al. Genetic defects are common in myopathies with tubular aggregates. *Annals of Clinical and Translational Neurology.* 2022;9(1):4-15. https://doi.org/10.1002/acn3.51477. Epub 2021 Dec 15. PMID: 34908252; PMCID: PMC8791796.
14. Samaha FJ, Quinlan JG. Myalgia and cramps: dystrophinopathy with wide-ranging laboratory findings. *Journal of Child Neurology.* 1996;11:21-24.
15. Malapart D, Recan D, Leturcq F, et al. Sporadic lower limb hypertrophy, and exercise induced myalgia in a woman with dystrophin gene deletion. *Journal of Neurology, Neurosurgery, and Psychiatry.* 1995;59:552-554.
16. Rosenberg H, Sambuughin N, Riazi S, et al. Malignant hyperthermia susceptibility. (December 19, 2003). In: Adam MP, Mirzaa GM, Pagon RA, et al., eds. *GeneReviews®.* University of Washington; 1993–2023. https://www.ncbi.nlm.nih.gov/books/NBK1146/. Updated January 16, 2020.

17. Beggs AH, Agrawal PB. Multiminicore disease. In: Adam MP, Ardinger HH, Pagon RA, et al., eds. *GeneReviews®*. University of Washington; 1993–2019. https://www.ncbi.nlm.nih.gov/books/NBK1290.

18. Moghadaszadeh B, Petit N, Jaillard C. Mutations in SEPN1 cause congenital muscular dystrophy with spinal rigidity and restrictive respiratory syndrome. *Nature Genetics*. 2001;29:17-18.

19. Bruno C, Sotgia F, Gazzerro E, et al. Caveolinopathies. In: Adam MP, Ardinger HH, Pagon RA, et al., eds. *GeneReviews®*. University of Washington; 1993–2019. https://www.ncbi.nlm.nih.gov/books/NBK1385.

20. Schara U, Vorgerd M, Popovic N, et al. Rippling muscle disease in children. *Journal of Child Neurology*. 2002;17:483-490.

Sensory and Autonomic Disturbances

OUTLINE

Sensory Symptoms, 249
Painful Limb Syndromes, 250
   Complex Regional Pain Syndrome I, 250
   SCN9A Neuropathic Pain Syndromes, 251
Familial Episodic Pain Syndromes, 252
Central Congenital Insensitivity To Pain, 252
Hereditary Sensory and Autonomic
   Neuropathies, 252
   Hereditary Sensory and Autonomic Neuropathy
      Type I, 252
   Hereditary Sensory and Autonomic Neuropathy
      Type II, 253
   Hereditary Sensory and Autonomic Neuropathy
      Type III, 253

Hereditary Sensory and Autonomic Neuropathy
   Type IV (Congenital Insensitivity to Pain With
   Anhidrosis), 253
Hereditary Sensory and Autonomic Neuropathy
   Type V, 254
Metabolic Neuropathies, 254
   Acute Intermittent Porphyria, 254
   Hereditary Tyrosinemia Type I, 255
Spinal Disorders, 255
   Foramen Magnum Tumors, 255
   Lumbar Disk Herniation, 255
   Syringomyelia, 256
Thalamic Pain, 257
References, 257

This chapter deals primarily with sensory disturbances of the limbs and trunk. Autonomic dysfunction is often associated with sensory loss but sometimes occurs alone. Chapter 17 considers sensory disturbances of the face.

SENSORY SYMPTOMS

Pain, dysesthesias, and loss of sensibility are the important symptoms of disturbed sensation. Peripheral neuropathy is the most common cause of disturbed sensation at any age. As a rule, hereditary neuropathies are more likely to cause loss of sensibility without discomfort, whereas acquired neuropathies are more likely to be painful. Discomfort is more likely than numbness to bring a patient to medical attention.

Nerve root pain generally follows a dermatomal distribution. Ordinarily it is described as deep and aching. The pain is more proximal than distal and may be constant or intermittent. When intermittent, the pain may radiate in a dermatomal distribution. The most common cause of root pain in adults is sciatica associated with lumbar disk disease. Disk disease also occurs in adolescents, usually because of trauma. In children radiculitis is a more common cause of root pain. Examples of radiculitis are the migratory aching of a limb preceding paralysis in the acute inflammatory demyelinating polyradiculoneuropathy/Guillain-Barré syndrome (see Chapter 7), and the radiating pain in a C5 distribution that heralds an idiopathic brachial neuritis (see Chapter 13).

Polyneuropathy involving small nerve fibers causes dysesthetic pain. This pain differs from previously experienced discomfort and is described as pins and needles, tingling, or burning. It compares with the abnormal sensation felt when dental anesthesia is wearing off. The discomfort is superficial, distal, and usually symmetric.

Loss of sensibility is the sole initial feature in children with sensory neuropathy. Because of the associated

TABLE 9.1   Patterns of Sensory Loss

Pattern	Site
All limbs	Spinal cord or peripheral nerve
Both legs	Spinal cord or peripheral nerve
Glove-and-stocking	Peripheral nerve
Legs and trunk	Spinal cord
One arm	Plexus
One leg	Plexus or spinal cord
Unilateral arm and leg	Brain or spinal cord

BOX 9.1   Disturbances of Sensation

- Brachial neuritis
  - Neuralgic amyotrophy (see Chapter 13)
  - Recurrent familial brachial neuropathy (see Chapter 13)
- Complex regional pain syndrome I (reflex sympathetic dystrophy)
- Congenital insensitivity (indifference) to pain
  - Lesch-Nyhan syndrome
  - Hereditary sensory and autonomic neuropathy Type IV (HSAN IV)
  - Central congenital insensitivity to pain
- Foramen magnum tumors
- Hereditary metabolic neuropathies
  - Acute intermittent porphyria
  - Hereditary tyrosinemia
- HSAN
  - HSAN I
  - HSAN II
  - HSAN III (familial dysautonomia)
  - HSAN IV (with anhidrosis)
- Lumbar disk herniation
- Syringomyelia
- Thalamic syndromes

clumsiness, delay in establishing a correct diagnosis is common. Strength and tests of cerebellar function are normal and tendon reflexes are absent. The combination of areflexia and clumsiness should suggest a sensory neuropathy.

Table 9.1 summarizes the pattern of sensory loss as a guide to the anatomical site of abnormality and Box 9.1 lists a differential diagnosis of conditions with sensory deficits.

PAINFUL LIMB SYNDROMES

Three painful arm syndromes are as follows: acute idiopathic brachial neuritis (also called neuralgic amyotrophy or brachial plexitis), familial recurrent brachial neuritis, and complex regional pain syndrome (CRPS) (reflex sympathetic dystrophy [RSD]). In the first two syndromes muscle atrophy follows a transitory pain in the shoulder or arm. Monoplegia is the prominent feature (see Chapter 13). Although muscle atrophy also occurs in CRPS, pain is the prominent feature. A discussion of CRPS follows.

Complex Regional Pain Syndrome I

The presence of regional pain and sensory changes following a noxious event defines CRPS. A working group of the International Association for the Study of Pain developed a new terminology that separates RSD from causalgia.[1] CRPS I replaced the term RSD; CRPS 2 replaced the term causalgia. The differentiating feature is the presence of definite nerve injury, which is absent in CPRS I but present in CPRS 2.

The definition of CRPS I is defined as "a pain syndrome that develops after an injury, is not limited to the distribution of a single peripheral nerve, and is disproportional to the inciting event." Although CPRS can occur in children and adolescents, it is most common in adults and has a female preponderance. Surgery, minor trauma, and fractures are common inciting events.

Clinical features. The essential feature of CRPS I is sustained burning pain in a limb combined with vasomotor and sudomotor dysfunction, leading to atrophic changes in skin, muscle, and bone following trauma. The pain is of greater severity than expected for the inciting injury. The mechanism remains a debated issue. Catecholamine hypersensitivity may account for the decreased sympathetic outflow and autonomic features in the affected limb.[2] There is a decrease in C-type and A-delta-type fibers in the affected limb, possibly due to imperceptible nerve injury at the time of the inciting event, with a subsequent increase in aberrant nociceptive fibers that are thought to function improperly.[3] The central and peripheral nervous systems demonstrate an enhanced response to pain and perpetuate the symptoms. Genetic and psychological factors likely play a role.

The mean age at onset in children is 11 years, and girls are more often affected than boys. CRPS I frequently follows trauma to one limb, with or without fracture. The trauma may be relatively minor, and the clinical syndrome is so unusual that a diagnosis of "hysteria" or "malingering" is common. Time until onset after injury is usually within 1 or 2 months, but the average interval from injury to diagnosis is 1 year.

The first symptom is pain at the site of injury, which progresses either proximally or distally without regard for dermatomal distribution or anatomical landmarks. Generalized swelling and vasomotor disturbances of the limb occur in 80% of children. Pain is intense, described as burning or aching, and is out of proportion to the injury. It may be maximally severe at onset or may become progressively worse for 3–6 months. Movement or dependence exacerbates the pain, causing the patient to hold the arm in a position of abduction and internal rotation as if swaddled to the body. The hand becomes swollen and hyperesthetic and feels warmer than normal.

Children with CRPS I do better than adults. Reported outcomes vary widely, probably based on the standard of diagnosis. In our experience most begin recovering within 6–12 months. Long-term pain is unusual, as are the trophic changes of the skin and bones that often occur in adults. Recovery is usually complete, and recurrence is unusual.

Diagnosis. The basis for diagnosis is the clinical features; laboratory tests are not confirmatory. Because the syndrome follows accidental or surgical trauma, litigation is commonplace and requires careful documentation of the clinical features examination. In recent years CRPS I has become a popular topic online and is often self-diagnosed incorrectly by patients with other types of chronic pain syndromes or conversion disorders.

One simple test is to immerse the affected limb in warm water. Wrinkling of the skin of the fingers or toes requires intact sympathetic innervation. The absence of wrinkling is evidence of a lesion in either the central or the peripheral sympathetic pathway. The other unaffected limb serves as a control. Note that while this is an adjunctive test, it does not necessarily prove or disprove the diagnosis.

Management. Utilize a multidisciplinary approach. Physical therapy and activity are vital to recovery. Because the limb is painful, there is a strong temptation to limit use; however, disuse further reduces blood flow and exacerbates muscle atrophy, joint contractures, and trophic changes. Nonsteroidal antiinflammatory drugs are standard and may reduce ongoing inflammation. More severe cases may benefit from steroids, gabapentin, or pregabalin. Adrenergic receptor antagonists or alpha-2 receptor agonists (phenoxybenzamine, clonidine) may be useful in managing sympathetically mediated pain. Calcium channel blockade with nifedipine can decrease vasoconstriction. Sympathectomy, implanted neurostimulators, transcranial magnetic stimulation (tMS), and intrathecal infusions can be considered for refractory cases. Many patients develop secondary psychological complications including anxiety, depression, and posttraumatic stress disorder. These conditions can further heighten pain awareness and worsen functioning. Treatment with counseling and selective serotonin reuptake inhibitors (SSRIs) is often required.

SCN9A Neuropathic Pain Syndromes

The *SCN9A* pain syndromes comprise three distinct disorders: erythromelalgia (EM), paroxysmal extreme pain disorder (PEPD), and small fiber neuropathy (SFN). *SCN9A*-associated SFN is an adult-onset disorder and will not be discussed here.

Clinical features. Erythromelalgia. EM is characterized by recurrent episodes of bilateral burning pain, usually in the feet, sometimes associated with redness, warmth, and swelling. Severe cases may involve the hands, face, and ears. Triggers include spicy foods, alcohol, exposure to heat, and prolonged standing.

Paroxysmal extreme pain disorder. PEPD presents in infancy with mainly autonomic symptoms including harlequin skin change, skin flushing, nonepileptic episodes of tonic stiffening, and syncope with bradycardia. Older children describe episodes of severe, deep pain involving the eyes, rectum, and submandibular region, usually associated with skin flushing. Cold wind, strong emotion, eating, and defecation can all trigger attacks.

Diagnosis. Molecular genetic testing reveals a heterozygous pathogenic variant of the *SCN9A* gene. Multigene panels for peripheral neuropathy and single-gene testing are available.[4]

Management. EM and PEPD both respond to carbamazepine, although relief of symptoms may be incomplete. PEPD may also respond to lamotrigine, topiramate, and valproic acid. Avoid triggers as much as possible. For EM, cooling the extremities provides relief. Patients with PEPD should be on a bowel regimen to avoid straining and worsening pain with defecation.

FAMILIAL EPISODIC PAIN SYNDROMES

There are at least four distinct subtypes of familial episodic pain syndromes, of which FEPS3 is by far the most common. All subtypes are the result of cation channel mutations affecting the dorsal root ganglion. FEPS3 is an autosomal dominant disorder caused by pathogenic changes in the *SCN11A* gene; the other subtypes are due to mutations in *TRPA1* (FEPS1), *SCN10A* (FEPS2), and *SCN9A* (FEPS4).

Clinical features. Episodic pain attacks beginning in infancy or early childhood characterize all the FEPS subtypes. Attacks typically involve the distal extremities and are difficult to identify in affected infants who may simply cry excessively. As children grow older, they are better able to describe their symptoms. Attacks often occur at night, involve both muscles and joints, and have no clear trigger.[5] Episodes last anywhere from minutes to hours and may occur several times per week, sometimes in conjunction with autonomic changes such as hyperhidrosis, tachycardia, and breathing difficulty. Although the pain is significant, motor skills are intact between episodes. Attacks may lessen or even stop with age.[6]

Diagnosis. Inflammatory markers are not elevated, and rheumatologic workup is negative. Imaging studies of the affected limbs are usually normal but may show small nonspecific joint effusions. Skin biopsy may be normal or have variable findings depending on the FEPS subtype. Molecular genetic testing confirms the diagnosis.

Management. The usual antiinflammatory pain medications are ineffective. Nonselective sodium channel blockers such as carbamazepine, mexiletine, and lidocaine are helpful in some patients.

CENTRAL CONGENITAL INSENSITIVITY TO PAIN

At least seven distinct genetic mutations lead to the phenotype of congenital insensitivity to pain. All the implicated mutations cause either failure of nociceptor development or nociceptors that are present but nonfunctional. Inheritance may be autosomal dominant or autosomal recessive, and there is some overlap with the hereditary sensory and autonomic neuropathies (HSANs), discussed here. The classification of such disorders is expected to evolve over time as we gain a greater understanding of their etiologies. Of note,

Lesch-Nyhan syndrome is a specific metabolic disorder characterized by self-mutilation and intellectual disability without evidence of sensory neuropathy (see Chapter 5).

Clinical features. Children with congenital insensitivity to pain come to medical attention when they begin to crawl or walk, or when they begin to inflict injuries on their lips or fingers while teething. Their parents recognize that injuries do not cause crying and that the children fail to learn the potential of injury from experience. The result is repeated bruising, fractures, ulcerations of the fingers and toes, and mutilation of the tongue. Sunburn and frostbite are common. Intellectual disability may or may not be present, depending on the underlying genetic change. Many children experience poor wound healing, anhidrosis, or reduced tear production. Some have increased susceptibility to *Staphylococcus aureus* infections.

Examination shows the absence of the corneal reflex and insensitivity to pain and temperature, but relative preservation of touch and vibration sensations. Tendon reflexes are present, an important differential point from sensory neuropathy.

Diagnosis. Molecular genetic testing is available.

Management. No treatment is available for the underlying insensitivity, but repeated injuries require supportive care. Injuries and recurrent infections reduce longevity and can lead to significant disability.

HEREDITARY SENSORY AND AUTONOMIC NEUROPATHIES

The classification of HSAN attempts to synthesize information based on natural history, mode of inheritance, and electrophysiological characteristics.

Hereditary Sensory and Autonomic Neuropathy Type I

HSAN I has subtypes HSAN1A-HSAN1E depending on the causative genetic mutation.

Clinical features. The clinical features and age at onset vary depending on the subtype but often begin in the second decade or later. The major clinical features are lancinating pains in the legs and ulcerations of the feet. However, initial symptoms are usually insidious, and the precise onset is often difficult to date. A callus develops on the sole of the foot, usually in the skin overlying a weight-bearing bony prominence. The callus blackens, becomes necrotic, and breaks down into an ulcer that is difficult to heal. Sensory loss precedes the ulcer, but often it is the ulcer, and not the sensory loss, that first brings the patient to medical attention. Although plantar ulcers are an important feature, they are not essential for diagnosis. When the proband has typical features of plantar ulcers and lancinating pain, other family members may have sensory loss in the feet, mild pes cavus, or peroneal atrophy, and loss of the ankle tendon reflex.

Sensory loss in the hands is variable and never as severe as in the feet. Finger ulcers do not occur. Distal muscle weakness and wasting are present in all advanced cases.

Diagnosis. Molecular genetic testing is available.

Electrophysiological studies show the slowing of sensory nerve conduction velocity and the absence of sensory nerve action potentials. Sural nerve biopsy reveals a marked decrease or absence of myelinated fibers and a mild-to-moderate reduction of small myelinated fibers.

Management. No treatment is available for the neuropathy, but good foot care prevents plantar ulcers. Patients must avoid tight-fitting shoes and activities that traumatize the feet and discontinue weight-bearing at the first sign of a plantar ulcer. Much of the foot mutilation reported in previous years was due to secondary infection of the ulcers. Warm soaks, elevation, and antibiotics prevent infection from mutilating the foot.

Hereditary Sensory and Autonomic Neuropathy Type II

HSAN II is transmitted by autosomal recessive inheritance and involves mutations in one of four genes: *KIF1A, RETREG1, SCN9A,* or *WNK1.*[7]

Clinical features. Symptoms probably begin during infancy and possibly at the time of birth. Infantile hypotonia is common (see Chapter 6). The distal extremities and feet are affected first, but sensory loss may spread with time. The result is a diffuse loss of all sensation; diminished touch and pressure are probably earlier and greater in extent than temperature and pain. Affected infants and children are constantly hurting themselves without a painful response. The absence of the protection that pain provides against injury results in ulcerations and infections of the fingers and toes, stress fractures, and injuries to long bones. Loss of deep sensibility causes injury and swelling of joints, and loss of

touch makes simple tasks, such as tying shoes, manipulating small objects, and buttoning buttons, difficult if not impossible. Tendon reflexes are absent throughout. Patients exhibit varying degrees of autonomic dysfunction including slow pupillary light reflexes, hyperhidrosis, and urinary incontinence.

Diagnosis. EMG demonstrates variably reduced compound muscle action potentials, and nerve conduction studies show reduced or absent sensory nerve potentials. Molecular genetic testing confirms the diagnosis.

Management. No treatment is available for the neuropathy. Parents must be vigilant for painless injuries. Discoloration of the skin and swelling of joints or limbs should raise the possibility of fracture. Children must learn to avoid activities that might cause injury and to examine themselves for signs of superficial infection.

Hereditary Sensory and Autonomic Neuropathy Type III

The usual name for HSAN III is *familial dysautonomia* or *the Riley-Day syndrome.* This disorder is present at birth. Cardinal features are hypotonia, feeding difficulties, and poor control of autonomic function. It occurs almost exclusively in patients with Jewish Ashkenazi ancestry and is associated with an absence of fungiform papillae on the tongue. A mutation in the gene encoding an IjB kinase complex-associated protein (*IKBKAP* mutation) is present in this condition. Because neonatal hypotonia is the most common presenting feature, this disorder is addressed more comprehensively in Chapter 6.

Hereditary Sensory and Autonomic Neuropathy Type IV (Congenital Insensitivity to Pain With Anhidrosis)

Genetic transmission of HSAN IV is by autosomal recessive inheritance. The abnormal gene site is 1q21-22.[8] Several point mutations in the nerve growth factor 1 receptor gene (*TRKA1*) have been associated with the clinical phenotype of HSAN IV. The major features are congenital insensitivity to pain, anhidrosis, and intellectual disability. All the clinical abnormalities are present at birth, and while complications of the pain-free state are a continuous problem, the underlying disease may not be progressive.

Clinical features. Anhidrosis, rather than insensitivity to pain, causes the initial symptoms. Patients with HSAN

IV frequently have bowel problems, recurrent syncope, and crises of hyperthermia. Affected infants have repeated episodes of fever, sometimes associated with seizures. These episodes usually occur during the summer; the cause is an inability to sweat in response to exogenous heat. Sweat glands are present in the skin but lack sympathetic innervation. Most infants are hypotonic and areflexic. Attainment of developmental milestones is slow, and, by 2 or 3 years of age, the child has had several self-inflicted injuries caused by pain insensitivity. Injuries may include ulcers of the fingers and toes, stress fractures, self-mutilation of the tongue, and Charcot joints.

Sensory examination shows widespread absence of pain and temperature sensation. Touch, vibration, and stereognosis are intact in some patients. Tendon reflexes are absent or hypoactive. The cranial nerves are intact and the corneal reflex and lacrimation are normal. Mild-to-moderate intellectual disability is present in almost every case. Other features, present in some children, are blond hair and fair skin, Horner syndrome, and aplasia of dental enamel.

Diagnosis. Familial dysautonomias, HSAN III, and HSAN IV have many features in common and are easily confused. However, insensitivity to pain is not prominent in HSAN III, and fungiform papillae of the tongue are present in HSAN IV. Molecular genetic testing is available for the disorders.

Management. No treatment is available for the underlying disease. Constant vigilance is required to prevent injuries to the skin and bones with secondary infection.

Hereditary Sensory and Autonomic Neuropathy Type V

This rare disorder is characterized by decreased numbers of small-diameter neurons in peripheral nerves and manifested by the absence of thermal and mechanical pain perception. Genetic studies show the role of nerve growth factor beta, which is also involved in the development of the autonomic nervous system and cholinergic pathways in the brain. HSAN V is not usually reported to cause intellectual disability or cognitive decline.

Clinical features. HSAN V is the least frequent of all the HSANs. It is characterized by a loss of thermal and mechanical pain perception and various milder autonomic dysfunctions. Anhidrosis is less marked than in patients with HSAN IV, along with an absence of the sympathetic skin response in nerve studies.

Both recessive and dominant modes of inheritance are possible for this condition. It was found to be associated with a mutation in the nerve growth factor beta gene (*NGFB*) in a Swedish family[9] and with a mutation in the neurotrophic tyrosine kinase receptor type 1 (*NTRK1*) in another report.[10]

Diagnosis. The diagnosis relies on the history and the absence of sympathetic skin responses. Molecular genetic testing is available.

Management. No treatment is available for the underlying disease. Constant vigilance is required to prevent injuries to the skin and bones with secondary infection.

METABOLIC NEUROPATHIES

Acute Intermittent Porphyria

Acute intermittent porphyria is an autosomal dominant disorder that results from an error in pyrrole metabolism due to a deficiency of porphobilinogen (PBG) deaminase. The gene location is 11q23.3, which encodes the *HMBS* gene. Individuals with similar degrees of enzyme deficiency may have considerable variation in phenotypic expression.[11]

Clinical features. Approximately 90% of individuals with acute intermittent porphyria never have clinical symptoms. Onset is rarely before puberty. Symptoms are periodic and occur at irregular intervals. Alterations in hormonal levels during a normal menstrual cycle or pregnancy, and exposure to certain drugs, especially barbiturates, trigger attacks. The most common clinical feature of acute intermittent porphyria is an attack of severe abdominal pain, often associated with vomiting, constipation, or diarrhea. Tachycardia, hypertension, and fever may be associated. Limb pain is common, and muscle weakness often develops. The weakness is a result of a motor neuropathy that causes greater weakness in proximal than distal muscles and in the arms more than the legs. Tendon reflexes are usually decreased and may be absent in weak muscles. Approximately half of the patients have cerebral dysfunction; mental status changes are particularly common, and seizures may occur. Chronic psychiatric symptoms, such as depression and anxiety, sometimes continue even between attacks.

Diagnosis. Suspect acute intermittent porphyria in people with acute or episodic neurological or psychiatric disturbances. Increased excretion of aminolevulinic acid and PBG occurs during attacks, but levels may be normal between attacks. The risk of attacks correlates with the excretion of PBG in the urine when the patient is free of symptoms. Molecular genetic diagnosis is definitive.

Management. The most important aspect of managing symptomatic disease is to prevent acute attacks by avoiding known precipitating factors. During an attack patients frequently require hospitalization because of severe pain. Carbohydrates are believed to reduce porphyrin synthesis and should be administered intravenously daily at a dose of 300–500 g as a 10% dextrose solution. Reports of benefits from hematin infusions, a specific feedback inhibitor of heme synthesis, are in the literature. However, hematin is neither readily available nor very soluble and may carry a risk of renal damage.

Hereditary Tyrosinemia Type I

Hereditary tyrosinemia type I is caused by deficiency of the enzyme fumarylacetoacetate hydrolase encoded by the *FAH* gene. Transmission of the genetic trait is by autosomal recessive inheritance and the gene map locus is 15q23-q25.

Clinical features. The major features are acute and chronic liver failure and renal Fanconi syndrome. However, recurrent attacks of painful dysesthesias or paralysis are a prominent feature of the disease in half of children. The attacks usually begin at 1 year of age and infection precedes the attack in half of the cases. Perhaps because of the child's age, pain localization is poor and referred to the legs and lower abdomen. Associated with the pain is axial hypertonicity that ranges in severity from mild neck stiffness to opisthotonos. Generalized weakness occurs in 30% of attacks and may necessitate respiratory support. Less common features of attacks are seizures and self-mutilation. Between attacks, the child appears normal.

Diagnosis. The basis for diagnosis is an increased blood concentration of tyrosine and a deficiency of fumarylacetoacetate hydrolase; many states include the disorder on neonatal screening tests. Molecular genetic testing confirms the diagnosis.

Management. A diet that restricts tyrosine and phenylalanine should be instituted as soon as possible. Nitisinone (Orfadin), 2-(2-nitro-4-trifluoro-methyl-benzyol)-1,3 cyclohexanedione, which blocks *p*-hydroxyphenylpyruvic acid dioxygenase, the second step in the tyrosine degradation pathway, prevents the accumulation of fumarylacetoacetate and its conversion to

succinylacetone.[12] Liver transplantation is the definitive treatment.

SPINAL DISORDERS

Foramen Magnum Tumors

Extramedullary tumors in and around the foramen magnum are known for false localizing signs and for mimicking other disorders, especially syringomyelia and multiple sclerosis. In children neurofibroma caused by neurofibromatosis is the only tumor found in this location.

Clinical features. The most common initial symptom is unilateral or bilateral dysesthesias of the fingers. Suboccipital or neck pain occurs as well. Ignoring such symptoms is common early in the course. Numbness and tingling usually begin in one hand and then migrate to the other. Dysesthesias in the feet are a late occurrence. Gait disturbances, incoordination of the hands, and bladder disturbances generally follow the sensory symptoms and are so alarming that they prompt medical consultation.

Many patients have café au lait spots, but few have evidence of subcutaneous neuromas. The distribution of weakness may be one arm, one side, or both legs; 25% of patients have weakness in all limbs. Atrophy of the hands is uncommon. Sensory loss may involve only one segment or may have a "cape" distribution. Diminished pain and temperature sensations are usual and other sensory disturbances may be present. Tendon reflexes are brisk in the arms and legs. Patients with neurofibromatosis may have multiple neurofibromas causing segmental abnormalities in several levels of the spinal cord.

Diagnosis. Magnetic resonance imaging (MRI) is the best method for showing abnormalities at the foramen magnum.

Management. Surgical excision of a C2 root neurofibroma relieves symptoms.

Lumbar Disk Herniation

Trauma is the usual cause of lumbar disk herniation in children. Almost all cases occur after age 10 years. They are more common in boys than in girls and are frequently sports related. Delays in diagnosis are commonplace because lumbar disk herniation is so unusual in children.

Clinical features. The initial features are pain and inability to function normally because of decreased range of motion, and discomfort in the back. Straight leg raising and bending forward from the waist are impaired. Frequently the pain has been present for a long time because most children will accommodate their disability. Examination reveals diminished sensation to pinprick in the distribution of the L5 and S1 dermatome and diminished or absent ankle tendon reflexes in more than half of patients.

Diagnosis. Radiographs of the lumbosacral spine reveal minor congenital anomalies (hemivertebra, sacralization of the lumbar spine) in an unusually large number of cases. MRI of the spine confirms the diagnosis.

Management. Rest and antiinflammatories provide relief in most patients. The indication for surgical treatment is pain that persists and limits function in spite of adequate medical measures.

Syringomyelia

Syringomyelia is a generic term for a fluid-filled cavity within the substance of the spinal cord. The cavity varies in length and may extend into the brainstem. A brainstem extension is termed *syringobulbia*. The cavity, or syrinx, is central in the gray matter and may enlarge in all directions. The cervicothoracic region is a favorite site, but the thoracolumbar syrinx also occurs, and occasionally a syrinx extends from the brainstem to the conus medullaris.

The mechanism of syrinx formation is uncertain. Cavitation of the spinal cord sometimes follows trauma and infarction, but these are not important mechanisms of syringomyelia in children. In childhood the cause of primary syringomyelia is either a congenital malformation (particularly associated with Chiari I malformation) or a cystic astrocytoma. Astrocytomas of the spinal cord, like those of the cerebellum, may have large cysts with only a nubbin of solid tumors. MRI has greatly enhanced the antemortem diagnosis of cystic astrocytoma by showing small areas of increased signal intensity in one or more portions of the cyst. Cystic astrocytoma is more likely to produce symptoms during the first decade, whereas congenital syringomyelia becomes symptomatic in the second decade or later and is usually associated with the Chiari anomaly. Chapters 12 and 13 consider cystic astrocytoma of the spinal cord; this section deals primarily with congenital syringomyelia.

Clinical features. The initial symptoms of syringomyelia depend on the cyst's location. Because the cavity is near the central canal, it first affects crossing fibers subserving pain and temperature. When the syrinx is in the cervical area, pain and temperature are typically lost in a "cape" or "vest" distribution. However, early involvement is often unilateral or at least asymmetric

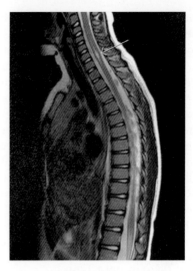

Fig. 9.1 Syrinx. T_2 sagittal magnetic resonance imaging of spine shows a dilated central canal/cervical syrinx (*arrow*).

and sometimes involves the fingers before the shoulders. Preservation of touch and pressure persists until the cyst enlarges into the posterior columns or the dorsal root entry zone. Loss of pain sensibility in the hands often leads to injury, ulceration, and infection, as seen in HSANs. Pain is prominent. Complaints include neck ache, headache, back pain, and radicular pain.

Scoliosis is common, and torticollis may be an initial sign in children with cervical cavities. As the cavity enlarges into the ventral horn, weakness and atrophy develop in the hands and may be associated with fasciculations; pressure on the lateral columns causes hyperreflexia and spasticity in the legs. Very long cavities may produce lower motor neuron signs in all limbs. Sphincter control is sometimes impaired. The posterior columns are generally the last to be affected so that vibration sense and touch are preserved until relatively late in the course. The progress of symptoms is extremely slow and insidious. The spinal cord accommodates well to the slowly developing pressure within. Thus, at the time of consultation, a long history of minor neurological handicaps such as clumsiness or difficulty running is common.

Bulbar signs are relatively uncommon and usually asymmetric. They include hemiatrophy of the tongue with deviation on protrusion, facial weakness, dysphasia, and dysarthria. Disturbances of the descending pathway of the trigeminal nerve cause loss of pain and temperature sensations on the same side of the face as facial weakness and tongue hemiatrophy.

Diagnosis. MRI is the diagnostic study of choice (Fig. 9.1).

Management. Syrinxes occurring with hydrocephalus and communicating with the fourth ventricle do well following a ventriculoperitoneal shunt. Syrinxes associated with Chiari I malformations collapse after shunting from the syrinx to the cerebellopontine angle, and noncommunicating syrinxes often collapse after the excision of an extramedullary obstruction.

THALAMIC PAIN

The thalamic pain syndrome occurs almost exclusively in adults following infarction of the thalamus. Similar symptoms sometimes occur in patients with thalamic glioma. The location of the lesion is usually the ventroposterolateral nucleus of the thalamus. Thalamic-type pain also occurs with lesions of the parietal lobe, medial lemniscus, and dorsolateral medulla.[13]

Clinical features. Touching the affected limb or part of the body produces intense discomfort described as "sharp," "crushing," or "burning." Suffering is considerable, and the quality of the pain is unfamiliar to the patient. Several different modes of stimulation, such as changes in ambient temperature, auditory stimulation, and even changes in emotional state, can accentuate pain. Despite the severity of these dysesthesias, the affected limb is otherwise anesthetic to ordinary sensory testing.

Diagnosis. The presence of thalamic pain should prompt imaging studies to determine the presence of a tumor, infarction, or demyelinating disease.

Management. Due to the severity of the pain, opioids are sometimes used but are not a suitable long-term treatment option. Antidepressants including SSRIs and amitriptyline, and anticonvulsants such as gabapentin or pregabalin are often used. The combination of levodopa and a peripheral decarboxylase inhibitor may be helpful. Deep brain stimulation and spinal cord stimulators have been used with variable success, and some smaller studies have examined the role of tMS to relieve pain, with suggestive although not definitive results.[14]

REFERENCES

1. Rowbotham MC. Complex regional pain syndrome type I (reflex sympathetic dystrophy). More than a myth. *Neurology.* 1998;51:4-5.
2. Wasner G, Schattschneider J, Heckmann K, et al. Vascular abnormalities in reflex sympathetic dystrophy (CRPS I): mechanisms and diagnostic value. *Brain.* 2001;124:587-599.
3. Albrecht PJ, Hines S, Eisenberg E, et al. Pathologic alterations of cutaneous innervation and vasculature in affected limbs from patients with complex regional pain syndrome. *Pain.* 2006;120(3):244-266.
4. Hisama FM, Dib-Hajj SD, Waxman SG. SCN9A neuropathic pain syndromes (May 6, 2006). In: Adam MP, Mirzaa GM, Pagon RA, et al., eds. *GeneReviews®*: University of Washington; 1993–2023. https://www.ncbi.nlm.nih.gov/books/NBK1163/. Updated January 23, 2020.
5. Zhang P, Xiao F, Li X, et al. Familial episodic pain syndrome: a case report and literature review. *Annals of Translational Medicine.* 2022;10(4):238. https://doi.org/10.21037/atm-22-102. PMID: 35280382; PMCID: PMC8908130.
6. Shen Y, Zheng Y, Hong D. Familial episodic pain syndromes. *Journal of Pain Research.* 2022;15:2505-2515. https://doi.org/10.2147/JPR.S375299. PMID: 36051609; PMCID: PMC9427007.
7. Kurth I. Hereditary sensory and autonomic neuropathy type II (November 23, 2010). In: Adam MP, Mirzaa GM, Pagon RA, et al., eds. *GeneReviews®*. University of Washington; 1993–2023. https://www.ncbi.nlm.nih.gov/books/NBK49247/. Updated April 1, 2021.
8. Bonkowski JL, Johnson J, Carey JC, et al. An infant with primary tooth loss and palmar hyperkeratosis: a novel mutation in the NTRK1 gene causing congenital insensitivity to pain with anhidrosis. *Pediatrics.* 2003;112:e237-e241.
9. Einarsdottir E, Carlsson A, Minde J, et al. A mutation in nerve growth factor beta gene (NGFB) causes loss of pain perception. *Human Molecular Genetics.* 2004;13:799-805.
10. Houlden H, King RH, Hashemi-Nejad A, et al. A novel TRK A (NTRK1) mutation associated with hereditary sensory and autonomic neuropathy type V. *Annals of Neurology.* 2001;49:521-525.
11. Anderson KE, Bloomer JR, Bonkovsky HL, et al. Recommendations for the diagnosis and treatment of the acute porphyrias. *Annals of Internal Medicine.* 2005;142:439-450.
12. Holme E, Lindstedt S. Nontransplant treatment of tyrosinemia. *Clinical Liver Disease.* 2000;4:805-814.
13. MacGowan DGL, Janal MN, Clark WC, et al. Central poststroke pain and Wallenberg's lateral medullary infarction. Frequency, character, and determinants in 63 patients. *Neurology.* 1997;49:120-125.
14. Rollnik JD, Wustefeld S, Dauper J, et al. Repetitive transcranial magnetic stimulation for the treatment of chronic pain – a pilot study. *European Neurology.* 2002;48:6-10.

Ataxia

OUTLINE

Acute and Recurrent Ataxias, 258
Brain Tumor, 259
Conversion Reaction, 259
Dominant Recurrent Ataxias, 260
Drug Ingestion, 261
Encephalitis (Brainstem or Limbic Encephalitis), 261
Inborn Errors of Metabolism, 262
Migraine, 263

Postinfectious/Immune-Mediated Disorders, 264
Trauma, 267
Vascular Disorders, 268
Chronic or Progressive Ataxia, 269
Brain Tumors, 269
Congenital Malformations, 272
Progressive Hereditary Ataxias, 274
References, 278

The term *ataxia* denotes disturbances in the fine control of posture and movement. The cerebellum and its major input systems from the frontal lobes and the posterior columns of the spinal cord provide this control. The initial and most prominent feature is usually an abnormal gait. The ataxic gait is wide based, lurching, and staggering, and it provokes disquiet in an observer for fear that the patient is in danger of falling. One observes a similar gait in people who are attempting to walk in a vehicle that has several directions of motion at once, such as a railroad train.

When an abnormality occurs in the vermis of the cerebellum, the child cannot sit still but constantly moves the body to-and-fro and bobs the head (titubation). In contrast, disturbances of the cerebellar hemispheres cause a tendency to veer in the direction of the affected hemisphere, with dysmetria and hypotonia in the ipsilateral limbs. Bifrontal lobe disease may produce symptoms and signs that are indistinguishable from those of cerebellar disease.

Loss of sensory input to the cerebellum, because of peripheral nerve or posterior column disease, necessitates constant looking at the feet to know their location in space (due to loss of proprioception). The gait is also wide based, but it is not so much lurching as careful. The foot raises high with each step and slaps down heavily

on the ground. Station and gait are considerably worse with the eyes closed, and the patient may actually fall to the floor (Romberg sign). Sensory ataxia is more likely to cause difficulty with fine finger movements than with reaching for objects.

Other features of cerebellar disease are a characteristic speech that varies in volume and has an increased separation of syllables (scanning speech), hypotonia, limb and ocular dysmetria, and tremor. The differential diagnosis of a child with acute ataxia or recurrent attacks of ataxia (Box 10.1) is quite different from that of a child with chronic static or progressive ataxia (Box 10.2). Therefore the discussion of these two presentations is separate in the text. However, one may "suddenly" become aware of what had been a slowly progressive ataxia, and children with recurrent ataxia may never recover to baseline function after each attack. Progressive ataxia superimposes on the acute attacks.

ACUTE AND RECURRENT ATAXIAS

The two most common causes of ataxia among children who were previously healthy and then suddenly have an ataxic gait are drug ingestion and acute postinfectious cerebellitis. Migraine, brainstem encephalitis, and an underlying neuroblastoma are the next considerations.

BOX 10.1 Acute or Recurrent Ataxia

Brain tumor
Conversion reaction
Drug ingestion
Encephalitis (brainstem)
Genetic disorders
Dominant recurrent ataxia
Episodic ataxia type 1
Episodic ataxia type 2
Hartnup disease
Maple syrup urine disease
Pyruvate dehydrogenase deficiency
Migraine with brainstem aura
Benign paroxysmal vertigo
Postinfectious/immune

Acute postinfectious cerebellitis
Miller Fisher syndrome
Multiple sclerosis
Myoclonic encephalopathy and neuroblastoma
Progressive cavitating leukoencephalopathy
Pseudoataxia (epileptic)
Trauma
Hematoma (see Chapter 2)
Postconcussion
Vertebrobasilar occlusion
Vascular disorders
Cerebellar hemorrhage
Kawasaki disease

BOX 10.2 Chronic or Progressive Ataxia

Brain Tumors
Cerebellar astrocytoma
Cerebellar hemangioblastoma (Von Hippel-Lindau disease)
Ependymoma
Medulloblastoma
Supratentorial tumors (see Chapter 4)

Congenital Malformations
Basilar impression
Cerebellar aplasia
Cerebellar hemisphere aplasia
Chiari malformation
Dandy-Walker malformation (see Chapter 18)
Vermal aplasia

Hereditary Ataxias
Autosomal dominant inheritance (see Table 10.1)
Autosomal recessive inheritance
Abetalipoproteinemia

Ataxia telangiectasia
Ataxia without oculomotor apraxia
Ataxia with episodic dystonia
Friedreich ataxia
Hartnup disease
Juvenile GM$_2$ gangliosidosis
Juvenile sulfatide lipidoses
Maple syrup urine disease
Marinesco-Sjögren syndrome
Pyruvate dehydrogenase deficiency
Ramsay Hunt syndrome
Hereditary motor and sensory neuropathies (HMSN IV) (see Chapter 7)
Respiratory chain disorders (see Chapter 8)

X-Linked Inheritance
Adrenoleukodystrophy (for infantile form, see Chapter 5)
Leber optic neuropathy (see Chapter 16)
X-linked hereditary ataxias (multiple)

Brain Tumor

Primary brain tumors ordinarily cause chronic progressive ataxia, and their discussion can be found later in this chapter. However, ataxia may be acute if the brain tumor bleeds or causes hydrocephalus. In addition, early clumsiness may not become apparent until it becomes severe enough to cause an obvious gait disturbance. Brain imaging is therefore a recommendation for most children with acute cerebellar ataxia.

Conversion Reaction

Clinical features. Psychogenic gait disturbances are relatively common in children, especially in adolescents. All conversion disorders have a female predominance but can be seen in males as well. Psychogenic symptoms are involuntary and usually protective against an overwhelming stressor. In contrast, malingering is a voluntary act. Psychogenic gait disturbances are often extreme. The child appears to sit without difficulty but when brought to standing immediately begins to sway from the waist. Stance is not wide to improve stability as it would occur in an organic ataxia. Instead, the child lurches, staggers, and otherwise travels across the room from object to object. The lurching maneuvers are often complex and require extraordinary balance. Strength, tone, sensation, and tendon reflexes are normal.

Diagnosis. The diagnosis of psychogenic gait disturbances is by observation; laboratory tests or imaging studies are not ordinarily required to exclude other possibilities.

Management. Determination of the precipitating stress is important. Conversion may represent a true call for help in a desperate situation such as sexual or physical abuse or severe depression with suicidality. Such cases require referral to a multispecialty team able to deal with the whole family. Fortunately, most children with psychogenic gait disturbances are responding to an immediate and less serious life stressor. Identifying possible stressors, modifying surrounding circumstances and activities, and improving coping mechanisms are necessary for the improvement and prevention of further psychogenic symptoms.

Dominant Recurrent Ataxias

There are at least eight recognized forms of episodic ataxia, the most common of which are episodic ataxia type 1 (EA1) and episodic ataxia type 2 (EA2). Both are the result of ion channel mutations. Mutations in a potassium channel gene underlie EA1 and mutations in a voltage-dependent calcium channel underlie EA2.[1]

EA1 (Paroxysmal Ataxia and Myokymia)

EA1 results from a mutation of the potassium channel gene *KCNA1* on chromosome 12p. The additional feature of continuous motor unit activity (see Chapter 8) suggests a defect in membrane stability affecting the central nervous system (CNS) and peripheral nervous system.

Clinical features. The onset of attacks is usually between 5 and 7 years of age. Abrupt postural change, startle, exercise, and stress may provoke an attack. The child becomes aware of attack onset by the sensation of spreading limpness or stiffness lasting for a few seconds. Incoordination, trembling of the head or limbs, and blurry vision often follow. Some children feel warm and perspire. Some can continue standing or walking, but most sit down. Attacks usually last for less than 10 minutes but can be as long as 6 hours. Seizures may occur. Myokymia of the face and limbs begins at about 12 years of age. Physical findings include large calves, normal muscle strength, and widespread myokymia of face, hands, arms, and legs, with a hand posture resembling carpopedal spasm. Electromyography (EMG) at rest shows continuous spontaneous activity.[2]

Diagnosis. The basis for clinical diagnosis is the history of typical attacks and the family history. EMG confirms the diagnosis by showing continuous motor unit activity, most often in the hands but also the proximal arm muscles and sometimes in the face. Molecular genetic testing is available, either for *KCNA1* specifically or in large ataxia panels.

Management. Some patients respond to daily antiepileptic drugs. When these fail, acetazolamide is helpful for some, but not all patients.

EA2 (Acetazolamide-Responsive Ataxia)

EA2, one form of spinocerebellar ataxia (SCA6), and one type of familial hemiplegic migraine all represent allelic mutations in the same calcium channel gene *CACNA1A* on chromosome 19p. About half of patients have migraine headaches; some episodes may be typical of migraine with brainstem aura.[2,3]

Clinical features. Clinical heterogeneity is considerable despite genetic localization to the 19p site. The onset is generally during school age or adolescence. The child first becomes unsteady and is then unable to maintain posture because of vertigo and ataxia. Vomiting is frequent and severe. Jerk nystagmus, sometimes with a rotary component, occurs during attacks. One to three attacks may occur each month, with symptoms lasting from 1 hour to 1 day. Attacks become milder and less frequent with age. Slowly progressive truncal ataxia and nystagmus may persist between attacks. In some patients ataxia is the only symptom, others have only vertigo, and still others have only nystagmus. Most affected individuals are normal between attacks, but some are phenotypically indistinguishable from those with SCA6 (see discussion in the "Progressive Hereditary Ataxias" section).

Diagnosis. The clinical features and the family history are the basis for diagnosis. Molecular diagnosis is available. Magnetic resonance imaging (MRI) may show selective atrophy of the cerebellar vermis. Basilar artery migraine and benign paroxysmal vertigo can be distinguished from dominant recurrent ataxia because in these conditions older family members have migraines but do not have recurrent ataxia. Further, attacks of benign paroxysmal vertigo rarely last more than a few minutes.

Management. Daily oral acetazolamide prevents the recurrence of attacks in almost every case. The mechanism of action is unknown. The dose is generally 125 mg twice a day in young children and 250 mg twice a day in older children. Flunarizine, 5–10 mg/day, may serve as an alternative therapy for children with acetazolamide intolerance. Antiepileptic and antimigraine medications are without value.

Other Episodic Ataxias

Multiple other types of episodic ataxias have been described, from episodic ataxia type 3 (EA3) through episodic ataxia type 8 (EA8). These ataxias are infrequent and have only been reported in a handful of families. Some patients present with phenotypes consistent with episodic ataxia but no genetic cause is ever found, suggesting that additional subtypes may be identified in the future.

Drug Ingestion

The incidence of accidental drug ingestion is greatest in children between 1 and 4 years of age.

Clinical features. An overdose of most psychoactive drugs causes ataxia, disturbances in personality or sensorium, and sometimes seizures. Toxic doses of antiepileptic drugs, especially phenytoin, may cause marked nystagmus and ataxia without an equivalent alteration in sensorium. Excessive use of antihistamines in the treatment of an infant or young child with allergies or an upper respiratory tract infection may cause ataxia. This is especially true in children with otitis media, who may have underlying unsteadiness because of middle ear infection and possible inner ear dysfunction.

Diagnosis. Carefully question the parents or care providers of every child with acute ataxia concerning drugs intentionally administered to the child and other drugs accessible in the home. Specific inquiry concerning the use of anticonvulsants or psychoactive drugs by family members is mandatory. Screen urine for drug metabolites and send blood for analysis when suspecting intoxication with a specific drug.

Management. Treatment depends on the specific drug ingested and its blood concentration. In most cases of ataxia caused by drug ingestion the drug can be safely eliminated spontaneously if vital function is not compromised, if acid-base balance is not disturbed, and if liver and kidney function is normal. In life-threatening situations dialysis may be necessary while supporting vital function in an intensive care unit. Gastric emptying has limited value when ataxia is already present.

Encephalitis (Brainstem or Limbic Encephalitis)

Ataxia may be the initial feature of an infectious encephalitis affecting primarily the structures of the posterior fossa. Potential etiological agents include echoviruses, coxsackieviruses, adenoviruses, *Mycoplasma pneumoniae*, and *Coxiella burnetti*.[4] Autoimmune encephalitis with anti-*N*-methyl-D-aspartate (NMDA) and voltage-gated potassium channel autoantibodies cause limbic encephalitis more frequently than infectious agents.[5]

Clinical features. Cranial nerve dysfunction is often associated with the ataxia. Generalized encephalitis characterized by declining consciousness and seizures may develop later. Meningismus is sometimes present. Children with autoimmune encephalitis typically experience significant psychiatric symptoms, including psychosis, aggression, agitation, and catatonia. The course is variable, and, although most children recover completely, some suffer considerable neurological impairment. Those who have only ataxia and cranial nerve palsies, with no disturbance of neocortical function, tend to recover best. Such cases are indistinguishable from the Miller Fisher syndrome on clinical grounds alone.

Diagnosis. Diagnosis requires showing a cellular response, primarily mononuclear leukocytes, in the cerebrospinal fluid (CSF), with or without some elevation of the protein content. Prolonged interpeak latencies of the brainstem auditory evoked response are the evidence of an abnormality within the brainstem parenchyma and not the peripheral sensory input system. The electroencephalogram (EEG) is usually normal in children with infectious brainstem encephalitis who have a normal sensorium, but seizures may be present and difficult to manage in autoimmune encephalitis. Adolescents with autoimmune encephalitis may have the "extreme delta brush" pattern on EEG or nonspecific slowing.[6]

Management. No specific treatment is available for the viral infection. Treatment with immune modulators is needed for autoimmune encephalitis, sometimes long term. Anti-NMDA receptor encephalitis can be associated with ovarian teratomas, and in those cases removal of the tumor may be curative.

Inborn Errors of Metabolism

Hartnup Disease

Hartnup disease is a rare disorder transmitted by autosomal recessive inheritance. The abnormal gene is *SLC6A19* and localizes to chromosome 5p15.[7] The basic error is a defect of amino acid transport in the kidney and small intestine. The result is aminoaciduria and the retention of amino acids in the small intestine. Tryptophan conversion is to nonessential indole products instead of nicotinamide.

Clinical features. Affected children are normal at birth but may be slow in attaining developmental milestones. Most achieve only borderline intelligence; others are normal. Affected individuals are photosensitive and have a severe pellagra-like skin rash after exposure to sunlight. Nicotinamide deficiency causes the rash. Many patients have episodes of limb ataxia, sometimes associated with nystagmus. Mental changes, ranging from emotional instability to delirium or states of decreased consciousness, may occur. Examination reveals hypotonia and normal or exaggerated tendon reflexes. Stress or intercurrent infection triggers the neurological disturbances, which may be due to the intestinal absorption of toxic amino acid breakdown products. Most patients have both rash and neurological disturbances, but each can occur without the other. Symptoms progress over several days and last for a week to a month before recovery occurs.

Diagnosis. The constant feature of Hartnup disease is aminoaciduria involving neutral monoamino monocarboxylic amino acids. These include alanine, serine, threonine, asparagine, glutamine, valine, leucine, isoleucine, phenylalanine, tyrosine, tryptophan, histidine, and citrulline.

Management. Daily oral administration of nicotinamide, 50–300 mg, may reverse the skin and neurological complications. A high-protein diet helps make up for the amino acid loss and the disease is rare in populations with an adequate diet.

Maple Syrup Urine Disease (Intermittent)

Maple syrup urine disease is a disorder of branched-chain amino acid metabolism caused by deficiency of the enzyme branched-chain keto acid dehydrogenase. The result of the deficiency is a neonatal organic acidemia. Transmission of the defect is by autosomal recessive inheritance. Three phenotypes are associated, depending on the percentage of enzyme deficiency. The classic form begins as seizures in the newborn (see Chapter 1), the intermediate form causes progressive intellectual disability (see Chapter 5), and the intermittent form causes recurrent attacks of ataxia and encephalopathy.

Clinical features. Affected individuals are normal at birth. Between the ages of 5 months and 2 years, minor infections, surgery, or a diet rich in protein provokes episodes of ataxia, irritability, and progressive lethargy. The length of an attack is variable; most children recover spontaneously, but some die of severe metabolic acidosis. Psychomotor development remains normal in survivors.

Diagnosis. The urine has a maple syrup odor during the attack, and the blood and urine have elevated concentrations of branched-chain amino acids and ketoacids. Between attacks, the concentrations of branched-chain amino acids and ketoacids are normal in both blood and urine. Newborn screening identifies most cases; molecular genetic testing demonstrates biallelic pathogenic variants in *BCKHA*, *BCKHB*, or *DBT*.[8]

Management. Children with intermittent maple syrup disease need a protein-restricted diet. Specifically, they must limit dietary leucine. Specialized medical diets free of branched-chain amino acids are indicated; consensus nutritional guidelines are available. Some have a thiamine-responsive enzyme defect, and 1 g of thiamine a day treats acute attacks. If this is successful, a recommended maintenance dose is 100 mg/day. The main objective during an acute attack is to reverse ketoacidosis. Peritoneal dialysis may be helpful in life-threatening situations.

Pyruvate Dehydrogenase Deficiency

The pyruvate dehydrogenase (PDH) complex is responsible for the oxidative decarboxylation of pyruvate to carbon dioxide and acetyl-coenzyme A (acetyl-CoA). Disorders of the complex are associated with several neurological conditions, including subacute necrotizing encephalomyelopathy (Leigh syndrome), mitochondrial myopathies, and lactic acidosis. The complex contains three main components that are termed E1, E2, and E3. E1 consists of two alpha subunits encoded on the X chromosome and two beta subunits. Episodes of intermittent ataxia and lactic acidosis characterize the X-linked form of PDH-E1 deficiency.[9] Mutations in the *PDHA1* gene, which encodes the E1 subunit, account for approximately 80% of cases.

Clinical features. The clinical features range from severe neonatal lactic acidosis and death to episodic ataxia with lactic and pyruvic acidosis and spinocerebellar degeneration. Most patients show mild developmental delay during early childhood. Episodes of ataxia, dysarthria, and sometimes lethargy usually begin after 3 years of age. In more severely affected patients episodes may begin during infancy and are associated with generalized weakness and states of decreased consciousness. Some attacks are spontaneous, but intercurrent infection, stress, or a meal high in carbohydrate provokes others. Attacks recur at irregular intervals and may last for periods ranging from 1 day to several weeks.

The severity of neurological dysfunction in any individual probably reflects the level of residual enzyme activity. Those with generalized weakness are also areflexic and have nystagmus or other disturbances in ocular motility. Ataxia is the predominant symptom. Intention tremor and dysarthria may be present. Hyperventilation is common and metabolic acidosis may be the cause. Patients with almost complete PDH deficiency die of lactic acidosis and central hypoventilation during infancy.

Diagnosis. PDH deficiency should be suspected in children with lactic acidosis, hypotonia, progressive or episodic ataxia, the Leigh disease phenotype, and recurrent polyneuropathy. The pyruvic acid concentration is elevated, and the lactate-to-pyruvate ratio is low. The blood concentration of lactate may be elevated between attacks; lactate and pyruvate concentrations are always elevated during attacks. Some children have hyperalaninemia as well. Analysis of enzyme activity in cultured fibroblasts, leukocytes, or muscle establishes the diagnosis. Molecular genetic testing is available.

Management. The ketogenic diet is a rational treatment for PDH-complex deficiency.[10] Patients are usually treated with thiamine (100–600 mg/day) and a high-fat (>55%), low-carbohydrate diet. In addition, daily oral acetazolamide, 125 mg twice a day in small children and 250 mg twice a day in older children, may significantly abort the attacks. Unfortunately, current treatments do not prevent disease progression in most patients.

Migraine
Migraine With Brainstem Aura

The term *migraine with brainstem aura* (formerly termed *basilar migraine*) characterizes recurrent attacks of brainstem or cerebellar dysfunction that occur as symptoms of a migraine attack. Despite its name, brainstem involvement is controversial, and several authors argue that cortical spreading depression is a more reasonable explanation for the "brainstem" symptoms in many cases.[11] Children who experience migraine with brainstem aura have typical migraines with an aura at other times.[12] Females are more often affected than are males. The peak incidence is during adolescence, but attacks may occur at any age. Infant-onset cases are more likely to present as benign paroxysmal vertigo.

Clinical features. Gait ataxia occurs in approximately 50% of patients. Other symptoms include hemianopsia, dysarthria, vertigo, tinnitus, alternating hemiparesis, and paresthesias of the fingers, toes, and corners of the mouth. An abrupt loss of consciousness may occur, usually lasting for only a few minutes. Cardiac arrhythmia and brainstem stroke are rare, life-threatening complications. A severe, throbbing, occipital headache usually follows the neurological disturbances. Nausea and vomiting occur less frequently than in other types of migraine.

Diagnosis. EEG distinguishes basilar migraines from benign occipital epilepsy. MRI and magnetic resonance angiogram (MRA) demonstrate normal brain and blood vessel architecture.

Management. Treatment of migraine with brainstem aura is the same as for other forms of migraine (see Chapter 3). Frequent attacks require a prophylactic agent.

Benign Paroxysmal Vertigo of Childhood

Benign paroxysmal vertigo of childhood is primarily a disorder in toddlers and young children but may occur in older children.

Clinical features. Recurrent attacks of vertigo are characteristic. Vertigo is maximal at onset. True cerebellar ataxia is not present, but vertigo is so profound that standing is impossible. The child either lies motionless on the floor or wants to be held. Consciousness is maintained throughout the event and there is no associated headache. The predominant symptoms are pallor, nystagmus, and fright. Episodes last only for minutes and may recur at irregular intervals. With time, attacks decrease in frequency and stop completely or evolve into more typical migraines. Migraines develop in 21% of patients.[13]

Diagnosis. The diagnosis is primarily clinical, and laboratory tests are useful only to exclude other possibilities. A family history of migraines, though not necessarily paroxysmal vertigo, is positive in 40% of cases. Some parents indicate that they experience vertigo with their attacks of migraine. Only in rare cases does a parent have a history of benign paroxysmal vertigo.

Management. The attacks are so brief that acute treatment is impossible. Migraine prophylaxis may be considered when attacks are frequent.

Postinfectious/Immune-Mediated Disorders

In many conditions discussed in this section the underlying cause of cerebellar dysfunction and some other neurological deficits is an altered immune state. Preceding viral infections are usually incriminated but documentation is limited to only half of cases. Natural varicella infections and the varicella vaccine are definite preceding causes. No other vaccine links to acute cerebellar ataxia.

Acute Cerebellar Ataxia

Acute cerebellar ataxia usually affects children between 2 and 7 years of age, but it may occur as late as 16 years of age. The disorder affects both sexes equally, and the incidence among family members is not increased. In the past acute cerebellar ataxia occurred most often following varicella infection. The widespread use of varicella vaccine has made the syndrome uncommon. However, it is a potential complication of live, inactivated vaccine administration.

Clinical features. The onset is explosive. A previously healthy child awakens from a nap and cannot stand. Ataxia is maximal at onset. Some worsening may occur during the first hours, but a longer progression, or a waxing and waning course, negates the diagnosis. Ataxia varies from mild unsteadiness while walking to complete inability to stand or walk. Even when ataxia is severe, mental status remains normal. Tendon reflexes may be present or absent; their absence suggests Miller Fisher syndrome. Nystagmus, when present, is usually mild. Chaotic movements of the eyes (opsoclonus) should suggest the myoclonic encephalopathy/neuroblastoma syndrome.

Symptoms begin to remit after a few days, but recovery of normal gait may take weeks to months. Patients with pure ataxia of the trunk or limbs and only mild nystagmus are likely to recover completely. Marked nystagmus or opsoclonus (see the "Myoclonic Encephalopathy/

Neuroblastoma Syndrome" section), tremors of the head and trunk, or moderate irritability are usually followed by persistent neurological sequelae.

Diagnosis. The diagnosis of acute postinfectious cerebellitis is one of exclusion. Every child should have a drug screening, and most will have a brain imaging study. Lumbar puncture is indicated when encephalitis is suspected.

Management. Acute postinfectious cerebellitis is a self-limited disease. Treatment is not required. Physical and occupational therapy may facilitate activities during the recovery phase.

Miller Fisher Syndrome

Ataxia, ophthalmoplegia, and areflexia characterize Miller Fisher syndrome. A similar disorder with ataxia and areflexia but without ophthalmoplegia is termed *acute ataxic neuropathy*. Miller Fisher syndrome is most likely a variant of Guillain-Barré syndrome, and *Campylobacter jejuni* serotype O:19 is a causative agent in both syndromes.[14]

Clinical features. A viral illness precedes the neurological symptoms by 5–10 days in 50% of cases. Either ophthalmoparesis or ataxia may be the initial feature. Both are present early in the course. The initial ocular motor disturbance is the paralysis of upgaze, followed by loss of lateral gaze, and then downgaze. Recovery takes place in the reverse order. Preservation of the Bell phenomenon sometimes occurs despite the paralysis of voluntary upward gaze, suggesting the possibility of supranuclear palsy. Ptosis occurs but is less severe than the vertical gaze palsy.

Decreased peripheral sensory input probably causes areflexia and more prominent limb than trunk ataxia. Weakness of the limbs may be noted. Unilateral or bilateral facial weakness occurs in a significant minority of children. Recovery generally begins within 2–4 weeks after symptoms become maximal and is complete within 6 months.

Diagnosis. The clinical distinction between Miller Fisher syndrome and brainstem encephalitis can be difficult. Altered mental status, multiple cranial nerve palsies, an abnormal EEG, or prolongation of the interpeak latencies of the brainstem auditory evoked response suggest brainstem encephalitis. The CSF profile in Miller Fisher syndrome parallels that of Guillain-Barré syndrome. A cellular response occurs early in the course, and protein elevation occurs later.

Management. Intravenous immunoglobulin to block antibodies and plasmapheresis to remove antibodies may be beneficial. The dose of immunoglobulin is 2 g/kg over 2–5 days. The outcome is usually good.

Multiple Sclerosis

Multiple sclerosis (MS) is usually a disease of young adults, but 3%–5% of cases occur in children less than 6 years.[15] The childhood forms of MS are similar to the adult forms.

In a prospective study of 296 children with acute demyelination 81 presented with focal involvement, 119 with acute disseminated encephalomyelitis (ADEM), and 96 with symptoms that suggest already established MS. Long-tract (motor, sensory, or sphincter) dysfunction was the most common finding in 226 children (76%), followed by symptoms localized to the brainstem in 121 children (41%), optic neuritis in 67 children (22%), and transverse myelitis in 42 children (14%).[16] Monofocal presentation was more common in adolescents. Recovery from acute demyelination is variable: 85% of children with optic neuritis recover full visual acuity but those with transverse myelitis suffer a higher rate of long-term sequelae.

Clinical features. Pediatric MS is exclusively the relapsing-remitting form. Prior to puberty, the female-to-male ratio is equal, but following puberty females outnumber males. Ataxia, concurrent with a febrile episode, is the most common initial feature in children, followed by encephalopathy, hemiparesis, or seizures.

Intranuclear ophthalmoplegia, unilateral or bilateral, develops in one-third of patients (see Chapter 15).

The clinical features that occur in MS are sufficiently variable that no single prototype is valid. The essential feature is repeated episodes of demyelination in noncontiguous areas of the CNS. Focal neurological deficits that develop rapidly and persist for weeks or months characterize an episode. Afterward the child has partial or complete recovery. Months or years separate recurrences, which are often concurrent with fever, but not with a specific febrile illness. Lethargy, nausea, and vomiting sometimes accompany the attacks in children but rarely in adults. The child is usually irritable and shows truncal and limb ataxia. Tendon reflexes are generally brisk throughout. Long-term difficulty with learning and persistent or progressive cognitive impairment is frequently seen.

Diagnosis. MS may be the suspected diagnosis at the time of the first attack, but definitive diagnosis requires recurrence to establish a polyphasic course. Examination of the CSF at the time of exacerbation reveals fewer than 25 lymphocytes/mm³, a normal or mildly elevated protein content, and sometimes the presence of oligoclonal bands.

MRI is the technique of choice for the diagnosis of MS and shows occult disease in up to 80% of affected individuals at the time of first presentation (Fig. 10.1). The finding of three or more white matter lesions on a T_2-weighted image MRI scan, especially if one of these lesions is in the perpendicular plane to the

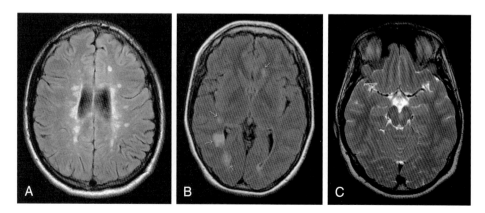

Fig. 10.1 Multiple Sclerosis. (A) T_2 flair axial magnetic resonance imaging (MRI) shows multiple demyelinating lesions. (B) Axial flair showing multiple demyelinating lesions (*arrows*). (C) T_2 axial MRI showing midbrain central demyelination.

corpus callosum, is a sensitive predictor of definite MS.[17] However, the extent and severity of lesions may not correlate with the clinical syndrome. After repeated attacks, the MRI reveals thalamic gray matter loss.[18]

Management. Although pediatric MS tends to progress more slowly than the adult-onset form and children recover from individual attacks more rapidly, children still reach disability sooner due to the earlier age of onset. The treatment of MS in children is similar to that in adults. Acute exacerbations require a short course of corticosteroids. Following an initial administration of methylprednisolone, 500–1000 mg, depending on the age, a tapering dose schedule is used. In 2018 the Food and Drug Administration (FDA) approved fingolimod for the treatment of MS in pediatric patients aged 10 years and older. Additional disease-modifying therapies are being studied, and many are used off-label in pediatric patients.

Provide physical, occupational, and speech therapies as needed following relapse. Cognitive rehabilitation may be helpful to aid in the recovery of executive function. Baseline neuropsychological testing is recommended, and educational accommodations are often required.

Myoclonic Encephalopathy/Neuroblastoma Syndrome

Myoclonic encephalopathy is a syndrome characterized by opsoclonus (chaotic irregular eye movements), myoclonic ataxia (irregular shock-like muscle contractions), and encephalopathy. The pathophysiological mechanism is an altered immune state. Initially, the syndrome was attributed either to the presence of occult neuroblastoma or to an unknown cause. With improved imaging techniques, the majority of cases appear to be neuroblastoma related. Two to three percent of children with neuroblastoma develop a myoclonic encephalopathy. A specific causal antibody is not established but a neuronal surface antibody is a suspect.[19] In a small percentage of cases a cause is never identified.

Clinical features. The mean age at onset is 18 months, with a range from 1 month to 4 years.[20] Unlike acute postinfectious cerebellitis and Miller Fisher syndrome, in which neurological symptoms are fully expressed within 1–2 days, the evolution of symptoms in myoclonic encephalopathy may take 1 week or longer.

Either ataxia or chaotic eye movements may bring the child to medical attention. Almost half of affected children show personality change or irritability, suggesting the presence of a more diffuse encephalopathy. Gait instability may be secondary to ataxia, myoclonus, or a combination of the two. Opsoclonus is a disorder of ocular muscles that is similar to myoclonus. Spontaneous, conjugate, irregular jerking of the eyes in all directions is characteristic. The movements are most prominent with attempts to change fixation and are then associated with blinking or eyelid flutter. Opsoclonus persists even in sleep and becomes more severe with agitation. The inability to focus contributes to gait disturbance and irritability.

Diagnosis. The clinical features are the basis for the diagnosis of myoclonic encephalopathy. Laboratory investigation is required to determine the underlying cause. Occult neuroblastoma is the suspected cause in all children with recurrent ataxia or the myoclonic encephalopathy syndrome. Neuroblastoma is also the likely cause when an acute ataxia progresses over several days or waxes and wanes.

The occult neuroblastoma is equally likely to be in the chest or the abdomen. In contrast, only 10%–15% of neuroblastomas are in the chest when myoclonic encephalopathy is absent. A small number may be present in the neck. The usual studies to detect neuroblastoma are an MRI of the chest and abdomen (Fig. 10.2)

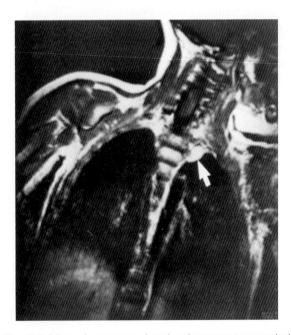

Fig. 10.2 Magnetic resonance imaging demonstrates an apical neuroblastoma (*arrow*) in a child with normal radiographs and computed tomography of the chest.

and a measurement of the urinary excretion of homovanillic acid and vanillylmandelic acid. CSF studies show B-cell expansion, a hallmark of the disease.[21]

Management. Long-term neurological outcome is variable despite the presence or absence of a tumor. In most children a prolonged course follows, with the waxing and waning of neurological dysfunction. Either adrenocorticotropic hormone (ACTH) or oral corticosteroids provide partial or complete relief of symptoms in 80% of patients. Rituximab is increasingly used instead of ACTH, and trazodone 25–50 mg nightly helps with rage attacks and sleep disturbance. Despite a dramatic initial response to therapy, relapses often occur either after discontinuing therapy or while treatment is in progress. The majority of affected children will have long-term residual deficits, although most are mild.[22] A small percentage experience significant long-term cognitive and physical sequelae.

Childhood Ataxia With Central Nervous System Hypomyelination/Vanishing White Matter

Vanishing white matter disease is one of the most prevalent inherited childhood leukoencephalopathies. Characteristics of this disorder are recurrent attacks of demyelination similar to ADEM and triggered by febrile illnesses, minor head injury, or acute fright, often leading to severe neurological deterioration and coma. The classical phenotype is characterized by early childhood onset of chronic neurological deterioration, dominated by cerebellar ataxia. Females may have coexistent ovarian dysgenesis. Most patients die a few years after onset. The defect resides in one of the five genes (*EIF2B1, EIF2B2, EIF2B3, EIF2B4, or EIF2B5*)[23] encoding the subunits of eukaryotic translation initiation factor eIF2B, which is an essential factor in all cells of the body for protein synthesis and its regulation under different stress conditions.

Clinical features. There are multiple phenotypes including a prenatal/congenital form, a subacute infantile form, an early childhood-onset form, a late childhood-/juvenile-onset form, and an adult-onset form. Motor symptoms predominate in the childhood forms, while cognitive decline and personality change characterize the adult form. The congenital type is often associated with severe encephalopathy; however, most children are developmentally normal or only mildly delayed before the first attack. Gait disturbances are usually the initial feature, usually ataxia but sometimes dystonia or spasticity. Repeated attacks cause neurological deterioration and shortened life span.

Diagnosis. This disorder is readily confused with ADEM at onset. However, the cranial MRI, which shows a patchy leukoencephalopathy with cavitation in affected areas, is not consistent with ADEM. With time, the cavities coalesce to form large white matter cysts that spare gray matter until late in the course. Chemical abnormalities such as elevated lactate in the brain, blood, and CSF are inconsistent. Molecular genetic testing confirms biallelic pathogenic variants in one of the five genes mentioned earlier.

Management. Make every effort to avoid fever and head trauma. Low-dose prophylactic antibiotics may be considered, as well as the use of a helmet to minimize the effects of normal childhood minor head traumas. The child should be closely monitored following any sort of stress, including illness, injury, surgery, or significant emotional stress or fright.

Pseudoataxia (Epileptic Ataxia)

Clinical features. Ataxia and other gait disturbances may be the only clinical features of seizure activity. Both limb and gait ataxia may be present, and the child's epilepsy may be undiagnosed. If the child is already taking antiepileptic drugs, a toxic drug effect is often the initial diagnosis. During the ataxic episode, the child may appear inattentive or confused. Like other seizure manifestations, ataxia is sudden in onset and episodic.

Diagnosis. The absence of nystagmus suggests that ataxia is a seizure manifestation and not caused by drug toxicity. The usual EEG findings concurrent with ataxia are prolonged, generalized, 2–3 Hz spike-wave complexes that have a frontal predominance. This is the typical EEG finding in Lennox-Gastaut syndrome (see Chapter 1). Such discharges are ordinarily associated with myoclonic jerks or akinetic seizures. Either one occurring briefly, but repeatedly, could interrupt smooth movement and produce ataxia.

Management. Pseudoataxia usually responds to anticonvulsant drugs.

Trauma

Mild head injuries are common in children and are an almost daily occurrence in toddlers. Recovery is always complete despite considerable parental concern. More serious head injuries, associated with loss of consciousness, seizures, and cerebral contusion, are less common but still account for several thousand deaths in children annually. Ataxia may follow even mild head injuries. In most cases ataxia is part of the so-called postconcussion syndrome, in which imaging studies do not show any structural derangement of the nervous system. In others a cerebellar contusion or posterior fossa hematoma may be present (see Chapter 2). Ataxia may also follow cervical injuries, especially during sports.

Postconcussion Syndrome

Clinical features. Many adults complain of headache, dizziness, and mental changes following even a mild head injury. Some of these symptoms also occur after head injury in children and probably represent a transitory derangement of cerebral function caused by the trauma. Even mild head trauma can cause a cerebral axonopathy, which may explain the persistence of symptoms.

In infants and small children the most prominent postconcussive symptom is ataxia. This is not necessarily a typical cerebellar ataxia but maybe only an unsteady gait. No limb dysmetria is present, and other neurological functions are normal.

In older children with postconcussive syndromes headache and dizziness are as common as ataxia. The headache is usually low grade and transient. When the headache worsens and becomes chronic it is usually an *analgesic-induced headache* (see Chapter 3). Gait is less disturbed, possibly because an older child better compensates for dizziness, but still the sensation of unsteadiness is present.

Diagnosis. The clinical syndrome is the basis for diagnosis. Cranial computed tomography (CT) at the time of injury to exclude intracranial hemorrhage is normal but MRI may show foci of high-signal intensity on T_2-weighted images, indicating axonal injury.

Management. Ataxia usually clears completely within 1 month and always within 6 months. Decreased activity and caution to prevent falls during the time of ataxia is the only treatment needed.

Vascular Disorders
Cerebellar Hemorrhage

Spontaneous cerebellar hemorrhage in children in the absence of coagulopathy is due to arteriovenous malformation, even though less than 10% of intracranial arteriovenous malformations in children are in the cerebellum. The two major features of cerebellar hemorrhage

are ataxia and headache. Even small bleeds may lead to hydrocephalus due to the location in the posterior fossa. Neurosurgery consultation is indicated as shunting, evacuation of blood, or posterior fossa decompression may be acutely needed.

Kawasaki Disease

Kawasaki disease is a systemic vasculitis that occurs predominantly in infants and children. The incidence of the disease is seasonal and higher in children of Asian descent, suggesting that both environmental and genetic factors play a role in pathogenesis.

Clinical features. Five of the following six criteria are required for diagnosis: fever, conjunctival injection, reddening of the oropharynx and lips, indurative edema of the limbs, polymorphic exanthems, and lymphadenopathy. Arthralgia, carditis, and aseptic meningitis may be associated features. Kawasaki disease is identical to childhood polyarteritis nodosa.

Multiple infarcts may occur in the brain. Acute ataxia, facial palsy, ocular motor palsies, and hemiplegia may occur. The neurological and coronary artery complications make Kawasaki disease a serious illness with a guarded prognosis.

Diagnosis. Clinical features of multisystem disease are essential for diagnosis. Abnormal laboratory findings include an increased sedimentation rate, a positive test for C-reactive protein, and increased serum complement and globulin levels. Skin biopsy shows the typical histopathological changes of arteritis.

Management. Intravenous immune globulin, 2 g/kg over 2–5 days, and high-dose aspirin in the acute phase are an effective method of treatment.

Vertebrobasilar Occlusion

Trauma to the vertebrobasilar arteries may occur with childhood injuries including sports and chiropractic manipulation. Bony canals encase the vertebral arteries from C2 to the foramen magnum. Sudden stretching of the arteries by hyperextension or hyperflexion of the neck causes endothelial injury and thrombosis.

Clinical features. The onset of symptoms is within minutes or hours of injury. Vertigo, nausea, and vomiting are the initial symptoms of brainstem ischemia. Occipital headache may be present as well. Ataxia is due to incoordination of the limbs on one side. It may be maximal at onset or progress over several days. Examination shows some combination of unilateral brainstem disturbances (diplopia, facial weakness) and ipsilateral cerebellar dysfunction.

Diagnosis. CT or MRI shows a unilateral infarction in the cerebellar hemisphere. Infarction of the lateral medulla may occur as well. Computed tomography angiography or MRA may falsely appear normal, but conventional arteriography localizes the arterial thrombosis.

Management. Many children recover completely in the months that follow injury. The benefit of antiplatelet versus anticoagulation is not well established, and treatment varies among academic medical centers. Unfractionated heparin or low-molecular-weight heparin can be used as a bridge to oral anticoagulation. Stenting or other intervention may be indicated in certain cases. If a clear traumatic etiology is not found, evaluation of the cervical skeleton to assess for bony abnormalities is indicated, as bony abnormalities are vastly more common in children with arterial dissections than in adults.[24] The clinician should make note of skin laxity or unusual joint flexibility, as these could be signs of a connective tissue disorder. Follow-up imaging 3–6 months after the injury is recommended.

CHRONIC OR PROGRESSIVE ATAXIA

A brain tumor is always an initial concern when progressive ataxia develops in previously normal children, especially if a headache is present as well (see Box 10.2). Congenital abnormalities that cause ataxia are often associated with some degree of cognitive impairment. The onset of symptoms may occur during infancy or be delayed until adult life. Friedreich ataxia (FRDA) is the most common hereditary form of progressive ataxia. The causes of chronic or progressive ataxia are usually easy to diagnose, and many are treatable. Failure to establish a diagnosis can have unfortunate consequences for the child.

Brain Tumors

Approximately 85% of primary brain tumors in children 2–12 years of age occur in the posterior fossa. Supratentorial tumors predominate in children less than 2 years and older than 12 years. Seventy percent of primary brain tumors are gliomas; only 5% of CNS tumors arise from the spinal cord. Neuroectodermal tumors are the second most common malignancy of childhood and the most common solid tumors. The four major tumors of the posterior fossa are cerebellar astrocytoma, brainstem glioma, ependymoma, and primitive neuroectodermal tumors (PNETs; medulloblastoma). The initial feature of brainstem glioma is cranial nerve dysfunction and not ataxia (see Chapter 15). Although this discussion is limited to tumors of the posterior fossa, it is important to remember that supratentorial brain tumors may also cause ataxia. Approximately one-quarter of children with supratentorial brain tumors have gait disturbances at the time of their first hospitalization, and many show signs of cerebellar dysfunction. Gait disturbances occur with equal frequency whether supratentorial tumors are in the midline or the hemispheres, whereas cerebellar signs are more common with midline tumors.

Cerebellar Astrocytoma

Cerebellar astrocytomas comprise 12% of brain tumors in children. The tumor usually grows slowly in the cerebellar hemisphere and consists of a large cyst with a mural nodule. It may be in the hemisphere, in the vermis, in both the hemisphere and vermis, or may occupy the fourth ventricle. Midline tumors are likely to be solid.

Clinical features. Occurrence is equal in both sexes. The peak incidence is at 5–9 years of age but may be as early as infancy. Headache is the most common initial complaint in school-age children, whereas unsteadiness of gait and vomiting are the initial symptoms in preschool children. Headache can be insidious and intermittent; typical morning headache and vomiting are rare. The first complaints of headache and nausea are nonspecific and often attributed to a flu-like illness. Only when symptoms persist is the possibility of increased intracranial pressure considered. In infants and small children separation of cranial sutures often relieves the symptoms of increased intracranial pressure. For this reason, gait disturbances without headache or vomiting are the common initial signs of cerebellar astrocytoma in infants.

Papilledema is present in most affected children at initial examination but is often absent in infants with separation of cranial sutures. Ataxia is present in three-quarters, dysmetria in half, and nystagmus in only a quarter. Ataxia varies in severity from a wide-based, lurching gait to a subtle alteration of gait observed only with tandem walking or quick turning. Its cause is partly the cerebellar location of the tumor and partly hydrocephalus. When the tumor is in the cerebellar hemisphere, ipsilateral or bilateral dysmetria may be present. Other neurological signs sometimes present in children with cerebellar astrocytoma are abducens palsy, multiple cranial nerve palsies, stiff neck, and head tilt.

Diagnosis. MRI is the best imaging study for diagnosis.

Management. Children with life-threatening hydrocephalus should undergo a shunting procedure as the first step in treatment. The shunt relieves many of the symptoms and signs, including ataxia. Corticosteroids are sufficient to relieve pressure in many children with less severe hydrocephalus.

The 5-year survival rate after surgical removal approaches 95%. The mural nodule must be located and removed or the tumor may recur. The amount of tumor resected is difficult to determine at the time of resection, and postoperative imaging studies improve upon the surgeon's estimate. The need for adjuvant radiotherapy is not established.

The total removal of deeper tumors that involve the floor of the fourth ventricle is rare. Local recurrence is common after partial resection. Repeat surgery may be curative in some cases, but postoperative radiation therapy appears to offer a better prognosis following partial resection. The overall disease-free survival rates following either surgery alone or surgery and radiotherapy are 92% at 5 years and 88% at 25 years. Low-grade cerebellar astrocytomas never require chemotherapy, regardless of the degree of surgical resection.

High-grade cerebellar astrocytoma (glioblastoma) is rare in children. More than 30% of childhood patients have dissemination of tumor through the neuraxis (spinal cord drop metastases). Examination of CSF for cytological features and complete myelography always follow surgical resection in patients with glioblastoma. An abnormal result in either indicates whole-axis radiation therapy.

Cerebellar Hemangioblastoma (Von Hippel-Lindau Disease)

Von Hippel-Lindau (VHL) disease is a multisystem disorder transmitted by autosomal dominant inheritance.[25] The most prominent features are hemangioblastomas of the cerebellum, spinal cord, and retina as well as pancreatic cysts. The expression of VHL disease is variable even within the same kindred, and there are no formal diagnostic criteria. The most common features are cerebellar and retinal hemangioblastoma (59%), renal carcinoma (28%), and pheochromocytoma (7%). Both simplex and inherited cases occur.

Clinical features. Mean age at onset of cerebellar hemangioblastoma in VHL disease is 32 years; onset before age 15 is unusual. The initial features are headache and ataxia. Retinal hemangioblastomas occur at a younger age and may cause visual impairment from hemorrhage as early as the first decade. They may be multiple and bilateral and appear on ophthalmoscopic examination as a dilated artery leading from the disk to a peripheral tumor with an engorged vein. Spinal hemangioblastomas are intramedullary in location and lead to syringomyelia. Pheochromocytomas occur in 7%–19% of patients and may be the only clinical manifestation.

Diagnosis. Suspect the diagnosis in individuals with any of the following: more than one hemangioblastoma of the CNS, an isolated hemangioblastoma associated with a visceral cyst or renal carcinoma, or any known manifestation with a family history of disease. Molecular genetic testing of the *VHL* gene detects mutations in nearly 100% of patients and is useful if the clinical picture is ambiguous. The gene for VHL disease is a tumor-suppressor gene that maps to chromosome 3p25. Clinical testing allows the identification of asymptomatic, affected family members who need annual examinations to look for treatable abnormalities. Such examinations should include indirect ophthalmoscopy and renal ultrasound, as well as gadolinium-enhanced MRI of the brain, total spine, and abdomen every 2 years.[26]

Management. Cryotherapy or photocoagulation of smaller retinal lesions can lead to complete tumor regression without visual loss. The treatment of cerebellar hemangioblastoma is surgical and total extirpation is the rule. Genetic counseling, testing, and monitoring of affected family members are recommended.

Ependymoma

The derivation of posterior fossa ependymoma is the cells that line the roof and floor of the fourth ventricle. These tumors can extend into both lateral recesses and grow out to the cerebellopontine angle. They account for approximately 10% of primary brain tumors in children.

Clinical features. The peak incidence in children is from birth to 4 years with an equal incidence in males and females. The clinical features evolve slowly and are often present for several months before initial consultation. Symptoms of increased intracranial pressure are the first feature in 90% of children. Disturbances of gait and coordination, neck pain, or cranial nerve dysfunction are the initial features in the remainder. Half of the affected children have ataxia, usually of the vermal type, and one-third have nystagmus. Head tilt or neck stiffness is present in one-third of children and indicates the extension of the tumor into the cervical canal.

Although steady deterioration is expected, some children have an intermittent course. Episodes of headache and vomiting, ataxia, and even nuchal rigidity last for days or weeks and are then followed by periods of well-being. The cause of the intermittent symptoms is transitory obstruction of the fourth ventricle or aqueduct by the tumor acting in a ball-valve fashion.

Diagnosis. Only two grades of ependymoma are recognized: classic (benign) and anaplastic (malignant). Because ependymomas typically arise in the ependymal linings of ventricles, tumors may spread through the entire neuraxis. A typical MRI appearance of a fourth ventricular ependymoma is a homogeneously enhancing solid mass that extends out of the foramina of Luschka or Magendie with associated obstructive hydrocephalus. Marked dilation of the ventricular system is usual. Evaluation includes contrast-enhanced MRI scans of the brain and entire spinal cord as well as cytological evaluation of the CSF.

Management. The single most important factor determining prognosis is the degree of resection.[27] The goals of surgery are to relieve hydrocephalus and to remove as much tumor as possible without damaging the fourth ventricle. Irradiation to the posterior fossa usually follows surgery, but not neuraxis radiation, unless the diagnosis of leptomeningeal spread is established. Poor prognostic features include an age of less than 2–5 years at diagnosis, brainstem invasion, and a radiation dose of less than 4500 cGy.[28]

Medulloblastoma

Medulloblastoma is a PNET of the posterior fossa with the capacity to differentiate into neuronal and glial tissue. Most tumors are in the vermis or fourth ventricle, with or without extension into the cerebellar hemispheres. Approximately 10% are in the hemisphere alone. Medulloblastomas represent approximately 85% of intracranial neuroepithelial tumors and 20% of all pediatric brain tumors. Data from the National Cancer Institute's Surveillance, Epidemiology, and End Results (SEER) registry indicate an increasing incidence of medulloblastoma.[29]

Clinical features. Ninety percent of cases have their onset during the first decade and the remainder during the second decade. Medulloblastoma is the most common primary brain tumor with onset during infancy.

The tumor grows rapidly, and the interval between onset of symptoms and medical consultation is generally brief: 2 weeks in 25% of cases and less than 1 month in 50%. Vomiting is an initial symptom in 58% of children, headache in 40%, an unsteady gait in 20%, and torticollis or stiff neck in 10%. The probable cause of prominent vomiting, with or without headache, as an early symptom is tumor irritation of the floor of the fourth ventricle. Gait disturbances are more common in young children, usually secondary to refusal to stand or walk rather than ataxia.

Two-thirds of children have papilledema at the time of initial examination. Truncal ataxia and limb ataxia are equally common, and both may be present. Only 22% of children have nystagmus. Tendon reflexes are hyperactive when hydrocephalus is present and hypoactive when the tumor is causing primarily cerebellar dysfunction.

Diagnosis. CT or MRI easily identifies medulloblastoma (Fig. 10.3). The tumors are vascular and become enhanced when contrast medium is used.

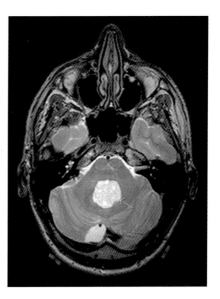

Fig. 10.3 Medulloblastoma. T_2 axial magnetic resonance imaging shows (*arrow*) a heterogeneous cystic mass in the vermis of cerebellum and an incidental subarachnoid cyst.

Management. The combined use of surgical resection, radiation therapy, and chemotherapy greatly improves the prognosis for children with medulloblastoma. The role of surgery is to provide histological identification, debulk the tumor, and relieve obstruction of the fourth ventricle. Ventriculoperitoneal shunting reduces intracranial pressure even before decompressive resection.

The overall 5-year survival rate ranges from 50% to 90% and is dependent on multiple factors including tumor burden at the time of diagnosis, cytogenetic and copy number variants. Survival is better in children who have gross total tumor resection compared with partial resection or biopsy. Craniospinal radiation increases survival better than local field radiation. The use of adjuvant chemotherapy significantly improves survival. Most initial recurrences occur at the primary site. One histological variant, anaplastic large cell medulloblastoma, carries a poorer prognosis because of a higher risk for early metastatic involvement and recurrence.[30] The presence of dissemination is the single most important factor that correlates with outcome.[31]

Congenital Malformations
Basilar Impression

Basilar impression is a disorder of the craniovertebral junction. Posterior displacement of the odontoid process compresses the spinal cord or brainstem.

Clinical features. The first symptoms are often head tilt, neck stiffness, and headache. Minor trauma to the head or neck frequently precipitates the onset of symptoms. Examination shows ataxia, nystagmus, and hyperreflexia.

Diagnosis. MRI is the best method to visualize both the cervicomedullary junction and an associated Chiari malformation or syringobulbia.

Management. Surgical decompression of the foramen magnum usually relieves symptoms.

Cerebellar Malformations

Congenital hemisphere hypoplasia. Congenital hypoplasia of the cerebellum can be unilateral or bilateral. More than half of patients with bilateral disease have an identifiable genetic disorder transmitted by autosomal recessive inheritance. The common histological feature is the absence of granular cells, with the relative preservation of Purkinje cells. Unilateral cerebellar hypoplasia is not associated with genetic disorders. In some hereditary forms granular cell degeneration may continue postnatally and cause progressive cerebellar dysfunction during infancy.

Clinical features. Developmental delay and hypotonia are the first features suggesting a CNS abnormality in the infant. Titubation of the head is a constant feature, and some combination of ataxia, dysmetria, and intention tremor is noted. A jerky, coarse nystagmus is usually present. Tendon reflexes may be increased or diminished. Those with hyperactive reflexes probably have congenital abnormalities of the corticospinal tract in addition to cerebellar hypoplasia. Seizures occur in some hereditary and some sporadic cases. Other neurological signs and symptoms may be present, depending on associated malformations. Cognitive impairment is typically present and ranges from mild to severe.

Diagnosis. MRI is diagnostic of the disorder (Fig. 10.4). It shows not only the extent of cerebellar hypoplasia but also associated anomalies. The folial pattern of the cerebellum is prominent, and there is compensatory enlargement of the fourth ventricle, cisterna magna, and vallecula.

Management. No treatment is available.

Vermal aplasia. Aplasia of the vermis is relatively common and often associated with other midline cerebral malformations. All or part of the vermis may be missing, and, when the vermis is incomplete, the caudal portion is usually lacking. Dominantly inherited aplasia of the anterior vermis is a rare condition.

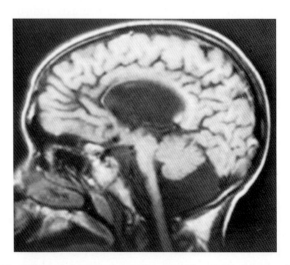

Fig. 10.4 Aplasia of the cerebellum associated with thinning of the corpus callosum.

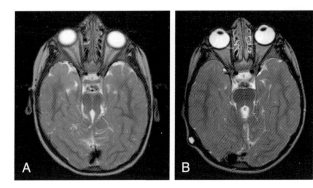

Fig. 10.5 Joubert Syndrome. T$_2$ axial magnetic resonance images of siblings with the molar tooth sign.

Clinical features. Partial agenesis of the cerebellar vermis may be asymptomatic. Symptoms are nonprogressive and vary from only mild gait ataxia and upbeating nystagmus to severe ataxia.

Complete agenesis causes titubation of the head and truncal ataxia. Vermal agenesis is frequently associated with other cerebral malformations, producing a constellation of symptoms and signs referable to neurological dysfunction. Two such examples are *Dandy-Walker malformation* (see Chapter 18) and *Joubert syndrome* (Fig. 10.5).

Joubert syndrome comprises hypotonia, developmental delay, and a distinctive cerebellar and brainstem abnormality known as the *molar tooth sign*. At least 34 genes may cause Joubert syndrome; 33 of these are autosomal recessive and one is X-linked.[32]

Diagnosis. MRI shows agenesis of the vermis of the cerebellum with enlargement of the cisterna magna (molar tooth sign). Other cerebral malformations, such as agenesis of the corpus callosum, may occur.

Management. No treatment is available.

X-Linked cerebellar ataxias. Multiple distinct abnormalities of the X chromosome cause cerebellar dysgenesis or hypoplasia with resultant ataxia. This is a rapidly expanding group of disorders whose classification is likely to evolve over the next several years.

Clinical features. Ataxia and motor milestone delays are consistent features. Hypotonia, mild dysphagia, and delayed motor development may be present from birth and often evolve into action tremors of the upper limbs and slow eye movements by early childhood. By adult life, neurological symptoms may include intellectual disability, moderate dysarthria, unsteady gait with truncal and locomotor ataxia, intention tremor, and limitation

of vertical gaze with slow conjugate eye movements. However, a wide variation in phenotypes exists depending on the specific mutation.

Diagnosis. Brain MRI shows atrophy of the cerebellar vermis and/or hemispheres. Some affected males have other associated cerebral malformations. Extraneurological manifestations may occur.

Management. Treatment is supportive.

Chiari Malformations

The *type I Chiari malformation* is a displacement of the cerebellar tonsils and posterior vermis of the cerebellum through the foramen magnum, compressing the spinomedullary junction. The *type II Chiari malformation* has an additional downward displacement of a dysplastic lower medulla and a lumbosacral meningomyelocele (see Chapter 12). A molecular genetic hypothesis of ectopic expression of a segmentation gene in the rhombomeres explains the several cerebellar and brainstem anomalies, as well as the defective basioccipital and supraoccipital bone formation.[33]

Clinical features. The widespread use of MRI has shown that Chiari I malformations are often an incidental finding in neuroimaging studies in children with epilepsy or migraines. When symptomatic, the onset is frequently during adolescence or adult life. Major clinical features are headache, head tilt, pain in the neck and shoulders, ataxia, and lower cranial nerve dysfunction. Physical signs vary among patients and may include weakness of the arms, hyperactive tendon reflexes in the legs, nystagmus, and ataxia. Children with chronic headaches and Chiari I often suffer from migraines and analgesic-induced headaches. The physical finding should be considered an incidental finding in children

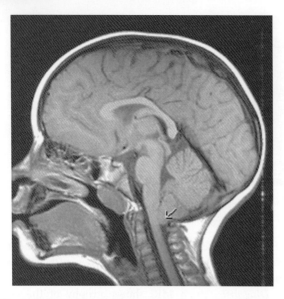

Fig. 10.6 Chiari Type I Malformation. T_1 sagittal magnetic resonance imaging shows downward displacement of the cerebellar tonsils (*arrow*).

with a normal neurological exam and lack of symptoms other than headaches.

Diagnosis. MRI provides the best visualization of posterior fossa structures. The distortion of the cerebellum and the hindbrain is precisely identified (Fig. 10.6). Obtain a cervical spine MRI as well, to assess for coexistent syrinx.

Management. Surgical decompression of the foramen magnum to at least the C3 vertebra is the recommended treatment in symptomatic individuals. Significant improvement occurs in more than half of patients.

Progressive Hereditary Ataxias
Autosomal Dominant Inheritance

Spinocerebellar degenerations. A genotypic classification of the dominantly inherited ataxias has replaced the phenotypic classification that included *Marie ataxia*, *olivopontocerebellar atrophy*, and *SCAs*.[34] Table 10.1 lists some of the more common progressive autosomal dominant ataxias with onset in childhood. There are over 40 currently identified dominantly inherited SCAs, and the number continues to grow. The most common subtypes are SCA1, SCA2, SCA3, and SCA6. SCA3, formerly known as *Machado-Joseph disease*, is the most common type overall.

TABLE 10.1   Autosomal Dominant Cerebellar Ataxias: Clinical Characteristics

Disease	Average Onset (Range in Years)	Clinical Features (All Include Ataxia)
SCA1	4th decade (<10 to >60)	Pyramidal signs, peripheral neuropathy
SCA2	3rd–4th decade (<10 to >60)	Slow saccadic eye movement, peripheral neuropathy, decreased DTRs, dementia
SCA3	4th decade (10–70)	Pyramidal and extrapyramidal signs; lid retraction, nystagmus, decreased saccade velocity; amyotrophic fasciculations, sensory loss
SCA4	4th–5th decade (19–59)	Sensory axonal neuropathy
SCA5	3rd–4th decade (10–68)	Early onset, slow course
SCA7	3rd–4th decade (1/2–60)	Visual loss with retinopathy
SCA12	3rd (8–55)	Early tremor, late dementia
DRPLA	Rare (United States) (8–20) 20% (Japan) (40–60s)	Early onset correlates with shorter duration; chorea, seizures, dementia, myoclonus

DRPLA, Dentatorubral-pallidoluysian atrophy; *DTRs*, deep tendon reflexes; *SCA*, spinocerebellar ataxia.
Adapted from Bird TD. Ataxia overview. In: *GeneClinics: Medical Genetics Knowledge Base [database online]*. University of Washington. Available from: http://www.geneclinics.org.

Clinical features. The clinical features overlap, and genetic testing is the best method for diagnosis. Common but not universal symptoms include decreased reflexes, peripheral neuropathy with sensory loss, and cognitive decline or impairment. Table 10.1 indicates a few distinguishing clinical features.

Diagnosis. Multigene panels are available. Since many SCAs are trinucleotide repeat disorders, anticipation may cause the child to experience significant symptoms before the parent is aware that he or she carries the disease.

Management. Treatment is symptomatic and, depending on the disease, may include anticonvulsants, muscle relaxants, and assistive devices.

Hypobetalipoproteinemia.

Clinical features. Several different disorders are associated with hypocholesterolemia, and reduced, but not absent, concentrations of apolipoprotein B and apolipoprotein A. Some patients with this lipid profile have no neurological symptoms; others have severe ataxia beginning in infancy. Malabsorption does not occur, but the infant fails to thrive and has progressive fatty cirrhosis of the liver. Severe hypotonia and absence of tendon reflexes are present in the first months.

Diagnosis. The diagnosis is a consideration in children with unexplained progressive ataxia. The total serum lipid content is normal, but the concentration of triglycerides is increased. Reduced concentrations of total high- and low-density lipoprotein cholesterol concentrations and apolipoproteins are characteristic.

Management. Administration of 100–300 mg/kg/day of DL-α-tocopherol prevents many of the complications of hypobetalipoproteinemia. Vitamins A and K supplements are also required.

Autosomal Recessive Inheritance

Ataxia is a feature of many degenerative disorders but is a presenting or cardinal feature in the disorders discussed in this section.

Abetalipoproteinemia.

Molecular defect(s) in the gene for the microsomal triglyceride transfer protein (MTTP) at chromosome 4q22-q24 cause abetalipoproteinemia. Transmission is by autosomal recessive inheritance. Other terms for the disorder are *acanthocytosis* and *Bassen-Kornzweig syndrome*. MTTP catalyzes the transport of triglycerides, cholesteryl esters, and phospholipids from phospholipid surfaces. The results are fat malabsorption and a progressive deficiency of vitamins A, E, and K.

Clinical features. Fat malabsorption is present from birth, and most newborns come to medical attention because of failure to thrive, vomiting, and large volumes of loose stool. A correct diagnosis is possible at that time.

Delayed psychomotor development occurs during infancy. Cerebellar ataxia develops in one-third of children during the first decade and in almost every child by the end of the second decade. Tendon reflexes are usually lost by 5 years of age. Progressive gait disturbances, dysmetria, and difficulty performing rapid alternating movements characterize the limb ataxia, which progresses until the third decade and then becomes stationary. Proprioceptive sensation in the hands and feet is lost, while pinprick and temperature sensations are less severely affected. Sensory loss results from demyelination in the posterior columns of the spinal cord and the peripheral nerves.

Retinitis pigmentosa is an almost constant feature. The age at onset is variable but is usually during the first decade. The initial symptom is night blindness. Nystagmus is common, and its cause may be either cerebellar disturbance or the loss of central vision.

Diagnosis. Severe anemia, with hemoglobin levels less than 8 g/dL (5 mmol/L), is common in young children but not in adults. The anemia, which may result from malabsorption, corrects with parenteral supplementation of iron or folate. Plasma cholesterol levels are less than 100 mg/dL (2.5 mmol/L), and triglyceride levels are less than 30 mg/dL (0.3 mmol/L). The absence of apolipoprotein B in plasma confirms the diagnosis. Measure the parents' plasma apolipoprotein B concentrations as well as the child's. In abetalipoproteinemia the heterozygote is normal; if partial deficiency of apolipoprotein B is present, the diagnosis of familial hypobetalipoproteinemia is more likely.

Management. The cause of the neurological complications of abetalipoproteinemia is chronic vitamin E deficiency. Dietary fat restriction and large oral doses of vitamin E (100 mg/kg/day) prevent the onset of symptoms or arrest their progression.

Ataxia telangiectasia.

Ataxia telangiectasia (AT) primarily affects the nervous and immune systems.[35] The associated gene, *ATM*, is a large gene located at chromosome 11q22-23. The gene product is involved in cell-cycle progression and the checkpoint response to DNA damage. Transmission is by autosomal recessive inheritance.

Clinical features. The principal feature is a progressive truncal ataxia that begins during the first year. In infants choreoathetosis develops instead of, or in addition to, ataxia. The ataxia begins as clumsiness and progresses so slowly that cerebral palsy is often diagnosed erroneously. Oculomotor apraxia is present in 90% of patients but may be mild at first and overlooked (see Chapter 15). Many children have reduced facial expressions. Cognitively, children develop normally at first, but many (up to one-third) develop mild intellectual disability over time. Telangiectasia usually develops after 2 years of age and sometimes as late as age 10. It first appears on the bulbar conjunctivae, giving the eyes a bloodshot appearance. Similar telangiectasia appears on the upper half of the ears, on the flexor surfaces of the limbs, and in a butterfly distribution on the face. Sun exposure or irritation exacerbates telangiectasias.

Recurrent sinopulmonary infection is one of the more serious features of the disease and reflects an underlying immunodeficiency. The synthesis of antibodies and certain immunoglobulin subclasses is disturbed because of disorders of B-cell and helper T-cell function. Serum and salivary IgA is absent in 70%–80% of children with telangiectasia, and IgE is absent or diminished in 80%–90%. The IgM concentration may be elevated in compensation for the IgA deficiency. The thymus has an embryonic appearance, and the α-fetoprotein concentration is elevated in most patients.

Taken together, the many features of this disease suggest a generalized disorder of tissue differentiation and cellular repair. The result is a malignancy risk of 38%, usually lymphoma and lymphocytic leukemia. Life expectancy is reduced, with mean survival in two large cohorts averaging in the early 20s, with a wide range.[36] Infection is the most common cause of death, and neoplasia is second.

Diagnosis. Suspect the diagnosis in infants with some combination of ataxia, chronic sinopulmonary infections, and oculomotor apraxia. As the child gets older, the addition of telangiectasia to the other clinical features makes the diagnosis a certainty. Complete studies of immunocompetence are required. Ninety percent of patients with AT have an elevated α-fetoprotein concentration and approximately 80% have decreased serum IgA, IgE, or IgG. Especially characteristic is a selective deficiency of the IgG_2 subclass. Molecular genetic testing is available in children with a compatible clinical syndrome and normal serum concentrations of α-fetoprotein and immunoglobulin.

Management. Treat all infections vigorously. Intravenous antibiotics are sometimes required for what would otherwise be trivial sinusitis in a normal child. Patients with AT are exquisitely sensitive to radiation, which produces cellular and chromosomal damage. Radiation may be a precipitant in the development of neoplasia. Therefore despite the frequency of sinopulmonary infections, minimize radiation exposure.

Ataxia with oculomotor apraxia type 1. This disorder may be mistaken for AT but is a different genetic disorder.[37]

Clinical features. Development is normal during the first year, but a slowly progressive ataxia develops during childhood. The onset of progressive gait imbalance is usually 7 years but ranges from 2 to 16 years. Dysarthria, dysmetria, and mild intention tremor follow. Oculomotor apraxia is a late feature and progresses to external ophthalmoplegia. A severe, progressive neuropathy results in generalized areflexia, quadriplegia, and atrophy of the hands and feet. Chorea and arm dystonia are common. Intellect is normal in some and impaired in others.

Diagnosis. Molecular genetic testing is clinically available.

Management. Treatment is supportive.

Ataxia with oculomotor apraxia type 2. This disorder may be mistaken for AT but is a different genetic disorder.[38]

Clinical features. The onset of symptoms is between age 3 and 30 years. The features include ataxia caused by cerebellar atrophy, axonal sensorimotor neuropathy, and oculomotor apraxia.

Diagnosis. The serum concentration of α-fetoprotein is elevated. Molecular genetic testing is clinically available.

Management. Treatment is supportive.

Friedreich ataxia. FRDA is the most common recessively inherited ataxia. The cause is an unstable triplet repeat of the frataxin gene *FXN* on chromosome 9q13.[39] The size at which the expansion causes disease is not established.

Clinical features. The onset is usually between 2 and 16 years of age, but symptoms may begin later. The initial feature is ataxia or clumsiness of gait in 95% of cases and scoliosis in 5%. The ataxia is slowly progressive and is associated with dysarthria, depressed tendon reflexes, extensor plantar responses, foreshortening of the foot creating a high arch, and loss of position and vibration senses. Two-thirds of patients have hypertrophic cardiomyopathy and 10% have diabetes mellitus. An atypical presentation occurs in 25%. These atypical syndromes include any of the following features: (1) onset after age

25 years, (2) present tendon reflexes, and (3) spastic paraparesis without ataxia.

Diagnosis. The clinical features suggest the diagnosis and molecular genetic testing provides confirmation. Motor nerve conduction velocities in the arms and legs are slightly slower than normal. In contrast, sensory action potentials are absent or markedly reduced in amplitude. Spinal somatosensory evoked responses are usually absent. Common changes on the electrocardiogram (ECG) are reduced amplitude of T waves and left or right ventricular hypertrophy. Arrhythmias and conduction defects are uncommon.

Management. The FDA recently approved omaveloxolone (Skyclarys) to treat Friedreich ataxia in adolescents and adults over 16 years. Omaveloxolone activates the antioxidative transcription factor Nrf2 and inhibits the proinflammatory transcription factor NF-κB, leading to improved cellular responses to stress. Clinical trials and post hoc analysis demonstrate moderate overall clinical improvement in treated patients.[40] Surgical stabilization prevents severe scoliosis. Regular ECG and chest radiographs to determine heart size are useful to monitor the development of cardiomyopathy. Chest pain on exertion responds to propranolol, and congestive heart failure responds to digitalis. Patients with diabetes require insulin treatment.

Juvenile GM$_2$ gangliosidosis. The transmission of all juvenile forms of both α- and β-hexosaminidase-A deficiency is by autosomal recessive inheritance. Some, like *Tay-Sachs disease,* mainly occur in Ashkenazi Jews, whereas others occur in individuals of non-Jewish descent (see Chapter 5). In all of these conditions GM$_2$ gangliosides are stored within the CNS.

Clinical features. A progressive ataxic syndrome occurs in patients with late-onset hexosaminidase-A deficiency. Symptom onset is usually before 15 years. Family members may believe that affected children are only clumsy before neurological deterioration becomes evident. Intention tremor, dysarthria, and limb and gait ataxia are prominent.

Diagnosis. Any child with an apparent "spinocerebellar degeneration" may have juvenile GM$_2$ gangliosidosis. Diagnosis requires confirmatory molecular genetic testing or the measurement of α- and β-hexosaminidase activity in fibroblasts.

Management. Specific treatment is not available.

Juvenile sulfatide lipidosis. Sulfatide lipidosis (*metachromatic leukodystrophy*) is a disorder of central and peripheral myelin metabolism usually caused by deficient activity of the enzyme arylsulfatase A. The defective gene is on chromosome 22q. Discussion of the late infantile form is in Chapters 5 and 7. The usual cause of the juvenile form is arylsulfatase deficiency, but a secondary cause is saposin B deficiency.

Clinical features. Juvenile sulfatide lipidosis begins later and has a slower course than the late infantile disease. Onset is usually between 4 and 12 years of age. Initial symptoms are poor school performance, behavioral change, and gait disturbance. Spasticity, progressive gait and limb ataxia, seizures, and cognitive deterioration follow. Peripheral neuropathy is not a prominent clinical feature, but prolonged motor conduction velocities are usually late in the course. Protein concentration in the CSF may be normal or only slightly elevated.

Progression is relatively rapid. Most children deteriorate into a vegetative state and die within 10 years. The time from onset to death ranges from 3 to 17 years and the age at onset does not predict the course.

Diagnosis. MRI shows widespread demyelination of the cerebral hemispheres. Late-onset disease may resemble MS. Diagnosis requires confirmatory molecular genetic testing or the demonstration of reduced or absent arylsulfatase A in peripheral leukocytes. Those with reduced amounts require testing for saposin B deficiency.

Management. Allogeneic bone marrow transplantation, when used early in the course, slows the rate of progression.

Marinesco-Sjögren syndrome. Cerebellar ataxia, congenital cataracts, myopathy, and intellectual disability are the characteristic features of Marinesco-Sjögren syndrome. Mutations of the *SIL1* gene cause two-thirds of cases; the remaining one-third lack a known etiology.

Clinical features. A constant feature is cataracts, which may be congenital or develop during infancy. The type of cataract varies and is not specific. Dysarthria, nystagmus, and ataxia of the trunk and limbs characterize the cerebellar dysfunction during infancy. Strabismus and hypotonia are frequently present in childhood. Developmental delay is a constant feature but varies from mild to severe. Other features include short stature, delayed sexual development, pes valgus, and scoliosis.

Although the onset of symptoms is in infancy, progression is slow or stationary. Ataxia leads to wheelchair confinement by the third or fourth decade and the shortening of life span is significant.

Diagnosis. The basis of diagnosis is clinical and neuroimaging studies. *SIL1* is the only known gene associated with Marinesco-Sjögren syndrome. Molecular genetic testing is possible, but some patients with the clinical syndrome have no genetic defect on sequence analysis.

Management. Treatment is supportive.

Other metabolic disorders. Descriptions of *Hartnup disease* and *maple syrup urine disease* are in the section on acute or recurrent ataxia. After an acute attack of these diseases, some patients never return to baseline but instead have chronic progressive ataxia. Such patients require screening for metabolic disorders (Table 10.2). *Refsum disease* is an inborn error of phytanic acid metabolism and transmission is by autosomal recessive inheritance. The cardinal features are retinitis pigmentosa, chronic or recurrent polyneuropathy, and cerebellar ataxia. Affected individuals usually have either night blindness or neuropathy (see Chapter 7).

TABLE 10.2 Metabolic Screening in Progressive Ataxias

Disease	Abnormality
Blood	
Abetalipoproteinemia	Lipoproteins, cholesterol
Adrenoleukodystrophy	Very long-chain fatty acids
Ataxia telangiectasia	IgA, IgE, α-fetoprotein
Hypobetalipoproteinemia	Lipoproteins, cholesterol
Mitochondrial disorders	Lactate, glucose-lactate tolerance
Sulfatide lipidoses	Arylsulfatase A
Urine	
Hartnup disease	Amino acids
Maple syrup urine disease[a]	Amino acids
Fibroblasts	
Carnitine acetyltransferase deficiency[a]	Carnitine acetyltransferase
GM$_2$ gangliosidosis	Hexosaminidase
Refsum disease	Phytanic acid
Bone Marrow	
Neurovisceral storage	Sea-blue histiocytes

[a]The most common conditions and the ones with disease-modifying treatments.

IGA, Immunoglobulin A; *IgE,* immunoglobulin E.

Disorders of pyruvate metabolism and the respiratory chain enzymes cause widespread disturbances in the nervous system and are described in Chapters 5, 7, and 8. The common features among the several disorders of mitochondrial metabolism include lactic acidosis, ataxia, hypotonia, ophthalmoplegia, intellectual disability, and peripheral neuropathy. A raised concentration of blood lactate or the production of lactic acidosis by administration of a standard glucose tolerance test suggests a mitochondrial disorder. Deficiency of PDH may produce acute, recurrent, or chronic ataxias and is discussed in the section on acute or recurrent ataxia. Respiratory chain disorders produce a combination of ataxia, dementia, myoclonus, and seizures.

X-Linked Inheritance

The childhood cerebral form of *X-linked adrenoleukodystrophy* begins with learning difficulty and behavioral problems starting between ages 4 and 10 that may mimic attention deficit hyperactivity disorder. Mutations in the *ABCD1* gene cause defective transport and breakdown of very long-chain fatty acids (VLCFAs) and subsequent neurotoxicity. The clinical features can mimic an SCA and require consideration in any family with only males affected.

Clinical features. The presenting symptoms are usually behavioral or learning problems. Additional clinical features include dysphagia, ataxia, vision problems, apraxia, regression of fine motor skills (including handwriting), and receptive language impairment. All affected boys should be monitored for adrenocortical insufficiency. The disease course is variable but may rapidly progress to disability and death within a few years.

Diagnosis. Affected boys have elevated levels of VLCFAs. MRI of the brain demonstrates a characteristic pattern of white matter volume loss and increased signal intensity in the posterior regions, with sparing of the anterior white matter. Genetic testing is available.

Management. Treatment includes corticosteroids and supportive therapies.

REFERENCES

1. Subramony SH, Schott K, Raike RS, et al. Novel CACNA1A mutation causes febrile episodic ataxia with interictal cerebellar deficits. *Annals of Neurology.* 2003;54:725-731.
2. De Vries B, Mamsa H, Stam AH, et al. Episodic ataxia associated with EAAT1 mutation C186S affecting glutamate reuptake. *Archives of Neurology.* 2009;66(1):97-101.

3. Perlman S. Hereditary ataxia overview. 1998 Oct 28 [Updated 2023 Nov 16]. In: Adam MP, Feldman J, Mirzaa GM, et al., eds. *GeneReviews*®. University of Washington; 1993-2024. https://www.ncbi.nlm.nih.gov/books/NBK1138/.

4. Sawaishi Y, Takahashi I, Hirayama Y, et al. Acute cerebellitis caused by *Coxiella burnetii*. *Annals of Neurology*. 1999;45:124-127.

5. Pillai SC, Hacohen Y, Tantsis E. Infectious and autoantibody-associated encephalitis: clinical features and long- term outcome. *Pediatrics*. 2015;135(4): e974-e984.

6. Schmitt SE, Pargeon K, Frechette ES, Hirsch LJ, Dalmau J, Friedman D. Extreme delta brush: a unique EEG pattern in adults with anti-NMDA receptor encephalitis. *Neurology*. 2012;79(11):1094-1100. https://doi.org/10.1212/WNL.0b013e3182698cd8. Epub 2012 Aug 29. PMID: 22933737; PMCID: PMC3525298.

7. Nozaki J, Dakeishi M, Ohura T, et al. Homozygosity mapping to chromosome 5p15 of a gene responsible for Hartnup disorder. *Biochemical and Biophysical Research Communications*. 2001;284:255-260.

8. Strauss KA, Puffenberger EG, Carson VJ. Maple syrup urine disease. 2006 Jan 30 [Updated 2020 Apr 23]. In: Adam MP, Mirzaa GM, Pagon RA, et al., eds. *GeneReviews*®. University of Washington; 1993-2023. https://www.ncbi.nlm.nih.gov/books/NBK1319/.

9. Head RA, Brown RM, Zolkipli Z, et al. Clinical and genetic spectrum of pyruvate dehydrogenase deficiency: dihydrolipoamide acetyltransferase (E2) deficiency. *Annals of Neurology*. 2005;58:234-241.

10. Klepper J, Leiendecker B, Bredahl R, et al. Introduction of a ketogenic diet in young infants. *Journal of Inherited Metabolic Disease*. 2002;25:449-460.

11. Yamani N, Chalmer MA, Olesen J. Migraine with brainstem aura: defining the core syndrome. *Brain*. 2019;142(12): 3868-3875. https://doi.org/10.1093/brain/awz338. PMID: 31789370.

12. Kirchmann M, Thomsen LL, Oleson J. Basilar type migraine: clinical, epidemiologic, and genetic features. *Neurology*. 2006;66:880-886.

13. Lindskog U, Odkvist L, Noaksson L, et al. Benign paroxysmal vertigo in childhood: a long-term follow-up. *Headache*. 1999;39:33-37.

14. Jacobs BC, Endtz H, van der Meche FG, et al. Serum anti-GQ1b IgG antibodies recognize surface epitopes on *Campylobacter jejuni* from patients with Miller Fisher syndrome. *Annals of Neurology*. 1995;37: 260-264.

15. Ruggieri M, Polizzi A, Pavone L, et al. Multiple sclerosis in children less under 6 years of age. *Neurology*. 1999;53:478-484.

16. Mikaeloff Y, Suissa S, Vallee L, et al. First episode of acute CNS inflammatory demyelination in childhood: prognostic factors for multiple sclerosis and disability. *Journal of Pediatrics*. 2004;144:246-252.

17. Frohman EM, Goodin DS, Calabresi PA, et al. The utility of MRI in suspected MS: report of the Therapeutics and Technology Assessment Subcommittee of the American Academy of Neurology. *Neurology*. 2003;61:602-611.

18. Mesarus S, Rocco MA, Absinto A, et al. Evidence of thalamic grey matter loss in pediatric multiple sclerosis. *Neurology*. 2008;70:1107-1113.

19. Blaes F, Fuhlhuber V, Korfei M, et al. Surface-binding autoantibodies to cerebellar neurons in opsoclonus syndrome. *Annals of Neurology*. 2005;58:313-317.

20. Russo C, Cohen SL, Petruzzi J, et al. Long-term neurological outcome in children with opsoclonus-myoclonus associated with neuroblastoma: a report of the Pediatric Oncology Group. *Medical and Pediatric Oncology*. 1997;29:284-288.

21. Pranzatelli M, Travelstead A, Tate E, et al. CSF B-cell expansion in opsoclonus-myoclonus syndrome: a biomarker of disease activity. *Movement Disorders*. 2004;19(7):770-777.

22. Hayward K, Jeremy RJ, Jenkins S, et al. Long-term neurobehavioral outcomes in children with neuroblastoma and opsoclonus-myoclonus-ataxia syndrome: relationship to MRI findings and anti-neuronal antibodies. *Journal of Pediatrics*. 2001;139:552-559.

23. van der Knaap MS, Fogli A, Boespflug-Tanguy O, et al. Childhood ataxia with central nervous system hypomyelination/vanishing white matter. 2003 Feb 20 [Updated 2019 Apr 4]. In: Adam MP, Mirzaa GM, Pagon RA, et al., eds. *GeneReviews*®. University of Washington; 1993-2023. https://www.ncbi.nlm.nih.gov/books/NBK1258/.

24. Hasan I, Wapnick S, Tenner MS. Vertebral artery dissection in children: a comprehensive review. *Pediatric Neurosurgery*. 2002;37:168-177.

25. Van Leeuwaarde RS, Ahmad S, Links TP, et al. Von Hippel-Lindau syndrome. In: Adam MP, Ardinger HH, Pagon RA, et al., eds. *GeneReviews*®. University of Washington; 1993-2019. https://www.ncbi.nlm.nih.gov/books/NBK1463.

26. van Leeuwaarde RS, Ahmad S, Links TP, et al. Von Hippel-Lindau syndrome. 2000 May 17 [Updated 2018 Sep 6]. In: Adam MP, Mirzaa GM, Pagon RA, et al., eds. *GeneReviews*®. University of Washington; 1993-2023. https://www.ncbi.nlm.nih.gov/books/NBK1463/.

27. Perilongo G, Massimino M, Sotti G, et al. Analyses of prognostic factors in a retrospective review of 92 children with ependymoma: Italian Pediatric Neuro-Oncology Group. *Medical and Pediatric Oncology*. 1998;29:79-85.

28. Paulino AC, Wen BC, Buatti JM, et al. Intracranial ependymomas: an analysis of prognostic factors and patterns of failure. *American Journal of Clinical Oncology.* 2002;25:117-122.

29. McNeil DE, Cote TR, Clegg L, et al. Incidence and trends in pediatric malignancies medulloblastoma/primitive neuroectodermal tumor: a SEER update. *Medical and Pediatric Oncology.* 2002;39:190-194.

30. Eberhart CG, Kepner JL, Goldthwaite PT, et al. Histopathologic grading of medulloblastomas: a Pediatric Oncology Group study. *Cancer.* 2002;94:552-560.

31. Helton KJ, Gajjar A, Hill DA, et al. Medulloblastoma metastatic to the suprasellar region at diagnosis: a report of six cases with clinicopathologic correlation. *Pediatric Neurosurgery.* 2002;38:111-117.

32. Parisi M, Glass I. Joubert syndrome. 2003 Jul 9 [Updated 2017 Jun 29]. In: Adam MP, Mirzaa GM, Pagon RA, et al., eds. *GeneReviews®.* University of Washington; 1993-2023. https://www.ncbi.nlm.nih.gov/sites/books/NBK1325/.

33. Sarnat HB, Benjamin DR, Siebert JR, et al. Agenesis of the mesencephalon and metencephalon with cerebellar hypoplasia: putative mutation in the EN2 gene. Report of 2 cases in early infancy. *Pediatric and Developmental Pathology.* 2002;5:54-68.

34. Bird TD. Hereditary ataxia overview. In: Adam MP, Ardinger HH, Pagon RA, et al., eds. University of Washington; 1993-2019. https://www.ncbi.nlm.nih.gov/books/NBK1138.

35. Gatti R, Perlman S. Ataxia-telangectasia. In: Adam MP, Ardinger HH, Pagon RA, et al., eds. University of Washington; 1993-2019. https://www.ncbi.nlm.nih.gov/books/NBK26468.

36. Crawford TO, Skolasky RL, Fernandez R. Survival probability in ataxia-telangiectasia. *Archives of Disease in Childhood.* 2006;91(7):610-611.

37. Coutinho P, Barbot C. Ataxia with oculomotor apraxia type 1. In: Adam MP, Ardinger HH, Pagon RA, et al., eds. *GeneReviews®.* University of Washington; 1993-2019. https://www.ncbi.nlm.nih.gov/books/NBK1456.

38. Moreira M-C, Koenig M. Ataxia with oculomotor apraxia type 2. In: Adam MP, Ardinger HH, Pagon RA, et al., eds. *GeneReviews®.* University of Washington; 1993-2019. https://www.ncbi.nlm.nih.gov/books/NBK1154.

39. Bidichandani SI, Delatycki MB. Friedrich ataxia. In: Adam MP, Ardinger HH, Pagon RA, et al., eds. *GeneReviews®.* University of Washington; 1993-2019. https://www.ncbi.nlm.nih.gov/books/NBK1281.

40. Lynch DR, Chin MP, Delatycki MB, et al. Safety and efficacy of omaveloxolone in Friedreich ataxia (MOXIe Study). *Annals of Neurology.* 2021;89(2):212-225. https://doi.org/10.1002/ana.25934. Epub 2020 Nov 5. PMID: 33068037; PMCID: PMC7894504.

11

Hemiplegia

OUTLINE

Hemiplegic Cerebral Palsy, 281
   Congenital Malformations, 282
   Neonatal Hemorrhage, 283
Approach to Acute Hemiplegia in Children, 283
   Childhood Stroke, 284
   Diabetes Mellitus, 287
   Epilepsy, 287
   Heart Disease, 288
   Hypercoagulable States, 289

Hypocoagulable States (Bleeding Diathesis), 290
Infections, 295
Migraine, 295
Trauma, 296
Tumors, 296
Chronic Progressive Hemiplegia, 296
   Sturge-Weber Syndrome, 296
References, 297

Hemiplegia may be congenital or acquired, acute or chronically progressive. Cerebral palsy is the most common cause of hemiplegia in the pediatric population. Childhood stroke is underrecognized and may occur in the setting of vasculopathy, prothrombotic states, or congenital heart disease. Genetic diseases, including hemiplegic migraine and alternating hemiplegia of childhood (AHC), are less common causes.

The approach to children with hemiplegia must distinguish between acute hemiplegia, in which weakness develops within a few hours, and chronic progressive hemiplegia, in which weakness evolves over days, weeks, or months. The distinction between an acute and an insidious onset should be easy but can be problematic. In children with a slowly evolving hemiplegia, missing early weakness is possible until an obvious level of functional disability is attained, by which time the hemiplegia seems new and acute.

An additional presentation of hemiplegia found in infants who come to medical attention because of developmental delay is slowness in meeting motor milestones and early establishment of hand preference. Children should not establish a hand preference until the second year. Such children may have a static structural problem from birth (*hemiplegic cerebral palsy*), but the clinical features are not apparent until the child is old enough to use the affected limbs.

Magnetic resonance imaging (MRI) is the diagnostic modality of choice for investigating all forms of hemiplegia. It is especially informative to show migrational defects in hemiplegic cerebral palsy associated with seizures. Magnetic resonance arteriography (MRA) is sufficiently informative in visualizing the vascular structures to obviate the need for arteriography in most children.

HEMIPLEGIC CEREBRAL PALSY

The term *hemiplegic cerebral palsy* comprises several pathological entities that result in limb weakness on one side of the body. In premature infants, the most common cause is periventricular hemorrhagic infarction (see Chapter 4). In term infants the underlying causes are often cerebral malformations, cerebral infarction, and intracerebral hemorrhage. Imaging studies of the brain are useful to provide the family with a definitive diagnosis.

The usual concern that brings infants with hemiplegia from birth for a neurological evaluation is delayed crawling or walking. Abnormalities of the legs are the focus of attention. Unilateral facial weakness is never associated, probably because bilateral corticobulbar innervation of the lower face persists until birth. Epilepsy occurs in approximately half of children with hemiplegic cerebral palsy.

Infants with injury to the dominant hemisphere can develop normal speech in the nondominant hemisphere, but it is at the expense of visuoperceptual and spatial skills. Infants with hemiplegia and early-onset seizures are an exception; they often show cognitive disturbances of verbal and nonverbal skills.

Congenital Malformations

Migrational defects comprise the majority of congenital malformations causing infantile hemiplegia (Fig. 11.1). The affected hemisphere is often small and may show a unilateral perisylvian syndrome in which the sylvian fissure is widened.[1] Chapter 17 describes a bilateral perisylvian syndrome with speech disturbances. Seizures and intellectual disability are often associated. As a rule, epilepsy is more common when congenital malformations cause infantile hemiplegia than when the cause is stroke.

Perinatal Stroke

Perinatal stroke is typically defined as infarct or hemorrhage occurring anywhere from 28 weeks gestation to 28 days of life, excluding subarachnoid and intraventricular hemorrhages of prematurity. *Acute* perinatal stroke occurs within the first 7 days of life. Arterial ischemic infarction comprises approximately 80% of perinatal strokes, with the remainder consisting

of cerebral sinovenous thrombosis or hemorrhagic infarction. Perinatal stroke is significantly more common than stroke later in childhood. Middle cerebral artery (MCA) infarcts occur the most frequently, followed by venous periventricular infarcts with basal ganglia involvement.

Clinical features. The infant may appear normal for the first several days. Seizures occur in almost all neonates with stroke (although they may not be clinically recognized) and are usually focal motor involving the contralateral arm or leg. At times, encephalopathy, lethargy, or irritability are present, prompting evaluation for HIE and sepsis. Some patients do not come to medical attention until later in infancy, when early handedness or delayed motor milestones are noted.

Diagnosis. Identification of risk factors aids in diagnosis, and includes several common pregnancy complications such as preeclampsia, maternal thrombophilia, chorioamnionitis, oligohydramnios, and premature rupture of membranes. Certain illicit substances such as cocaine and methamphetamine are associated with neonatal hemorrhagic stroke. As expected, delivery complications requiring emergency cesarean section and the need for vacuum extraction or high forceps delivery are associated with higher risk. Neonatal risk factors include inherited thrombophilia, asphyxia, congenital cardiac disease, polycythemia, dehydration, disseminated intravascular coagulation, and infection.

Head ultrasound is usually the initial imaging study but MRI with MRA/MRV is preferred if possible. Hematologic and cardiac workup may be indicated

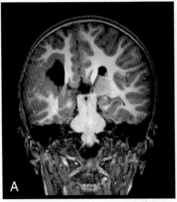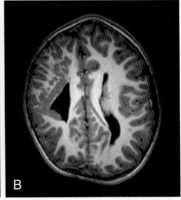

Fig. 11.1 Closed Lip Schizencephaly With Periventricular Heterotopias. (A) T$_1$ coronal magnetic resonance imaging (MRI) and (B) axial MRI.

if the etiology of stroke is unclear; however, be aware that hematologic evaluation is challenging due to poorly defined normative values for the neonatal population, and any abnormalities require confirmatory testing later in life. Certain genetic variants, such as *COL4A1*, cause abnormal angiogenesis and may predispose to perinatal stroke.

Follow-up imaging studies may show either unilateral enlargement of the lateral ventricle or porencephaly in the distribution of the MCA contralateral to the hemiparesis. Hemiatrophy of the pons contralateral to the abnormal hemisphere may be an associated feature.

Management. Provide supportive care, including adequate oxygenation, correction of dehydration and anemia, and management of seizures. Thrombolytics are virtually never used, both due to lack of evidence in neonates and because the time of symptom onset is often unclear. Mechanical thrombectomy is limited by infants' small size. Babies with known thrombophilia or congenital cardiac disease may benefit from the use of low-molecular-weight heparin (LMWH). Patients with cerebral sinovenous thrombosis appear to tolerate and benefit from LMWH, and most institutions utilize LMWH in this scenario once cerebral sinus venous thrombosis is discovered or at least once thrombus propagation occurs.[2]

Neonatal Hemorrhage

Intracranial hemorrhage affects 1% of full-term neonates.[3] Small, unilateral, parietal, or temporal hemorrhages occur almost exclusively in term newborns and are not associated with either trauma or asphyxia. Larger hemorrhages into the temporal lobe sometimes result when obstetric forceps apply excessive force to the lateral skull, but more often they are idiopathic. Intraventricular hemorrhage may be an associated feature. Hemorrhagic disease of the newborn is a consideration in areas in which vitamin K is not routinely administered or not given due to parental refusal.

Clinical features. Newborns with small hemorrhages are normal at birth and seem well until seizures begin any time during the first week. The symptoms of larger hemorrhages may be apnea, seizures, or both. Seizures are usually focal, and hemiplegia or hypotonia is present on examination. Some infants recover completely, whereas others show residual hemiplegia and cognitive deficits.

Diagnosis. Seizures and apnea usually prompt lumbar puncture to exclude the possibility of sepsis. The cerebrospinal fluid is grossly bloody. Head ultrasound, computed tomography (CT), or MRI shows hemorrhage, and follow-up studies show focal encephalomalacia.

Management. Correction of significant thrombocytopenia, replacement of coagulation factors when applicable, vitamin K for all neonates and higher doses for certain factor deficiencies (maternal use of warfarin, phenobarbital, or phenytoin), and ventricular drain sometimes followed by ventriculoperitoneal (VP) shunt are needed for intraventricular bleeds with hydrocephalus. Correct anemia and dehydration when present and treat seizures when they coexist.

APPROACH TO ACUTE HEMIPLEGIA IN CHILDREN

The sudden onset of an acute, focal neurological deficit suggests either a vascular, epileptic, or migraine mechanism (Box 11.1). Strokes manifest as abrupt onset of weakness within seconds, seizures within a couple of minutes, and migraines tend to manifest their neurological signs over several minutes. Infants and children who have acute hemiplegia are divided into two groups according to whether or not epilepsia partialis continua precedes the hemiplegia. Both groups may have seizures on the paretic side after hemiplegia is established. Cerebral infarction, usually in the distribution of the MCA, accounts for one-quarter of cases in which seizures precede hemiplegia and more than half of cases in which hemiplegia is the initial feature. Whatever the cause, the probability of a permanent motor deficit is almost 100% when the initial feature is epilepsia partialis continua and about 50% when it is not.

> ## BOX 11.1 Differential Diagnosis of Acute Hemiplegia
>
> - Alternating hemiplegia
> - Cerebrovascular disease[a]
> - Diabetes mellitus
> - Epilepsy
> - Hypoglycemia (see Chapter 2)
> - Kawasaki disease (see Chapter 10)
> - Migraine[a]
> - Trauma
> - Tumor[a]
>
> [a]The most common conditions and the ones with disease modifying treatments.

Childhood Stroke

Childhood stroke is less frequent than perinatal stroke but is an important and underrecognized consideration in any child with acute-onset hemiplegia (Box 11.2). Boys outnumber girls even when controlling for trauma, and the incidence is higher in Black children even when controlling for sickle cell disease (SCD). The cause of these discrepancies remains unclear. Acute ischemic stroke is more common in children with congenital cardiac disease, malignancy, or inherited thrombophilia (Box 11.3); strokes due to dissection of the posterior circulation are more common in children who have recently suffered neck or head trauma. More detailed discussions of arteritis, thrombophilia, SCD, congenital cardiac disease, and vascular trauma are found later in this chapter.

Clinical features. The affected child presents with speech or language dysfunction, unilateral weakness, visual disturbance, or ataxia. Altered mental status, headache, and seizures may or may not be present.

Diagnosis. MRI with MRA is the imaging modality of choice; many institutions offer "stroke-protocol"

MRIs with only the most salient sequences, allowing for more rapid evaluation. Formal angiography is often not required, but if indicated allows for acute intervention, and offers more detailed vascular evaluation.

BOX 11.3 Inherited States Promoting Cerebral Infarction

1. Activated Protein C Resistance
   - Factor V Leiden mutation
2. Deficiencies
   - Antithrombin III
   - Protein C
   - Protein S
3. Other Genetic Factors
   - Elevated antiphospholipid antibodies and lupus anticoagulant
   - Elevated factor VIII levels, and low plasminogen or high fibrinogen
   - Elevated lipoprotein(a)
   - Plasminogen activator inhibitor promoter polymorphism (PAI 1)
   - Prothrombin gene *20210* mutation

BOX 11.2 Causes of Stroke

Cerebrovascular Malformations
- Arteriovenous malformation
- Fibromuscular dysplasia
- Hereditary hemorrhagic telangiectasia
- Sturge-Weber syndrome

Coagulopathies/Hemoglobinopathies
- Antiphospholipid antibodies/lupus anticoagulant
- Congenital coagulation defects[a]
- Disseminated intravascular coagulation
- Drug-induced thrombosis
- Malignancy
- Sickle cell anemia/disease[a]
- Thrombocytopenic purpura

Heart Disease
- Arrhythmia
- Atrial myxoma
- Bacterial endocarditis
- Cardiac catheterization
- Cardiomyopathy
- Cyanotic congenital defects[a]
- Mitral valve prolapse[a]
- Prosthetic heart valve
- Rhabdomyoma
- Rheumatic heart disease

Trauma
- Arterial dissection[a]
- Blunt trauma to neck
- Intraoral trauma
- Vertebral manipulation

Vasculitis
- Carotid infection
- Drug abuse (amphetamines and cocaine)
- Hemolytic-uremic syndrome (see Chapter 2)
- Hypersensitivity vasculitis
- Isolated angiitis
- Kawasaki disease (see Chapter 10)
- Meningitis[a] (see Chapter 4)
- Mixed connective tissue disease
- Systemic lupus erythematosus
- Takayasu arteritis
- Varicella infection

Vasculopathies
- Fabry disease
- Homocystinuria[a] (see Chapter 5)
- Mitochondrial encephalopathy, lactic acidosis, and stroke (MELAS)
- Moyamoya disease

[a]The most common conditions and the ones with disease modifying treatments.

Neck imaging is required if there is high suspicion for posterior circulation infarct or cervical carotid artery occlusion.

Management. The management of acute stroke in children remains controversial with few evidence-based protocols. In general, children recover from acute ischemic stroke more completely than adults, and supportive care rather than intervention is recommended for children with smaller strokes and minimal symptoms. For children with large, symptomatic infarcts, consider thrombolytic therapy with intravenous tissue plasminogen activator (tPA), endovascular tPA, or thrombectomy. Exact tPA doses for children are not well established. The child's size is an important consideration, as there are technical limitations regarding catheterization of smaller arteries. In addition children are more likely to suffer strokes as a result of arteriopathy such as moyamoya disease or inflammatory arteritis (see "Moyamoya Disease" and "Vasculopathies" later in this chapter), and catheterizing inflamed arteries carries its own risks. Such decisions are best made in a recognized stroke center with the assistance of pediatric stroke specialists.[2]

Arteriovenous Malformations

Supratentorial malformations may cause acute or chronic progressive hemiplegia. Intraparenchymal hemorrhage causes acute hemiplegia. The major clinical features of hemorrhage into a hemisphere are loss of consciousness, seizures, and hemiplegia. Large hematomas cause midline structures to shift and increase intracranial pressure. Chapter 4 contains the discussion of arteriovenous malformations. MRA, CT angiogram, or direct angiogram are the best techniques to visualize the malformation.

Carotid and Vertebral Artery Disorders

Cervical infections. Unilateral and bilateral occlusions of the cervical portion of the internal carotid arteries may occur in children with a history of chronic tonsillitis and cervical lymphadenopathy. Whether this is cause and effect or coincidence is uncertain. Tonsillitis may cause carotid arteritis.

Unilateral cerebral infarction may occur in the course of cat-scratch disease (see Chapter 2) and mycoplasma pneumonia. In both diseases, the presence of submandibular lymph node involvement is associated with arteritis of the adjacent carotid artery. Necrotizing fasciitis is a serious cause of inflammatory arteritis with

subsequent occlusion of one or both carotid arteries. The source of parapharyngeal space infection is usually chronic dental infection. Mixed aerobic and anaerobic organisms are isolated on culture.

Clinical features. The usual sequence in cervical arteritis is fever and neck tenderness followed by sudden hemiplegia. Bilateral hemiplegia may occur when both sides are infected.

Diagnosis. Culture of the throat or lymph node specimens is required to identify the offending organism or organisms. Arteriography, CT angiogram, or MRA identifies the site and extent of carotid occlusion.

Management. An aggressive course of antibiotic therapy, especially for necrotizing fasciitis, is mandatory. The outcome is variable, and recovery may be partial or complete.

Fibromuscular dysplasia. Fibromuscular dysplasia (FMD) is an idiopathic, segmental, nonatheromatous disorder of the renal arteries and the extracranial segment of the internal carotid artery within 4 cm of its bifurcation. Seven percent of patients also have intracerebral aneurysms.

Clinical features. Transitory ischemic attacks and stroke are the only clinical neurological features of FMD. Hypertension occurs in patients with renal artery involvement. FMD is primarily a disease of women over 50 years but can occur in children.

Diagnosis. Arteriography shows an irregular contour of the internal carotid artery in the neck resembling a string of beads. Suspect concomitant FMD of the renal arteries if hypertension is present.

Management. Either operative transluminal balloon angioplasty or carotid endarterectomy are options to treat the stenosis. The long-term prognosis in children is unknown.

Trauma to the carotid artery. Children may experience carotid thrombosis and dissection from seemingly trivial injuries, such as during exercise and sports, and these can also occur without known cause in otherwise normal children.[4] They also occur in child abuse (grabbing and shaking the neck) or from injuries to the carotid artery during a fall, when the child has a blunt object (e.g., pencil, lollipop) in the mouth. Other risk factors for carotid dissection include FMD, Ehlers-Danlos syndrome type IV, Marfan syndrome, coarctation of the aorta, cystic medial necrosis, autosomal dominant polycystic kidney disease, osteogenesis imperfecta, atherosclerosis, extreme arterial tortuosity, moyamoya syndrome, and pharyngeal infections (see "Cervical Infections" earlier in this chapter).[5]

Clinical features. Usually, a delay of several hours and sometimes days separates the injury from the onset of symptoms. The delay probably represents the time needed for thrombus to form within the artery. Clinical features may include hemiparesis, hemianesthesia, hemianopia, and aphasia when the dominant hemisphere is affected. Deficits may be transitory or permanent, but most children recover at least partially. Seizures are rare.

Diagnosis. MRA and CT angiography safely visualize carotid dissection and occlusion. Formal angiography should be considered if clinical suspicion is high and standard imaging is negative. Arterial wall imaging is an emerging diagnostic modality that may be useful in the future.

Management. In children with cervicocephalic arterial dissection (CCAD), use either unfractionated heparin (UFH) or LMWH. It is common and reasonable to treat a child with CCAD with either subcutaneous LMWH or warfarin for 3–6 months. Alternatively, an antiplatelet agent may be used. Continue therapy beyond 6 months when symptoms recur or when there is radiographic evidence of a residual abnormality of the dissected artery. Surgery such as bypass or extracranial to intracranial shunts may be considered in patients who continue to have symptoms from a CCAD while on medical therapy. Do not give anticoagulation medication to children with an intracranial dissection or with subarachnoid hemorrhage from CCAD.[6]

Trauma to the vertebral artery. Vertebral artery thrombosis or dissection may follow minor neck trauma, especially rapid neck rotation. The site of occlusion is usually at the C1–C2 level. Boys are more often affected than girls.

Clinical features. The usual features of vertebral artery injury are headache and brainstem dysfunction. Repeated episodes of hemiparesis associated with bitemporal throbbing headache and vomiting may occur and maybe misdiagnosed as a migraine variant. As with other types of vascular trauma, most children recover at least partially but permanent neurologic deficits are possible.

Diagnosis. Clinical symptoms lead the clinician to order an imaging study (often a stroke-protocol MRI), which may show areas of restricted diffusion in the posterior circulation. The possibility of stroke leads to vascular imaging, which reveals vertebral artery occlusion

or dissection. Importantly, the neck must be included in vascular imaging studies in order to adequately assess the vertebral arteries. If a clear history of trauma is lacking, then further evaluation of the cervical vertebrae is required to rule out bony abnormalities predisposing to injuries of the posterior circulation. Note any unusual joint flexibility or skin laxity, as this may indicate an underlying connective tissue disorder.

Management. Treatment is not well established and varies among institutions. LMWH or oral anticoagulants are typically continued for 3–6 months. Long-term aspirin prophylaxis is a common recommendation. Repeat imaging after 3–6 months is recommended.

Alternating Hemiplegia of Childhood

AHC is one phenotypic manifestation of the spectrum of *ATP1A3* disorders. The *ATP1A3* gene regulates the sodium-potassium ATPase protein complex. Other *ATP1A3* disorders include rapid-onset dystonia-parkinsonism, cerebellar ataxia, areflexia, pes cavus, optic atrophy, and sensorineural hearing loss (CAPOS) syndrome.[7]

Clinical features. Onset is from birth to 18 months with a mean of 8 months. The initial features are mild developmental delay and abnormal eye movements. Motor attacks may comprise hemiplegia, dystonia, or choreoathetosis. Some children become dyspneic during episodes if the tongue is involved. Autonomic dysregulation is rare but potentially serious. Some individuals identify triggers associated with the attacks; common triggers include heat, illness, sleep deprivation, and stress. As a rule, young infants have more dystonic features and older children are more likely to have flaccid hemiplegia. Brief episodes of monocular or binocular nystagmus, lasting for 1–3 minutes, are often associated with both dystonic and hemiplegic attacks. Because the attack onset is abrupt, dystonia is often mistaken for a seizure and hemiplegia for a stroke. Most reports of epileptic seizures in infants with this syndrome are probably dystonic attacks; however, up to 50% of affected individuals develop epilepsy later in life.

The duration of hemiplegia varies from minutes to days, and intensity waxes and wanes during a single episode. During long attacks, hemiplegia may shift from side to side or both sides may be affected. If both sides are affected, one side may recover more quickly than the other. The arm is usually weaker than the leg, and walking may not be impaired. Hemiplegia disappears during sleep and reappears on awakening but not immediately.

Dystonic episodes may primarily affect the limbs on one side, causing hemidystonia, or affect the trunk, causing opisthotonic posturing. Some children scream during attacks as if in pain. Headache may occur at the onset of an attack but not afterward. Writhing movements that suggest choreoathetosis may be associated. Mental slowing occurs early in the course and mental regression follows later. Stepwise neurological impairment occurs as well, as if recovery from individual attacks is incomplete, and mild to severe cognitive impairment is the norm.

Diagnosis. MRI is normal. The diagnosis relies mainly on clinical features; molecular genetic testing demonstrates heterozygous pathogenic variants in the *ATP3A1* gene.

Management. Treatment focuses on avoidance of triggers and symptom management. Anticonvulsant and antimigraine medications generally fail to prevent attacks or prevent progression. However, topiramate prophylaxis may prevent recurrent attacks. Flunarizine, a calcium channel blocking agent, reduces the frequency of attacks, but its efficacy is not established and it is not available in the United States. Other calcium channel blocking agents and anticonvulsant drugs have not been useful for prophylaxis. Benzodiazepines reduce discomfort and assist with sleep during dystonic attacks.

Alternating hemiplegia and dopa-responsive dystonia (see Chapter 14) share the feature of episodic dystonia with diurnal variation, and infants with attacks of dystonia should receive a trial of carbidopa-levodopa or dopamine agonists.

Brain Tumors

The usual cause of acute hemiplegia from brain tumor is hemorrhage into or around the tumor. Hemorrhage may hide the underlying tumor on CT and MRI is more informative (see Chapter 4). Tumors may also cause a slowly progressive hemiparesis with or without increased intracranial pressure, disk edema, or seizures.

Diabetes Mellitus

Acute but transitory attacks of hemiparesis occur in children with insulin-dependent diabetes mellitus. Hypoglycemia is the likely mechanism as opposed to cerebrovascular accident.

Clinical features. Attacks occur during sleep in a diabetic child stressed by illness or are induced by exercise. Hemiparesis is present on awakening; weakness is often greater in the face and arm than in the leg. Sensation is intact, but aphasia is present if the dominant hemisphere is affected. Tendon reflexes may be depressed or brisk in the affected arm, and an extensor plantar response is usually present. Headache is a constant feature and may be unilateral or generalized. Some patients are nauseated. Attacks last for 3–24 hours, and recovery is complete.

Diagnosis. Stroke is not a complication of juvenile insulin-dependent diabetes except during episodes of severe, sustained hypoglycemia or ketoacidosis (see Chapter 2). MRI in children with transitory hemiplegia does not show infarction.

Management. Prevention of hypoglycemia limits the possibility of recurrence.

Epilepsy
Postictal Hemiparesis and Hemiparetic Seizures

Todd paralysis is a term used to describe hemiparesis that lasts for minutes or hours and follows a focal motor seizure. It occurs most often following prolonged seizures, especially those caused by an underlying structural abnormality.

Hemiparesis may be a seizure manifestation as well as a postictal event. Such seizures are *hemiparetic* or *focal inhibitory* seizures. Todd paralysis may be difficult to distinguish from hemiparetic seizures because it is not always clear whether a seizure preceded the hemiparesis or whether the hemiparesis is ictal.

Clinical features. The initial feature may be a brief focal seizure followed by flaccid hemiparesis or the abrupt onset of flaccid monoparesis or hemiparesis. This may occur with or without altered mentation and awareness. The severity and distribution of weakness vary, affecting one limb more than the other and sometimes the face. Tendon reflexes are normal in the hemiparetic limbs, but the plantar response may be extensor.

Diagnosis. Postictal electromyography (EEG) does not show ongoing seizures but may show epileptiform discharges or slowing over the hemisphere contralateral to the weakness. A radioisotope scan (positron emission tomography scan) shows increased focal uptake in the affected hemisphere during the ictal phase and decreased uptake between seizures. Results of MRI, CT, and cerebral arteriography may be normal or may demonstrate cerebral malformations of the epileptogenic hemisphere.

Management. No treatment other than patience is needed for postictal hemiparesis; however, acute seizure management with benzodiazepines or others may be needed for an ictal event (see Chapter 1).

Heart Disease
Congenital Heart Disease

Cerebrovascular complications of congenital heart disease are most likely in children with cyanotic heart conditions, who are at risk for cardioembolic stroke, thrombotic stroke, and watershed infarcts from drops in perfusion pressure. The rates of stroke in children with complex congenital heart disease vary with (1) the severity of the malformation, (2) the number of corrective surgeries required, (3) anesthetic techniques during surgery, (4) patient selection, and (5) length of follow-up. The greatest risk for children with congenital heart disease occurs at the time of surgery or cardiac catheterization[8] or if the child requires extracorporeal membrane oxygenation. Cerebral dysgenesis is an important consideration in children with congenital heart disease. Postmortem studies show a 10%–29% prevalence of associated cerebral malformations. Children with hypoplastic left heart syndrome are especially at risk for associated brain dysgenesis.

Clinical features. Venous thrombosis occurs most often in infants with cyanotic heart disease who are dehydrated and polycythemic. One or more sinuses may occlude. Failure of venous drainage always increases intracranial pressure. Hemiparesis is a major clinical feature and may occur first on one side and then on the other with sagittal sinus obstruction. Seizures and decreased consciousness are associated features. The mortality rate is high in infants with thrombosis of major venous sinuses, and most survivors have neurological morbidity.

Children with cyanotic heart disease are at risk for arterial embolism when vegetations are present within the heart or because of the right-to-left shunt, which allows peripheral emboli to bypass the lungs and reach the brain. The potential for cerebral abscess formation increases in children with a right-to-left shunt because decreased arterial oxygen saturation lowers cerebral resistance to infection.

The initial feature is sudden onset of hemiparesis associated with headache, seizures, and loss of consciousness. Seizures are at first focal and recurrent but later become generalized.

Diagnosis. MRI/MRV is the preferred procedure for the detection of venous thrombosis and emboli. A pattern of hemorrhagic infarction occurs adjacent to the site of venous thrombosis, and multiple areas of infarction are associated with embolization.

The CT appearance may be normal during the first 12–24 hours following embolization. By the next day, the study shows a low-density lesion. Although the sequence is consistent with a sterile embolus, the possibility of subsequent abscess formation is a consideration. Repeat enhanced CT or MRI studies within 1 week reveal ring enhancement if an abscess developed.

Management. Treatment for congestive heart failure may reduce the possibility of cardiogenic embolism and stroke. Repairing the congenital heart defect reduces the risk of subsequent stroke (this is unknown with patent foramen ovale [PFO]). UFH or LMWH is given until oral anticoagulants are adjusted for children with a cardiac embolism unrelated to a PFO who are judged to have a high risk for recurrent embolism. Alternatively, it is reasonable to use LMWH exclusively. In children with a risk of cardiac embolism, continue either LMWH or oral anticoagulants for at least 1 year or until the lesion responsible for the risk has been corrected. If the risk of recurrent embolism is judged to be high, continue anticoagulation indefinitely provided it is well tolerated. For children with a suspected cardiac embolism unrelated to a PFO with a lower or unknown risk of stroke, begin aspirin and continue it for at least 1 year. Surgical repair or transcatheter closure should be considered in individuals with a major atrial septal defect both to reduce the stroke risk and to prevent long-term cardiac complications. Anticoagulant therapy is not used for individuals with native valve endocarditis. Antibiotics are important to decrease the possibility of transformation into abscess in cases of endocarditis.

Supportive treatment includes correcting dehydration and controlling increased intracranial pressure. Although data are limited, current guidelines support the use of UFH or LMWH in the treatment of cerebral venous sinus thrombosis (CVST). In addition, the administration of endovascular tPA or mechanical thrombectomy may be considered if the clot progresses despite anticoagulation. The question of how to treat CVST with coexistent hemorrhage is complex with limited published data, and generally relies on expert opinion and treatment at a pediatric stroke center.[9]

Mitral Valve Disease

Mitral valve disease may be congenital or acquired, and includes mitral valve stenosis, regurgitation, and/or prolapse. The most common cause of acquired mitral valve disease is rheumatic fever (see "Rheumatic Heart Disease"). Severe congenital mitral stenosis causes inadequate cardiac output and is a medical emergency that may cause significant ischemic brain injury. Mitral valve prolapse and regurgitation increase the risk of stroke either by causing cardiac arrhythmias or via emboli that may be thrown from the abnormal valve leaflets.

Clinical features. Neurologic dysfunction is rarely the presenting sign of mitral valve disease in children. When such an event does occur, symptoms may range from relatively minor transient ischemic attacks to larger strokes with permanent neurologic sequelae.

Diagnosis. Patients may have late systolic murmurs or a mid-systolic click; however, the absence of these does not rule out valvular disease. A full cardiac evaluation including echocardiography is required to establish the diagnosis.

Management. Treatment of mitral valve disease in children remains controversial but typically involves balloon valvuloplasty for mitral stenosis, and repair versus valve replacement for prolapse and regurgitation. Once a child has suffered TIA or stroke, surgical intervention should be considered in addition to the initiation of an antiplatelet agent such as low-dose aspirin.

Rheumatic Heart Disease

The frequency and severity of rheumatic fever and rheumatic heart disease in North America have been decreasing for several decades. Unfortunately, a mini epidemic of acute rheumatic fever recurs every 5–10 years in the United States. Rheumatic heart disease involves the mitral valve in 85% of patients, the aortic valve in 54%, and the tricuspid and pulmonary valves in less than 5%. The source of cerebral emboli is either valvular vegetations or septic emboli due to infective endocarditis.

Clinical features. The main features of mitral valve disease are cardiac failure and arrhythmia. Aortic valve disease is often asymptomatic. Neurological complications are always due to bacterial endocarditis except in the immediate postoperative period when embolization is the likely explanation. Symptoms are much the same as in congenital heart disease.

Diagnosis. Rheumatic heart disease is an established diagnosis long before the first stroke. Multiple blood cultures identify the organism and select the best drug for intravenous antibiotic therapy.

Management. Bacterial endocarditis requires vigorous intravenous antibiotic therapy. A diagnosis of rheumatic fever with cardiac involvement requires lifelong antibiotic prophylaxis prior to invasive procedures to minimize the risk of developing endocarditis/septic emboli.

Hypercoagulable States

A prothrombotic condition is frequently seen in children presenting with arterial ischemic stroke and is especially common in children with CVST.[10]

Abnormalities of blood cells or blood cell concentration may place the child at risk for hemorrhagic or ischemic stroke. Low platelet count due to autoimmune thrombocytopenia or bone marrow suppression may lead to hemorrhage. Anything that increases blood viscosity, such as sickled cells, polycythemia, or chronic hypoxia, may predispose a child to arterial or venous infarct. Dehydration is associated with arterial strokes and cerebrovascular thrombosis (CVT), possibly because it increases viscosity. Anemia is a risk factor for arterial ischemic infarction and CVT, possibly due to alterations in hemodynamics or imbalances in thrombotic pathways.

Risk factors for an ongoing prothrombotic state include recurrent episodes of deep vein thrombosis or pulmonary emboli, especially if they occur at a young age, or a family history of thrombotic events. The likelihood of stroke from most prothrombotic states seems to be relatively low, but the stroke risk increases when other risk factors are present. Thus it is reasonable to test for the most common prothrombotic states even when another explanation for the stroke is present. Hypercoagulable states include antithrombin III, protein C, or protein S deficiencies, activated protein C resistance, factor V Leiden mutation, prothrombin gene mutation (*G20210A*), antiphospholipid antibody syndrome, and elevated levels of lipoprotein A and homocysteine. Protein C deficiency and the genetic polymorphisms collectively (factor V Leiden, prothrombin gene mutation) may be independent risk factors in children for recurrent arterial stroke. Cerebral venous and, less often, cerebral arterial thromboses may occur in patients with paroxysmal nocturnal hemoglobinuria. Polycythemia rubra vera, essential thrombocythemia, and disseminated intravascular coagulation may lead to cerebral infarction or intracranial hemorrhage.

Thrombosis also accompanies secondary to transitory hematological abnormalities associated with intercurrent illness. For example, idiopathic nephrotic syndrome is associated with decreased antithrombin and CVT.[11]

Clinical features. The typical features of venous thrombosis are headache and obtundation caused by increased intracranial pressure, seizures, and successive hemiplegia on either side. Suspect an inherited hypercoagulable state in children with recurrent venous thromboses, a family history of venous thrombosis, or thrombosis at an unusual site. Arterial thromboses usually cause ischemic stroke in the distribution of a single cerebral artery.

Diagnosis. Suspect venous thrombosis when hemiplegia and increased intracranial pressure develop suddenly. The diagnosis of sagittal sinus thromboses is suggested when parasagittal hemorrhage or infarction is associated with absence of the normal flow void in the sagittal sinus on MRI/MRV. Cerebral arteriography is the definitive procedure. Table 11.1 summarizes laboratory studies.

Management. Provide supportive care for all types of strokes. Correct dehydration and anemia when present. In prothrombotic states, the child may benefit from the use of UFH or LMWH.

Ventricular drain sometimes followed by VP shunt is needed for intraventricular bleeds with hydrocephalus. Correct anemia and dehydration when present. Remove risk factors such as smoking and oral contraception when possible. Symptomatic treatment includes decreasing intracranial pressure, treating seizures when present, and rehydrating the patient without increasing cerebral edema.

Hypocoagulable States (Bleeding Diathesis)

Common congenital coagulation factor deficiencies include deficiencies of coagulation factor VIII (hemophilia A), coagulation factor IX (hemophilia B), and von Willebrand factor. A deficiency of any factor that regulates coagulation places the child at risk for hemorrhage.

Management. Correction of significant thrombocytopenia, replacement of coagulation factors when applicable, vitamin K for all neonates and higher doses for certain factor deficiencies (maternal use of warfarin, phenobarbital or phenytoin), and ventricular drain sometimes followed by VP shunt is needed for intraventricular bleeds with hydrocephalus. Correct anemia and dehydration when present and treat seizures when they coexist.

TABLE 11.1 Evaluation of Cerebral Infarction

Blood	
Activated protein C resistance, antiphosphospholipid antibodies, apolipoproteins, cholesterol (high- and low-density lipoproteins), complete blood count, culture, erythrocyte sedimentation rate, factor V, free protein S, lactic acid, Leiden mutation, lupus anticoagulant, plasminogen, protein C, serum homocystine, triglycerides	Bacterial endocarditis, homocystinuria, hypercoagulable state, hyperlipidemia, leukemia, lupus erythematosus, MELAS, polycythemia, sickle cell anemia, vasculitis
Urine	
Drug/toxicology screen, urinalysis	Cocaine or methamphetamine abuse, homocystinuria, nephritis, nephrosis
Heart	
Echocardiography, electrocardiography	Bacterial endocarditis, congenital heart disease, mitral valve prolapse, rheumatic heart disease
Brain	
MRI, MRA head and neck, CTA, angiography	Arterial dissection, arterial thrombosis, arteriovenous malformation, fibromuscular hypoplasia, moyamoya disease, vasculitis

CTA, Computed tomography angiography; *MELAS*, mitochondrial encephalomyopathy, lactic acidosis, and stroke-like episodes; *MRI*, magnetic resonance imaging; *MRA*, magnetic resonance angiography.

Lipoprotein Disorders

Familial lipid and lipoprotein abnormalities may cause premature cerebrovascular disease in infants and children. Genetic transmission of these disorders is typically by autosomal dominant inheritance.

Clinical features. Ischemic episodes cause transitory or permanent hemiplegia, sometimes associated with hemianopia, hemianesthesia, and aphasia. Affected families have a history of cerebrovascular and coronary artery disease developing at an early age.

Diagnosis. Most children have low plasma concentrations of high-density lipoprotein cholesterol, high plasma concentrations of triglycerides, or elevated levels of lipoprotein A. The mechanism of arteriosclerosis is lipoprotein-mediated endothelial damage with secondary thrombus formation.

Management. Dietary treatment, lipid-lowering medications, and daily aspirin administration comprise the management program.

Mitochondrial Encephalopathy, Lactic Acidosis, and Stroke

The most common mutation in mitochondrial encephalopathy, lactic acidosis, and stroke (MELAS) is in the mitochondrial gene *MTTL1* encoding tRNA (Leu-UUR).[12]

Clinical features. MELAS is a multisystem disorder with onset between 2 and 10 years. Early psychomotor development is usually normal, but short stature is common. The most common initial symptoms are generalized tonic-clonic seizures, recurrent headaches, anorexia, and recurrent vomiting. Exercise intolerance or proximal limb weakness can be the initial feature. Seizures are often associated with stroke-like episodes of transient hemiparesis or cortical blindness. These stroke-like episodes may be associated with altered consciousness and may be recurrent. The cumulative residual effects of the stroke-like episodes gradually impair motor abilities, vision, and mentation, often by adolescence or young adulthood. Sensorineural hearing loss is common.

Affected children are usually normal at birth. Failure to thrive, growth retardation, and progressive deafness are characteristic of onset during infancy. In later-onset cases, the main neurological features are recurrent attacks of prolonged migraine-like headaches and vomiting, seizures (myoclonic, focal, generalized) that often progress to status epilepticus, the sudden onset of focal neurological defects (hemiplegia, hemianopia, aphasia), and encephalopathy. Mental deterioration, when present, occurs anytime during childhood. Neurological abnormalities are initially intermittent and then become progressive.

Diagnosis. MRI shows multifocal infarction-like areas that do not conform to definite vascular territories. The initial lesions are often in the occipital lobes; progressive disease affects the cerebral and cerebellar cortices, the basal ganglia, and the thalamus. The concentration of lactate in the blood and cerebrospinal fluid is elevated; magnetic resonance spectroscopy shows a lactate peak. Muscle biopsy specimens show *ragged-red fibers*. Molecular diagnosis is commercially available. The blood leukocyte DNA reveals the A3243G mutation in 80% of MELAS patients.

Management. Treat acute stroke-like episodes with a bolus of intravenous arginine, 500 mg/kg, within 3 hours of symptom onset followed by additional 500 mg/kg doses given as continuous 24-hour infusions over the next three to five days. Following the initial stroke-like event, start the child on daily arginine prophylaxis (150–300 mg/kg/day in three divided doses), which decreases the risk of recurrence. Because illness can trigger a crisis, all affected patients should be fully vaccinated. Avoid mitochondrial toxins including valproic acid, aminoglycoside antibiotics, metformin, linezolid, and dichloroacetate (which increases the risk of peripheral neuropathy). Due to increased incidence of deafness, visual deficits, cardiac abnormalities, and diabetes, annual screening is recommended including hearing and vision tests, cardiac evaluation, and urinalysis and fasting blood glucose.[13]

Moyamoya Disease

Moyamoya is not a disease, but rather a chronic, noninflammatory vasculopathy secondary to several other disorders which results in slowly progressive, bilateral occlusion of the internal carotid arteries starting at the carotid siphon. Occlusion of the basilar artery may occur as well. Associated conditions include sickle cell anemia (SCA), trisomy 21, neurofibromatosis 1, ventricular septal defect, mitral valve stenosis, and tetralogy of Fallot. Because the occlusion is slowly progressive, multiple anastomoses form between the internal and external carotid arteries. The result is a new vascular network at the base of the brain composed of collaterals from the anterior or posterior choroidal arteries, the basilar artery, and the meningeal arteries. On angiography, these telangiectasias produce a hazy appearance, as if a puff of smoke, from which is derived the Japanese word moyamoya (Fig. 11.2). The disorder is worldwide in distribution, with a female-to-male bias of 3:2.

Clinical features. The initial symptoms vary from recurrent headache to abrupt hemiparesis. Infants and young children may have an explosive onset

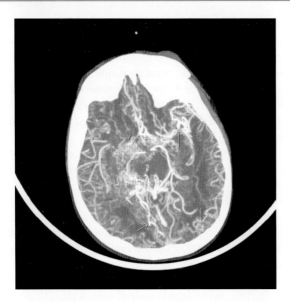

Fig. 11.2 Moyamoya Disease. Computed tomography angiogram shows narrowing of vessels, leptomeningeal and basilar collaterals, and tortuous vessels (*arrows*).

characterized by the sudden development of complete hemiplegia affecting the face and limbs. The child is at least lethargic and sometimes comatose. When the child is sufficiently alert, examination may reveal hemianopia, hemianesthesia, and aphasia. Some children have chorea of the face and of all limbs, which is worse on one side. Recovery follows, but before it is complete, new episodes of focal neurological dysfunction occur on either the same or the opposite side. These episodes include hemiparesis, hemianesthesia, or aphasia, alone or in combination. The outcome in such cases is generally poor. Most children will have chronic weakness on one or both sides, epilepsy, and intellectual disability. Mortality is significant.

Recurrent transient ischemic attacks are an alternative manifestation. Characteristic of the attacks are episodic hemiparesis and dysesthesias lasting for minutes or hours, not associated with loss of consciousness. Frequently, hyperpnea or excitement triggers attacks, which may recur daily. After 4 or 5 years, the attacks cease but residual deficits persist.

Repeated episodes of monoparesis or symptoms of subarachnoid hemorrhage are other possible features of moyamoya disease. Monoparesis generally occurs after infancy and subarachnoid hemorrhage after 16 years.

Diagnosis. The typical "puff of smoke" may be seen by MRA, CT angiogram, or catheter angiogram. CT or MRI may show a large cerebral infarction caused by stenosis in the internal carotid artery. Definitive diagnosis requires arteriographic demonstration of bilateral stenosis in the distal internal carotid arteries and the development of collaterals in the basal ganglia and meninges. Studies should include a search for an underlying vasculopathy or coagulopathy.

Management. Treatment is mainly surgical and involves direct and indirect cerebrovascular bypass or a combination of the two approaches. Children who undergo surgery or suffer a stroke are typically treated with a lifelong aspirin regimen.

Sickle Cell Disease

SCD is a genetic disorder with several distinct genotypes, encompassing a group of disorders associated with mutations in the *HBB* gene and defined by the presence of hemoglobin S (HbS). SCA (caused by HbSS) accounts for 60%–70% of SCD in the United States. The other forms of SCD result from coinheritance of HbS with other abnormal globin β-chain variants.[14] It is the most common hematological disorder associated with stroke, with those suffering from SCA at particular risk.

Silent infarcts occur in the distribution of small vessels. The most common underlying lesion is intracranial arterial stenosis or obstruction, often seen in the proximal middle cerebral and anterior cerebral arteries. Sickled erythrocytes cause chronic injury to the vessel endothelium, resulting in a narrow lumen. Subarachnoid hemorrhage and intraparenchymal hemorrhage can also occur.

Prior to modern therapy, neurological complications occurred in up to 25% of patients with SCA. Abnormal erythrocytes clog large and small vessels, decreasing total, hemispheric, or regional blood flow. Cerebral infarction often occurs in the region of arterial border zones.

Clinical features. The major systemic features of untreated SCA are jaundice, pallor, weakness, and fatigability from chronic hemolytic anemia. Approximately 50% of children with SCA show symptoms by 1 year, and virtually all have symptoms by 5 years of age. The incidence of cerebral infarction varies among studies but previous estimates put the number as high as 46%; fortunately, this has decreased with improved screening and treatment strategies.[15] Strokes occur at the time of a thrombotic, vaso-occlusive crisis. Dehydration or anoxia is often the cause of a crisis. Fever with abdominal and chest pain are characteristic. Focal or generalized seizures are the initial neurological feature in 70% of patients, and long-term epilepsy may result from vasculopathy and hypoperfusion.[16] After the seizures have ended, hemiplegia and other focal neurological deficits are noted. Some recovery follows, but there is a tendency for recurrent strokes, epilepsy, and cognitive impairment. Strokes affecting both hemispheres produce a pseudobulbar palsy with brainstem dysfunction.

Children with SCA often autoinfarct their spleens and are therefore at risk for severe infections due to encapsulated bacteria. Meningitis is a significant concern, particularly if the child has not been fully vaccinated or is not receiving antibiotic prophylaxis.

Diagnosis. Screening for HbSS disease and associated variants is standard in newborns. High-performance liquid chromatography, isoelectric focusing, or hemoglobin electrophoresis are used to quantify HbS. Mutation analysis is available. Most affected children have an established diagnosis long before experiencing vaso-occlusive crisis with concern for stroke. CT or MRI documents the extent of cerebral infarction and hemorrhage. If several such crises have occurred, cortical atrophy may be present. Formal angiography is not standard but can be considered if suspicion for moyamoya disease exists (see "Moyamoya Disease" earlier in this chapter).

Management. Routine screening and prophylaxis are essential to prevent acute complications, and standardized guidelines are readily available online through the National Institutes of Health. In order to prevent invasive pneumococcal infection, treat all children with SCA with prophylactic oral penicillin until age 5 or until they have completed their pneumococcal vaccines. Monitor for hypertension and treat as per the standard pediatric recommendations. To assess stroke risk, screen children with SCA annually with transcranial doppler (TCD) starting at age 2 through at least age 16. Children with conditional or elevated TCD results should be referred for chronic transfusion therapy, which offers the best chance of preventing stroke.

Any child with SCD who presents with fever and altered mental status or focal neurologic signs should be treated immediately with empiric antibiotics to cover *Streptococcus pneumoniae* and gram-negative organisms.

For children with SCD and acute stroke confirmed by neuroimaging, initiate urgent exchange transfusion.

Once a child has suffered a stroke, they should receive monthly simple or exchange transfusions. If this is not possible, treat with hydroxyurea, which induces HbF synthesis. HbF synthesis decreases sickling, improves red cell survival, lowers the white blood cell count, and acts as a vasodilator.

Stem cell transplantation from a normal matched sibling stem cell donor or one with a sickle cell trait can be curative.[17]

CRISPR-Cas9 gene editing presents a new therapeutic option for treating SCD and beta thalassemia that results in high levels of fetal hemoglobin and a significant decrease in the number of vaso-occlusive crises.[18]

Vasculopathies

Hypersensitivity vasculitis. The term *hypersensitivity vasculitis* covers several disorders that have a known underlying cause (drugs, infection), characteristic purpura of the legs, and vascular inflammation. Neurological complications occur only in Henoch-Schönlein purpura, for which an antecedent infection is the probable cause.

Clinical features. The systemic features of Henoch-Schönlein purpura are fever, palpable purpura on the extensor surfaces of the limbs, and abdominal pain with nausea and vomiting. Joint pain and renal involvement are common. Neurologic involvement is seen less frequently, but when present it may be severe. Many affected children have headaches and abnormalities on EEG. Focal neurological deficits occur in one-third of patients, with hemiplegia accounting for half of these cases. A seizure may precede hemiplegia. Associated with hemiplegia are hemianesthesia, hemianopia, and aphasia. These deficits may be permanent.

Diagnosis. CT or MRI shows infarction, hemorrhage, or both.

Management. Corticosteroids treat the underlying disease.

Isolated angiitis of the central nervous system. Isolated angiitis, or primary angiitis of the central nervous system (CNS), is an inflammation of small- to medium-sized vessels of the brain, meninges, and spinal cord without associated systemic signs or symptoms. It is rare in children, and the exact immunological mechanism is poorly understood. The clinical features are recurrent headache, sometimes of a migrainous type, encephalopathy, and stroke. Arteriography shows multiple areas of irregular narrowing of the cerebral vessels. Diagnosis is challenging due to the lack of formal diagnostic criteria and the fact that the disease is patchy, meaning that even brain biopsy is falsely negative in approximately 25% of cases; many cases are only diagnosed on postmortem examination. Corticosteroid therapy may be beneficial, but additional treatment with pulse cyclophosphamide or rituximab is often required.

Systemic lupus erythematosus. Several collagen vascular disorders can cause neurological disturbances in adults, but systemic lupus erythematosus (SLE) is the main cause in children. SLE is an episodic multisystem, autoimmune disease, characterized by the presence of various autoantibodies and altered complement levels. The presence of antinuclear antibodies (ANAs) is sensitive but not specific, as most patients with a positive ANA do not have lupus. SLE accounts for 4.5% of patients seen in pediatric rheumatology clinics. The onset of SLE is uncommon before adolescence. In childhood, the ratio of affected girls to boys is 4.5:1. Mixed connective tissue disease is a rare cause of either large-vessel occlusion or hemorrhage secondary to fibrinoid necrosis.

Clinical features. Most children have fever, arthralgia, and skin rash at the time of diagnosis. The clinical features of lupus in children are generally similar to those in adults, except for a higher incidence of hepatosplenomegaly, chorea, nephritis, and avascular necrosis.

Neurological features are present in one-quarter of children at the time of diagnosis and in 30%–60% sometime during the course. CNS involvement usually indicates a severe clinical course. Neuropsychiatric abnormalities are almost a constant feature. The prevalence of recurrent headaches is 71%, migraine 36%, cognitive disorders 55%, isolated seizures 47%, epilepsy 15%, acute confusional state 35%, dysesthesia or paresthesia 14%, transient ischemic attacks 12%, and CVA 8%. Chorea and myositis are rare complications. Unlike systemic complaints, neurological disturbances are likely to progress or develop anew even after initiating treatment.

Vasculitis in SLE is rare and affects small arterioles and venules. Perivasculitis is more common. Cerebral infarcts occur mainly in patients with hypertension or severe renal and cardiac disease. They are associated with positive results on serological tests for syphilis and the presence of lupus anticoagulant.

Hemiplegia may follow a seizure, and may be caused by postictal Todd paralysis, cerebral infarction, or hemorrhage.

Diagnosis. The diagnosis of lupus requires a compatible clinical syndrome and the detection of an abnormal titer of ANA. ANA is present in almost all patients. Antibodies to double-stranded DNA are pathognomonic for SLE and present in almost all patients with active disease. Antibodies to extractable nuclear antigen (Sm, Ro/SS-A, La/SS-B, RNP) and antihistone antibodies are strongly associated with SLE. Anti-Sm is highly specific for the disease. Rheumatoid factor is present in 10%–30% of cases. The presence of anticardiolipin antibodies is associated with hemolytic anemia and thrombotic events. CT or MRI of the head is useful to determine the presence of hemorrhage or infarction. Results of cerebral arteriography may be normal.

Management. The usual treatment of the CNS manifestations of SLE is high-dose oral or intravenous corticosteroids after excluding an infectious process. Several studies support the use of both steroids and cyclophosphamide in treating CNS lupus. In patients with antiphospholipid antibodies and a platelet count greater than 70,000/mm³, low-dose aspirin therapy is recommended. Anticoagulation with LMWH followed by oral anticoagulants is required for children with stroke and antiphospholipid antibodies.

Takayasu arteritis. Takayasu arteritis, also known as *the pulseless disease*, is a chronic inflammatory, large-vessel vasculitis affecting the aorta and its major branches. The cause is unknown.

Clinical features. The disease typically presents in women of childbearing age but may occur as early as infancy. It is defined by granulomatous inflammation of the aorta and its major branches. Ninety percent of patients are female, and most are of Japanese ethnicity. The most common features are fever, weight loss, myalgias, arthralgia, absent pulses, and vascular bruits. Renal artery stenosis leads to renovascular hypertension. The cause of neurological manifestations of the disease is cerebral hypoperfusion secondary to stenosis of the carotid and vertebral arteries, and complications of hypertension. Stroke occurs in only 5%–10% of patients and may be associated with seizures. Examination reveals loss of radial pulses, and sometimes a carotid bruit.

Diagnosis. CT or MRI reveals infarction. Arteriography shows involvement of the ascending aorta and its major branches. Cardiac catheterization is necessary to define the full extent of arteritis. Some vessels have a beaded appearance; others terminate abruptly and have prestenotic dilatation.

Management. Treatment consists of corticosteroids and other immunosuppressive agents. Management of hypertension is critical, and antiplatelet agents are useful in preventing thrombosis. Surgical intervention, angioplasty, and stent placement are sometimes required.

Early diagnosis and treatment can lead to full recovery, but neurological sequelae are common.

Infections

Hemiplegia occurs during the course of bacterial meningitis, resulting from vasculitis or venous thromboses, and during the course of viral encephalitis, especially herpes simplex, resulting from parenchymal necrosis. In both bacterial and viral infections, prolonged or repetitive focal seizures often precede hemiplegia. Brain abscess may cause hemiplegia, but evolution is usually slowly progressive rather than acute.

Varicella

Arterial ischemic strokes may occur during the course of varicella infection, 1 week to several months after the appearance of a rash.[19] The infarcts are small and located in the basal ganglia and internal capsule.

Migraine

Migraine is a hereditary disorder associated with, but not caused by, paroxysmal alterations in cerebral blood flow. Transitory neurological abnormalities may accompany the attack. The cause is a primary neuronal disturbance rather than cerebral ischemia. However, cerebral infarction may occur in adolescents during a prolonged attack and may represent something more than ordinary migraine. Mitochondrial disorders and channelopathies are possible mechanisms. The occurrence of transient focal motor deficits, usually hemiplegia or ophthalmoplegia (see Chapter 15), during an occasional migraine attack is called complicated migraine. In some families, hemiplegic migraine is a familial trait and may be due to multiple different mutations.

Complicated Migraine

Clinical features. The family has a history of migraine, but usually other family members have not experienced hemiplegia during an attack. The evolution

of symptoms is variable but may include scintillating or simple scotomas, unilateral dysesthesias of the hand and mouth, and unilateral weakness of the arm and face usually sparing the leg. Occurring concurrently with hemiparesis is a throbbing frontotemporal headache contralateral to the affected hemisphere. Nausea and vomiting follow. The patient falls asleep and usually recovers function on awakening. Hemiparesis lasts for less than 24 hours.

Diagnosis. Migraine is a clinical diagnosis that relies on a positive family history of the disorder. During an attack of hemiplegic migraine, EEG may demonstrate polymorphic delta activity in the hemisphere contralateral to the weakness. Neuroimaging studies are unnecessary if the patient has a history of previous attacks but are recommended initially to rule out stroke.

Management. See Chapter 3 for a summary of migraine management.

Familial Hemiplegic Migraine

Familial hemiplegic migraine (FHM) differs from complicated migraine because weakness is a required symptom and other family members are similarly affected. Transmission is autosomal dominant involving pathogenic variants in *CACNA1A* (most common), *ATP1A2*, or *SCN1A20*.[20]

PRRT2 proline-rich transmembrane protein mutations were recently discovered to cause a minority of cases. In many cases the cause remains undetermined, leading to suspicion that additional mutations have yet to be identified.

Clinical features. Hemiplegia is an essential symptom and may be prolonged, lasting 72 hours or more. Associated features may include visual disturbance, sensory loss, such as numbness or paresthesias of the face or a limb, and difficulty with speech. Attacks are stereotyped, occur primarily in childhood or adolescence, and in some instances occur in the absence of headache. The hemiplegia, although more severe in the face and arm, also affects the leg, and always outlasts the headache. Hemianesthesia of the hemiplegic side is a prominent feature. Aphasia occurs when the dominant hemisphere is affected. Confusion, stupor, or psychosis may be present during an attack. The psychosis includes both auditory and visual hallucinations, as well as delusions. Executive dysfunction, such as difficulty with attention, may persist for months, however stroke or permanent neurologic sequelae are extremely rare and should prompt an expanded diagnostic evaluation.

Symptoms last for 2 or 3 days. Acute deficits usually resolve completely, but certain neurologic abnormalities may be present in between attacks depending on the patient's specific genotype. Gaze-evoked nystagmus and progressive ataxia may be seen in children with *CACNA1A1* mutations. Epilepsy is a known comorbidity and is most often seen in patients with pathogenic variants in *ATP1A2* and can be associated with intellectual disability. Certain rare *ATP1A2* mutations cause a rare but severe phenotype presenting with seizures, coma, and hyperthermia. Diagnosis may be complicated by significant clinical overlap with episodic ataxia, spinocerebellar ataxia, infantile-onset epilepsies, and mitochondrial disease.

Diagnosis. The basis for diagnosis is the clinical findings and family history. The diagnostic criteria are: (1) fulfills criteria for migraine with aura; (2) the aura includes transient, possibly prolonged but fully reversible hemiparesis as well as fully reversible visual, sensory, and/or speech/language symptoms; and (3) at least one first-degree relative has similar attacks. Molecular testing is available on a clinical basis, but negative genetic testing does not rule out the diagnosis. Children with *CACNA1A1* mutations may have atrophy of the cerebellar vermis on imaging, but this is an inconsistent and nonspecific finding.

Management. Acetazolamide is a useful prophylactic agent in several channelopathies and is the first-line treatment for *CACNA1A1*-FHM. A trial of standard migraine prophylactic drugs (tricyclic antidepressants, beta-blockers, calcium channel blockers) is reasonable. Triggers include standard migraine precipitants (bright lights, odors, stress) but also include minor head trauma and cerebral angiography. Affected children should avoid contact sports.

Trauma

Trauma accounts for half of all deaths in children. Approximately 10% of traumatic injuries in children are not accidental. Head injury is the leading cause of death from child abuse, and half of survivors have permanent neurological handicaps.

Epidural hematoma, subdural hematoma, cerebral laceration, and intracerebral hemorrhage can produce focal signs such as hemiplegia. However, brain swelling is such a prominent feature of even trivial head injury in

> ### BOX 11.4   Progressive Hemiplegia
> - Adrenoleukodystrophy (see Chapter 5)
> - Arteriovenous malformation (see Chapter 4)
> - Brain abscess (see Chapter 4)
> - Cerebral hemisphere tumor (see Chapter 4)
> - Demyelinating diseases
> - Late-onset globoid leukodystrophy (see Chapter 5)
> - Multiple sclerosis (see Chapter 10)
> - Sturge-Weber syndrome

children that diminished consciousness and seizures are the typical clinical features (see Chapter 2).

Tumors

The initial clinical feature of primary tumors of the cerebral hemispheres is more likely to be chronic progressive hemiplegia than acute hemiplegia. However, tumors may cause acute hemiplegia when they bleed or provoke seizures and are a consideration in the evaluation of acute hemiplegia.

CHRONIC PROGRESSIVE HEMIPLEGIA

The important causes of chronic progressive hemiplegia are brain tumor, brain abscess, and arteriovenous malformations. Increased intracranial pressure is the initial feature of all three. Their discussion is in Chapter 4. Progressive hemiplegia is sometimes an initial feature of demyelinating diseases (see Chapters 5 and 10; see Box 11.4).

Sturge-Weber Syndrome

The Sturge-Weber syndrome (SWS) is a sporadic neurocutaneous disorder characterized by the association of a venous angioma of the pia mater with a port-wine stain of the face. Other findings include cognitive impairment, contralateral hemiparesis and hemiatrophy, and homonymous hemianopia. The syndrome occurs sporadically and in all races.

Clinical features. The clinical features are highly variable, and individuals with cutaneous lesions and seizures but with normal intelligence and no focal neurological deficit are common. The cutaneous angioma is usually present at birth. It is flat and variable in size but usually involves the upper lid. The size of the cutaneous angioma does not predict the size of the intracranial angioma. It is unilateral in 70% of children and ipsilateral to the venous angioma of the pia. Even when the facial nevus is bilateral, the pial angioma is usually unilateral. The characteristic neurological and radiographic features of SWS may be present without the cutaneous angioma. Only 10%–20% of children with a port-wine nevus of the forehead have a leptomeningeal angioma. Bilateral brain lesions occur in a minority of children.

Seizures occur in 80% of children with SWS, typically characterized by focal motor seizures starting within the first year of life. Focal or generalized status epilepticus may occur (see Chapter 1). Severe seizures are associated with poorer cognitive outcomes.

Hemiparesis, contralateral to the facial angioma, occurs in up to 50% of children. Hemiparesis often appears after a focal-onset seizure and progresses in severity after subsequent seizures. Transitory episodes of hemiplegia, not related to clinical or EEG evidence of seizure activity, may occur and cause stepwise deterioration. Some episodes are associated with migraine-like headache, and others occur in the absence of other symptoms and cerebral ischemia may be the cause. Glaucoma occurs in 71% of children with SWS, usually developing in the first decade.

Diagnosis. The association of neurological abnormalities and a port-wine stain of the face should suggest SWS. The pial angioma is best visualized by a contrast-enhanced MRI and only rarely by angiography.

Management. The seizures are often difficult to control with anticonvulsant medications. Hemispherectomy is an option in cases of epilepsy refractory to medical treatment and may promote improved neurodevelopment outcome by limiting the child's seizure burden. A limited resection suffices for some children. In general, the surgical considerations in children with SWS are similar to those used with other epileptic patients. Early hemispherectomy is the recommended procedure when refractory focal seizure onset is in infancy. Low-dose aspirin should be considered for children whose MRI demonstrates progressive calcifications. Yearly ophthalmology examinations with glaucoma screening are required.

REFERENCES

1. Sebire G, Husson B, Dusser A, et al. Congenital unilateral perisylvian syndrome: radiological basis and clinical correlations. *Journal of Neurology, Neurosurgery, and Psychiatry.* 1996;61:52-56.
2. Ferriero DM, Fullerton HJ, Bernard TJ, American Heart Association Stroke Council and Council on Cardiovascular and Stroke Nursing. Management of stroke in neonates and children: a scientific statement from the American Heart Association/American Stroke Association. *Stroke.* 2019;50(3):e51-e96. https://doi.org/10.1161/STR.0000000000000183. PMID: 30686119.
3. Gradnitzer E, Urlesberger B, Maurer U, et al. Cerebral hemorrhage in term newborn infants: an analysis of 10 years (1989–1999). *Wien Klinische Wochenschr.* 2002;152:9-13.
4. Rafay MF, Armstrong D, Deveber G, et al. Craniocervical arterial dissection in children: clinical and radiographic presentation and outcome. *Journal of Child Neurology.* 2006;21:8-16.
5. Roach ES, Golomb MR, Adams R, et al. Management of stroke in infants and children: a scientific statement from a special writing group of the American Heart Association Stroke Council and the Council on Cardiovascular Disease in the young. *Stroke.* 2008;39:2644-2691.
6. Rawanduzy CA, Earl E, Mayer G, Lucke-Wold B. Pediatric stroke: a review of common etiologies and management strategies. *Biomedicines.* 2022;11(1):2. https://doi.org/10.3390/biomedicines11010002. PMID: 36672510; PMCID: PMC9856134.
7. Brashear A, Sweadner KJ, Cook JF, et al. ATP1A3-related neurologic disorders (February 7, 2008). In: Adam MP, Mirzaa GM, Pagon RA, et al., eds. *GeneReviews®.* University of Washington; 1993–2023. https://www.ncbi.nlm.nih.gov/books/NBK1115/. Updated February 22, 2018.
8. Roach ES. Etiology of stroke in children. *Seminars in Pediatric Neurology.* 2002;7:244-260.
9. Marcela Torres, Tyler Hamby, Sarah Philip, Jo Ann Tilley. Catheter directed thrombolytic therapy for pediatric cerebral sinus vein thrombosis. *Blood.* 2019;134(Supplement_1):3666. https://doi.org/10.1182/blood-2019-132082.
10. Barnes C, Deveber G. Prothrombotic abnormalities in childhood ischaemic stroke. *Thrombosis Research.* 2006;118:67-74.
11. Fluss J, Geary DG, deVeber G. Cerebral sinovenous thrombosis and idiopathic nephrotic syndrome in childhood: report of four new cases and review of the literature. *European Journal of Pediatrics.* 2006;165:709-716.
12. El-Hattab AW, Almannai M, Scaglia F. Melas. In: Adam MP, Ardinger HH, Pagon RA, et al., eds. *GeneReviews®.* University of Washington; 1993–2019. https://www.ncbi.nlm.nih.gov/books/NBK1233.
13. El-Hattab AW, Almannai M, Scaglia F. Melas (February 27, 2001). In: Adam MP, Mirzaa GM, Pagon RA, et al.,

eds. *GeneReviews®*. University of Washington; 1993–2023. https://www.ncbi.nlm.nih.gov/books/NBK1233/. Updated November 29, 2018.

14. Bender MA. Sickle cell disease. In: Adam MP, Ardinger HH, Pagon RA, et al., eds. *GeneReviews®*. University of Washington; 1993–2019. https://www.ncbi.nlm.nih.gov/books/NBK1377.

15. Steen RG, Xiong X, Langston JW, et al. Brain injury in children with sickle cell disease: prevalence and etiology. *Annals of Neurology*. 2003;54:564-572.

16. Prengler M, Pavlakis SG, Boyd S, et al. Sickle cell disease: ischemia and seizures. *Annals of Neurology*. 2005;58:290-302.

17. Walters MC, Storb R, Patience M, et al. Impact of bone marrow transplantation for symptomatic sickle cell disease: an interim report. Multicenter investigation of bone marrow transplantation for sickle cell disease. *Blood*. 2000;95:1918-1924.

18. Frangoul H, Altshuler D, Cappellini MD, et al. CRISPR-Cas9 gene editing for sickle cell disease and β-thalassemia. *New England Journal of Medicine*. 2021;384(3):252-260. https://doi.org/10.1056/NEJMoa2031054. Epub 2020 Dec 5. PMID: 33283989.

19. Sebire G, Meyer L, Chabrier S. Varicella as a risk factor for cerebral infarction in childhood: a case-control study. *Annals of Neurology*. 1999;45:679-680.

20. Jen JC. Familial hemiplegic migraine (July 17, 2001). In: Adam MP, Mirzaa GM, Pagon RA, et al., eds. *GeneReviews®*. University of Washington; 1993–2023. https://www.ncbi.nlm.nih.gov/books/NBK1388/. Updated April 29, 2021.

12

Paraplegia and Quadriplegia

OUTLINE

Approach to Paraplegia, 299
Spinal Paraplegia and Quadriplegia, 299
    Symptoms and Signs, 300
    Congenital Malformations, 300
    Hereditary Spastic Paraplegia, 305
    Metabolic Disorders, 308

Neonatal Cord Infarction, 308
Transverse Myelitis, 309
Trauma, 310
Tumors of the Spinal Cord, 312
Cerebral Paraplegia and Quadriplegia, 313
References, 315

In this text the term *paraplegia* denotes partial or complete weakness of both legs and the term *quadriplegia* denotes partial or complete weakness of all limbs, thereby obviating need for the terms *paraparesis* and *quadriparesis*. Many conditions described fully in this chapter are abnormalities of the spinal cord. The same spinal abnormality can cause paraplegia or quadriplegia, depending on the location of the injury. Therefore the discussion of both is together in this chapter.

APPROACH TO PARAPLEGIA

Weakness of both legs, without any involvement of the arms, suggests an abnormality of either the spinal cord or the peripheral nerves. Ordinarily, a pattern of distal weakness and sensory loss, muscle atrophy, and absent tendon reflexes provides recognition of peripheral neuropathies. In contrast, spinal paraplegia causes spasticity, exaggerated tendon reflexes, and a dermatomal level of sensory loss. Disturbances in the conus medullaris and cauda equina, especially congenital malformation, may produce a complex of signs in which spinal cord or peripheral nerve localization is difficult. Indeed, both may be involved. Spinal paraplegia may be asymmetric at first, and then the initial feature is monoplegia (see Chapter 13). When anatomical localization between the spinal cord and peripheral nerves is difficult, electromyography (EMG) and nerve conduction studies are useful in making the distinction.

Cerebral abnormalities sometimes cause paraplegia. In such a case the child's arms as well as the legs are usually weak. However, leg weakness is so much greater than arm weakness that paraplegia is the chief complaint. Mesial frontal lobe lesions can cause isolated weakness of both legs but typically also cause seizures or alterations in mental status. It is important to remember that both the brain and the spinal cord may be abnormal and that the abnormalities can be in continuity (syringomyelia) or separated (Chiari malformation and myelomeningocele).

SPINAL PARAPLEGIA AND QUADRIPLEGIA

Box 12.1 lists conditions that cause acute, chronic, or progressive spinal paraplegia. In the absence of trauma spinal cord compression and myelitis are the main causes of an acute onset or rapidly progressive paraplegia. Acute spinal cord compression from any cause is a medical emergency requiring rapid diagnosis and therapy to avoid permanent paraplegia. Corticosteroids have the same antiinflammatory effect on the spinal cord as on the brain and temporarily decrease swelling while awaiting definitive surgical treatment.

299

BOX 12.1   **Spinal Paraplegia**

- Congenital malformations
  - Arachnoid cyst
  - Arteriovenous malformations
  - Atlantoaxial dislocation
  - Caudal regression syndrome
  - Dysraphic states
  - Chiari malformation
  - Myelomeningocele
  - Tethered spinal cord
  - Syringomyelia (see Chapter 9)
- Familial spastic paraplegia
- Infections
  - Diskitis
  - Epidural abscess
  - Herpes zoster myelitis
  - Polyradiculoneuropathy (see Chapter 7)
  - Tuberculous osteomyelitis
- Lupus myelopathy
- Metabolic disorders
- Adrenomyeloneuropathy (adrenoleukodystrophy)
- Argininemia
- Krabbe disease
- Neonatal cord infarction
- Transverse myelitis
  - Neuromyelitis optica
  - Acute disseminated encephalomyelitis
  - Myelin oligodendrocyte glycoprotein (MOG) antibody disease
  - Multiple sclerosis
- Concussion
  - Epidural hematoma
  - Fracture dislocation
- Neonatal cord trauma (see Chapter 6)
- Tumors
  - Astrocytoma
  - Ependymoma
  - Ewing sarcoma
  - Neuroblastoma

Several techniques are available to visualize the spinal cord. Each has its place, and sometimes the use of more than one technique achieves a comprehensive picture of the disease process. Magnetic resonance imaging (MRI) is clearly the procedure of choice to visualize the spine and should be used first. Computed tomography (CT) and radioisotope bone scanning are useful for visualizing the vertebral column, especially when osteomyelitis is a consideration. Isotope bone scans localize the process but rarely provide an etiology.

Symptoms and Signs

Clumsiness of gait, refusal to stand or walk, and loss of bladder or bowel control are the common complaints of spinal paraplegia. Clumsiness of gait is the usual feature of slowly progressive disorders. When functional decline is sufficiently insidious, the disturbance may go on for years without raising concern. Refusal to stand or walk is a symptom of an acute process. When a young child refuses to support weight, the underlying cause may be weakness, pain, or both.

Scoliosis is a feature of many spinal cord disorders. It occurs with neural tube defects, spinal cord tumors, and several degenerative disorders. It also occurs when the paraspinal muscles are weaker on one side of the spine than on the other side. The presence of scoliosis, in females before puberty and in males of all ages, should strongly suggest either a spinal cord disorder or a neuromuscular disease (see Chapters 6 and 7).

Abnormalities in the skin overlying the spine, such as an abnormal tuft of hair, pigmentation, a sinus opening, or a mass, may indicate an underlying dysraphic state. Spina bifida is usually an associated feature.

Foot deformities and especially stunted growth of a limb are malevolent signs of lower spinal cord dysfunction. The usual deformity is foreshortening of the foot (pes cavus). In such cases disturbances of bladder control are often an associated feature.

Brief, irregular contractions of small groups of muscles that persist during sleep characterize *spinal myoclonus*. Myoclonic contractions are often mistaken for seizure activity or fasciculations. The cause of myoclonus is irritation of pools of motor neurons and interneurons, usually by an intramedullary tumor or syrinx. The dermatomal distribution of the myoclonus localizes the site of irritation within the spinal cord. Alternatively, spinal myoclonus can present as sequelae from severe traumatic or hypoxic brain injury, due to disinhibition of anterior horn cells or multifocal cortical hyperexcitability.[1]

Congenital Malformations

Some congenital malformations, such as caudal regression syndrome and myelomeningocele, are obvious at birth. Many others do not cause symptoms until adolescence or later. Congenital malformations are always a consideration when progressive paraplegia appears in childhood.

Arachnoid Cysts

Arachnoid cysts of the spinal cord, like those of the brain (see Chapter 4), are usually asymptomatic and discovered incidentally on imaging studies. Familial cases should suggest neurofibromatosis type 2 (see Chapter 5).

Clinical features. Arachnoid cysts may be single or multiple and are usually thoracic. Symptomatic arachnoid cysts are unusual in childhood and encountered more often in adolescents and young adults. The features are back pain or radicular pain and paraplegia. Standing intensifies symptoms, and changes in position may relieve or exacerbate symptoms. The pain tends to increase in severity with time.

Diagnosis. MRI is the diagnostic modality of choice. The cyst has the same MRI characteristics as cerebrospinal fluid (CSF).

Management. Shunting of a symptomatic cyst is curative. However, it is common to blame a subarachnoid cyst for symptoms that have another cause.

Arteriovenous Malformations

Arteriovenous malformations of the spinal cord are uncommon in childhood and even rarer in infancy, although case reports do exist.[2]

Clinical features. The progression of symptoms is usually insidious, and the time from onset to diagnosis may be several years. Subacute or chronic pain is the initial feature in one-third of patients and subarachnoid hemorrhage in one-quarter. Paraplegia is an early feature in only one-third, but monoplegia or paraplegia is present in almost all children at the time of diagnosis. Most children have slowly progressive spastic paraplegia and loss of bladder control.

When subarachnoid hemorrhage is the initial feature, the malformation is more likely to be in the cervical portion of the spinal cord. Blunt trauma to the spine may be a precipitating factor. The onset of paraplegia or quadriplegia is then acute and associated with back pain. Back pain and episodic weakness that improve completely or in part may be initial features in some children, but impairment is progressive. This type of presentation is misleading and the diagnosis is often delayed.

Diagnosis. MRI/magnetic resonance angiography is the first step in diagnosis. It distinguishes intramedullary from dural and extramedullary locations of the malformation and may allow recognition of thrombus formation. Formal arteriography is often necessary to demonstrate the intramedullary extent of the malformation and all the feeding vessels.

Management. The potential approaches to therapy for intraspinal and intracranial malformations are similar (see Chapter 4).

Atlantoaxial Dislocation

The odontoid process is the major factor preventing the dislocation of C1 onto C2. True aplasia of the odontoid process is rare and leads to severe instability. Hypoplasia of the odontoid process can occur alone or as part of Morquio syndrome, other mucopolysaccharidoses, Klippel-Feil syndrome (see Chapter 18), several types of genetic chondrodysplasia, and some chromosomal abnormalities.[3] Asymptomatic atlantoaxial subluxation may occur in 20% of children with Down syndrome secondary to congenital hypoplasia of the articulation of C1 and C2; symptomatic dislocation is much less common.

Clinical features. Congenital atlantoaxial dislocation produces an acute or slowly progressive quadriplegia that may begin any time from the neonatal period to adult life. When the onset is in a newborn, the clinical features resemble an acute infantile spinal muscular atrophy (see Chapter 6). The infant has generalized hypotonia with preservation of facial expression and extraocular movement. The tendon reflexes are absent at first but then become hyperactive.

Dislocations during childhood frequently follow a fall or head injury. In such cases symptoms may begin suddenly and include not only those of myelopathy but also those related to vertebral artery occlusion.

Morquio syndrome is primarily a disease of the skeleton, with only secondary abnormalities of the spinal cord. It is also known as mucopolysaccharidosis type IV. Mutations in the *GALNS* and *GLB1* genes result in defective breakdown of glycosaminoglycans (formerly called mucopolysaccharides). Beginning in the second year or thereafter, the following features develop in affected children: prominent ribs and sternum, knock knees, progressive shortening of the neck, and dwarfism. The odontoid process is hypoplastic or absent. Acute, subacute, or chronic cervical myelopathy develops, sometimes precipitated by a fall. Loss of endurance, fainting attacks, and a "pins and needles" sensation in the arms characterize an insidious onset of symptoms. Corneal clouding, respiratory symptoms, hepatomegaly, and heart valve defects may also occur. Intelligence is usually normal, but life expectancy may be shortened depending on the severity of symptoms.

The essential feature of *Klippel-Feil syndrome* is a reduced number and abnormal fusion of cervical vertebrae. Mutations in the *GDF6*, *GDF3*, and *MEOX1* genes lead to defective bone formation. As in Morquio syndrome, the head appears to rest directly on the shoulders, the posterior hairline is low, and head movement in all directions is limited. Children often suffer from chronic headaches and neck pain. Elevation of the scapulae and deformity of the ribs (*Sprengel deformity*) are often present. Weakness and atrophy of the arm muscles and mirror movements of the hands are features of evolving paraplegia. Associated abnormalities may be present in the genitourinary, cardiac, and musculoskeletal systems.

Symptomatic atlantoaxial dislocation in children with Down syndrome may occur anytime from infancy to the 20s. Females are more often affected than males. Symptoms include neck pain, torticollis, and an abnormal gait. Spinal cord compression is progressive and leads to quadriplegia and urinary incontinence.

Diagnosis. C1 usually moves anteriorly to C2. Flexion radiographs assess the separation between the dens and the anterior arch of C1. MRI is best to view the relationship between the cord and the subluxing bones. Flexion-extension plain films of the cervical spine are often used to make the diagnosis, but CT or MRI may be more useful to assess for associated abnormalities. *The neck of children with trisomy 21 should not be forcefully flexed for lumbar puncture as this may dislocate the atlantoaxial joint and cause acute spinal cord compression.*

Management. Surgical stabilization of the atlantoaxial junction is a consideration in any child with evidence of spinal cord compression. The choice of surgical procedure depends on the mechanism of compression.

Caudal Regression Syndrome

The term *caudal regression syndrome* covers several malformations of the caudal spine that range from sacral agenesis to sirenomelia, in which the legs are fused together (also known as mermaid syndrome). The mechanism of caudal regression is incompletely understood, but some cases are clearly genetic in origin, while approximately 20% of mothers of children with caudal dysgenesis have insulin-dependent diabetes mellitus.[4] Although the name implies regression of a normally formed cord, defects in neural tube closure and prosencephalization are often associated features. The clinical spectrum varies from absence of the lumbosacral spinal cord, resulting in small, paralyzed legs, to a single malformed leg associated with malformations of the rectum and genitourinary tract.

Chiari Malformation

The type I Chiari malformation is an extension of the cerebellar tonsils through the foramen magnum, sometimes with associated syringomyelia. The type II malformation combines the cerebellar herniation with distortion and dysplasia of the medulla and occurs in more than 50% of children with lumbar myelomeningocele. The herniated portion may become ischemic and necrotic and can cause compression of the brainstem and upper cervical spinal cord.

Ectopic expression of a segmentation gene in the rhombomeres may explain the Chiari malformation and the brainstem anomalies, myelodysplasia, and the defective bone formation that results in a small posterior fossa.[5]

Clinical features. Most Chiari I malformations are discovered as an incidental finding on an MRI ordered because of headache. The malformation itself is rarely the cause of the headache. The initial features of a *symptomatic* Chiari malformation are usually insidious. Oropharyngeal dysfunction is a presenting feature in 35% of children less than 6 years of age, followed by scoliosis (23%) and head and neck pain (23%).[6] Among older children, headache and neck pain are the first features in 38% and weakness in 56%. Eighty percent show motor deficits on examination, usually atrophy and hyporeflexia in the arms and spasticity and hyperreflexia in the legs. Sensory loss and scoliosis are each present in half of the cases.

Type II malformation should be suspected in every child with myelomeningocele. The child may have hydrocephalus secondary to aqueductal stenosis or by an obstruction of the outflow of CSF from the fourth ventricle due to herniation. Respiratory distress is the most important feature of the Chiari II malformation. Rapid respirations, episodes of apnea, and Cheyne-Stokes respirations may occur. Other evidence of brainstem compression includes poor feeding, vomiting, dysphagia, and paralysis of the tongue. Sudden cardio-respiratory failure may lead to death if the underlying abnormality is not addressed.

Diagnosis. MRI is the best method to visualize the posterior fossa and cervical cord. CT is useful to further delineate bony abnormalities.

Management. Posterior fossa decompression is the usual technique to manage newborns with myelomeningocele and respiratory distress caused by the Chiari II malformation. Unfortunately, permanent deficits are the rule. Posterior fossa decompression is usually successful in relieving symptoms of cord compression in older children without myelomeningocele. Associated hydrocephalus requires ventriculoperitoneal shunting in many cases.

Fetal myelomeningocele repair is possible and is performed in several specialized centers. Fetal outcomes are encouraging, with significantly decreased need for ventriculoperitoneal shunting and increased ambulation following in utero surgical correction. Maternal morbidity is an ongoing concern; fetoscopic repair allows for vaginal delivery and fewer uterine complications than open repair, which requires subsequent caesarian delivery and risk for uterine scar thinning and dehiscence. Fetal outcomes for both types of surgery are similar.[7]

Myelomeningocele

Dysraphia comprises all defects in the closure of the neural tube and its coverings. Closure occurs during the third and fourth weeks of gestation. The mesoderm surrounding the neural tube gives rise to the dura, skull, and vertebrae but not to the skin. Therefore defects in the final closure of the neural tube and its mesodermal case do not preclude the presence of a dermal covering.

Despite extensive epidemiological studies, the causes of myelomeningocele remain unclear. Both genetic and environmental factors play a role. Folate deficiency is one likely cause. Maternal *MTHFR* mutations, which impair folate metabolism, are another associated risk factor, as are certain anticonvulsant medications and maternal diabetes mellitus. Females who have previously had a child with dysraphia have an approximate 2% risk of recurrence, and prenatal diagnosis is available.

α-Fetoprotein, the principal plasma protein of the fetus, is present in amniotic fluid. The concentration of α-fetoprotein in the amniotic fluid increases when plasma proteins exude through a skin defect. Prenatal diagnosis is possible by the combination of measuring the maternal serum concentration of α-fetoprotein and ultrasound examination of the fetus.

The incidence of dysraphic defects has been declining in the United States and the United Kingdom. Antenatal screening alone does not explain the decline; changes in critical environmental factors may be important. Because the ingestion of folic acid supplements during early pregnancy reduces the incidence of neural tube defects, the consumption of 0.4 mg of folic acid daily is advisable for all females of childbearing age. Females with a prior history of delivering a child with a neural tube defect, or with any of the risk factors listed earlier, should take 4 mg/day of folic acid from at least 4 weeks before conception through the first 3 months of pregnancy.

Clinical features. Spina bifida cystica, the protrusion of a cystic mass through the defect, is an obvious deformity of the newborn's spine. More than 90% are thoracolumbar. Among newborns with spina bifida cystica, the protruding sac is a meningocele without neural elements in 10%–20% and is a myelomeningocele in the rest. Meningoceles tend to have a partial dermal covering and are often pedunculated, with a narrow base connecting the sac to the underlying spinal cord. Myelomeningoceles usually have a broad base, lack epithelial covering, and ooze a combination of CSF and serum. Portions of the dome contain exposed remnants of the spinal cord.

In newborns with spina bifida cystica it is important to determine the extent of neurological dysfunction caused by the myelopathy, the potential for the development of hydrocephalus, and the presence of other malformations in the nervous system and in other organs. When myelomeningocele is the only deformity, the newborn is alert and responsive and has no difficulty in feeding. Diminished consciousness or responsiveness and difficulty in feeding should suggest perinatal asphyxia or cerebral malformations such as hydrocephalus. Cyanosis, pallor, or dyspnea suggests associated malformations in the cardiovascular system. Multiple major defects are present in approximately 30% of cases.

The spinal segments involved can be determined by locating the myelomeningocele with reference to the ribs and iliac crest. Several patterns of motor dysfunction are observable depending on the cyst's location. Motor dysfunction results from interruption of the corticospinal tracts and from dysgenesis of the segmental innervation. At birth, the legs are flaccid, the hips are dislocated, and arthrogryposis of the lower extremities is present. Spastic paraplegia, a spastic bladder, and a level of sensory loss develop in infants with a thoracic lesion. Segmental withdrawal reflexes below the level of the lesion, which indicate the presence of an intact but isolated spinal cord segment below the cyst, are present in half of patients. Infants with deformities of the conus medullaris maintain a flaccid paraplegia, have lumbosacral sensory loss, lack a withdrawal response in the legs, and have a distended bladder with overflow incontinence.

Only 15% of newborns with myelomeningocele have clinical evidence of hydrocephalus at birth, but ultrasound detects hydrocephalus in 60% of affected newborns. Hydrocephalus eventually develops in 80%. The first clinical features of hydrocephalus often follow the repair of the myelomeningocele, but the two are not related. Aqueductal stenosis and the Chiari II malformation are the cause of hydrocephalus in the majority of infants with myelomeningocele.

Diagnosis. Examination alone establishes the diagnosis of spina bifida cystica. EMG may be useful to clarify the distribution of segmental dysfunction. Cranial ultrasound to look for hydrocephalus is required for every newborn. MRI is useful to define malformations of the brain, especially the Chiari malformation (see Fig. 10.6). Therapeutic decisions may require such information. Even in the absence of hydrocephalus at birth, repeat ultrasound examinations in 2–4 weeks are required to evaluate ventricular size.

Management. The chance of surviving the first year is poor without back closure shortly after birth. However, closure is not a surgical emergency, and delays of a week or longer do not influence the survival rate. Other factors associated with increased mortality are a high spinal location of the defect and clinical hydrocephalus at birth. The long-term outcome depends on the degree of neurological deficit from the spinal defect and any associated brain abnormalities.

Tethered Spinal Cord

A thickened filum terminale, a lipoma, a dermal sinus, or diastematomyelia may anchor the conus medullaris to the base of the vertebrae. Spina bifida occulta is usually an associated feature. As the child grows, the tether causes the spinal cord to stretch and the lumbosacral segments to become ischemic. The mitochondrial oxidative metabolism of neurons is impaired, and neurological dysfunction follows.

Dermal sinus is a midline opening of the skin usually marked by a tuft of hair or port-wine stain. An abnormal invagination of ectoderm into the posterior closure site of the neural tube causes the problem. Most sinuses terminate subcutaneously as a blind pouch or dermoid cyst. Others extend through a spina bifida to the developing neuraxis, at which point they attach to the dura or the spinal cord as a fibrous band or dermoid cyst. Such sinuses tether the spinal cord and serve as a route for bacteria from the skin to reach the subarachnoid space and cause meningitis.

Diastematomyelia consists of a bifid spinal cord (also called *diplomyelia*) that is normal in the cervical and upper thoracic regions and then divides into lateral halves (Fig. 12.1). Two types of diastematomyelia occur with equal frequency. In one type a dural sheath surrounds each half of the cord and a fibrous or bony septum separates the two halves. Once the cord separates, it never rejoins. In the other type a single dural sheath surrounds both halves and a septum is not present. The two halves rejoin after one or two segments. Therefore the cause of spinal cord splitting is not the presence of a septum, but rather a primary disturbance in the formation of luminal borders caused by faulty closure of the neural tube. It is usually associated with other dysraphic disturbances such as spina bifida occulta or cystica.

Clinical features. The initial features of a tethered spinal cord occur at any age from infancy to young adulthood. The clinical features vary with age. External signs of spinal dysraphism (tuft of hair, subcutaneous lipoma, and dermal sinus) are present in more than half of patients, and spina bifida occulta or sacral deformity is present in almost 90%.

Infants and young children are most likely to show clumsiness of gait, stunted growth, or deformity of one foot or leg, and disturbances in bladder or bowel function. These may occur alone or in combination. Consequently, the first specialist consulted may be an orthopedic surgeon, urologist, neurologist, or neurosurgeon. The progression of symptoms and signs is insidious, and a static problem is the first diagnosis in most children. Children with only a clumsy gait or disturbances in urinary control tend to have normal or exaggerated tendon reflexes and an extensor plantar response. In some children diminished or absent ankle tendon reflexes are noted on one or both sides. Children with foot deformity usually have pes cavus and stunted growth of the entire leg. The other leg may

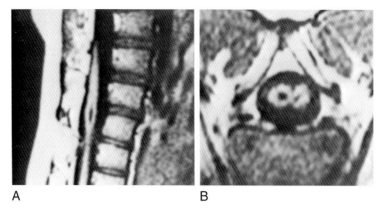

Fig. 12.1 Diplomyelia. Magnetic resonance imaging (MRI) shows two cords with two central canals. (A) Longitudinal MRI shows a spinal cord with an enlarged segment and cystic center. (B) Cross-section of the same cord shows two segments with two central canals.

appear normal or have a milder deformity without a growth disturbance. Diminished tendon reflexes in the deformed foot are more likely than increased reflexes.

The initial feature of tethered spinal cord in older children and adolescents is either clumsiness of gait or scoliosis. Bilateral, but mild, foot deformities are sometimes present, and urinary incontinence and constipation are reported. Exaggerated knee and ankle tendon reflexes are usual, and the plantar response is usually extensor.

Diagnosis. EMG is not a useful screening procedure, as the results are usually abnormal. Radiographs of the spine may show a spina bifida, but MRI is the appropriate diagnostic test and is particularly useful in the detection of lumbosacral lipoma. The essential feature of a tethered spinal cord is a low-lying conus medullaris. At 28 weeks' gestation, the tip of the conus is at the L3 vertebral level. It generally raises one level by 40 weeks' gestation. A conus that extends below the L2 to L3 interspace in children 5 years and older is always abnormal.

Management. Surgical relief of the tethering prevents further deterioration of neurological function and improves preexisting deficits in up to 50% of children.[8]

Hereditary Spastic Paraplegia

Hereditary spastic paraplegia (HSP) is a heterogeneous group of over 80 distinct genetic disorders in which the prominent clinical feature is either static or progressive spastic paraplegia. Most cases are *uncomplicated* HSP, in which neurological impairment is limited to progressive spastic paraplegia, a hypertonic urinary bladder

disturbance, and mild diminution of vibration and position sense. Others have *complicated* or *complex* HSP in which the spastic paraplegia is associated with other neurological findings such as seizures, dementia, amyotrophy, extrapyramidal disturbance, or peripheral neuropathy. Terminology is confusing because the diseases were initially named SPG (for *sp*astic para*g*legia) followed by a number according to the order in which they were discovered. As our genetic understanding improves, the HSPs are increasingly referred to by their causative genetic variant. The literature contains both terminologies.

The majority of HSPs are autosomal dominant (AD), comprising 75%–80% of cases. Pathogenic variants in *SPAST* cause most cases of AD HSP overall, but *ATL1* mutations are the most common cause of early-onset disease seen in children.[9]

Autosomal recessive types are highly variable and often extremely rare; many are described only in single families. X-linked and mitochondrial types exist but are the rarest forms and are typically *complicated*.

Clinical features. The age at onset ranges from infancy to late adulthood. Early- and late-onset cases may occur among members of the same family. Motor milestones are normal in affected infants except for toe walking. Frequently, the diagnosis in such children is diplegic cerebral palsy (CP), especially if spasticity presents early and appears nonprogressive. Increased tone is more prominent than weakness, which may or may not be present. Tone typically increases slowly for several years and then stabilizes. At this point, the child may have minimal stiffness of gait or be unable to stand or walk.

Usually, tendon reflexes are brisk in the legs and arms, and ankle clonus may be present. However, some children have absent or diminished ankle tendon reflexes due to an associated length-dependent axonal neuropathy. Increased reflexes are usually the only sign of involvement of the arms. Vibratory and position sense are diminished in half of patients. Urinary symptoms, usually in the form of frequency and urgency, and pes cavus deformities each occur in one-third of affected children.

Diagnosis. MRI of the brain and spinal cord is usually normal; any abnormalities found (such as thin corpus callosum) tend to be nonspecific and nondiagnostic. The differential diagnosis includes multiple sclerosis (MS), structural abnormalities involving the spinal cord, B_{12} deficiency, adrenomyeloneuropathy (AMN) and other leukodystrophies, and dopa-responsive dystonia. The diagnosis of HSP is suspect in any child with very slowly progressive spastic paraplegia. Laboratory studies are not helpful except to exclude other conditions such as adrenoleukodystrophy and argininemia. Due to the wide genetic and phenotypic variability, a multigene panel is often the most expedient way to arrive at a diagnosis.

Management. There is no cure, and treatment focuses on symptom management. Oral agents such as baclofen or Botox injections are used to relieve spasticity. Many children require ankle-foot orthoses to improve gait. Consultation with urology may assist with treating urinary urgency. Children with complicated HSP require management of associated issues such as epilepsy, cognitive impairment, and sensory neuropathy. Genetic counseling is recommended for all affected families.

Diskitis (Disk Space Infection)

Disk space infection is a relatively uncommon disorder of childhood in which one disk space is infected secondary to subacute osteomyelitis of the adjacent vertebral bodies. The cause is bacterial infection. *Staphylococcus aureus* is the organism most often grown on cultures of disk material removed by needle biopsy and is probably the major cause. Blood cultures are often negative, likely because the infection is subacute. Biopsy is typically unnecessary.

Clinical features. The initial feature is either difficulty walking or back pain. Difficulty walking occurs almost exclusively in children less than 3 years of age.

The typical child has a low-grade or no fever, is observed to be limping, and may refuse to stand or walk. This symptom complex evolves over 24–48 hours. Affected children prefer to lie on their sides rather than to rest supine, resist standing, and then seem uncomfortable and walk with a shuffling gait. Examination shows loss of lumbar lordosis and absolute resistance to flexion of the spine. The hips or back are sometimes tender.

Pain as an initial feature occurs more often after 3 years of age. The pain may be vertebral, or rarely, abdominal. When abdominal, the pain gradually increases in intensity and may radiate from the epigastrium to the umbilicus or pelvis. Abdominal pain in association with low-grade fever and an elevated peripheral white blood cell count invariably suggests the possibility of appendicitis or other intraabdominal disease. Fortunately, abdominal pain is the least common presenting feature.

Back pain is the most common complaint. Older children may indicate a specific area of pain and tenderness. Younger children may have only an abnormal posture intended to splint the painful area. Back pain usually leads to prompt diagnosis because attention immediately directs to the spine. Examination reveals loss of lumbar lordosis and decreased movement of the spine, especially flexion.

Diagnosis. Disk space infection is a consideration in all children who have sudden back pain or refuse to walk, and in whom there are no specific neurological abnormalities. Strength, tone, and tendon reflexes in the legs are normal. Radiographs of the spine reveal narrowing of the affected intervertebral space, most often in the lumbar region but sometimes as high as the C5 to C6 positions. MRI is the best method to demonstrate inflammation within the disk. It shows osteomyelitis of the surrounding vertebrae as well as of the disk space (Fig. 12.2).

Management. Initiate intravenous antibiotics as soon as diagnostic confirmation is complete. Immobilization is not necessary because most children are nearly asymptomatic when discharged from the hospital.

Herpes Zoster Myelitis

Immunosuppressed individuals may experience reactivation of the varicella-zoster virus that had been latent in sensory ganglia following primary chickenpox infection.

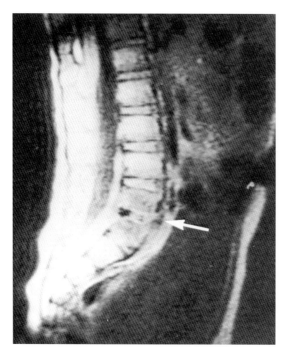

Fig. 12.2 Diskitis. Magnetic resonance imaging reveals collapse of the disk space (*arrow*) and demineralization of the adjoining vertebral bodies.

Clinical features. The spinal cord becomes involved within 3 weeks after a truncal rash appears. Myelopathy usually progresses for 3 weeks, but progression may last as long as 6 months in immunocompromised patients. Cord involvement is bilateral in 80% of cases.

Diagnosis. Diagnosis depends on recognition of the characteristic herpetic rash at the dermatomal level of the myelitis. Unfortunately, myelitis sometimes precedes the onset of rash. Images of the spine are required to exclude other causes. The CSF shows a pleocytosis and protein elevation that is greatest at the time of maximal neurological deficit.

Management. Treatment with corticosteroids and acyclovir is a standard practice, although their benefit is uncertain. In general, those treated promptly have the best response.

Tuberculous Osteomyelitis

Tuberculosis causes vertebral infection by hematogenous dissemination. Any level of the vertebral column may be affected. The infection usually begins in one vertebral body and then spreads to adjacent vertebrae and

the surrounding soft tissue. Fewer than 20% of patients with tuberculous osteomyelitis have symptoms of spinal cord dysfunction. The pathophysiological mechanisms include epidural abscess, arteritis, and vertebral collapse. In addition, tuberculous granuloma of the spine may occur in the absence of vertebral disease.

Clinical features. Tuberculosis of the vertebrae and spine, also known as Pott disease or tuberculous spondylitis, is primarily a disease of children and young adults in countries with high rates of tuberculosis infection, although in the United States it is more typically seen in immunocompromised adults. Young children with vertebral osteomyelitis not extending to the spinal cord may refuse to walk because of pain, and their symptoms may mimic paraplegia. The prominent features are fever, anorexia, and back pain. In children less than 10 years of age, infection is generally diffuse, affecting several vertebrae and adjacent tissues. Older children tend to have localized infection but with a higher incidence of spinal cord compression. The symptoms and signs of spinal cord compression from tuberculosis are similar to those described for an epidural abscess, except that progression is slower.

Diagnosis. The CSF is usually under pressure and shows a pleocytosis with polymorphonuclear leukocytes predominating early in the course and lymphocytes predominating in the later stages. The total cell count rarely exceeds 500 cells/mm^3. Protein concentrations are elevated, and glucose concentrations are depressed. Stained smears show acid-fast organisms and the organism can be isolated on cultures of the CSF.

MRI is the most useful modality to detect osteomyelitis. As the disease progresses, radiographs reveal the collapse of adjacent vertebrae and gibbus formation (structural kyphosis).

Management. Treatment of tuberculous osteomyelitis and meningitis are similar, although the length of treatment differs. For tuberculous osteomyelitis in children, the Centers for Disease Control and Prevention recommends isoniazid, rifampin, and pyrazinamide for 8 weeks, followed by 4–7 months of isoniazid and rifampin. In situations where isoniazid resistance is suspected, the addition of ethambutol should be considered, although this is not always used in children. In cases of tuberculous meningitis and disseminated tuberculosis treatment needs to be continued for 9–12 months. Directly observed therapy should be used in all children with tuberculosis. Corticosteroids, either dexamethasone or prednisolone, have been shown to decrease mortality and should be part of the treatment regimen for tuberculous meningitis.[10]

Lupus Myelopathy

Transverse myelopathy is a rare complication of systemic lupus erythematosus, occurring in 1%–2% of patients. The usual features are back pain, rapidly progressive paraplegia, and bowel and bladder dysfunction. Most patients exhibit a sensory level on examination, and many have coexistent optic neuritis that may raise concern for neuromyelitis optica (NMO) (see the following section). The protein concentration of the CSF is elevated, and MRI of the spine is abnormal. Treatment is with intravenous methylprednisolone and immunosuppressants. Recovery is variable, and patients who present with dense motor deficits are less likely to recover completely. Approximately 20% have no recovery or deteriorate.

Metabolic Disorders

Adrenomyeloneuropathy

AMN is the most common phenotype of adrenoleukodystrophy accounting for 40%–50% of cases.[10] The etiology is impaired ability to oxidize very-long-chain fatty acids (see Chapter 5). The causative mutation is in the *ABCD1* gene and genetic transmission is by X-linked inheritance.

Clinical features. Paraplegia begins after age 20 and is slowly progressive throughout adult life. Intellectual impairment is common and prolonged survival is the rule.[11] Most patients develop Addison disease, which predates paraplegia almost half of the time. Sensory neuropathy may be associated. Approximately 20% of female heterozygotes develop clinical disease.

Diagnosis. MS is a common misdiagnosis among female heterozygotes. The demonstration of increased plasma concentrations of very-long-chain fatty acids is essential for diagnosis.

Management. Symptomatic males require regular assessment of adrenal function and corticosteroid replacement therapy for adrenal insufficiency. Unfortunately, corticosteroid replacement therapy has no effect on nervous system involvement. Bone marrow transplantation is an option for boys and adolescents who are in the early stages of symptom development with evidence of brain involvement on MRI. Recently, the Food and Drug Administration in the United States

approved the use of Skysona, a one-time gene therapy directed specifically toward children with cerebral adrenoleukodystrophy. Significant side effects may occur with treatment, including cancers of the blood and bone marrow. Treatment is available at a few highly specialized centers within the United States.

Arginase Deficiency

Arginase catalyzes the metabolism of arginine to ornithine and urea in the urea cycle. Arginase deficiency is the least common of all urea cycle disturbances. Genetic transmission is as an autosomal recessive trait.[12]

Clinical features. Motor and cognitive development slows in early childhood and then regresses. Most children develop progressive spastic paraplegia or quadriplegia. Other features may include recurrent vomiting and seizures.

Diagnosis. The serum concentration of arginine is elevated, and 90% of children have elevated blood concentrations of ammonia. There is typically no detectable arginase activity in red blood cells. In the United States, most infants are diagnosed based on the expanded newborn screen. Molecular genetic testing is available.

Management. Dietary protein restriction may slow the progression of the disorder and sometimes cause improvement.

Krabbe Disease

The early infantile form of Krabbe disease (globoid leukodystrophy) causes psychomotor regression (see Chapter 5) and a peripheral neuropathy (see Chapter 7). The disorder is due to mutations of the gene encoding glycosylceramidase (*GALC*) at chromosome site 14q31.[13]

A late-onset form of the disease, with onset from childhood to adolescence, may show only spastic paraplegia or more often spastic paraplegia and visual loss. Many patients with late-onset disease are compound heterozygotes, having one copy of two different mutations associated with enzyme deficiency. Hematopoietic stem cell transplantation in presymptomatic infants and older individuals with mild symptoms may improve and preserve cognitive function, but peripheral nervous system function may deteriorate.

Neonatal Cord Infarction

Infarction of the spinal cord is a hazard in newborns undergoing umbilical artery catheterization. The artery of Adamkiewicz arises from the aorta at the level of T10 to T12 and is the major segmental artery to the thoracolumbar spinal cord. Placing the catheter tip between levels T10 and T11 may cause embolization of the artery resulting in acute and sometimes irreversible paraplegia. A similar syndrome occurs among premature or small-for-date newborns in the absence of catheterization. The mechanism in such cases is unknown but hypotension may be causal.

Transverse Myelitis

Transverse myelitis is an acute, inflammatory, demyelinating disorder of the spinal cord that evolves in hours or days. Transverse myelitis was previously considered an idiopathic or cryptogenic condition distinct from autoimmune disorders, however, with improved diagnostic testing, it has become clear that the vast majority of cases are associated with the presence of autoantibodies, either at the time of the initial event or discovered following subsequent flares.

Transverse myelitis is part of the constellation of symptoms in NMO, acute disseminated encephalomyelitis (ADEM), MS, and myelin oligodendrocyte glycoprotein antibody disease (MOGAD).

Clinical features. Mean age at onset is 9 years but varies depending on the specific etiology. Symptoms progress rapidly, attaining maximal deficit within 2 days. The level of myelitis is usually thoracic and demarcated by sensory loss; it may be limited to one or two levels or may extend longitudinally through the majority of the cord. Asymmetric leg weakness is common. The bladder fills and does not empty voluntarily. Tendon reflexes may be increased or reduced. Recovery typically begins

after several days but is often incomplete, and permanent deficits may occur.

NMO consists of transverse myelitis and optic neuritis. The two do not necessarily occur simultaneously. Myelitis precedes optic neuritis in 13% of patients and follows it in 76%; myelitis and neuritis occur simultaneously in 10%. Involvement of the cerebrum is rare but can occur. In addition to the symptoms referable to the spinal cord as described earlier the child complains of decreased visual acuity in one or both eyes, as well as pain with eye movements and decreased color saturation. Visual acuity testing, fundoscopic examination, and consultation with an ophthalmologist are required. Disk edema is common but often less pronounced than that seen in MOGAD (see the following). The pupillary responses are present but sluggish.

ADEM involves diffuse, often patchy inflammatory and demyelinating changes throughout the neuroaxis including the cerebral hemispheres and spinal cord. Children typically present with decreased level of consciousness, irritability, and personality changes in addition to focal neurologic symptoms; psychosis may be a prominent part of the encephalopathy. Cranial nerve palsies, dysphagia, fever, and irregular respirations indicate involvement of the brainstem.

MS causes demyelinating lesions of the optic nerves, brain, and spine (Fig 12.3). It has a wide range of presentations and is discussed in more detail in Chapter 10.

MOGAD presents similarly to MS but is caused by myelin oligodendrocyte glycoprotein (MOG) antibodies. Optic neuritis and transverse myelitis are common initial symptoms; disk edema associated with the optic

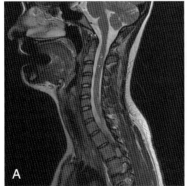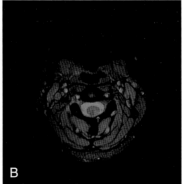

Fig. 12.3 Multiple Sclerosis. C2 to C3 segment demyelinating lesion in (A) sagittal and (B) transverse T_2 magnetic resonance imaging.

neuritis tends to be more pronounced than that seen in NMO. Seizures may occur. Visual recovery is complete or near-complete in most cases,[14] but motor recovery is less predictable.

Diagnosis. Children with suspected transverse myelitis should undergo MRI of the brain and total spine, with and without contrast, as well as immunologic evaluation. Lumbar puncture often demonstrates increased protein and may show the presence of oligoclonal bands or an elevated IgG index. Children with NMO have positive aquaporin-4 antibodies, while children with MOGAD demonstrate MOG antibodies. Cerebral white matter lesions are common in ADEM and MS, slightly less common in MOGAD, and rare in NMO.

Management. The recommended treatment protocol is high-dose intravenous methylprednisolone (20 mg/kg/day, maximum 1 g/day) for 3–5 days, followed by tapering doses of oral prednisone over 4–6 weeks (longer for children with MOG positive disease). Intravenous immunoglobulin and plasmapheresis are second-line interventions. When effective, immunoglobulins abort the progression of symptoms but do not result in immediate symptom improvement, which is due to self-healing mechanisms such as remyelination. Consider plasmapheresis if symptoms continue to worsen despite administering immunoglobulin. Physical and occupational therapies are almost always required; school accommodations are needed for visual, sensory, and motor deficits and, at times, to offer increased educational support in the setting of persistent cognitive symptoms. Antibodies that remain persistently positive despite treatment are associated with relapse. Such children should be under the care and supervision of a neuroimmunologist to determine if long-term immune suppression or disease-modifying agents are appropriate.

Trauma

Spinal cord injuries are fortunately rare in children, comprising approximately 5% of all spinal cord injuries treated in hospitals in the United States. Motor vehicle crashes are the primary cause, followed by falls, sports injuries, and violent injuries such as gunshot wounds. The cervical spine is particularly vulnerable and accounts for 65%–80% of childhood spine injuries as compared to only 30% in adults. Large head-to-body size ratio, more elastic connective tissues, and horizontal alignment of the vertebral facets at least partly explain the high incidence of cervical spine injuries in children under the age of 14. Once a child reaches adolescence, injury patterns more closely resemble those of adults.[15]

Diagnosis. MRI is the imaging modality of choice and the most appropriate study to evaluate the spinal cord. However, spinal cord injury without radiographic abnormality (SCIWORA) is a well-described entity in adults and is even more common in children. Children suffering from sports injuries or physical abuse have especially high rates of SCIWORA, and the treating physician must maintain a high index of suspicion for any child with an abnormal neck or neurological exam, high-risk mechanism of injury or distracting injury, even in the absence of radiographic evidence of damage.[16]

Management. Virtually no evidence-based guidelines exist for the treatment of spinal cord injury in children. There is no evidence to support the use of hypothermia or steroids in the pediatric population. Basic practices such as immobilization are the same as those for adults, and many institutions have standardized protocols for acute spine injury. Much of the care focuses on medical stabilization in preparation for rehabilitation. Physical and occupational therapies are the standard of care; most patients also require a bowel routine, evaluation for and management of neurogenic bladder, and feeding and nutrition evaluation. Late complications such as scoliosis and spasticity should be managed by an interdisciplinary team, including orthopedics, physical and rehabilitation medicine, and/or neurology. Children have been long thought to recover from spinal injuries more completely than adults; however, actual evidence for this is minimal.

Compressed Vertebral Body Fractures

Clinical features. Compression fractures of the thoracolumbar region occur when a child jumps or falls from a height greater than 10 feet and lands in a standing or sitting position; they also may occur more insidiously in children undergoing long-term steroid treatment. Transection of the spinal cord has not occurred, but spinal cord concussion may cause paraplegia. Back pain at the fracture site is immediate and intense. Nerve root compression causes pain that radiates into the groin and legs.

Diagnosis. Thoracolumbar radiographs reveal the fracture and MRI of the spinal cord is normal.

Management. Immobilization relieves back pain and promotes healing of the fracture. Physical therapy is standard. Children with steroid-related fractures need calcium and vitamin D supplementation; consider the addition of a bisphosphonate to treat symptomatic osteoporosis.

Fracture Dislocation and Spinal Cord Transection

Motor vehicle accidents are the usual cause of spinal cord transection from fracture dislocation of the vertebral column. A forceful flexion of the spine fractures the articular facets and allows the vertebral body to move forward or laterally, with consequent contusion or transection of the spinal cord. The common sites of traumatic transection are the levels C1 to C2, C5 to C7, and T12 to L2.

Clinical features. Neurological deficits at and below the level of spinal cord contusion or transection are immediate and profound. Many children with fracture dislocations sustained head injuries at the time of trauma and are unconscious.

Immediately after the injury, the child has flaccid weakness of the limbs below the level of the lesion associated with loss of tendon and cutaneous reflexes (spinal shock). In high cervical spinal cord lesions eliciting the knee and ankle tendon reflexes, anal reflex, and plantar response may be possible during the initial period of spinal shock. Spinal shock lasts for approximately 1 week in infants and young children and up to 6 weeks in adolescents.

First, the superficial reflexes return, then the plantar response becomes one of extension, and finally, massive withdrawal reflexes (mass reflex) appear. Trivial stimulation of the foot or leg triggers the mass reflex, usually in a specific zone unique to the patient. The response at first is dorsiflexion of the foot, flexion at the knees, and flexion and adduction at the thighs. Later, contractions of the abdomen, sweating, piloerection, and emptying of the bladder and bowel occur. During this time of heightened reflex activity, the tendon reflexes return and become exaggerated.

Below the level of injury, the sensation is lost to a variable degree, depending on the completeness of the transection. When the injury is incomplete, sensation begins to return within weeks and may continue to improve for up to 2 years. Patients with partial or complete transections may complain of pain and tingling below the level of injury.

In addition to the development of a small, spastic bladder autonomic dysfunction includes constipation,

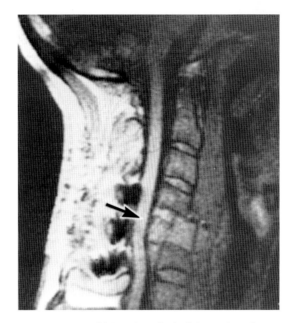

Fig. 12.4 Fracture Dislocation. C4 is dislocated on C5, causing compression (*arrow*) of the cord.

lack of sweating, orthostatic hypotension, and disturbed temperature regulation.

Diagnosis. Radiographs of the vertebrae readily identify fracture dislocations. MRI of the spinal cord produces further information on the presence of compressive hematomas and the structural integrity of the spinal cord (Fig. 12.4).

Management. The immediate treatment of fracture dislocation is to reduce the dislocation and prevent further damage to the cord by the use of corticosteroids, surgery, and immobilization. An intravenous infusion of methylprednisolone, 30 mg/kg within the first 8 hours after injury followed by 4 mg/kg/h for 23 hours, significantly reduces neurological morbidity. A discussion of the long-term management of spinal cord injuries is beyond the scope of this text. Specialized centers provide the best results.

Spinal Cord Concussion

A direct blow to the back may produce a transitory disturbance in spinal cord function. The cause of dysfunction is edema (spinal shock); the spinal cord is intact.

Clinical features. Most injuries occur at the level of the cervical cord or the thoracolumbar juncture. The major clinical features are flaccid paraplegia or quadriplegia, a sensory level at the site of injury, loss of tendon reflexes, and urinary retention. Recovery begins within a few hours and is complete within a week.

Diagnosis. At the onset of weakness, spinal cord compression syndrome, such as epidural hematomas, is a consideration, and an imaging study of the spine is necessary.

Management. The indications for methylprednisolone treatment are given in the "Fracture Dislocation and Spinal Cord Transection" section.

Spinal Epidural Hematoma

Spinal epidural hematoma usually results from direct vertebral trauma and is especially common in children with an underlying bleeding tendency. The hematoma causes symptoms by progressive compression of the cord, and the clinical features are like any other extradural mass lesion. MRI is usually the basis for diagnosis. Treatment is surgical evacuation.

Tumors of the Spinal Cord

Ewing's sarcoma accounts for nearly 20% of cases of spinal cord compression in children over 5 years of age, while neuroblastoma is the most common cause in younger children. Astrocytoma and ependymoma are the main primary tumors. Motor deficits, usually paraplegia, are an early feature in 86% of spinal cord tumors and back pain in 63%.

Astrocytoma

Chapter 9 discusses the problems of differentiating cystic astrocytoma of the spinal cord from syringomyelia (see the "Syringomyelia" section).

Clinical features. Astrocytomas have a highly variable presentation depending on the grade and location of the tumor. They can be long and may extend from the lower brainstem to the conus medullaris. The initial features of multiple-segment spinal astrocytomas may occur in the arms or legs; weakness of one arm is characteristic in many cases. Neck pain is not always present, and bowel and bladder function are usually normal. Examination shows mild spastic weakness of the legs. The solid portion of the tumor is often in the neck with cystic caudal extension.

Alternatively, children may present with progressive spastic paraplegia, sometimes associated with thoracic pain and scoliosis. When a solid tumor extends into the conus medullaris, tendon reflexes in the legs may be diminished or absent, and bowel and bladder function are impaired.

Intraaxial tumors of the cervicomedullary junction are often low-grade and have an indolent course. They may cause cranial nerve dysfunction or spinal cord compression. Difficulty swallowing and nasal speech are the main features of cranial nerve dysfunction (see Chapter 17).

Diagnosis. MRI is the definitive diagnostic procedure. It allows visualization of both the solid and cystic portions of the tumor (Fig. 12.5). Biopsy and genetic studies aid in classification and the formulation of treatment plans.

Management. Treatment depends largely on the tumor grade, location, genetics, and associated symptoms. Surgery followed by radiation treatment and chemotherapy is recommended for aggressive cases. Low-grade astrocytomas causing minimal symptoms can usually be treated conservatively with close monitoring.

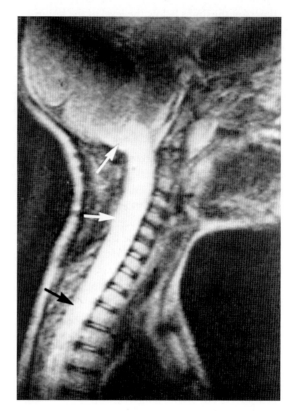

Fig. 12.5 Astrocytoma of the Cervical Cord. The tumor demonstrates an intense signal (*arrows*) on T_2-weighted images.

Ependymoma

Ependymomas are composed primarily of ependymal cells and arise from the lining of the ventricular system or central canal. They are more often intracranial than intraspinal in children. When intraspinal, they tend to be located in the lumbar region or in the cauda equina but may occur anywhere along the neuraxis.

Clinical features. Clinical features vary with the location of the tumor. Initial features may include scoliosis, pain in the legs or back, paresthesia, or weakness in one or both legs. Delay in diagnosis is frequent when scoliosis is the only sign. Eventually, the child develops difficulty walking, and this feature usually leads to appropriate diagnostic testing.

Stiff neck and cervical pain that is worse at night are the early features of cervical ependymomas. Tumors of the cauda equina may sometimes rupture and produce meningismus, fever, and pleocytosis mimicking bacterial meningitis. Spastic paraplegia is the usual finding on examination. Cervical tumors cause weakness of one arm as well. Tumors of the cauda equina produce flaccid weakness and atrophy of leg muscles associated with loss of tendon reflexes.

Diagnosis. MRI is the primary modality for imaging tumors of the spinal cord.

Management. Microsurgical techniques make possible the complete removal of intramedullary ependymomas, which are rarely infiltrative; however, recurrence is common in cases in which complete resection is not achieved. The role of postoperative local radiation therapy in treating benign tumors is uncertain. Malignant ependymomas of the spinal cord are unusual in children but require total neuraxis irradiation when present.

Neuroblastoma

Neuroblastoma is a neuroendocrine tumor derived from cells of the sympathetic chain and cranial ganglia and is the most common extracranial solid tumor of infancy and childhood. Neurological dysfunction results from direct invasion, metastasis, and distant "humoral" effects (see Chapter 10). Tumors in a paraspinal location may extend through a neural foramen and compress the spinal cord.

Clinical features. Paraplegia is the initial manifestation of neuroblastoma extending into the epidural space from a paravertebral origin. Because most affected children are infants or toddlers, the first symptom is usually refusal to stand or walk. Mild weakness may progress to complete paraplegia within hours or days. Examination generally reveals flaccid paraplegia, a distended bladder, and exaggerated tendon reflexes in the legs. Sensation may be difficult to test.

Diagnosis. Radiographs or CTs of the chest, abdomen, or pelvis usually show the extravertebral portion of the tumor, and MRI delineates the extent of spinal compression.

Management. In children with acute spinal cord compression high-dose corticosteroids, before surgical extirpation and radiation therapy, provide some symptomatic relief. Certain genetic markers are associated with a worse prognosis, but even high-risk disease now has a survival rate of 50% at 5 years.

Cerebral Paraplegia and Quadriplegia

Almost all progressive disorders of the brain that result in quadriplegia also have dementia as an initial or prominent feature (see Chapter 5). Pure paraplegia of cerebral origin is unusual. At the very least, the patient has impairment of fine finger movements and increased tendon reflex activity in the arms. Pure paraplegia should always direct attention to the spinal cord.

Cerebral Palsy

CP is a nonprogressive neurodevelopmental disorder resulting from lesions to the developing brain, typically during the fetal or perinatal period. The prevalence of moderately severe cases is approximately 2 per 1000 live births; the prevalence of CP has increased among very small premature infants, as more have survived. Reduced life expectancy is common in children with CP who are immobile, with profound cognitive impairment, or require special feeding.[17] Otherwise, children with CP may live well into adult life, and very mild CP may become virtually unnoticeable in older children and adults. Although the brain insult is static, symptoms continue to evolve throughout childhood which may falsely give the impression of a progressive disease. Conversely, several slowly progressive disorders may be misdiagnosed as CP (Table 12.1).

Risk factors include perinatal asphyxia, maternal infection, fetal stroke or disruption in fetal blood flow, prematurity, maternal hypercoagulable state, maternal substance abuse, preeclampsia, multiple gestation, or placental abnormalities. There is increasing evidence that genetic factors may play a role.

TABLE 12.1 **Slowly Progressive Disorders Sometimes Misdiagnosed as Cerebral Palsy**	
Condition	**Chapter**
Polyneuropathy	
GM$_1$ gangliosidosis type II	5
Hereditary motor and sensory neuropathies	7
Infantile neuroaxonal dystrophy	5
Metachromatic leukodystrophy	5
Ataxia	
Abetalipoproteinemia	10
Ataxia telangiectasia	10
Friedreich ataxia	10
Spasticity-Chorea	
Familial spastic paraplegia	12
Glutaric aciduria type I	14
Lesch-Nyhan syndrome	5
Niemann-Pick disease type C	5
Pelizaeus-Merzbacher disease	5
Rett syndrome	5

In general, a brain MRI is appropriate in every child with CP in order to identify the brain abnormality. Always consider a genetic or metabolic workup in children who appear to have CP but lack a consistent perinatal history or have significant clinical symptoms with normal head imaging.

Traditionally, the classification of CP is by the pattern of motor impairment. The spastic types are paraplegia or diplegia, quadriplegia, and hemiplegia (see Chapter 11). The hypotonic types are ataxic (see Chapter 10) and athetoid (see Chapter 14).

Spastic diplegia (Paraplegia). Diplegia means weakness of all four limbs, but the legs are weaker than the arms. The motor impairment in the arms may be limited to increased responses of tendon reflexes; the classification of such children is *paraplegia*. Periventricular leukomalacia is the usual cause of spastic diplegia in children born prematurely. In neonates and especially in premature infants the periventricular white matter represents a watershed area and is vulnerable to hypoxic insults. Cystic lesions in the white matter are often unilateral or at least asymmetric, causing hemiplegia superimposed on spastic diplegia.

Clinical features. Many children with spastic diplegia have normal tone, or even hypotonia, during the first 4 months. The onset of spasticity in the legs is insidious and slowly progressive during the first year. Four-point creeping is impossible because of leg extension. Either rolling or crawling on the floor with the belly on the ground achieves movement. The milestone of sitting up alone develops late or is never achieved. From the supine position, the infant pulls to a standing rather than a sitting position. Later, bending forward at the waist, to compensate for the lack of flexion at the hip and knee, and placing one hand on the floor for balance accomplishes sitting posture. Most children with spastic diplegia stand on their toes, with flexion at the knees and an increased lumbar lordosis. Leg spasticity makes walking difficult but is achievable by throwing the body forward or from side to side to transfer weight.

Examination shows spasticity in the legs and less spasticity in the arms. All limbs show exaggerated tendon reflexes. Reflex sensitivity and responsiveness are increased; percussion at the knee causes a crossed adductor response. Ankle clonus and an extensor plantar response are usually present. When vertically suspended, the legs cross at the thigh because of strong adductor muscle contractions (*scissoring*).

Subluxation or dislocation of the hips is relatively common in children with severe spasticity; the cause, in part, is from the constant adduction of the thighs and insufficient development of the hip joint resulting from delayed standing or inability to stand.

Diagnosis. Spastic diplegia is a clinical diagnosis. MRI easily identifies abnormalities in the deep white matter secondary to periventricular leukomalacia, but children with a known history of perinatal distress secondary to prematurity do not require follow-up imaging studies. It is important not to mistake CP for a progressive disease of the brain or cervical portion of the spine. Features that suggest a progressive disease are a family history of spasticity or weakness, cognitive regression, loss of motor skills previously obtained, atrophy of muscles, and sensory loss.

Management. Appropriate treatment of CP requires a multidisciplinary approach involving neurology; orthopedics; nutrition and gastroenterology; developmental and educational supports; vision and hearing evaluations; and some combination of physical, occupational, speech, and feeding therapies. Early introduction of therapies is standard of care and is believed to improve long-term outcomes, although controlled clinical trials are lacking. Certain specific interventions, such as constraint-induced movement therapy for unilateral CP, do have some objective evidence of efficacy.[18] It is possible that the main benefit of physical therapy is to maintain range of motion over the long term. Baclofen and tizanidine are often used to treat spasticity. Tizanidine causes more sedation than baclofen; both decrease tone throughout the entire body which can worsen baseline axial hypotonia. Gabapentin treats spasticity and may be helpful for neuro-irritability, insomnia, or autonomic dysreflexia.[19]

Injections of botulinum toxin and placement of a baclofen pump are useful procedures for the treatment of spasticity. Pump placement is just below the skin at the waistline. The pump connects to a small catheter through which the baclofen releases. Because baclofen naturally moves downward in the thecal space, pumps are most useful for patients with diplegia as opposed to quadriplegia. The pump releases medication at prescribed intervals, which adjusts through an external programmer. Refills, needed every 2–3 months, require a return visit to the doctor. The refill is injected by syringe through the skin and into the pump. After 5–7 years, the battery life ends and the pump is surgically removed to replace the battery. Children with baclofen pumps should always have a supply of enteral baclofen to give as needed in case of pump failure, as abrupt baclofen withdrawal may precipitate seizures, respiratory distress, blood pressure instability, and delirium.

Spastic quadriplegia. All limbs are affected, the legs often more severely than the arms. The term *double hemiplegia* may be applied if the arms are worse than the legs. Intrauterine disease, usually malformations, is the cause of most spastic quadriplegia. Hypoxic-ischemic encephalopathy of the term newborn accounts for a minority of cases.

Clinical features. Developmental delay is profound, and the infant quickly comes to medical attention. Failure to meet motor milestones, abnormal posturing of the head and limbs, and seizures are the common reasons for neurological evaluation. In severely affected children the characteristic supine posture is retraction of the head and neck, flexion of the arms at the elbows with the hands clenched, and extension of the legs. Infantile reflexes (Moro and tonic neck) are obligatory and stereotyped and persist after 6 months of age. Microcephaly is frequently an associated feature.

Because of damage to both hemispheres, supranuclear bulbar palsy (dysphagia and dysarthria) is common. Disturbances in vision and ocular motility are frequently associated features, and seizures occur in 50% of affected children.

Diagnosis. The clinical findings are the basis for diagnosis. Laboratory studies are useful when the underlying cause is not obvious or the possibility of a genetically transmitted defect exists. MRI of the brain is especially useful to show malformations.

Management. Treatment is the same as described in the "Spastic Diplegia (Paraplegia)" section.

REFERENCES

1. Werhahn KJ, Brown P, Thompson PD, et al. The clinical features and prognosis of chronic posthypoxic myoclonus. *Movement Disorders.* 1997;12(2):216-220.
2. Barrow DL, Colohan AR, Dawson R. Intradural perimedullary arteriovenous fistulas (type IV spinal cord arteriovenous malformations). *Journal of Neurosurgery.* 1994;81(2):221-229.
3. Crockard HA, Stevens JM. Craniovertebral junction anomalies in inherited disorders: part of the syndrome or caused by the disorder? *European Journal of Pediatrics.* 1995;154:504-512.
4. Lynch SA, Wang Y, Strachan T, et al. Autosomal dominant sacral agenesis: Currarino syndrome. *Journal of Medical Genetics.* 2000;37:561-566.
5. Sarnat HB. Regional ependymal upregulation of vimentin in Chiari II malformation, aqueductal stenosis, and hydromyelia. *Pediatric and Developmental Pathology.* 2004;7(1):48-60.
6. Greenlee JDW, Donovan KA, Hasan DM, et al. Chiari I malformation in the very young child: the spectrum of presentations and experience in 31 children under age 6 years. *Pediatrics.* 2002;110:1212-1219.
7. Sanz Cortes M, Chmait RH, Lapa DA, et al. Experience of 300 cases of prenatal fetoscopic open spina bifida repair: report of the International Fetoscopic Neural Tube Defect Repair Consortium. *American Journal of Obstetrics and Gynecology.* 2021;225(6):678.e1-678.e11. https://doi.org/10.1016/j.ajog.2021.05.044. Epub 2021 Jun 3. PMID: 34089698.
8. Cornette L, Verpoorten C, Lagae L, et al. Tethered cord syndrome in occult spinal dysraphism. Timing and outcome of surgical release. *Neurology.* 1998;50:1761-1765.
9. Hedera P. Hereditary spastic paraplegia overview. 2000 Aug 15 [Updated 2021 Feb 11]. In: Adam MP, Mirzaa GM, Pagon RA, et al., eds. *GeneReviews®.* University of Washington; 1993-2023. https://www.ncbi.nlm.nih.gov/books/NBK1509/.

10. Raymond GV, Moser AB, Fatemi A. X-linked adreno-leukodystrophy. In: Adam MP, Ardinger HH, Pagon RA, et al., eds. *GeneReviews*®. University of Washington; 1993-2019. https://www.ncbi.nlm.nih.gov/books/NBK1315.

11. van Geel BM, Assies J, Wanders RJA, et al. X linked adrenoleukodystrophy: clinical presentation, diagnosis, and therapy. *Journal of Neurology, Neurosurgery, and Psychiatry*. 1997;63:4-14.

12. Wong D, Cederbaum S, Crombez EA. Arginase deficiency. In: Adam MP, Ardinger HH, Pagon RA, et al., eds. *GeneReviews*®. University of Washington; 1993-2019. https://www.ncbi.nlm.nih.gov/books/NBK1159.

13. Orsini JJ, Escolar ML, Wasserstein MP, et al. Krabbe disease. In: Adam MP, Ardinger HH, Pagon RA, et al., eds. *GeneReviews*®. University of Washington; 1993-2019. https://www.ncbi.nlm.nih.gov/books/NBK1238.

14. Havla J, Pakeerathan T, Schwake C, et al. Age-dependent favorable visual recovery despite significant retinal atrophy in pediatric MOGAD: how much retina do you really need to see well? *Journal of Neuroinflammation*. 2021;18(1):121. https://doi.org/10.1186/s12974-021-02160-9. PMID: 34051804; PMCID: PMC8164737.

15. Benmelouka A, Shamseldin LS, Nourelden AZ, Negida A. A review on the etiology and management of pediatric traumatic spinal cord injuries. *Advanced Journal of Emergency Medicine*. 2019;4(2):e28. https://doi.org/10.22114/ajem.v0i0.256. PMID: 32322796; PMCID: PMC7163256.

16. Parent S, Mac-Thiong JM, Roy-Beaudry M, Sosa JF, Labelle H. Spinal cord injury in the pediatric population: a systematic review of the literature. *Journal of Neurotrauma*. 2011;28(8):1515-1524. https://doi.org/10.1089/neu.2009.1153. Epub 2011 Jun 9. PMID: 21501096; PMCID: PMC3143390.

17. Strauss DJ, Shavelle RM, Anderson TW. Life expectancy of children with cerebral palsy. *Pediatric Neurology*. 1998;18:143-149.

18. Hoare BJ, Wallen MA, Thorley MN, Jackman ML, Carey LM, Imms C. Constraint-induced movement therapy in children with unilateral cerebral palsy. *Cochrane Database of Systematic Reviews*. 2019;4(4):CD004149. https://doi.org/10.1002/14651858.CD004149.pub3. PMID: 30932166; PMCID: PMC6442500.

19. Rabchevsky AG, Patel SP, Duale H. Gabapentin for spasticity and autonomic dysreflexia after severe spinal cord injury. *Spinal Cord*. 2011;49:99-105.

13

Monoplegia

OUTLINE

Approach To Monoplegia, 317
Monomelic Amyotrophy (Hirayama Disease), 317
Plexopathies, 318
    Acute Idiopathic Plexitis, 318

Acute Symptomatic Plexitis, 319
Plexus Tumors, 322
Mononeuropathies, 322
References, 324

Weakness or paralysis of a limb is usually due to pathology of the spine and the proximal portion of nerves. Monoplegia may also be the initial presentation of hemiplegia, paraplegia, or quadriplegia. Therefore one must also consult the differential diagnosis of spinal paraplegia provided in Box 12.1 and the table and boxes in Chapter 11 referring to the differential diagnosis of cerebral hemiplegia.

APPROACH TO MONOPLEGIA

Either pain or weakness may cause refusal to use a limb. The cause of most painful limbs is orthopedic or rheumatological (arthritis, infection, and tumor). A trivial pull on an infant's arm may dislocate the radial head and causes an apparent monoplegia. Pain followed by weakness is a feature of plexitis.

Box 13.1 summarizes the differential diagnosis of acute monoplegia. Plexopathies and neuropathies are the leading causes of pure monoplegia. Stroke often affects one limb more than others, usually the arm more than the leg. The presentation may suggest monoplegia, but careful examination often reveals increased tendon reflexes and an extensor plantar response in the seemingly unaffected limb. Any suggestion of hemiplegia rather than monoplegia, or increased tendon reflexes in the paretic limb, should focus attention on the brain and cervical cord as the pathological site.

Chronic, progressive brachial monoplegia is uncommon. When it occurs, one should suspect syringomyelia and tumors of the cervical cord or brachial plexus. Chronic, progressive weakness of one leg suggests a tumor of the spinal cord or a neurofibroma of the lumbar plexus. A monomelic form of spinal muscular atrophy, affecting only one leg or one arm, should be considered when progressive weakness is unaccompanied by sensory loss.

MONOMELIC AMYOTROPHY (HIRAYAMA DISEASE)

Monomelic amyotrophy is a rare disorder that is more common in people of Asian descent. It is presumed to have a genetic cause, but a pathogenic genetic variant has not been identified. While trauma and immobilization of the limb may precede the onset of atrophy by several months, a cause-and-effect relationship is not established; it may be that this is a triggering factor in those with an underlying genetic predisposition.

Clinical features. The disorder occurs in males between the ages of 15 and 25. The initial features are weakness and atrophy in one limb, usually the arm. The tongue may be affected but other cranial nerves are spared. Tendon reflexes in the involved limb are hypoactive or absent. Sensation is normal. Tremor of one or both hands is often associated with wasting; the appearance of fasciculations heralds weakness and atrophy. Progression is slow, and spontaneous arrest within 5 years is the rule, but in rare cases the contralateral limb is affected after a gap of several years.

Diagnosis. Needle electromyography (EMG) studies of all limbs are essential to show the extent of involvement. The studies are often normal at onset and show a denervation pattern 3–4 weeks later. Motor conduction is normal. Magnetic resonance imaging (MRI) of the spine and plexus is required to exclude a tumor.

Management. Physical therapy, occupational therapy, splinting, and bracing are the main supportive treatment options.

PLEXOPATHIES

Acute Idiopathic Plexitis

Acute plexitis is a demyelinating disorder of the brachial or lumbar plexus thought to be immune mediated. Brachial plexitis is far more common than lumbar plexitis.

Brachial Plexitis (Parsonage-Turner syndrome)

Brachial plexitis (*brachial neuritis, neuralgic amyotrophy,* or *Parsonage-Turner syndrome*) occurs from infancy to adult life with a male predominance. Risk factors include underlying autoimmune disease, recent vaccination, connective tissue disorders, and recent surgery

or anesthesia. Cases may occur after seemingly mild upper respiratory infections, and symptoms may overlap with asthmatic amyotrophy (described later in this chapter). Coxsackie B virus, parvovirus B19, mumps, human immunodeficiency virus, cytomegalovirus, SARS-CoV2, and several others have been implicated.

Clinical features. The onset of symptoms is usually explosive. Pain is the initial feature in 95% of patients. Pain localization is to the shoulder but may be more diffuse or limited to the lower arm, and tends to be severe. It may awaken the patient, and the description is "sharp, stabbing, throbbing, or aching." The duration of pain, which is frequently constant, varies from several hours to 3 weeks. As the pain subsides, weakness appears. Weakness is in the distribution of the upper plexus alone in half of patients and the entire plexus in most of the rest. Lower plexitis alone is unusual. Although the initial pain abates, paresthesias may accompany the weakness. Two-thirds of people report improved strength during the month after onset. Upper plexus palsies improve faster than lower plexus palsies. Among all patients, one-third recovers within 1 year, three-quarters by 2 years, and 90% by 3 years. After 3 years, further improvement may occur, but permanent residua are expected. Recurrences are unusual and less severe than the initial episode. In rare instances both arms are affected.

Diagnosis. Pain and weakness in one arm are also symptoms of spinal cord compression, indicating the need for spinal cord imaging studies. MRI is often used to rule out other causes of shoulder pain and weakness such as rotator cuff tear or impingement syndrome; the earliest sign of denervation is diffusely increased T2 signal within the affected muscles.[1] Lumbar puncture is usually not indicated, but if done the cerebrospinal fluid is normal or shows a slight lymphocytosis and mild elevation in protein. EMG and nerve conduction studies are helpful in showing the extent of plexopathy. Electrical evidence of bilateral involvement may be present even in patients with unilateral symptoms.

Management. Treatment is mainly supportive and focused on pain management. Nonsteroidal antiinflammatory drugs may decrease inflammation; corticosteroids and intravenous immune globulin (IVIG) have little supporting evidence other than anecdotal reports of efficacy.[2] Gabapentin between 20 and 60 mg/kg/day divided into three or four doses and pregabalin, a more effective choice, at 3–10 mg/kg/day divided into two doses, are helpful in controlling neuropathic pain but not the paresthesias or weakness associated with the plexopathy. Carbamazepine and amitriptyline are other options for pain management. Keep the affected arm in a sling to avoid traction injuries and encourage physical and occupational therapies.

Lumbar Plexitis

Lumbar plexitis occurs at all ages and is similar to brachial plexitis, except that it affects the leg instead of the arm. The mechanism is probably the same as in brachial plexitis.

Clinical features. Fever is often the first symptom as well as pain in one or both legs. The pain has an abrupt onset and may occur in a femoral or sciatic distribution. Sciatica, when present, suggests disk disease. Young children refuse to stand or walk, and older children limp. Weakness may develop concurrently with pain or be delayed for as long as 3 weeks. The onset of weakness is insidious and often difficult to date, but usually, it begins 8 days after the onset of pain. Weakness progresses for a week and then stabilizes. Tendon reflexes are absent in the affected leg but are present in other limbs.

Recovery is characterized first by abatement of pain and then by increasing strength. The average time from onset of pain to maximal recovery is 18 weeks, with a range of 8 weeks to several years. Functional recovery is almost universal, but mild weakness may persist.

Diagnosis. The sudden onset of pain and weakness in one leg suggests spinal cord or disk disease. MRI of the spine is a means of excluding other disorders; the results are invariably normal in lumbar plexitis, but denervated muscles in the leg may show diffusely increased T2 signal. The cerebrospinal fluid is normal except for a mild elevation of the protein concentration. EMG performed 3 weeks after onset shows patchy denervation.

Management. Management is like that for brachial plexitis. Gabapentin, pregabalin, carbamazepine, and amitriptyline help control pain. Corticosteroids or IVIG may be used although evidence of their efficacy is weak. Recommend range of motion exercises until strength recovers and occupational therapy to deal with any possible deficit.

Acute Symptomatic Plexitis

Asthmatic Amyotrophy (Hopkins Syndrome)

Sudden flaccid paralysis of one or more limbs, resembling poliomyelitis, may occur during recovery from status asthmaticus requiring glucocorticoid treatment. The etiological mechanism for this syndrome is unknown but appears to result from localized damage to anterior horn cells.

Clinical features. Age at onset is from 1 to 11, and the male-to-female ratio is 7:4. The interval between the asthmatic attack and the paralysis is 1–11 days, with an average of 5 days. Monoplegia occurs in 90% of cases, with the arm involved twice as often as the leg. The other 10% have hemiplegia or diplegia. Meningeal irritation is not present. Sensation is intact, but the paralyzed limb is painful in half of cases. Recovery is incomplete, and most affected children have some degree of permanent paralysis.

Diagnosis. Asthmatic amyotrophy is primarily a clinical diagnosis based on the sequence of events. The diagnosis requires distinction from paralytic poliomyelitis and idiopathic brachial neuritis. The basis for excluding paralytic poliomyelitis is normal cerebrospinal fluid in asthmatic amyotrophy. A few white blood cells may be present in the cerebrospinal fluid but never to the extent encountered in poliomyelitis, and the protein concentration is normal. EMG during the acute phase shows active denervation of the paralyzed limb, but the pattern of denervation does not follow the radicular distribution expected in a brachial neuritis.

Management. Gabapentin and pregabalin may be helpful in controlling neuropathic pain. Other analgesia may be needed. As with plexitis, physical and occupational therapies are required.

Hereditary Brachial Plexopathy (Hereditary Neuralgic Amyotrophy)

The two major phenotypes of *focal familial recurrent neuropathy* are hereditary brachial plexopathy (also called *hereditary neuralgic amyotrophy*) and hereditary neuropathy with liability to pressure palsies (see the "Mononeuropathies" section). The phenotypes can be confused because isolated nerve palsies may occur in hereditary brachial plexopathy, and brachial plexopathy occurs in patients with hereditary neuropathy with a liability to pressure palsies. Transmission of both disorders is by autosomal dominant inheritance, but the underlying mutations are at different sites on chromosome 17. The mutation responsible for hereditary brachial plexopathy is *SEPT9* located in chromosome 17q25.[3,4]

Clinical features. Hereditary brachial plexopathy may be difficult to distinguish from idiopathic brachial plexitis in the absence of a family history or a patient's history of similar episodes. Events that may trigger an attack are similar to those seen in brachial plexitis and include infection, immunization, emotional stress, strenuous use of the affected limb, and childbirth. However, patients with hereditary brachial plexopathy often have minor dysmorphisms such as hypotelorism or cleft palate, as well as a positive family history.

Two different courses exist with only one type per family, suggesting the possibility of genetic heterogeneity.[5] Characteristics of the *classic course* are severe attacks with relatively symptom-free intervals. Patients with the *chronic course* experience interictal persistence of pain and weakness. The initial attack usually occurs during the second or third decade but may appear at birth. Attributing palsies at birth to trauma is common despite the positive family history. Weakness resolves completely, only to recur later.

Severe arm pain exacerbated by movement characterizes the attack. Weakness follows in days to weeks, which is usually maximal within a few days and always by 1 month. The entire plexus may be involved, but more often only the upper trunk is affected. Even with total plexus involvement, the upper plexus is weaker than other parts. Examination shows proximal arm weakness. Distal weakness may be present as well. Tendon reflexes are absent from affected muscles. Weakness persists for weeks to months and is associated with atrophy and fasciculations. Pain, which is frequently the only sensory finding, subsides after the first week.

Recovery begins weeks to months after attaining maximal weakness. Return of function is usually complete, although some residual weakness may persist after repeated attacks. The frequency of attacks is variable; several attacks may occur within a single year, but the usual pattern is two or three attacks per decade.

Occasionally children have an episode of lumbar plexopathy. Pain in the thigh and proximal weakness are characteristic. Brachial and lumbar plexopathies are almost never concurrent, although bilateral brachial plexopathy is a relatively common event. Isolated cranial nerve palsies may occur in families with hereditary brachial plexopathy. The vagus nerve is the one most often affected and causes hoarseness and dysphagia. Other cranial neuropathies result in transitory facial palsy and unilateral hearing loss.

Diagnosis. The family history, early age at onset, unique triggering events, recurrences, and involvement of other nerves differentiate hereditary brachial plexopathy from idiopathic brachial neuritis. EMG shows a diffuse axonopathy in the affected arm and some evidence of denervation in the asymptomatic arm. Asymptomatic legs are electrically normal.

Management. Treatment is the same as for idiopathic brachial and lumbar plexitis.

Neonatal Traumatic Brachial Neuropathy

The incidence of neonatal brachial plexus birth injuries is estimated at 1:1000 live births. The cause of obstetric brachial plexus palsies is excessive traction on the plexus. Upper plexus injuries occur when pulling the head and arm away from each other. This occurs in the vertex position when the head is pulled forcefully to deliver the aftercoming shoulder or when normal contractions force the head and neck downward with the shoulder trapped by the pelvis. Injuries in the breech position occur when pulling the arm downward to free the aftercoming head or when rotating the head to occipitoanterior when the shoulder is fixed. Complete (upper and lower) plexus injuries occur during vertex deliveries when traction is exerted on a prolapsed arm and in breech deliveries when the trunk is pulled downward but an aftercoming arm is fixed.

Clinical features. Most neonatal brachial plexus injuries occur in large, full-term newborns of primiparous mothers, especially when the fetus is malpositioned and the delivery is long and difficult. Shoulder dystocia is the strongest modifiable risk factor.[6] The traditional division of brachial plexus injuries is into those involving the upper roots (named for *Erb* and *Duchenne*) and those involving the lower roots (named for *Klumpke*). However, solitary lower root injuries are unusual. In 88% of cases the palsy affects only the C5 through C7 cervical roots and 12% have a complete plexus palsy. Bilateral, but not necessarily symmetrical, involvement occurs in 8% of cases.

Because the upper plexus (C5–C7) is always involved, the posture of the arm is typical and reflects weakness of the proximal muscles. The arm is adducted and internally rotated at the shoulder and is extended and pronated at the elbow, so that the partially flexed fingers face backward. Extension of the wrist is lost and the fingers fisted. The biceps and triceps reflexes are absent. Injuries that extend higher than the C4 segment result in ipsilateral diaphragmatic paralysis.

Newborns with complete brachial plexus palsies have flaccid, dry limbs with neither proximal nor distal movement. Horner syndrome (ptosis, miosis, and anhidrosis) is sometimes associated. Sensory loss to pinprick is present with partial or complete palsies but may not conform to the segmental pattern of weakness.

Diagnosis. Recognition of brachial plexus palsy is by the typical posture of the arm and by failure of movement when the Moro reflex is tested. Because the injury often takes place during a long and difficult delivery, asphyxia may be present as well. In such cases generalized hypotonia may mask the focal arm weakness. Approximately 10% of newborns with brachial plexus injuries have facial nerve palsy and fractures of the clavicle or humerus.

Management. The spontaneous recovery rate is approximately 70%. One goal of therapy is to prevent the development of contractures. Range of motion exercises prevent contractures, while splinting, or other forms of immobilization, causes them. Significant recovery occurs throughout the first year, but infants who show no improvement in strength at the end of 6 months are unlikely to show functional improvement later. Infants who have shown no improvement by 1 month of age should be referred to a multidisciplinary brachial plexus clinic. Surgical reconstruction of the plexus (nerve grafts, nerve reattachment, neuroma excision, etc.) is a consideration in infants with no evidence of some spontaneous recovery at 3–6 months. Although surgery can be quite effective for certain injuries, secondary surgeries are often required due to asymmetric growth around the area of nerve injury.

Osteomyelitis-Neuritis

Apparent limb weakness caused by pain is a well-recognized phenomenon. However, true brachial neuritis may occur in response to osteomyelitis of the shoulder. Ischemic nerve damage caused by vasculitis is the assumed mechanism.

Clinical features. Osteomyelitis-neuritis occurs predominantly during infancy. The initial feature is a flaccid arm without pain or tenderness. Body temperature may be normal at first but soon becomes elevated. Pain develops on movement of the shoulder, and tenderness to palpation follows. No swelling is present. The biceps and triceps reflexes may be depressed or absent.

Diagnosis. Suspect osteomyelitis of the proximal humerus when brachial plexitis develops during infancy. Radiographs of the humerus become abnormal at the end of the first week, when they show destruction of the lateral margin of the humerus, but

MRI or radioisotope bone scan shows a focal area of uptake in the proximal humerus, the scapula, or both shortly after onset. After 3 weeks, EMG shows patchy denervation in the muscles innervated by the upper plexus. These results support the idea that this is a true plexitis and not just a painful limb.

Aspirates from the shoulder joint or blood culture identify the organism. Group B *Streptococcus* is often isolated in specimens from young infants. Older children have other bacterial species.

Management. Three to four weeks of intravenous antibiotics is the recommended treatment. Recovery of arm strength may be incomplete.

Postnatal Injuries

Brachial plexus. Traction and pressure injuries of the brachial plexus are relatively common because of its superficial position. Motor vehicle and sports accidents account for the majority of severe injuries. However, mild injuries also occur in the following situations: (1) when an adult suddenly yanks a child's arm, either protectively or to force movement; (2) by a blow to the shoulder, such as in a football scrimmage or from the recoil of a rifle; (3) because of prolonged wearing of a heavy backpack; (4) when the arm is kept hyperextended during surgery; and (5) by pressure in the axilla from poorly positioned crutches.

Clinical features. Mild injuries do not affect all portions of the plexus equally. Diffuse weakness is uncommon. Pain may be an important initial feature, and sensory loss is uncommon. Recovery begins within days or weeks and is complete. Atrophy does not occur.

More severe injuries are usually associated with fractures of the clavicle and scapula, and dislocation of the humerus. The upper plexus is generally affected more severely than the lower plexus, but complete paralysis may be present at the onset. Sensory loss is less marked than weakness, and the two may not correspond in distribution. Pain is common not only from the plexopathy but also from the bone and soft tissue injuries. The most painful injuries are those associated with root avulsion.

Tendon reflexes are absent, and atrophy develops in denervated muscle. Recovery progresses from proximal to distal and Tinel sign plots the recovery: tingling in the distal part of a limb caused by tapping over the regenerating segment of a nerve. Complete reinnervation, when it occurs, may take several months or years. The completeness of recovery depends on the severity and nature of the injury. Pressure and traction injuries in which anatomical integrity is not disturbed recover best, whereas injuries that tear the nerve or avulse the root do not recover at all without surgical intervention.

Diagnosis. MRI demonstrates signal change within and surrounding the plexus. EMG is useful in identifying the pattern of nerve injury and in providing information on the prognosis. Even with mild traction injuries, the amplitude of motor and sensory action potentials attenuates, and motor and sensory conduction slows.

Management. Mild injuries do not require treatment other than range of motion exercises. For more severe traction injuries, resting the limb for the first month is usually necessary. During that time, provide analgesia as needed for pain and electrically stimulate muscles away from the site of injury to maintain tone. Initiate range of motion exercises once pain subsides.

Promptly correct fractures and dislocations that cause pressure on the brachial plexus. Lacerated nerves require surgical restoration of anatomical integrity.

Lumbar plexus. Injuries of the lumbar plexus are much less common than injuries of the brachial plexus. The pelvis and the heavy muscles of the hip provide considerable protection from direct trauma.

Clinical features. Lumbar plexus injuries are usually associated with fracture dislocation of the pelvis. Motor vehicle accidents or falls from a considerable height are required to produce sufficient force to fracture the pelvis. Therefore the patient usually has multiple injuries, and the lumbar plexus injury may be the last identified. Lumbar plexus injuries produce a patchy weakness that is difficult to differentiate from mononeuritis multiplex.

Diagnosis. MRI adequately identifies many plexus injuries, although milder or more subtle injuries may be missed. EMG helps distinguish plexus injuries and nerve injuries.

Management. Fracture-dislocations require treatment to relieve pressure on the plexus. As with brachial plexus injuries, the completeness of recovery depends on the anatomical integrity of the nerves.

Plexus Tumors

Plexus tumors in childhood are rare. The most common primary tumor is the plexiform neurofibroma (Fig. 13.1). These can affect either the brachial or the lumbar plexus. They grow very slowly and cause progressive but selected weakness over several years.

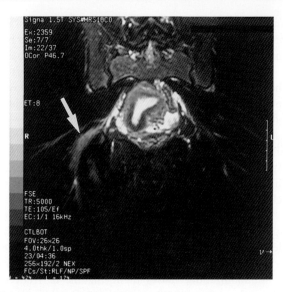

Fig. 13.1 Neurofibroma of the Lumbar Plexus. Magnetic resonance imaging of the plexus using a subtraction technique shows enlargement of the sciatic nerve (*arrow*).

Secondary tumors of the brachial plexus are the neuroblastoma and primitive neuroectodermal tumors arising in the chest.

MRI visualizes plexus tumors when fat subtraction techniques are used.

Mononeuropathies
Radial Neuropathy

Radial nerve injuries usually occur in the spinal groove of the humerus, just below the takeoff of the motor branch to the triceps muscle. Injury may occur with fractures of the humerus or by external pressure. Such pressure usually results when a sleeping or sedated patient is in a position that compresses the nerve between the humerus and a hard surface, such as an operating room table or chair.

Isolated radial nerve injuries may occur in newborns with a history of failure of progression of labor. These may result from prolonged radial nerve compression.[7]

Clinical features. Wrist and finger drop are characteristic of injuries to the radial nerve within the spiral groove. The brachioradialis muscle may be weak and its tendon reflex lost. Sensory disturbances are restricted to the back of the hand near the base of the thumb. With the wrist dropped, a fist is mechanically difficult to make but the finger flexors are not weak.

Diagnosis. Electrophysiological studies are useful for locating the site of injury and assessing the anatomical integrity of the nerve and the prognosis for recovery.

Management. Pressure injuries recover completely in 6–8 weeks. During that time, a splint is useful for placing the wrist in extension so that the patient can flex the fingers.

Ulnar Neuropathy

The most common site of ulnar injury is the elbow. This injury may result from external pressure, recurrent dislocation of the nerve from its groove, and fracture of the distal humerus. Mild ulnar neuropathies are frequently caused by the patient resting the elbow on the edge of a car window or sitting with their head in their hand and the elbow propped on a hard surface.

Clinical features. Paresthesias on the ulnar side of the hand, the little finger, and the ring finger are experienced. Tapping the ulnar groove increases discomfort. Hand strength is lost, and the intrinsic muscles become wasted. The little finger and the adjacent side of the ring finger have diminished or absent sensation.

Diagnosis. Electrophysiological techniques localize the injury along the course of the nerve.

Management. Minor pressure injuries do not require treatment, and recovery is complete within a few weeks. Advise the patient not to lean on the elbow (this is often a difficult habit to break). Injuries to the elbow that cause fracture or nerve dislocation require surgical repair.

Median Neuropathy

The cause of nontraumatic median neuropathies is compression of the nerve in the carpal tunnel and traumatic injuries at the elbow. In children a storage disease such as mucolipidosis may cause nerve compression in the carpal tunnel, but idiopathic cases occur as well. Fracture at the elbow is the usual cause of traumatic median neuropathy.

Clinical features. The most common features are numbness and pain in the hand. Nontraumatic median neuropathy is often bilateral. Weakness and atrophy are more likely to occur in traumatic injuries of the nerve than in carpal tunnel entrapment.

Diagnosis. EMG is useful to localize the lesion, especially when surgical decompression is an option.

Management. Surgical decompression may be beneficial for both nontraumatic and traumatic injuries. Immobilization is helpful in cases of repetitive injury.

Peroneal Neuropathy

The peroneal nerve lies in a superficial position adjacent to the fibula. External pressure readily compresses the nerve against the bone. This most often occurs in children who have undergone significant weight loss or trauma to the nerve. EMG documented a prenatal peroneal palsy, presumably caused by pressure, in one newborn.[8]

Clinical features. The prominent feature is an acute, painless foot drop, with weakness of both dorsiflexion and eversion of the foot. In young children parents may notice recurrent stumbling or "tripping over their toes" on the affected side. Sensation is usually intact, but sometimes there is numbness over the lower lateral leg and dorsum of the foot. When only the deep branch of the peroneal nerve is involved, sensory loss is restricted to a small triangle between the first two toes. Complete or significant spontaneous recovery is the rule except after considerable trauma.

Diagnosis. Electrodiagnosis is useful to discriminate peroneal nerve lesions from disturbances of the fifth lumbar root.

Management. A foot drop brace is a useful aid to walking until recovery is complete.

Hereditary Neuropathy With Liability to Pressure Palsy

The characteristic feature of hereditary neuropathy with liability to pressure palsy is the development of a mononeuropathy following trivial trauma. In some cases the brachial plexus is affected. Transmission is typically autosomal dominant but can be caused by novel mutations; molecular or sequence analysis demonstrates pathogenic variants in the *PMP22* gene.9

Clinical features. The first episode usually occurs during the second or third decade but may occur earlier. Typical precipitating factors include sleeping on a limb, body contact in sports, constrictive clothing, or positioning during surgery. Individuals quickly learn to avoid activities that provoke episodes. Superficial nerves (radial, ulnar, median, and peroneal) are the ones most commonly affected. The resulting mononeuropathy affects both motor and sensory fibers and may present with neuropathic pain. Tendon reflexes are lost. Recovery is complete within days to weeks; any residual deficits are mild.

Diagnosis. Except for the family history, the first episode might suggest ordinary pressure palsy, although the trivial nature of the trauma should alert the physician to the underlying neuropathy. Consider the diagnosis in children with repeated neuropathies or multifocal neuropathies even in the absence of a family history.

Molecular genetic testing or sequence analysis establishes the diagnosis. Electrophysiological studies show slow conduction time, not only in the affected limb but also in all limbs. Other family members may show generalized slowing of conduction between attacks.

Management. No treatment is available for the underlying neuropathy. Alterations in lifestyle may be needed to avoid pressure palsies. Rapid weight loss and the use of neurotoxic agents such as vincristine should be avoided if at all possible. A wrist splint is useful for carpal tunnel syndrome and an ankle-foot orthotic is for foot drop. Protective pads at elbows or knees may prevent pressure and trauma to local nerves. Advise patients against sitting with legs crossed, leaning on elbows, and activities requiring repetitive movements. Despite the best effort, some patients eventually develop a generalized motor and sensory neuropathy.

REFERENCES

1. Gaskin CM, Helms CA. Parsonage-Turner syndrome: MR imaging findings and clinical information of 27 patients. *Radiology*. 2006;240(2):501-507. https://doi.org/10.1148/radiol.2402050405. PMID: 16864674.
2. Jerath VP, Mahajan VK. Parsonage-Turner syndrome: a firsthand experience of an uncommon malady. *American Journal of Neurodegenerative Disease*. 2021;10(4):34-37. PMID: 34712516; PMCID: PMC8546633.
3. Hoque R, Schwendimann RN, Kelley RE, et al. Painful brachial plexopathies in SEPT9 mutations: adverse outcome related to comorbid states. *Journal of Clinical Neuromuscular Disease*. 2008;9:379-384.
4. Stögbauer F, Young P, Kuhlenbaumer G, et al. Hereditary recurrent focal neuropathies. Clinical and molecular features. *Neurology*. 2000;54:546-551.
5. van Alfen N, van Engelen BGM, Reinders JWC, et al. The natural history of hereditary neuralgic amyotrophy in the Dutch population. Two distinct types? *Brain*. 2000;123:718-723.
6. Shah V, Coroneos CJ, Ng E. The evaluation and management of neonatal brachial plexus palsy. *Paediatrics & Child Health*. 2021;26(8):493-497. https://doi.org/10.1093/pch/pxab083. PMID: 34992702; PMCID: PMC8711584.
7. Hayman M, Roland EH, Hill A. Newborn radial nerve palsy: report of four cases and review of published reports. *Pediatric Neurology*. 1999;21:648-651.
8. Jones Jr HR, Herbison GJ, Jacobs SR, et al. Intrauterine onset of a mononeuropathy: peroneal neuropathy in a newborn with electromyographic findings at age one day compatible with prenatal onset. *Muscle & Nerve*. 1996;19:88-91.
9. Chrestian N. Hereditary Neuropathy with Liability to Pressure Palsies (September 28, 1998). In: Adam MP, Mirzaa GM, Pagon RA, et al., eds. GeneReviews® University of Washington; 1993–2023. https://www.ncbi.nlm.nih.gov/books/NBK1392/. Updated August 27, 2020.

14

Movement Disorders

OUTLINE

Chorea, Tics, Tourette, Dystonia, Dyskinesia,
   Tremor, 325
Approach to the Patient, 325
Tics and Tourette Syndrome, 326
Stereotypies, 327
   Pediatric Autoimmune Neuropsychiatric
      Disorder Related to Streptococcal Infection, 328
Chorea and Athetosis, 328
   Choreoathetoid Cerebral Palsy, 329
   Cardiopulmonary Bypass Surgery, 330
   Drug-Induced Chorea, 330
   Genetic Disorders, 331
   Systemic Disorders, 333
Dystonia, 333
   Drug-Induced Dystonia, 333

Focal Dystonias, 334
Hemifacial Spasm, 335
Generalized Genetic (Hereditary)
   Dystonias, 336
Mirror Movements, 340
Myoclonus, 340
   Opsoclonus-Myoclonus-Ataxia Syndrome, 341
   Symptomatic Myoclonus, 342
Movement Disorders in Drowsiness and Sleep, 343
   Restless Legs Syndrome, 343
Tremor, 344
   Essential Tremor, 344
   Paroxysmal Dystonic Head Tremor, 345
References, 345

CHOREA, TICS, TOURETTE, DYSTONIA, DYSKINESIA, TREMOR

Involuntary movements are usually associated with abnormalities of the basal ganglia and their connections and occur in several different neurological disorders. Abnormal movements can be the main or initial features of disease, or they can occur as a late manifestation. Discussion of the former type is in this chapter, and the latter in other chapters.

APPROACH TO THE PATIENT

Movement disorders are difficult to describe; they require visualization. If abnormal movements are not present at the time of examination, instruct the parents to record the movements at home. Some relatively common movements are recognizable by description, but the rich variety of abnormal movements and postures that may occur defies classification. The most experienced observer will mistake, at times, one movement for another or will have difficulty conceptualizing the nature of an abnormal movement.

Many abnormal movements are paroxysmal or at least intermittent. Motion, excitement, startle, emotional upset, or sleep induces some movements. The physician should ask what makes the movement worse and if it is action induced. Ask children to perform the action during the examination. Paroxysmal movements raise the question of epilepsy. Indeed, the concurrent presence of seizures and involuntary movements characterize many neurological disorders of childhood. The following guidelines are useful to distinguish involuntary movements from seizures: (1) involuntary movements, with the exception of spinal myoclonus and movement disorders of drowsiness and sleep, abate or disappear during sleep while seizures persist or may worsen; (2) involuntary movements usually have a more stereotyped appearance and, with the exception of acute drug reactions, are more persistent than seizures; (3) loss of consciousness or awareness is characteristic of seizures but not involuntary movements; and (4) epileptiform activity on electroencephalography (EEG) accompanies seizures, but not involuntary movements.

There are various types of abnormal movements including myoclonus, tremor, tics, chorea, athetosis, ballismus, and dystonia. Any diffuse brain disorder can cause abnormal movements, often of multiple types. In general, consider movement disorders in the differential of any abnormal movement seen in the context of infectious, autoimmune, or metabolic CNS disease. Such disorders should be included in the differential of all the various types of movements discussed throughout this chapter.

TICS AND TOURETTE SYNDROME

Tics are stereotyped movements (motor tic) or utterances (verbal tic) that are sudden, brief, and purposeless. A tic can be accurately described and reproduced by an observer (e.g., "he blinks his eyes," "she clears her throat"). Tics are suppressible, but this requires significant effort and may result in an explosive outburst of movements once the child feels they can no longer "hold them in." Stress or excitement exacerbates tics, relaxation reduces tics, and sleep makes them stop.

Tourette syndrome is any combination of verbal and motor tics persisting for at least 1 year. It is not a separate disease, but rather part of a phenotypic spectrum that includes simple motor tics, attention-deficit disorder, and obsessive-compulsive behavior.[1] It is common for multiple family members to be affected to varying degrees, but the nature of genetic transmission remains unclear. Inheritance is likely complex, involving multiple genes in conjunction with environmental triggers.[2] Multiple environmental factors play a role in the development of tic disorders. Stimulants may provoke tics in predisposed children, and streptococcal infection may cause the sudden onset of severe tics or obsessive-compulsive disorder (OCD). The term PANDAS (*pediatric autoimmune neuropsychiatric disorders associated with streptococcal infection*) acknowledges the association between streptococcal infection and acute-onset chorea or tics (discussed later in this chapter).

Clinical features. Onset is between 2 and 15 years of age but most commonly around the age of 6–7. It is

unusual but not impossible to develop tics in adolescence or adulthood. Many such patients actually have psychogenic tics or had unrecognized tics as younger children.

The majority of tics involve simple movements of the neck, eyes, head or face; common motor tics include blinking, grimacing, lip smacking, and shrugging of one or both shoulders.

The initial vocal tics are usually clearing of the throat, a snorting or sniffing noise, and coughing. Many children who make sniffing or coughing noises will undergo an extensive evaluation for allergies and receive treatment that does not result in improvement. Grunting and hissing are other verbal tics. Uttering profanities (coprolalia) is rare in children but may occur.

Symptoms wax and wane spontaneously and in response to certain stimuli. A child may develop one tic which gradually worsens before plateauing and remitting; they may then develop a completely different tic or have recurrence of previous movements. Some children have multiple distinct tics at once. Common triggers include school, competitive sports, fatigue, and excitement. Tics often become markedly worse when attention is drawn to them, or the child feels self-conscious or embarrassed. Parents or teachers may unintentionally worsen tics by repeatedly telling the child to stop performing the movement. Most children with tics report a "premonitory urge," or an uncomfortable feeling of tension preceding the tic followed by a brief sensation of relief once the movement is performed. Therefore, while it is possible for the child to temporarily suppress the tics, this is uncomfortable and unsustainable for long periods of time.

A large percentage of children with tics have comorbid impulse control disorders, including attention-deficit hyperactivity disorder (ADHD), OCD, oppositional defiant disorder, or rage attacks. Anxiety and depression are common and often are related to impaired social relationships or bullying. Although most children with tics have normal intelligence, many experience educational challenges, including specific learning disabilities, poor handwriting, and ADHD. Such comorbidities are often more distressing and disabling than the tics themselves.

Diagnosis. The clinical features establish the diagnosis. Laboratory tests, EEGs, and imaging studies are not helpful and are unnecessary in obvious cases. Neuropsychological testing usually shows normal intelligence but may suggest inattentiveness or anxiety.

Management. Most children with tics and Tourette syndrome do not require drug treatment. The decision to prescribe medication depends on whether the tics bother the *child*; drug therapy is not required if the tics bother the parents but do not disturb the child's life. Tell the parents that the tics are not a sign of progressive neurological or mental illness, that they may worsen with stress, and will often diminish in frequency if ignored. Teachers must be advised that the child's abnormal movements are tics and are not intentionally disruptive; classmates and friends often benefit from a brief explanation of the disorder if the movements are prompting teasing or questioning.

Drug treatment is difficult to evaluate because the disorder's natural history is one of exacerbation and remission. Historically, the drugs most often used to control tics were pimozide, fluphenazine, ziprasidone, and haloperidol. These can be quite effective but can have unwanted side effects including sedation, irritability, and decreased appetite. Dystonia and akathisia are idiosyncratic reactions. Due to the unfavorable side effect profile of neuroleptics, we use clonidine or guanfacine as first-line treatment. They may not be as effective but are safer with more favorable side effect profiles. In addition they often help with ADHD symptoms. Dosing starts with clonidine 0.05 mg daily and may be increased up to 0.2 mg bid if tolerated, with sedation being the main side effect. Guanfacine is less sedating and just as effective. Begin with 0.5 mg daily and increase up to 2 mg bid as needed. Extended release guanfacine is also available with doses ranging from 1 to 4 mg daily. If tics cause physical pain or exhaustion, neuroleptics may be required. Deep brain stimulation (DBS) or targeted botulinum toxin injections have been used in rare, severe cases.[3]

Comprehensive behavioral intervention for tics (CBIT) is a safe and probably effective treatment[4] that allows patients to avoid pharmacologic treatments with their associated potential side effects. There are three types of CBIT: habit reversal training, relaxation therapy, and awareness training. Although large trials for CBIT are lacking, it is an attractive option for patients wishing to avoid medication. One drawback is the paucity of occupational therapists trained in the technique, which results in patients having to travel to large cities or major medical centers for weekly therapy sessions.

Many children with tics suffer from anxiety and OCD, which interferes with social skills and learning. Treating this component results in a more relaxed child, with secondary reduction in the frequency of tics. Fluoxetine, citalopram, or escitalopram is often our first choice in treating children with Tourette syndrome and comorbid anxiety or OCD. Start titration from 5 to 20 mg in the case of citalopram and fluoxetine, or from 2.5 to 10 mg in the case of escitalopram over 4 weeks. Some children may need higher doses. A few children develop anhedonia as a side effect of selective serotonin reuptake inhibitors (SSRIs). In those cases sertraline 25–100 mg/day may be a better choice. Fluvoxamine is helpful in children with prominent obsessive-compulsive tendencies. Pharmacogenomic testing is available and helps inform the choice of appropriate psychotropic drugs.

Caffeine ingestion may exacerbate tics and should be reduced or removed from the diet. Stimulants are often used to treat ADHD but may worsen tics; consider using nonstimulant treatment options for ADHD such as atomoxetine (Strattera) or viloxazine (Qelbree). Educational accommodations are vital for children with significant tics, especially since school is typically the largest stressor in a child's life. The Tourette Association of America provides helpful literature for educators and guidelines for creating educational plans.

The long-term outcome for children with tics is difficult to ascertain. Many reports indicate that tics improve and even stop during adult life, but a recent report indicates that tics were still present in 90% of adults with childhood-onset tics.[5]

STEREOTYPIES

Stereotypies in children are commonly not associated with underlying pathology. In these cases they tend to be transient and are often outgrown by adolescence, although may persist into adulthood. Stereotypies are repeated, purposeless movements that may be simple or complex. Simple stereotypies are foot or finger tapping and hair curling. Complex stereotypies range from shuddering attacks to sequential movements of the head, arms, and body. They appear intentional. Occasionally, a history of similar movements is present in other family members.

The main differential diagnosis is with seizures and complex tics. Seizures are not suppressible and are often associated with changes in awareness, postictal lethargy, or confusion. Complex tics are more difficult to differentiate. Stereotypies differ from tics in that suppression of the movement does not cause tension, and other features of Tourette syndrome are not present. Stereotypies tend to disappear as the child ages. Treatment is neither needed nor effective. The best management is to ignore the movements.

Pediatric Autoimmune Neuropsychiatric Disorder Related to Streptococcal Infection

Multiple variations of infection or autoimmune acute-onset neuropsychiatric disorders have been described in children. Pediatric autoimmune neuropsychiatric disorder related to streptococcal infection (PANDAS) is the most well-known entity, although the literature may also refer to pediatric acute-onset neuropsychiatric syndrome (PANS), childhood acute neuropsychiatric symptoms (CANS), and pediatric infection triggered autoimmune neuropsychiatric disorders (PITANDS). PANDAS and related disorders were described relatively recently, and the diagnosis remains controversial. There is no doubt that PANDAS as a diagnosis has been heavily publicized and marketed to concerned parents in the lay literature, resulting in large numbers of inappropriate diagnoses in children who are more likely suffering from tics with comorbid anxiety or OCD. Such misdiagnoses are concerning because they result in ineffective, invasive, or risky treatments while delaying appropriate care. However, it also appears clear that rare cases of PANDAS do occur and require prompt recognition and treatment in order to prevent long-term sequelae.

Clinical features. The most convincing cases consist of a previously healthy, typically developing child who presents with the acute onset of tics and psychiatric disturbances in the setting of acute streptococcal infection (usually strep throat). Tics are usually severe and multifocal, and psychiatric symptoms are profound; parents describe the onset as if the child "fell off a cliff" seemingly overnight. Obsessive-compulsive behaviors, anxiety, aggression, and emotional lability are the most common psychiatric manifestations, and frank psychosis may occur.

Diagnosis. The proposed criteria[6] for diagnosis of PANDAS are as follows:

1. Presence of diagnostic criteria for OCD and/or tic disorder;
2. Pediatric onset, between 3 years and the beginning of puberty;
3. Episodic course of symptom severity, characterized by acute, severe onset and dramatic symptom exacerbations;

4. Temporal relationship between symptom onset and/or exacerbation and group A b-hemolytic streptococcal infections (GABHS); and
5. Association with neurologic abnormalities, such as motor hyperactivity, tics, or choreiform movements.

PANS is similar but has distinct diagnostic criteria including severely restricted food intake; streptococcal infection is not required for diagnosis. CANS is a universal term meant to encompass PANDAS and PANS but without specific autoimmune or infectious criteria.

Preexisting tics, Tourette syndrome, OCD, or anxiety should prompt careful evaluation to ensure that the child is not simply experiencing an exacerbation of their baseline disorder. Streptococcal infections and carrier states are common in children, and the presence of positive antistreptolysin or anti-DNase B antibodies is not sufficient for diagnosis unless a convincing clinical picture also exists. It is important to note that currently, *there is no accepted biomarker* for PANDAS or PANS.

Most children with PANDAS will undergo a larger workup for suspected autoimmune encephalitis. Complete blood count, inflammatory markers such as ESR or CRP, assessment of hepatic and renal function, and autoimmune markers are all reasonable laboratory tests. Perform a lumbar puncture if there is concern for autoimmune encephalitis or acute CNS infection. *Mycoplasma pneumoniae*, influenza, Epstein-Barr virus, and *Borrelia burgdorferi* are potential infectious triggers for PANS. MRI and EEG are often obtained but offer no specific diagnostic clues.

Management. Virtually no rigorous evidence exists regarding the treatment of PANDAS. Small studies suggest benefits with the use of steroids, intravenous immunoglobulin (IVIG), and plasma exchange; symptomatic management with behavioral therapy and treatment of psychiatric symptoms is also recommended.[7] Tonsillectomy is performed in some cases, but we advise caution regarding any invasive surgical procedure, particularly in a disorder in which diagnostic and treatment guidelines are not well established.

CHOREA AND ATHETOSIS

Chorea is a random, rapid movement affecting any part of the body that is neither rhythmic nor stereotyped, and may migrate from side-to-side and limb-to-limb. Because patients may attempt to mask the involuntary movement with a voluntary movement, it gives the appearance of restlessness. *Akathisia*, an inward compulsion to move (discussed later), also causes the appearance of restlessness. Depending on the condition, chorea may be unilateral or bilateral and may affect the face and trunk as well as the limbs. An observer cannot precisely describe chorea because it has no fixed form.

Chorea is more readily observed when separated from any superimposed voluntary movement that may follow it. When the child lightly grips the examiner's fingers, the grip alternately tightens and loosens, as if the patient is "milking" the examiner's hands. Hypotonia is common in many conditions causing chorea. Children move their tongue constantly, in and out, when asked to maintain it protruded (motor impersistence).

Athetosis consists of low-amplitude, writhing movements of the limbs that may occur alone but are often associated with chorea (choreoathetosis). The usual cause of athetosis without chorea is perinatal brain injury. Kernicterus was once a major cause of choreoathetosis but is now a rare event. Perinatal asphyxia is now the predominant etiology. Many children with athetosis have atonic cerebral palsy, and others have spastic diplegia.

Ballismus is characterized by high-amplitude movements of the proximal musculature, causing flinging movements of the limbs or pelvis. In adults it may occur in limbs contralateral to a vascular lesion in the subthalamic nucleus; in children, it is usually associated with chorea and seen in cerebral palsy, kernicterus, Sydenham chorea, and lupus erythematosus.

Choreoathetoid Cerebral Palsy

By far the most common cause of congenital chorea is choreoathetoid cerebral palsy, also called dyskinetic cerebral palsy. Choreoathetoid CP comprises 10%–20% of total cerebral palsy cases.

Clinical features. Children with dyskinetic or choreoathetoid CP are more likely to have been full-term as opposed to premature infants, and usually suffered a brief but severe hypoxic event disproportionately affecting the basal ganglia and thalamus. As with other forms of CP, the features depend on the extent of the initial brain insult. Children who are severely affected often have spastic quadriparesis and intellectual disability in addition to near-continuous choreoathetoid movements. Such children have elevated caloric requirements and can present with malnutrition if their movement disorder is not considered when formulating a nutrition

plan. Ballismus is possible and may be confused with epileptic spasms or myoclonic seizures. In milder cases infants and toddlers present with abnormal tone and gross motor delays caused by uncontrollable movements and abnormal posturing interfering with the acquisition of normal motor skills.

Diagnosis. Diagnosis is based on clinical criteria, and specific assessment tools exist for the evaluation of children with dyskinetic CP. MRI of the brain shows evidence of prior injury to the deep gray matter including the basal ganglia and thalamus.

Management. Standard management of any child with cerebral palsy includes early assessment and prompt initiation of physical, occupational, and speech therapies as indicated. Monitor nutrition carefully, especially in those children with very active movement disorders. Supplemental tube feeding may be needed even in children who are able to eat by mouth. Levodopa may reduce abnormal movements and improves gait. Assistive devices and equipment can improve mobility and independence and reduce the risk of falls. Encourage the development of an educational plan with appropriate accommodations.

Sydenham (Rheumatic) Chorea

Sydenham chorea is an antineuronal antibody-mediated neuropsychiatric disease and is the most common cause of acquired chorea in children. It is a cardinal feature of rheumatic fever and is sufficient alone to make the diagnosis. Rheumatic chorea occurs primarily in populations with untreated group A, beta-hemolytic streptococcal infections; it represents an autoimmune disorder that occurs in genetically predisposed children. There is likely some overlap with PANDAS, described earlier.

Clinical features. The onset is less explosive than PANDAS. Chorea, hypotonia, dysarthria, and emotional lability are cardinal features. Difficulty in school may bring the child to medical attention. Chorea causes the child to be restless, and discipline by the teacher results in emotional stress. Obsessive-compulsive behavior may be present.

Examination reveals a fidgeting child with migratory chorea of limbs and face. Initially, the chorea may be unilateral, but eventually becomes generalized in most patients. Efforts to conceal chorea with voluntary movement only add to the appearance of restlessness. Gradual improvement occurs over several months. Most recover completely. Rheumatic valvular heart disease develops in one-third of untreated patients.

Diagnosis. The diagnosis is mainly clinical but is confirmed by the presence of anti-DNase B antibodies with an elevated ASO titer. Antineuronal antibodies are present. The differential diagnosis includes other pediatric autoimmune neuropsychiatric diseases such as PANDAS and PANS, lupus-associated chorea, and drug-induced chorea (Box 14.1). It may be necessary to examine the blood for lupus antinuclear antibodies and thyroid function. The onset of Sydenham chorea may be weeks after the provocative streptococcal infection, and the antistreptolysin O titer may be then back to normal or only slightly increased. During the time of illness, T_2-weighted MRI images may show increased signal intensity in the putamen and globus pallidus that resolves when the child has recovered.

> ## BOX 14.1 Differential Diagnosis of Chorea as an Initial or Prominent Symptom
>
> - Cardiopulmonary bypass surgery
> - Genetic disorders
>   - Abetalipoproteinemia (see Chapter 10)
>   - Ataxia-telangiectasia (see Chapter 10)
>   - Benign familial chorea
>   - Fahr disease
>   - Familial paroxysmal choreoathetosis (see Chapter 1)
>   - Glutaric aciduria
>   - Hepatolenticular degeneration (Wilson disease)
>   - Huntington disease (see Chapter 5)
>   - Lesch-Nyhan syndrome (see Chapter 5)
>   - Machado-Joseph disease (see Chapter 5)
>   - Neuroacanthocytosis
> - Drug-induced movement disorders
>   - Anticonvulsants
>   - Antiemetics[a]
>   - Oral contraceptives
>   - Psychotropic agents[a]
>   - Stimulants[a]
>   - Theophylline
> - Systemic conditions
>   - Hyperthyroidism[a]
>   - Lupus erythematosus[a]
>   - Pregnancy[a] (chorea gravidarum)
>   - Sydenham[a] (rheumatic) chorea
> - Tumors of cerebral hemisphere (see Chapter 4)

[a]The most common conditions and the ones with disease modifying treatments.

Management. Most importantly, evaluate the heart by echocardiogram as subclinical valvular involvement is common and requires treatment by a cardiologist. Severe chorea can be treated with benzodiazepines or risperidone. Steroids and IVIG have been used in some patients with severe cases.[8] The fundamental treatment of all children with Sydenham chorea is the same as for acute rheumatic fever: penicillin in high doses for 10 days to eradicate active streptococcal infection and prophylactic penicillin therapy until age 21.

Cardiopulmonary Bypass Surgery

Also referred to as "post-pump chorea," severe choreoathetosis previously was a complication of up to 10% of children with congenital heart disease following cardiopulmonary bypass surgery, although the number of affected children seems to be decreasing.[9] Circulatory arrest and prolonged, deep hypothermia are risk factors; the mechanism is not exactly known but may be due to reversible metabolic injury to the basal ganglia.

Clinical features. Most affected children are more than 1 year of age and have cyanotic heart disease with systemic to pulmonary collaterals. Choreoathetosis begins within 2 weeks postoperatively and may be associated with oral-facial dyskinesias, hypotonia, affective changes, and pseudobulbar signs. Some children have only mild chorea that resolves spontaneously within 2 months. Others may have severe exhausting chorea, unresponsive to treatment, which results in either death or severe neurological morbidity. Many survivors develop intellectual disabilities.[10]

Diagnosis. The clinical features are the primary basis for diagnosis. Magnetic resonance imaging (MRI) results are often normal or nonspecific.

Management. Sedation prevents exhaustion in severely affected children. Choreoathetosis is often resistant to drug therapy. Clonazepam, gabapentin, and pregabalin may prove useful to reduce movement. Tetrabenazine and trihexyphenidyl should be considered for refractory cases.

Drug-Induced Chorea

Choreiform movements and akathisia or dystonic posturing may occur as effects of drugs, especially dopamine antagonists. Chorea is more often a consequence of the abrupt discontinuation of a dopamine antagonist. Akathisia is more likely to be a dose-related effect, whereas dystonia is usually an idiosyncratic reaction (see the "Dystonia" section). Phenytoin and ethosuximide may induce chorea as a toxic or idiosyncratic manifestation. Oral contraceptives may induce chorea. The mechanism is unknown. Neuroleptics are associated with idiosyncratic dystonic reactions and tardive dyskinesia, and stimulant drugs (dextroamphetamine and methylphenidate) are associated with chorea, akathisia, and tics (see the "Tics and Tourette Syndrome" section).

Tardive Dyskinesia

The term *tardive dyskinesia* denotes drug-induced choreiform movements that occur late in the course of drug therapy. These movements are often limited to the lingual, facial, and buccal muscles. Drug-induced buccolingual dyskinesia is unusual in children.

Tardive dyskinesias are most often associated with drugs used to modify behavior (neuroleptics), such as phenothiazines, haloperidol, risperidone, quetiapine, or olanzapine, and antiemetics such as metoclopramide and prochlorperazine; they also occur rarely in children with status asthmaticus treated with theophylline. The estimated annual incidence of tardive dyskinesia in children taking neuroleptic drugs is less than 1%. The incidence after long-term exposure in children is reported to be as high as 9.8%, which is still less than the 23.4% reported in adults.[11] However, the overall risk to children may be greater due to longer drug exposures with higher cumulative doses.[12]

Clinical features. Tardive dyskinesia is a complex of stereotyped movements. It usually affects the mouth and face, resembles chewing, and includes tongue protrusion and lip smacking; the trunk may be involved in rocking movements and the fingers in alternating flexion and extension resembling piano playing. Limb chorea, dystonia, myoclonus, tics, and facial grimacing may be associated features. Stress exacerbates the movements and sleep relieves them.

Symptoms appear months to years after the start of therapy and are not related to changes in dosage. In children discontinuing the drug usually stops the movement, but persistent movements are possible.

Diagnosis. Drug-induced dyskinesia is suspected in any child who shows abnormal movements of the face or limbs while taking neuroleptic drugs. The distinction of tardive dyskinesia from facial tics is important in children with Tourette syndrome and the distinction of facial mannerisms from tics in adolescents with schizophrenia.

Management. Discontinue all neuroleptic drugs as quickly as possible when symptoms of dyskinesia develop. This may not be practical when psychosis or severe behavioral dysregulation requires drug therapy. In such circumstances the first step is to make sure the child is on a newer antipsychotic medicine with lower D2 affinity. If dyskinesia does not resolve once the offending agent has been stopped, consider treatment with tetrabenazine. New vesicular monoamine transporter 2 (VMAT) inhibitors such as deutetrabenazine and valbenzine are currently used to treat TD in adults and may be approved for use in children in the future.[13] DBS can be considered for severe, refractory cases.

Emergent Withdrawal Syndrome

Chorea and myoclonus may appear for the first time after abruptly discontinuing or reducing the dosage of neuroleptic drugs. Lingual-facial-buccal dyskinesia may be present as well. The symptoms are self-limited and cease in weeks to months. Slow tapering of neuroleptics reduces the possibility of this syndrome. Reintroduction of the medication with slower withdrawal may be helpful in cases triggered by abrupt removal of a dopamine-blocking agent.

Genetic Disorders

Cerebellar ataxia is often the initial feature of abetalipoproteinemia and ataxia-telangiectasia. Chorea may occur in both conditions, but only in ataxia-telangiectasia does chorea occur without ataxia. Huntington disease is an important cause of chorea and dystonia, but in children the initial feature is declining school performance. The discussion of Huntington disease in children is in Chapter 5.

NKX2.1-Related Choreiform Disorders

Pathogenic variants in the *NKX2.1* gene cause a range of phenotypes from benign hereditary chorea to full brain-lung-thyroid syndrome. Inheritance is autosomal dominant. Chorea is the most common symptom, but typically occurs with pulmonary and thyroid involvement (50%) or thyroid involvement without pulmonary manifestations (30%); only 13% experience chorea alone.[14]

Clinical features. Affected newborns with the brain-lung-thyroid phenotype come to medical attention due to neonatal respiratory distress and congenital hypothyroidism. Chorea presents during infancy (most common) or childhood and is nonprogressive and continuous. Other associated features include hypotonia and ataxia which usually resolve during childhood. Intelligence is typically normal, but some patients have developmental delays or cognitive impairments. Drop attacks are common, but EEG monitoring demonstrates that these are secondary to chorea and not seizures.

Diagnosis. Most patients have a positive family history although specific clinical manifestations may vary even within the same family. Imaging and EEG studies are normal. Sequence analysis or deletion/duplication analysis identifies the pathogenic variant.

Management. Patients have an increased risk of pulmonary and thyroid cancers and require annual screening for malignancies. Levodopa at doses of 7–9 mg/kg/day is often helpful, as is tetrabenazine. Trihexyphenidyl and clonazepam have been used in some cases. Physical therapy is recommended for all affected children. Avoid neuroleptics, which may worsen chorea.

Primary Familial Brain Calcification (Idiopathic Basal Ganglia Calcification or Fahr Disease)

Primary familial brain calcification syndrome (previously called idiopathic basal ganglia calcification or Fahr disease) is an autosomal dominant neurodegenerative disorder characterized by the combination of encephalopathy and progressive calcification of the basal ganglia. Psychiatric symptoms are common and often the first manifestation of disease. The patient goes on to develop clumsiness, dysarthria, dysphagia, movement disorders, and muscle cramping. Headaches, vertigo, and seizures are frequently associated.[15] Significant clinical heterogeneity exists.

Clinical features. Onset may be in childhood, but the usual age of onset is in the third to fifth decades. The core clinical features are neuropsychiatric and movement disorders. The expression frequently varies within a family.

Diagnosis. A family history of disease is often present. Diagnosis requires bilateral calcification of the basal ganglia associated with neurological deterioration and the absence of an underlying metabolic disorder. The most common area of calcification is the globus pallidus. However, additional areas of involvement include the putamen, caudate, dentate, thalamus, and cerebral white matter. Every child with basal ganglia calcification requires an assessment of parathyroid function to exclude the possibility of either hyperparathyroidism or

pseudohypoparathyroidism. Several causative genetic mutations have been identified, including in *PDGFB*, *PDGFRB*, *SLC20A2*, and *XPR1*. These mutations account for approximately 50% of cases.

Management. Specific treatment is not available. Symptoms may respond to drug therapy. Use neuroleptics cautiously, as these may worsen any underlying movement disorder.

VPS13A Disease (Choreoacanthocytosis)

The nonspecific term *neuroacanthocytosis* encompasses several disorders, including autosomal recessive choreoacanthocytosis (*VPS13A* disease) and X-linked McLeod syndrome.[16] The acanthocyte is an abnormal erythrocyte that has thorny projections from the cell surface. Acanthocytosis occurs in at least three neurological syndromes: McLeod syndrome (see Chapter 8), *VPS13A* disease, and abetalipoproteinemia (see Chapter 10). The clinical features in severe cases of McLeod syndrome may be similar to those of *VPS13A* disease.

Clinical features. Onset is usually in adult life but may occur as early as the first decade. The most consistent neurological findings are impairment of frontal lobe function and psychiatric symptoms. Tics, oromandibular dyskinesia and dystonia, and self-mutilation of the lips may be associated features. Phenotypic variability is considerable and may include axonal neuropathy, loss of tendon reflexes, dementia, seizures, and psychosis; "huntingtonism" refers to the triad of movement disorder, psychiatric symptoms, and decreased cognition. In fact the symptoms of *VPS13A* disease and Huntington's disease are nearly identical, apart from seizures which are much more common in *VPS13A* disease. Orofacial dystonia triggered by eating ("feeding dystonia") may cause weight loss and malnutrition.

Diagnosis. The association of acanthocytes or echinocytes (cells with rounded projections) and neurological disease in the absence of lipoprotein abnormality suggests the diagnosis. MRI demonstrates caudate atrophy. Serum concentrations of creatine kinase may be elevated. Molecular genetic testing shows biallelic pathogenic variants in *VPS13A*.[17]

Management. Only symptomatic treatment is available. Mouth guards may help protect the tongue and lips. DBS has been helpful in some patients. Death occurs 10–20 years after onset.

Systemic Disorders
Hyperthyroidism

Chapter 15 discusses the ocular manifestations of thyrotoxicosis. Tremor is the most common associated movement disorder. Chorea is unusual, but, when present, may affect the face, limbs, and trunk. The movements cease when the child becomes euthyroid.

Lupus Erythematosus

Clinical features. Lupus-associated chorea is uncommon but may be the initial feature of the disease. Onset of symptoms is 7 years before to 3 years after the appearance of systemic features. It is indistinguishable from Sydenham chorea in appearance. The average duration is 12 weeks, but one-quarter of patients have recurrences. Additional neurological features of lupus (ataxia, psychosis, and seizures) are common in children who have chorea but occur only after the appearance of systemic symptoms. Therefore chorea may be a solitary manifestation of disease.

Diagnosis. The diagnosis is clear in children with known lupus erythematosus. When chorea is the initial feature of lupus, the diagnosis is more problematic. The erythrocyte sedimentation rate may be elevated in both lupus and Sydenham chorea and is not a distinguishing feature. The presence of elevated concentrations of antinuclear antibodies and anti-DNA lupus antibodies is critical to diagnosis.

Management. The treatment of children with neurological manifestations of lupus erythematosus requires high-dose corticosteroids and cyclophosphamide. Rituximab, IVIG, and plasmapheresis are second-line treatments. The overall outcome for neuropsychiatric lupus is poor but may improve with increasing use of newer biologic agents.[18]

Pregnancy (Chorea Gravidarum)

Chorea of any cause beginning in pregnancy is chorea gravidarum. Rheumatic fever was once the most frequent cause but it is now the antiphospholipid antibody syndrome, with or without systemic lupus erythematosus that is the most common cause.

Clinical features. The onset of chorea is usually during the second to fifth month of pregnancy but may begin postpartum. Cognitive change may accompany the chorea. Symptoms usually resolve spontaneously within weeks to months.

Diagnosis. Women who develop chorea during pregnancy require studies for rheumatic fever, antiphospholipid antibody syndrome, and systemic lupus erythematosus.

Management. This is a self-limited condition, and drugs should be used cautiously so as not to harm the fetus.

DYSTONIA

Repetitive muscle contractions that are sustained at the peak and result in torsional postures characterize dystonia. The appearance is one of an abnormal posture rather than an involuntary movement. The muscle contractions can affect the limbs, trunk, or face (*grimacing*). Involvement may be of a single body part (*focal dystonia*), two or more contiguous body parts (*segmental dystonia*), the arm and leg on one side of the body (*hemidystonia*), or one or both legs and the contiguous trunk and any other body part (*generalized dystonia*).

Persistent focal dystonias are relatively common in adults but are unusual in children except when drug induced. Children with focal, stereotyped movements of the eyelids, face, or neck are much more likely to have a tic than focal dystonia. Box 14.2 lists childhood forms of focal dystonia.

Generalized dystonia usually begins in one limb. The patient has difficulty performing an act rather than a movement, so that the foot becomes dystonic when walking forward but may not be dystonic when sitting, standing, or running. Sensory tricks are maneuvers such as the patient touching their chin, which result in transient control of the dystonia.

Drug-Induced Dystonia
Acute Reactions

Focal or generalized dystonia may occur as an acute idiosyncratic reaction following a first dose of dopamine antagonist (antiemetics and antipsychotics). Possible reactions include trismus, opisthotonos, torticollis, and oculogyric crisis. Difficulty with swallowing and speaking may occur. Metoclopramide, a nonphenothiazine antiemetic that blocks postsynaptic dopamine receptors, may produce acute and delayed (tardive) dystonia, as may prochlorperazine or promethazine. The acute reactions are usually self-limited or respond to treatment with anticholinergics such as benztropine, but they may be prolonged and resistant to therapy. A dose of diphenhydramine may resolve the acute reaction. We always

---

BOX 14.2 Differential Diagnosis of Dystonia in Childhood

- Drug induced
  - Metoclopramide
  - Prochlorperazine
  - Promethazine
- Focal dystonia
  - Blepharospasm
  - Torticollis
  - Writer's cramp
  - Hemifacial spasm
- Hereditary (Genetic) dystonias
  - Dopa responsive
    - DYT-GCH1 (extremely sensitive to levodopa)
    - DYT-TH (partial sensitivity)
    - DYT-SPR (partial sensitivity)
  - Dopa unresponsive
    - Glutaric acidemia type I
    - Hepatolenticular degeneration (Wilson's disease)
    - Idiopathic torsion dystonia (DYT-TOR1A)
    - Bilateral striatal necrosis
    - Pantothenate kinase–associated neurodegeneration (PKAN)
    - Rapid-onset dystonia-parkinsonism (DYT-ATP1A3)
- Symptomatic generalized dystonias
  - Tumor
  - Active encephalopathy or encephalitis
  - Prior brain insult

BOX 14.3 Differential Diagnosis of Torticollis and Head Tilt

- Benign paroxysmal torticollis[a]
- Cervical cord syringomyelia (see Chapter 12)
- Cervical cord tumors (see Chapter 12)
- Cervicomedullary malformations[a] (see Chapters 10 and 18)
- Diplopia[a] (see Chapter 15)
- Dystonia
- Familial paroxysmal choreoathetosis (see Chapter 1)
- Juvenile rheumatoid arthritis
- Posterior fossa tumors (see Chapter 10)
- Sandifer syndrome
- Spasmus nutans[a] (see Chapter 15)
- Sternocleidomastoid injuries
- Tics and Tourette syndrome[a]

[a]The most common conditions and the ones with disease modifying treatments.

---

is not confused with dystonia. Focal dystonia involving eye closure in children is usually drug induced.

Baclofen, clonazepam, trihexyphenidyl, and injections of botulinum A toxin are often successful in treating blepharospasm and orofacial dystonia in adults.

Torticollis

Box 14.3 summarizes the differential diagnoses of torticollis and head tilt. The first step in diagnosis is to distinguish fixed from nonfixed torticollis. In fixed torticollis the neck is not moveable to the neutral position. The causation may be a structural disturbance of the cervical vertebrae or may occur when pain prevents movement.

Evidence of concurrent dystonia in the face or limbs indicates the need for further evaluation directed at underlying causes of dystonia. When torticollis and corticospinal tract signs (hyperactive tendon reflexes, ankle clonus, or extensor plantar responses) are associated, suspect a cervical spinal cord disturbance and order a cervical MRI. Symptoms of increased intracranial pressure indicate a posterior fossa tumor with early herniation. When torticollis is the only abnormal feature, the underlying causes may include focal dystonia, injury to the neck muscles, and inflammatory conditions such as juvenile rheumatoid arthritis.

Nonfixed torticollis that occurs in self-limited attacks suggests benign paroxysmal torticollis, familial paroxysmal choreoathetosis, or hereditary dystonia.[19] The

instruct our patients to have some diphenhydramine available when starting dopamine-blocking agents.

Tardive Dystonia

Usually, tardive dystonia has a generalized distribution in children, but occurs as a focal disturbance in adults. Tetrabenazine is helpful in most patients, and anticholinergic drugs offer relief in others.

Focal Dystonias

Blepharospasm

Blepharospasm is an involuntary spasmodic closure of the eyes. Box 14.3 summarizes the differential diagnosis for children. Essential blepharospasm, an incapacitating condition, is a disorder of middle or late adult life and never begins in childhood. Tics account for almost all cases of involuntary eye closure in children. Eye fluttering occurs during absence seizures (see Chapter 1) but combination of head tilt, head bobbing, and nystagmus in infants is termed *spasmus nutans* (see Chapter 15).

Benign paroxysmal torticollis. The underlying cause of benign paroxysmal torticollis is unknown. A migraine variant, closely related to benign paroxysmal vertigo (see Chapter 10), is the apparent cause in some infants but not in others.

Clinical features. Onset is usually in the first year. Head tilting to one side (not always the same side) and slight head rotation characterize the episodes. The child may resist efforts to return the head to a neutral position, but overcoming the resistance is possible. Some children have no other symptoms, whereas others have pallor, irritability, malaise, and vomiting. Most attacks last for 1–3 days, end spontaneously, and tend to recur three to six times a year. Children who are old enough to stand and walk become may ataxic during attacks.

With time, the attacks may evolve into episodes characteristic of cyclic vomiting, benign paroxysmal vertigo or migraine, or may simply cease without further symptoms. The disorder may occur in siblings, indicating a genetic factor, but usually the family history only reveals migraine.

Diagnosis. Suspect the disorder in any infant with attacks of torticollis that remit spontaneously and pursue a family history of migraine. Familial paroxysmal choreoathetosis and familial paroxysmal dystonia do not begin during early infancy. Sandifer syndrome, intermittent retrocollis associated with reflux, is an alternative consideration.

Management. No treatment is available or needed for acute attacks, but cyproheptadine may be helpful in children with associated nausea or vomiting.

Writer's Cramp

Writer's cramp is a focal, task-specific dystonia. It may occur only when writing, or when performing other specific manual tasks such as typing or playing the piano (occupational cramp). The cramp is more often isolated but may be associated with other focal dystonias, such as torticollis, or with generalized dystonia.

Clinical features. Onset is usually after 20 years of age but may be in the second decade. In writer's cramp or other task-specific dystonias the dystonic postures occur when the patient attempts to write or perform the task. The initial features are any of the following: aching in the hand when writing, loss of handwriting neatness or speed, and difficulty in holding writing

implements. All three symptoms are eventually present. Dystonic postures occur when the patient attempts to write. During writing, the hand and arm lift from the paper, and the fingers may flex or extend. Writing with the affected hand becomes impossible and the patient learns to write with the nondominant hand, which may also become dystonic.

Symptoms are at first intermittent and are especially severe when others observe the writing. Later the movement occurs with each attempt at writing. Some patients have lifelong difficulty with using the dominant hand for writing and may have difficulty with other manual tasks as well. Others experience remissions and exacerbations. Progression to generalized dystonia is rare.

Diagnosis. Diagnosis is based on the clinical history. Distinguish isolated focal dystonia and generalized dystonia with focal onset. Thoroughly explore the family history and repeat the examination to determine the presence of dystonia in other body parts.

Management. Botulinum toxin type A is used to treat focal dystonias. Oral medications are the same as those used to treat generalized dystonia (see the "Idiopathic Torsion Dystonia" section).

Hemifacial Spasm

Involuntary, irregular contractions of the muscles innervated by one facial nerve characterize hemifacial spasm. This is a very rare condition in children. The spasms may develop because of aberrant regeneration following facial nerve injury, secondary to posterior fossa tumor, or without apparent cause. Rare familial cases exist, suggesting a potential underlying genetic cause.

Clinical features. Spasms are embarrassing and disturbing but not painful. The orbicularis oculi muscles are the muscles affected first and most commonly, causing forced closure of the eye. As facial muscles on one side become affected, they pull the mouth to one side. Spasms may occur several times a minute, especially during times of stress. The subsequent course depends on the underlying cause.

Diagnosis. Hemifacial spasm in children may be mistaken for a focal seizure. The stereotyped appearance of the spasm and a concurrent normal EEG are distinguishing features. Suspect a posterior fossa tumor in every child with hemifacial spasm. Brain MRI is required in every instance unless symptoms are explained by a history of prior facial nerve injury.

Management. Some patients respond to treatment with carbamazepine at anticonvulsant doses (see Chapter 1), but most do not respond to medical therapy. Injection of botulinum toxin into the muscles in spasm is the treatment of choice. Surgical procedures to relieve pressure on the facial nerve from adjacent vessels are of questionable value.

Generalized Genetic (Hereditary) Dystonias

When describing genetic dystonias, it is helpful to consider the age of onset, body areas affected, temporal patterns, and any other associated features. Previously, the classification of autosomal dominant dystonias (DYTs) employed a numeric system based on which phenotypes were first described. Advances in genetic testing now allow us to categorize genetic dystonias based on the specific gene affected (e.g., instead of DYT1, the disorder is termed DYT-TOR1A).

Dopa-Responsive Dystonia

There are three genetic dopa-responsive dystonia syndromes affecting children, which are distinguished by age of onset, dystonia type, and the level of responsiveness to levodopa. GTP cyclohydrolase 1-deficient dopa-responsive dystonia (DYT-GCH1) is autosomal dominant with reduced penetrance and is exquisitely sensitive to low doses of levodopa. This is the disorder that most physicians refer to when speaking of "dopa-responsive dystonia." DYT-TH and DYT-SPR are autosomal recessive dystonias caused by tyrosine hydroxylase deficiency and sepiapterin-reductase deficiency, respectively. Both are partially responsive to levodopa.[20]

Clinical features. The onset of GTP cyclohydrolase 1-deficient dopa-responsive dystonia (DYT-GCH1) is approximately 6 years of age. The initial feature is usually foot dystonia, which causes a gait disturbance. Parkinsonian-like symptoms follow. Diurnal fluctuation in the severity of symptoms is common. Symptoms improve considerably on awakening and worsen later in the day. Arm dystonia with abnormal hand posturing and postural tremor sometimes appears first. Examination reveals brisk deep-tendon reflexes in the legs and ankle clonus. A gradual progression to generalized dystonia follows. Intellectual, cerebellar, sensory, or autonomic disturbances do not occur, but migraines, sleep disturbances, and mood disorders are common. Significant phenotypic variability is possible, even within the same family.[21]

Tyrosine hydroxylase deficiency (DYT-TH) often begins in infancy but may be as late as 6 years. Some have mild dystonia and others have a parkinsonian-like syndrome with bradykinesia and hypotonia. Autonomic disturbance, ptosis, and oculogyric crisis are possible. The initial feature is nearly always a gait disturbance caused by leg dystonia. Flexion at the hip and knee and plantar flexion of the foot cause toe walking. Both flexor and extensor posturing of the arms develop, finally parkinsonian features such as cogwheel rigidity, mask-like facies, and bradykinesia appear. The disease reaches a plateau in adolescence. Postural or intention tremor occurs in almost half of patients, but typical parkinsonian tremor is unusual.[22]

Sepiapterin deficiency (DYT-SPH) is rare and not well understood. Initial symptoms in infancy are nonspecific developmental delay and axial hypotonia, often leading to an incorrect diagnosis of cerebral palsy. As the child gets older, symptoms evolve to include weakness, dystonia, intellectual disability, oculogyric crisis, and parkinsonian features. Psychiatric disorders, autonomic disturbances, and disrupted sleep are common. As with the other disorders discussed here, diurnal fluctuations are the norm.

Diagnosis. Every child with dystonia should be treated with a trial of carbidopa-levodopa. For children with DYT-GCH1, the response is dramatic and often diagnostic. Genetic dystonia panels and single-gene testing are available on a clinical basis.

Management. Initiate carbidopa-levodopa therapy at the lowest possible dose and slowly increase it until a response is established. Long-term therapy is beneficial and required. Symptoms return after discontinuing the drug. DYT-TH and DYT-SPH are only partially responsive to levodopa; DYT-SPH may also respond to 5-hydroxytryptophan (5-HTP) in combination with carbidopa-levodopa. Children with DYT-TH and DYT-SPH may require additional drug therapy with dopamine agonists or anticholinergics.

Glutaric Acidemia Type I

Glutaric acidemia type I is a rare inborn error in the catabolism of lysine, hydroxylysine, and tryptophan. Transmission is by autosomal recessive inheritance of mutated forms of the *GCDH* gene. Deficiency of glutaryl-coenzyme-A dehydrogenase causes the disorder.

Clinical features. Megalencephaly is usually present at birth. Neurological findings may be otherwise normal.

Two patterns of illness occur in affected infants.[23] In two-thirds of infants, the initial feature is acute encephalopathy characterized by somnolence, irritability, and excessive sweating. Seizures sometimes occur. The prognosis in such cases is poor. Afterward, development regresses and progressive choreoathetosis and dystonia occur.

The other pattern is more insidious and the prognosis better. Affected infants are at first hypotonic and later have mild developmental delay and dyskinesias. Cerebral palsy is a common misdiagnosis (see Chapter 12).

Diagnosis. Metabolic acidosis may be present. Abnormal urinary concentration of glutaric, 3-hydroxyglutaric, 3-hydroxybutyric, and acetoacetic acids is detectable. Molecular genetic testing and prenatal diagnosis are available. MRI may show widening of the Sylvian fissures and cerebral atrophy, most marked in the frontal and temporal lobes. The presence of reduced brain tissue in an enlarged head has been termed *microcephalic megalencephaly* and is highly suspicious for glutaric acidemia type I.[24]

Management. Protein restriction, lysine-free formulas, and oral carnitine supplementation together with the immediate administration of fluids, glucose, electrolytes, and antipyretics during febrile illnesses may slow disease progression.[25]

Hepatolenticular Degeneration (Wilson Disease)

Genetic transmission of hepatolenticular degeneration is autosomal recessive inheritance, caused by mutations of the *ATP7B* gene regulating copper transport from the hepatocytes into the bile. Mutations that completely prevent function of the gene produce a more severe phenotype than certain types of missense mutations. Tissue damage occurs after excessive copper accumulation in the liver, brain, and cornea. *ATP7B* mutations are increasingly associated with other neurological diseases as well, including certain types of axonal neuropathies, Alzheimer disease, and Parkinson disease.[26]

Clinical features. Wilson disease can present with hepatic, neurological, or psychiatric disturbances, alone or in combination. The age at onset ranges from 3 to over 50.[27] *Hepatic failure is the prominent clinical feature in children less than 10 years of age, usually without neurological symptoms or signs.* Neurological manifestations with only minimal symptoms of liver disease are more likely when the onset of symptoms is in the second

decade. A single symptom, such as a disturbance of gait or speech, is often the initial feature and may remain unchanged for years. Eventually the initial symptoms worsen, and new features develop (dysarthria, dystonia, dysdiadochokinesia, rigidity, gait and postural abnormalities, tremor, and drooling). Dystonia of bulbar muscles is responsible for three prominent features of the disease: dysarthria, a fixed pseudosmile (risus sardonicus), and a high-pitched whining noise on inspiration.

Psychiatric disturbances precede neurological abnormalities in 20% of cases. They range from behavioral disturbances to paranoid psychoses. Dementia is not an early feature of the disease.

The Kayser-Fleischer ring, a yellow-brown granular deposit at the limbus of the cornea, is a certain indicator of disease. The cause is copper deposition in the Descemet membrane. It is present in almost all patients with neurological manifestations, although it may be absent in children with liver disease alone.

Diagnosis. Hepatolenticular degeneration is a consideration in any child with acquired and progressive dysarthria and dystonia. The association of chronic liver disease with neurological disturbances increases the probability of hepatolenticular degeneration. The detection of low serum copper and ceruloplasmin concentrations and increased urinary copper excretion or the demonstration of a Kayser-Fleischer ring by slit-lamp examination establishes the diagnosis. Ninety-six percent of patients will have a serum ceruloplasmin concentration of less than 20 mg/dL, corresponding to less than 56 g/dL of ceruloplasmin copper. Molecular genetic testing of the *ATP7B* gene is clinically available.

Management. Treatment is lifelong. Chelating agents (e.g., penicillamine or trientine) that increase urinary excretion of copper are the primary treatment for Wilson disease; however, these are not specific for copper, and formal management guidelines remain controversial. Copper-specific chelating agents are under investigation, but not currently approved for use in humans. The dose of D-penicillamine is 250 mg four times a day for children more than 10 years of age and half as much for younger children. Ingestion of penicillamine is always on an empty stomach together with a daily dose of 25 mg pyridoxine. Measures of 24-hour urine copper excretion confirm chelation. Urinary copper values should run 5–10 times normal. Improvement is slow, and neurological improvement frequently takes several months. Worsening may occur during the first months of therapy, but this should not be a cause for alarm. Early treatment is essential to decrease morbidity and mortality.

Oral administration of zinc interferes with absorption of copper and is useful after initial de-coppering with a chelating agent. Antioxidants, such as vitamin E, help to prevent tissue damage, particularly to the liver. Liver transplantation is required for patients who fail to respond or cannot tolerate medical therapy. All siblings of patients with Wilson disease require careful screening for disease and early treatment.

Idiopathic Torsion Dystonia

Early-onset idiopathic torsion dystonia (DYT-TOR1A, formerly known as DYT1) is transmitted by autosomal dominant inheritance with reduced penetrance (30%–40%) and variable expression. The gene *TOR1A*, located on chromosome 9q34, is causative.[28] The frequency of idiopathic torsion dystonia in Ashkenazi Jews is 5–10 times greater than in other groups. Nonfamilial cases probably represent autosomal dominant inheritance with incomplete penetrance.

Clinical features. Age at onset has a bimodal distribution; for early onset the median is 9 years, and for late onset the median is 45 years. The early-onset cases are more genetically homogeneous.

The limbs usually become dystonic before the trunk. The initial features may be in the arms, legs, or larynx. Early leg involvement is more common in children than in adults. Despite the focal features at onset, dystonia always generalizes in children, affecting the limbs and trunk. Spontaneous stabilization is the rule, but remission is unusual. The eventual outcome varies from complete disability to functional independence.

Other clinical features include dysarthria, orofacial movements, dysphagia, postural tremor, and blepharospasm. Cognitive deterioration does not occur, but, as a group, patients with familial disease have a lower IQ than those with sporadic cases.

Diagnosis. The clinical features of dystonic movements and postures and the family history suggest the diagnosis. Normal perinatal history, no exposure to drugs, no evidence of intellectual or corticospinal deterioration, and no demonstrable biochemical disorder exclude other possibilities. Molecular genetic testing confirms the diagnosis.

Management. Medical management is often ineffective. DBS of the bilateral globus pallidum is useful in many patients.[19] High-dose anticholinergic therapy (trihexyphenidyl, 30 mg/d) provides the best medical results. While children tend to tolerate higher doses than adults, confusion and memory impairment may limit usefulness. Other drugs that may be of value include baclofen, carbamazepine, and benzodiazepines. All juvenile-onset dystonic patients deserve a trial of L-dopa to exclude dopa-responsive dystonia (see discussion on dopa-responsive dystonia earlier in this chapter). Botulinum toxin is useful for selected focal problems.

Infantile Bilateral Striatal Necrosis

Bilateral striatal necrosis (BSN) occurs in several genetic disorders that share pathological features of bilateral, symmetric, spongy degeneration of the corpus striatum and degeneration of the globus pallidus.[29] *Familial infantile striatal degeneration* is rare, and inheritance can be autosomal recessive (caused by mutations of the *NUP62* gene) or mitochondrial (caused by *MTATP6* mutations). The familial form has an insidious onset and a slowly progressive course; the sporadic form is associated with acute systemic illness. Many features of BSN overlap with Leigh syndrome and metabolic disorders, such as glutaric acidemia I and methylmalonic aciduria. Onset is in infancy or early childhood.

Clinical features. Two clinical syndromes are associated with infantile BSN. The first has an insidious onset during infancy or early childhood and a long clinical course that includes dystonia, cognitive impairment, seizures, and death. A clinical and pathological overlap exists between progressive infantile BSN, subacute necrotizing encephalomyelopathy (see Chapter 5), and Leber hereditary optic neuropathy (see Chapter 16).

A second syndrome begins as acute encephalopathy, usually following a febrile illness with nausea and vomiting. The major features are dystonia and tremor. The severity of symptoms may fluctuate at the time of intercurrent illness. Some children recover spontaneously; others are permanently impaired.

Diagnosis. The observation of static or progressive striatal necrosis on serial MRI examinations suggests the diagnosis. Due to clinical overlap with other genetic syndromes, a chromosome microarray, mitochondrial genetic testing, and/or whole exome sequencing may be more useful than testing for specific genetic defects.

Management. All features of biotin-responsive BSN respond to administration of biotin, 5–10 mg/kg/day, but reappear within 1 month after biotin is discontinued. All children with evidence of BSN deserve a trial of biotin.

Pantothenate Kinase–Associated Neurodegeneration

PKAN, previously called *Hallervorden-Spatz syndrome*, is a neurodegeneration with brain iron accumulation.[30] It is a genetic disorder transmitted as an autosomal recessive trait via biallelic mutations of the *PANK2* gene. Other rare causes of neurodegeneration with brain iron accumulation include Woodhouse-Sakati syndrome, infantile and atypical neuroaxonal dystrophy, fatty acid hydroxylase–associated neurodegeneration, mitochondrial membrane protein–associated neurodegeneration, COASY protein–associated neurodegeneration, and beta-propeller protein–associated neurodegeneration.

Clinical features. The characteristic features of PKAN are progressive dystonia and basal ganglia iron deposition. The disorder becomes symptomatic between 2 and 10 years of age in more than half of patients but may appear as late as the third decade. The initial feature is progressive rigidity, first in the foot, causing an equinovarus deformity, and then in the hand. Other features are choreoathetosis, rigidity, and dysarthria. Two-thirds of patients have a pigmentary retinopathy.[31] Mental deterioration and spasticity follow. Previously, death occurred within 5–10 years, but with improvements in symptomatic management many patients now survive into adulthood.

Diagnosis. The MRI features and molecular genetic testing are the basis for antemortem diagnosis. T_2-weighted MRI shows low-intensity signal images from the globus pallidus with a central area of increased signal intensity, *the eye-of-the-tiger sign* (Fig. 14.1). Postmortem examination shows degeneration of the pallidum and substantia nigra with deposition of iron-containing material.

Management. Agents that chelate iron have not proved effective. Symptomatic treatment for dystonia includes intramuscular botulinum toxin, baclofen pump placement, oral trihexyphenidyl, and DBS.

Rapid-Onset Dystonia-Parkinsonism

Rapid-onset dystonia-parkinsonism (DYT-ATP1A3, formerly called DYT12) is a separate autosomal dominant form of dystonia characterized by an unusually rapid evolution of signs and symptoms.[31]

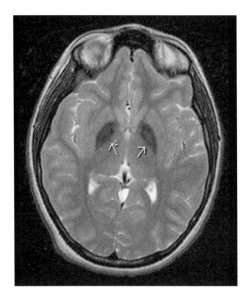

Fig. 14.1 Pantothenate Kinase–Associated Neurodegeneration (Hallervorden-Spatz Syndrome). T_2 axial magnetic resonance imaging (MRI) shows the characteristic iron deposition in the globus pallidus, the eye-of-the-tiger sign (*arrows*).

Clinical features. The disorder is characterized by the acute (hours) or subacute (days to weeks) development of generalized dystonia and parkinsonism that involves the face and arms more than the legs. Symptoms respond poorly to treatment with levodopa. Age at onset is 4–55 years. Severe bulbar symptoms such as dysarthria, drooling, and orofacial dystonia are associated. Some show hypertonicity and hyperreflexia.

Diagnosis. Diagnosis depends on the clinical features. Molecular genetic testing is available.

Management. A trial of levodopa is reasonable in any child with new-onset dystonia to rule out DYT-GCH1 but is not effective in this disorder. When levodopa fails, then high dosages of benzodiazepines or trihexyphenidyl may provide symptomatic relief. Children often tolerate high dosages when the dose is slowly increased; adults rarely tolerate such high dosages.

Symptomatic Generalized Dystonia

An underlying tumor, active encephalopathy, or prior brain damage can cause dystonia.

Clinical features. The onset of dystonia may be at the time of acute encephalopathy, after the acute phase is over, or several years later, when the encephalopathy is static. Delayed-onset chorea and dystonia in children with perinatal disturbances such as asphyxia or kernicterus usually begin by 2–3 years of age but may begin in adolescence. After involuntary movements appear, they tend to become progressively more severe, but intellectual decline is not an associated feature. Delayed-onset dystonia may have a generalized distribution.

Hemidystonia most often occurs after stroke or head injury but may be a symptom of neuronal storage diseases or tumors of the basal ganglia, alternating hemiplegia, and the antiphospholipid antibody syndrome (see Chapter 11). The dystonic limbs are contralateral to the damaged basal ganglia.

Diagnosis. Children with a known cause for the development of dystonia or chorea do not require extensive studies, although obtaining an MRI to rule out new injury is reasonable. The new symptoms are discouraging for patients and families who have adjusted to a fixed neurological deficit. Provide assurance that the new symptoms are not evidence of new brain degeneration, but only the appearance of new symptoms from old lesions. This sequence is most likely when injury is perinatal and brain maturation is required to manifest involuntary movements.

The appearance of hemidystonia, even with a known predisposing event, necessitates an MRI to look for localized changes that may require treatment, such as an expanding cyst. Consider the possibility of a tumor in children who had been neurologically intact before hemidystonia appeared.

Management. The drugs used to treat symptomatic dystonia are no different from those used for genetic dystonia, but the results may not be as favorable. Botulinum toxin may be useful when specific muscle contractions are causing severe disability.

MIRROR MOVEMENTS

Mirror movements are involuntary movements of one side of the body, usually the hands, which occur as mirror reversals of an intended movement on the other side of the body. They are normal during infancy and tend to disappear before 10 years of age, coincident with myelination of the corpus callosum. *Congenital mirror movements* persist into adulthood and are inherited in an autosomal dominant fashion with incomplete penetrance. The most common mutations are in the *DCC* gene, in which case they may be associated with agenesis of the corpus callosum and mild intellectual disability.[32]

Congenital mirror movements have also been reported, rarely, in Kallman syndrome, Klippel-Feil syndrome, Joubert syndrome, and Mobius syndrome. Early-onset and persistent mirror movements are sometimes a component of hemiplegic cerebral palsy.

Acquired mirror movements can be seen in neurodegenerative conditions or abnormalities of the cervicomedullary junction. Although more common in adults, any child with new-onset mirror movements requires imaging of the brain and cervical spine.

MYOCLONUS

The term *myoclonus* encompasses several involuntary movements characterized by rapid muscle jerks. They are less frequent and severe during sleep but may not disappear. Myoclonus may be rhythmic or nonrhythmic; focal, multifocal, or generalized; spontaneous or activated by movement (action myoclonus) or sensory stimulation (reflex myoclonus). In addition it may be cortical, subcortical, or spinal, and may be positive or negative. *Positive myoclonus* is the sudden contraction of muscles, while *negative myoclonus* is the abrupt cessation of muscle action; negative myoclonus causes sudden postural changes and may lead to falls.

The distinction of nonepileptic myoclonus from tic, chorea, tremor, and seizures can be challenging. Tics are usually more complex and stereotyped movements than myoclonus and can be briefly suppressed by voluntary effort; myoclonus is not voluntarily suppressible. Chorea is more random than myoclonus and is often incorporated into voluntary movement; myoclonus is never part of a larger movement. Rhythmic myoclonus and tremor look alike and are sometimes difficult to distinguish clinically. Tremor is a continuous to-and-fro movement, whereas rhythmic myoclonus has a pause between movements. Epileptic myoclonus (e.g., as seen in juvenile myoclonic epilepsy) and nonepileptic myoclonus can be extremely difficult to differentiate clinically and often require further evaluation with prolonged EEG monitoring (see Chapter 1 for a discussion of epileptic myoclonus).

Physiological myoclonus occurs in normal people during drowsiness and sleep (see the section on movement disorders that persist during sleep).

The causes of symptomatic myoclonus include drugs, electrolyte abnormalities, a cerebral injury, or part of a generalized progressive encephalopathy.

Opsoclonus-Myoclonus-Ataxia Syndrome

Opsoclonus-myoclonus-ataxia syndrome (OMAS) is an autoimmune, likely paraneoplastic disorder associated with neuroblastoma. "Tumor-negative" cases may represent the effects of tumors that are too small to detect with our current diagnostic tools; however, other autoimmune etiologies are possible.

Clinical features. Onset is typically around the age of 18–24 months but has been reported in infants and older children. Chaotic, multidirectional, and darting eye movements (*opsoclonus*) are often the presenting symptom. Multifocal myoclonus and ataxia then develop. Importantly, it is possible to present with myoclonus and ataxia alone, or with isolated opsoclonus. Irritability, sleep disturbances, inconsolable crying, and rage attacks are common. Regression in motor skills or speech may be seen, and many affected children suffer long-term intellectual disabilities and cognitive impairment.

Approximately 50% have peripheral neuroblastic tumors, usually neuroblastoma (73%). Ganglioneuroma and ganglioneuroblastoma are other common causes, and ovarian teratoma has been documented in rare cases. Tumors, when present, almost always occur peripherally along the sympathetic chain or in the adrenals. Primary brain tumors are not associated with the disorder.

Diagnosis. The rarity of OMAS makes establishing diagnostic criteria difficult. Current diagnosis is usually based on the presence of three out of four cardinal features: opsoclonus, myoclonus, ataxia, and neuroblastoma. Box 14.4 delineates an accepted rating scale for OMAS symptoms. Atypical cases are common, and MRI of the brain is often needed to rule out a posterior fossa lesion. All children with OMAS require whole body

---

BOX 14.4 Mitchell and Pike OMS Rating Scale

Mitchell and Pike OMS Rating Scale

Category	Score	Description
Stance	0	Standing and sitting balance normal for age
	1	Mildly unstable standing for age, slightly wide based
	2	Unable to stand without support but can sit without support
	3	Unable to sit without using hands to prop or other support
Gait	0	Walking normal for age
	1	Mildly wide-based gait for age, but able to walk indoors and outdoors independently
	2	Walks only or predominantly with support from person or equipment
	3	Unable to walk even with support from person or equipment
Arm/hand function	0	Normal for age
	1	Mild, infrequent tremor or jerkiness without functional impairment
	2	Fine motor function persistently impaired for age, but less precise manipulative tasks normal or almost normal
	3	Major difficulties in all age-appropriate fine motor and manipulative tasks
Opsoclonus	0	None
	1	Rare or only when elicited by change in fixation or squeeze test
	2	Frequent interferes intermittently with fixation or tracking
	3	Persistent, interfering continuously with function and tracking
Mood/behavior	0	Normal
	1	Mild increase in irritability but consolable and/or mild sleep disturbances
	2	Irritability and sleep disturbances interfering with child and family life
	3	Persistent severe distress
Speech	0	Normal for age. No loss
	1	Mildly unclear, plateaued in development
	2	Loss of some words or some grammatical constructs (i.e., from sentences to phrases) but still communicates verbally
	3	Severe loss of verbal communication and speech.

OMS, Opsoclonus-myoclonus syndrome.

MRI (neck to pelvis). When this is difficult to obtain, the provider may instead get chest X-ray, abdominal ultrasound, and MIBG scintigraphy, with whole body MRI if initial imaging is negative. Laboratory investigations for neuroblastoma include urine catecholamine metabolites, serum neuron-specific enolase, and lactate dehydrogenase. Perform lumbar puncture to rule out OMAS mimics such as autoimmune encephalitis; flow cytometry should be obtained to look for B-cell expansion, which is a marker of active OMAS and can be used as a baseline to assess response to B-cell depleting therapies.

There is no single established biomarker for OMAS. Some children have pleocytosis and many (58%) have oligoclonal bands in the CSF. Infectious triggers have been identified in some cases, and infectious workup can be considered on a case-specific basis; however all children require neuroblastoma evaluation even if an infectious agent is found.[33]

Management. Evidence suggests that more intensive treatment results in better cognitive outcomes. OMAS rarely remits on its own, and there is a high incidence of relapses with permanent neurologic sequelae, thus justifying early and aggressive management. Steroids, either ACTH or corticosteroids, as well as IVIG or plasma exchange are common initial steps. Rituximab is used for long-term immune suppression more often than cyclophosphamide. Trazodone helps with sleep and mitigates some of the behavioral outbursts. Specific treatment protocols vary between institutions.

Hereditary Essential Myoclonus (*SGCE* Myoclonus-Dystonia)

Essential myoclonus is an autosomal dominant genetic condition of focal, segmental, or generalized jerking aggravated by action or stress caused by *SGCE* gene mutations.

Clinical features. Onset is in the first or second decade. Both sexes are equally affected. The movements are predominantly in the face, trunk, and proximal muscles. While usually generalized, they may be restricted to one side of the body. Approximately 50% of affected patients also have focal or segmental dystonia such as writer's cramp; OCD or anxiety are common comorbidities. Life expectancy is normal.[34]

Diagnosis. Careful neurological examination, EEG, and brain imaging exclude symptomatic and epileptic myoclonus. Molecular genetic testing reveals pathogenic variants in the *SGCE* gene.

Management. Mild essential myoclonus does not require treatment. Botulinum toxin type A injection into the affected muscles often reduces the movement. There is good evidence supporting the use of zonisamide in the treatment of any disorder involving myoclonus. Interestingly, adult patients report dramatic improvement with alcohol consumption.

Symptomatic Myoclonus

Myoclonus is often a symptom of an underlying neurological disease. Generalized myoclonus is the rule when the cause is a diffuse, progressive encephalopathy (such as lysosomal storage diseases) and segmental when the lesion is focal in the brainstem or spinal cord. Multifocal myoclonus may occur as a side effect of gabapentin and SSRIs among others. Lamotrigine and carbamazepine may exacerbate preexisting myoclonus, for example in the treatment of juvenile myoclonic epilepsy.

Posthypoxic Myoclonus (Lance-Adams Syndrome)

Chronic posthypoxic myoclonus is a form of action myoclonus in patients who have suffered an episode of hypoxia. It is distinct from acute hypoxic myoclonus which portends a grim neurological outcome when seen in the intensive care unit. Chronic posthypoxic myoclonus was previously referred to as Lance-Adams syndrome. Chronic posthypoxic myoclonus does not follow hypoxic-ischemic encephalopathy of the newborn; it is more commonly seen in adults following cardiopulmonary resuscitation. Single or repetitive myoclonic jerks occur when voluntary movement is attempted. Facial and pharyngeal muscle myoclonus interferes with speech and swallowing. Cerebellar disturbances are usually associated findings.

Myoclonus usually begins during recovery from anoxic encephalopathy and once started never remits. Levetiracetam, zonisamide, valproate, and clonazepam are effective treatments in approximately 50%. DBS has been used in severe cases.[35]

Segmental (Focal) Myoclonus

Segmental myoclonus is an involuntary contraction of contiguous muscles innervated by the brainstem or spinal cord. It may be rhythmic or nonrhythmic. Rhythmic segmental myoclonus looks like a focal seizure. The underlying causes in children are limited mainly to demyelinating diseases and intrinsic tumors. Cystic astrocytoma of the spinal cord is the major cause of spinal myoclonus and may be the initial feature (see Chapter 12).

Palatal myoclonus is the most common segmental myoclonus of brainstem origin. Unilateral or bilateral rhythmic contractions of the palate (80–180 per minute) that usually persist during sleep are characteristic. It may be associated with rhythmic contractions of the eyes, larynx, neck, diaphragm, trunk, and limbs. Lesions in the central tegmental tract or the dentato-olivary pathways cause palatal myoclonus. The median interval between the precipitating cause and the onset of palatal myoclonus is 10–11 months. Clonazepam and tetrabenazine are the most useful drugs in the treatment of segmental myoclonus.

Dentatorubro Pallidoluysian Atrophy

Dentatorubro pallidoluysian atrophy presents in adolescence with progressive dementia, myoclonus, epilepsy, spasticity, and dystonia. It is discussed in Chapter 5.

MOVEMENT DISORDERS IN DROWSINESS AND SLEEP

The vast majority of movement disorders cease during sleep; this is one of the defining characteristics that helps differentiate movement disorders from other paroxysmal disorders such as seizures. Sleep disorders associated with abnormal movements are the exception, as are the rare primary movement disorders that persist in sleep. In general, the history of abnormal movements during wakefulness that do not resolve with sleep should prompt consideration of alternative diagnoses such as epilepsy or psychogenic movements during pseudo-sleep.

Restless Legs Syndrome

Once thought exclusively a disorder of adults, restless legs syndrome is now recognized to occur in up to 2% of children and may cause significant behavioral symptoms and educational challenges.[36] A combination of genetic, environmental, and medical issues can trigger the syndrome, which can range in severity from mild to disabling. Symptoms may be continuous or wax and wane; periods of spontaneous remission are common.

Clinical features. The essential elements of the syndrome are an urge to move the legs, usually accompanied by uncomfortable or unpleasant sensations in the legs. Young children may describe the sensation as "bugs" in their legs, or simply become irritable and restless when attempting to fall asleep. These elements begin or worsen during periods of rest or inactivity such as lying or sitting; they are partially or totally relieved by movement and worse in the evening or at night.[37] The movements cause an overall decrease in both quality and quantity of sleep, which then results in behavioral dysregulation, trouble with memory and focus, and school difficulty.

Diagnosis. The American Academy of Sleep Medicine and the International Restless Legs Syndrome Study Group have created diagnostic guidelines. Diagnosis is established based on the clinical features. A sleep laboratory study is useful to diagnose both RLS and any other associated sleep disorders. Eighty percent of affected children have deficient serum ferritin blood concentrations. Although genetic causes have been identified, genetic testing is usually not required.

Treatment. Oral iron is the mainstay of treatment for those with low ferritin levels. Intravenous iron has been used in adults although data in children are limited. Other potential treatments include gabapentin, pregabalin, clonazepam, and pramipexole.

Benign Physiologic Myoclonus of Drowsiness and Sleep

Myoclonic jerks commonly occur during drowsiness and sleep but may provoke parental concern in young infants and children, particularly when the movements are frequent or pronounced.

Clinical features. Benign myoclonus occurs in all age groups with a range of intensities. Since infants and young children are frequently observed during sleep, these are the age groups that are brought to medical attention, usually due to concern for seizures. Caretakers report that the child "twitches" or "jerks" during sleep. Careful questioning reveals that the movements are neither rhythmic nor sustained, and typically involve the arm or leg either unilaterally or bilaterally. Myoclonus is multifocal; sustained myoclonus in a single limb should prompt further evaluation to rule out epilepsy. Myoclonus ceases when the child awakens but may be present during drowsiness, particularly during the moments when transitioning into sleep.

Diagnosis. The history alone usually establishes the diagnosis. Nocturnal EEG is occasionally required to rule out epileptic myoclonus, particularly in children with epilepsy risk factors.

Management. Reassurance is all that is required in most cases. If myoclonus is massive or causing frequent awakenings, consider prescribing a small dose of clonazepam prior to bedtime.

Rhythmic Movement Disorder of Sleep

Rhythmic movements during transition from drowsiness to sleep or between sleep stages are common in infants and toddlers, and occasionally are seen in older children, adolescents, and adults. Movements become problematic when they consistently disrupt sleep or result in injuries. They are often mistaken for seizures.

Clinical features. A wide variety of movements may be seen. Some of the most common are head shaking (or, in more severe cases, head banging), rocking, or shaking of the limbs. It is more common in children with trisomy 21,[38] but occurs in approximately 1%–2% of all infants and toddlers.[39]

Diagnosis. Because the movements are rhythmic and can be violent, video EEG or polysomnogram are needed to confirm the diagnosis and rule out unusual forms of epilepsy such as nocturnal frontal lobe epilepsy or focal motor seizures.

Management. Rhythmic movements are a normal self-soothing mechanism in many young children, and do not require treatment unless they are disrupting sleep or causing injury. In such cases consider treating with clonazepam or gabapentin prior to bedtime. Since most sleep disorders worsen with excessive fatigue, it is important for the child's caregivers to encourage good sleep habits.

ADCY5 Dyskinesia. *ADCY5* dyskinesia is one of the rare movement disorders that is present during wakefulness but may persist during sleep. It is discussed in more detail in Chapter 1.

TREMOR

Tremor is an involuntary oscillating movement with a fixed frequency. The frequency and amplitude are constant; because frequency decreases with age, amplitude increases. Shuddering, cerebellar ataxia or dysmetria, and asterixis are not tremors because they lack rhythm. Myoclonus may be rhythmic but the movement interrupts between oscillations.

All normal people have a low-amplitude physiological tremor, inherent in maintaining a posture, which is easily observed when holding a laser pointer steady. Physiological tremor enhances to a clinically detectable level in some situations (anxiety, excitement, exercise, fatigue, and stress) and with the use of certain drugs (adrenergic agonists, nicotine, prednisone, thyroid hormone, and xanthines). Hyperthyroidism is routinely associated with enhanced physiological tremor.

Parkinsonism is a common cause of pathological tremors in adults, but rarely occurs in children except when drug induced or as part of a complex degenerative disorder. Typical parkinsonian tremor is seldom present in these situations. Essential tremor is the major cause of tremor in children.

Essential Tremor

Essential (familial) tremor is a monosymptomatic condition probably transmitted as an autosomal dominant trait. The exact genetic basis of inheritance is unknown; mutations in the *DRD3* gene may account for some cases.[40]

Clinical features. Childhood- and adult-onset cases are similar. The tremor usually appears in the second decade but can begin as early as 1 or 2 years of age. The child or parents first notice tremors upon awakening, or in the hands when attempting to perform fine motor movements. The head, face, and neck are sometimes affected. The head tremor is usually mild and has a "no-no" appearance. The tremor frequency in the limbs is typically between 4 and 8 Hz. Essential tremor may impair function, especially schoolwork, and therefore disturb the patient. Some children may simply appear restless or clumsy prior to developing clear *action tremor* symptomatology.

Greater precision of movement enhances the tremor. Therefore tremor appears first and most prominently in the hands. It is further enhanced by anxiety, concentrated effort to stop the tremor, and fatigue. Essential tremor is generally a lifelong condition.

Diagnosis. Essential tremor in children is often mistaken for cerebellar dysfunction because it occurs with action (intention). The two are easily differentiated because essential tremor is rhythmic and not dysmetric (does not become worse at the endpoint) and because it is not associated with other signs of cerebellar dysfunction.

Management. Not all children with essential tremor require treatment. Adaptive devices and accommodations are often just as helpful as medication, and include weighted utensils, wide/weighted writing implements, and school accommodations that allow for use of tablets or computers rather than writing by hand. Medication should be reserved for situations in which tremor impairs function. Propranolol, 1–2 mg/kg/day, or primidone, 2–10 mg/kg/day, are effective to control tremor in 70% of cases. Other options include topiramate[41] or gabapentin. Benzodiazepines are effective but typically not recommended due to their side effect profile. A surgical option for individuals with incapacitating essential tremor is DBS of the ventral intermediate nucleus of the thalamus.[42] Alcohol ingestion relieves essential tremor, but this treatment should be discouraged for obvious reasons.

Juvenile-Onset Parkinson Disease

Juvenile-onset Parkinson disease is defined as Parkinson disease with onset before the age of 20. It is extremely rare, and multiple causative genes have been identified (some present in only one family).[43] Various susceptibility genes and environmental factors also exist.

Clinical features. In general, the term *parkinsonism* refers to resting tremor, slowed movement (bradykinesia), muscle rigidity, and postural instability. It is a nonspecific term that applies to multiple distinct neurodegenerative processes. Specific genetic causes of juvenile-onset Parkinson disease often have unique symptomatology in addition to the standard parkinsonian symptoms, which may include seizures or psychiatric disturbances. The progressive, degenerative nature of juvenile-onset Parkinson disease distinguishes it from nonprogressive disorders such as hereditary dopa-responsive dystonia.

Diagnosis. A careful physical and mental examination in addition to a complete family history suggests the diagnosis. A thorough medical history is required to rule out medication toxicity as a cause of parkinsonism. Obtain MRI of the brain to evaluate for other causes of progressive tremor or rigidity. Molecular genetic testing is available. Due to the rarity of individual genetic etiologies, multigene panels are typically more helpful than single-gene testing, and most affected children undergo an extensive genetic workup.

Management. Clinical trials for gene-targeted therapies are ongoing for certain specific mutations. Otherwise, treatment is similar to that for adults with Parkinson disease, including levodopa, COMT inhibitors, and dopamine agonists. MAO-B inhibitors are often used but present difficulties due to significant interactions with various foods and medications.

Paroxysmal Dystonic Head Tremor

Clinical features. Paroxysmal dystonic head tremor is typically associated with cervical dystonia and is an uncommon syndrome in children. The major feature is attacks of horizontal head tremor (frequency 5–8 Hz), as if the person were saying "no." Onset occurs in adolescence, with a male preponderance. The attacks vary from 1 to 30 minutes, are not provoked by any single stimulus, and cannot be suppressed. A head tilt or clear cervical dystonia predates the onset of tremor by 5–10 years.

Diagnosis. Diagnosis is one of exclusion. Imaging studies of the brain show no abnormalities, and there are no other symptoms to suggest a degenerative process. In an infant the combination of head nodding and head tilt would be diagnosed as spasmus nutans even in the absence of nystagmus (see Chapter 15), and perhaps the underlying mechanism is similar.

Management. Treatment is the same as for cervical dystonia.

REFERENCES

1. Jankovic J. Tourette's syndrome. *New England Journal of Medicine*. 2001;345:1184-1192.
2. Dietrich A, Fernandez TV, King RA, et al. The Tourette International Collaborative Genetics (TIC Genetics) study, finding the genes causing Tourette syndrome: objectives and methods. *European Child & Adolescent Psychiatry*. 2015;24(2):141-151.
3. Seideman MF, Seideman TA. A review of the current treatment of Tourette syndrome. *Journal of Pediatric Pharmacology and Therapeutics*. 2020;25(5):401-412. https://doi.org/10.5863/1551-6776-25.5.401. PMID: 32641910; PMCID: PMC7337131.
4. Piacentini J, Woods DW, Scahill L, et al. Behavior therapy for children with Tourette disorder: a randomized controlled trial. *JAMA*. 2010;303(19):1929-1937. https://doi.org/10.1001/jama.2010.607. PMID: 20483969; PMCID: PMC2993317.
5. Pappert EJ, Goetz CG, Louis ED, et al. Objective assessments of longitudinal outcome in Gilles de la Tourette syndrome. *Neurology*. 2003;61:936-940.
6. Prato A, Gulisano M, Scerbo M, Barone R, Vicario CM, Rizzo R. Diagnostic approach to pediatric autoimmune neuropsychiatric disorders associated with streptococcal infections (PANDAS): a narrative review of literature

data. *Frontiers in Pediatrics.* 2021;9:746639. https://doi.org/10.3389/fped.2021.746639. PMID: 34778136; PMCID: PMC8580040.

7. Sigra S, Hesselmark E, Bejerot S. Treatment of PANDAS and PANS: a systematic review. *Neuroscience & Biobehavioral Reviews.* 2018;86:51-65. https://doi.org/10.1016/j.neubiorev.2018.01.001. Epub 2018 Jan 6. PMID: 29309797.

8. Walker KG, Wilmshurst JM. An update on the treatment of Sydenham's chorea: the evidence for established and evolving interventions. *Therapeutic Advances in Neurological Disorders.* 2010;3(5):301-309.

9. Menache C, du Plessis A, Wessel D, et al. Current incidence of acute neurologic complications after open-heart operations in children. *The Annals of Thoracic Surgery.* 2002;73(6):1752-1758.

10. du Plessis AJ, Bellinger DC, Gauvreau K, et al. Neurologic outcome of choreoathetoid encephalopathy after cardiac surgery. *Pediatric Neurology.* 2002;27:9-17.

11. Jankovic J, Mejia NI. Tardive dyskinesia and withdrawal emergent syndrome in children. *Expert Review of Neurotherapeutics.* 2010;10(6):893-901.

12. Correll CU, Kane JM. One-year incidence rates of tardive dyskinesia in children and adolescents treated with second-generation antipsychotics: a systematic review. *Journal of Child and Adolescent Psychopharmacology.* 2007;17(5):647-656. https://doi.org/10.1089/cap.2006.0117.

13. Ricciardi L, Pringsheim T, Barnes TRE, et al. Treatment recommendations for tardive dyskinesia. *The Canadian Journal of Psychiatry.* 2019;64(6):388-399. https://doi.org/10.1177/0706743719828968. Epub 2019 Feb 21. PMID: 30791698; PMCID: PMC6591749.

14. Patel NJ, Jankovic J. NKX2-1-related disorders (February 20, 2014). In: Adam MP, Mirzaa GM, Pagon RA, et al., eds. *GeneReviews®* University of Washington; 1993–2023. https://www.ncbi.nlm.nih.gov/books/NBK185066/. Updated June 29, 2023.

15. Ramos EM, Oliveira J, Sobrido MJ, et al. Primary familial brain calcification. In: Adam MP, Ardinger HH, Pagon RA, et al., eds. *GeneReviews.* University of Washington; 1993–2019. https://www.ncbi.nlm.nih.gov/books/NBK1421.

16. Walker RH, Jung HH, Dobson-Stone C, et al. Neurologic phenotypes associated with acanthocytosis. *Neurology.* 2007;68:92-98.

17. Peikert K, Dobson-Stone C, Rampoldi L, et al. VPS13A disease (June 14, 2002). In: Adam MP, Mirzaa GM, Pagon RA, et al., eds. *GeneReviews®.* University of Washington; 1993–2023. https://www.ncbi.nlm.nih.gov/books/NBK1387/. Updated March 30, 2023.

18. Magro-Checa C, Zirkzee EJ, Huizinga TW, Steup-Beekman GM. Management of neuropsychiatric systemic lupus erythematosus: current approaches and future perspectives. *Drugs.* 2016;76(4):459-483. https://doi.org/10.1007/s40265-015-0534-3. PMID: 26809245; PMCID: PMC4791452.

19. Volkmann J, Benecke R. Deep brain stimulation for dystonia: patient selection and evaluation. *Movement Disorders.* 2002;17(Suppl 3):S112-S115.

20. Furukawa Y. GTP cyclohydrolase 1-deficient dopa-responsive dystonia. In: Adam MP, Ardinger HH, Pagon RA, et al., eds. *GeneReviews.* University of Washington; 1993–2019. https://www.ncbi.nlm.nih.gov/books/NBK1508.

21. Klein C, Lohmann K, Marras C, et al. Hereditary dystonia overview. In: Adam MP, Ardinger HH, Pagon RA, et al., eds. *GeneReviews.* University of Washington; 1993–2019. https://www.ncbi.nlm.nih.gov/books/NBK1155.

22. Furukawa Y, Kish S. Tyrosine hydroxylase deficiency. In: Adam MP, Ardinger HH, Pagon RA, et al., eds. *GeneReviews.* University of Washington; 1993–2019. https://www.ncbi.nlm.nih.gov/books/NBK1437.

23. Bjugstad KB, Goodman SI, Freed CR. Age at symptom onset predicts severity of motor impairment and clinical outcome of glutaric acidemia type 1. *The Journal of Pediatrics.* 2000;137:681-686.

24. Hedlund GL, Longo N, Pasquali M. Glutaric acidemia type 1. *American Journal of Medical Genetics Part C: Seminars in Medical Genetics.* 2006;142C(2):86-94.

25. Strauss KA, Lazovic J, Wintermark M, et al. Multimodal imaging of striatal degeneration in Amish patients with glutaryl-CoA dehydrogenase deficiency. *Brain.* 2007;130:1905-1920.

26. Bandmann O, Weiss KH, Kaler SG. Wilson's disease and other neurological copper disorders. *Lancet Neurology.* 2015;14(1):103-113.

27. Weiss KH. Wilson disease. In: Adam MP, Ardinger HH, Pagon RA, et al., eds. *GeneReviews.* University of Washington; 1993–2019. https://www.ncbi.nlm.nih.gov/books/NBK1512.

28. Ozelius L, Lubarr N. DYT1 Early-onset isolated dystonia. In: Adam MP, Ardinger HH, Pagon RA, et al., eds. *GeneReviews.* University of Washington; 1993–2019. https://www.ncbi.nlm.nih.gov/books/NBK1492.

29. Straussberg R, Shorer Z, Weitz R, et al. Familial infantile bilateral striatal necrosis. Clinical features and response to biotin treatment. *Neurology.* 2002;59:983-989.

30. Gregory A, Hayflick S. Pantothenate kinase-associated neurodegeneration. In: Adam MP, Ardinger HH, Pagon RA, et al., eds. *GeneReviews.* University of Washing-

ton; 1993–2019. https://www.ncbi.nlm.nih.gov/books/NBK1490.

31. Brashear A, Sweadner KJ, Cook JF, et al. ATP1A3-related neurologic disorders. In: Adam MP, Ardinger HH, Pagon RA, et al., eds. *GeneReviews*. University of Washington; 1993–2019. https://www.ncbi.nlm.nih.gov/books/NBK1115.

32. Méneret A, Trouillard O, Dunoyer M, et al. Congenital mirror movements (March 12, 2015). In: Adam MP, Feldman J, Mirzaa GM, et al., eds. *GeneReviews*®. University of Washington; 1993–2023. https://www.ncbi.nlm.nih.gov/books/NBK279760/. Updated September 24, 2020.

33. Rossor T, Yeh EA, Khakoo Y, et al.; OMS Study Group. Diagnosis and management of opsoclonus-myoclonus-ataxia syndrome in children: an international perspective. *Neurology Neuroimmunology & Neuroinflammation*. 2022;9(3):e1153. https://doi.org/10.1212/NXI.0000000000001153. PMID: 35260471; PMCID: PMC8906188.

34. Raymond D, Saunders-Pullman R, Ozelius L. SGCE myoclonus-dystonia (May 21, 2003). In: Adam MP, Feldman J, Mirzaa GM, et al, eds. *GeneReviews*®. University of Washington; 1993–2023. https://www.ncbi.nlm.nih.gov/books/NBK1414/. Updated June 4, 2020.

35. Gupta HV, Caviness JN. Post-hypoxic myoclonus: current concepts, neurophysiology, and treatment. *Tremor and Other Hyperkinetic Movements*. 2016:6;409.

36. DelRosso LM, Mogavero MP, Bruni O, Ferri R. Restless legs syndrome and restless sleep disorder in children.

Sleep Medicine Clinics. 2023 Jun;18(2):201-212. https://doi.org/10.1016/j.jsmc.2023.01.008.

37. Allen RP, Picchietti D, Hening WA, et al. Restless legs syndrome diagnosis and epidemiology workshop at the National Institutes of Health: International Restless Legs Syndrome Study Group. *Sleep Medicine*. 2003;4:101-119.

38. Kose C, Wood I, Gwyther A, et al. Sleep-related rhythmic movement disorder in young children with down syndrome: prevalence and clinical features. *Brain Sci.* 2021;11:1326. https://doi.org/10.3390/brainsci11101326.

39. Gogo E, van Sluijs RM, Cheung T, et al. Objectively confirmed prevalence of sleep-related rhythmic movement disorder in pre-school children. *Sleep Med.* 2019;53:16–21. https://doi.org/10.1016/j.sleep.2018.08.021.

40. Louis ED. Essential tremor. *New England Journal of Medicine*. 2001;345:887-891.

41. Ondo WG, Jankovic J, Connor GS, et al. Topiramate in essential tremor: a double-blind, placebo-controlled trial. *Neurology*. 2006;66:672-677.

42. Vaillencourt DE, Sturman MM, Metmann LV, eds. Deep brain stimulation of the VIM thalamic nucleus modifies several features of essential tremor. *Neurology*. 2003;61:919.

43. Cook Shukla L, Schulze J, Farlow J, et al. Parkinson disease overview. 2004 May 25 [Updated 2019 Jul 25]. In: Adam MP, Feldman J, Mirzaa GM, et al., eds. *GeneReviews*®. University of Washington; 1993–2023. https://www.ncbi.nlm.nih.gov/books/NBK1223/.

Disorders of Ocular Motility

OUTLINE

Nonparalytic Strabismus, 348
    Esotropia, 348
    Exotropia, 349
Ophthalmoplegia, 349
    Congenital Ophthalmoplegia, 349
    Acute Unilateral Ophthalmoplegia, 352
    Postviral Cranial Nerve VI Palsy, 355
    Acute Bilateral Ophthalmoplegia, 357
    Chronic Bilateral Ophthalmoplegia, 358
    Gaze Palsies, 359
    Convergence Paralysis, 360

Nystagmus, 361
    Physiological Nystagmus, 362
    Congenital Nystagmus, 362
Acquired Nystagmus, 363
    Spasmus Nutans, 363
    Pendular Nystagmus, 363
    Downbeat Nystagmus, 364
    Upbeat Nystagmus, 365
    Dissociated Nystagmus, 365
References, 365

The maintenance of binocular vision requires harmonious function of the visual sensory system, gaze centers, ocular motor nerves, neuromuscular junction, and ocular muscles. This chapter deals with nonparalytic strabismus, paralytic strabismus (ophthalmoplegia), gaze palsies, ptosis, and nystagmus. The discussion of visual and pupillary disorders is in Chapter 16.

NONPARALYTIC STRABISMUS

Abnormal ocular alignment affects 3%–4% of preschool children. Many individuals have a latent tendency for ocular misalignment, termed *heterophoria*, which becomes apparent only under stress or fatigue. During periods of misalignment, the child may have diplopia or headache. Persistent ocular misalignment is *strabismus*. Children with strabismus suppress the image from one eye to avoid diplopia. If only one eye fixates continuously, visual acuity may be lost permanently in the other (*developmental amblyopia*).

Complementary pairs of ocular muscles are yoked together; for example, when the lateral rectus pulls the left eye to the left, the medial rectus simultaneously pulls the right eye to the right. Yoking allows for conjugate gaze. In nonparalytic strabismus caused by brain injury yoking is defective due to faulty fusion or faulty control of conjugate gaze mechanisms. Each eye moves through a normal range when tested separately (*ductions*), but the eyes are disconjugate when used together (*versions*). In neurologically normal children the most common cause of nonparalytic strabismus is an inherited trait.

Ocular alignment in the newborn is usually poor, with transitory shifts of alignment from convergence to divergence. Ocular alignment usually establishes by 3–4 weeks of age but may not occur until 5 months. Approximately 2% of newborns exhibit tonic downward deviation of the eyes during the waking state, despite having normal intracranial pressure. Constant ocular alignment usually begins after 3 months of age. The eyes assume a normal position during sleep and are able to move upward reflexively.

Esotropia

Esotropia is a constant inward deviation (convergence) of the eyes. It is called alternating esotropia when fixation occurs with both eyes. Unilateral esotropia is when fixation occurs continuously with the opposite eye. Early-onset esotropia presents before 6 months of age. The observation of accommodative esotropia is usually between 2 and 3 years of age and may be undetected until adolescence.

Clinical features. Children with infantile esotropia often alternate fixation between eyes and may cross-fixate (i.e., look to the left with the right eye and to the right with the left eye). The misalignment is sufficient for family members to see that a problem exists. Some children fixate almost entirely with one eye and are at risk for permanent loss of visual acuity, *developmental amblyopia*, in the other.

Accommodative esotropia occurs when accommodation compensates for hyperopia (farsightedness). Accommodation more sharply focuses the blurred image. Because convergence accompanies accommodation, one eye turns inward. Some children with accommodative esotropia cross-fixate and use each eye alternatively, while the other maintains fixation. However, if one eye is more hyperopic than the other eye, only the better eye fixates and the unused eye has a considerable potential for amblyopia.

Diagnosis. An ophthalmologist should examine the eyes to determine whether hyperopia is present.

Management. Eyeglasses correct hyperopic errors. The treatment of early-onset esotropia, in which only one eye fixates, consists of alternate eye patching to prevent amblyopia. Early corrective surgery is required for persistent esotropia. Esotropia presenting after 6 years of age raises concern for a posterior fossa disorder such as a Chiari malformation.

Exotropia

Exotropia is an outward divergence of the eyes. It may be intermittent (exophoria) or constant (exotropia).

Clinical features. Exophoria is a relatively common condition that begins before 4 years of age. It is most often evident when the child is fatigued and fixating on a far object or in bright sunlight. The natural history of the condition is unknown. Exotropia may be congenital but poor vision in the outward-turning eye is also a cause.

Diagnosis. Exotropia is an indication to examine the eye for intraocular disease.

Management. In children with intermittent exotropia the decision to perform corrective surgery depends on the frequency and degree of the abnormality. When exotropia is constant, treatment depends on the underlying cause of visual loss.

OPHTHALMOPLEGIA

The causes of paralytic strabismus include disorders of the ocular motor nerves, the ocular muscles, or the neuromuscular junction. Table 15.1 summarizes the muscles, the nerves, and their functions. The eyes no longer move together, and diplopia is experienced. Strabismus and diplopia worsen when the child looks in the direction of action of the paralyzed muscle.

Congenital Ophthalmoplegia

Testing of eye movements is uncommon in newborns and ophthalmoplegia is often missed. It is common for strabismus to remain unnoticed for several months and then discounted as transitory esotropia. Therefore consider congenital ophthalmoplegia even when a history of ophthalmoplegia at birth is lacking.

Oculomotor Nerve Palsy/III Cranial Nerve

Clinical features. Congenital oculomotor nerve palsy usually is unilateral and complete. Pupillary reflex paralysis is variable. Other cranial nerve palsies, especially abducens, may be associated. The palsy is often unrecognized at birth. Most oculomotor nerve palsies are idiopathic, but some are genetic or caused by orbital trauma. The affected eye is exotropic and usually amblyopic. Lid retraction on attempted adduction or downward gaze may be evidence of aberrant regeneration.

TABLE 15.1	The Extraocular Muscles	
Ocular Muscles	**Innervation**	**Functions**
Lateral rectus	Abducens	Abduction
Medial rectus	Oculomotor	Adduction
Superior rectus	Oculomotor	Elevation, intorsion, adduction
Inferior rectus	Oculomotor	Depression, extorsion, adduction
Inferior oblique	Oculomotor	Extorsion, elevation, abduction
Superior oblique	Trochlear	Intorsion, depression, abduction

Diagnosis. Magnetic resonance imaging (MRI) excludes the possibility of an intracranial mass compressing the nerve. Exophthalmos suggests an orbital tumor. A nonreactive, dilated pupil excludes the diagnosis of myasthenia gravis, but a normal pupil requires testing for myasthenia.

Management. Extraocular muscle surgery may improve the cosmetic appearance but rarely improves ocular motility or visual function.

Trochlear Nerve Palsy/IV Cranial Nerve

Clinical features. Congenital superior oblique palsy is usually unilateral. Birth trauma is usually the suspected cause, but the actual cause is rarely established. Most congenital cases are idiopathic. The head tilts away from the paralyzed side to keep the eyes in alignment and avoid diplopia. The major ocular features are hypertropia, greatest in the field of action of the involved superior oblique muscle; underactivity of the paretic superior oblique muscle and overactivity of the inferior oblique muscle; and increased hypertropia when the head tilts to the paralyzed side (positive *Bielschowsky test*).

Diagnosis. Head tilt, or *torticollis* (see Chapter 14), is not a constant feature. Once examination confirms a superior oblique palsy, important etiological considerations other than congenital include trauma, myasthenia gravis, and brainstem glioma.

Management. Prisms are effective for small angle deviations; otherwise, patients require surgery.

Abducens Nerve Palsy/VI Cranial Nerve

Clinical features. Congenital abducens nerve palsy may be unilateral or bilateral and is sometimes associated with other cranial nerve palsies. Lateral movement of the affected eye(s) is limited partially or completely. Most infants use cross-fixation and thereby retain vision in both eyes. In the few reported cases of congenital palsy with pathological correlation, the abducens nerve is absent and its nucleus is hypoplastic.

Möbius syndrome is the association of congenital facial diplegia and bilateral abducens nerve palsies (see Chapter 17). *Duane syndrome* is congenital, nonprogressive horizontal ophthalmoplegia caused by aplasia of one or both nuclei of the abducens nerve with innervation of the atrophic lateral rectus by fibers of the oculomotor nerve.[1] In most cases, the cause is unknown; however, a minority are caused by mutations of the *CHN1, MAFB,* or *SALL4* genes. The characteristic features are lateral rectus palsy, some limitation of adduction, and narrowing of the palpebral fissure because of globe retraction on attempted adduction. *Möbius* and *Duane syndromes* are rhombencephalic maldevelopment syndromes often associated with lingual, palatal, respiratory, or long-track motor and coordination deficits.[2]

Diagnosis. MRI excludes the possibility of an intracranial mass lesion and hearing testing is required.

Management. Surgical procedures may be useful to correct head turn and to provide binocular single vision, but they do not restore ocular motility.

Brown Syndrome

Brown syndrome results from congenital shortening of the superior oblique muscle or tendon. The result is mechanical limitation of elevation in adduction. Usually, only one eye is involved.

Clinical features. Elevation is limited in adduction but is relatively normal in abduction. Passive elevation (forced duction) is also restricted. Other features include widening of the palpebral fissure on adduction and backward head tilt.

Diagnosis. The diagnosis of Brown syndrome requires the exclusion of acquired shortening of the superior oblique muscle. The causes of acquired shortening of the superior oblique muscle include juvenile rheumatoid arthritis, trauma, and inflammatory processes affecting the top of the orbit (see the "Orbital Inflammatory Disease" section).

Management. Surgical procedures that extend the superior oblique muscle can be useful in congenital cases.

Congenital Fibrosis of the Extraocular Muscles

Congenital fibrosis of the extraocular muscles (CFEOM) refers to at least eight distinct strabismus syndromes, defined by ophthalmological and other associated findings.[3] The types are CFEOM1A, CFEOM1B, CFEOM2, CFEOM3A, CFEOM3B, CEFOM3C, Tukel syndrome, and CFEOM3 with polymicrogyria. Multiple different genetic variants have been implicated in the various forms, and inheritance may be autosomal dominant or recessive.

Clinical features. Affected children have congenital bilateral ptosis and restrictive ophthalmoplegia, with their eyes partially or completely fixed in a downward position. CFEOM is a relatively static disorder that is phenotypically homogeneous when completely penetrant. The head is tilted back to allow vision, and diplopia is not associated despite the severe misalignment of the eyes. Identifying the inheritance pattern and associated features such as cognitive impairment, microcephaly, or oligodactyly aids in differentiating various subtypes.

Diagnosis. The clinical findings and the family history are key for diagnosis. Genetic testing is available.

Management. The goal of treatment is improvement of vision by correcting ptosis.

Congenital Myasthenia Gravis

Several clinical syndromes of myasthenia gravis occur in the newborn (see Chapter 6) and child. Congenital myasthenic syndromes (CMSs) are genetic disorders of the neuromuscular junction. They are classified as presynaptic, synaptic, or postsynaptic. Multiple genetic defects have been associated with each subtype, and both autosomal dominant and autosomal recessive inheritance can be seen. Here, we will focus solely on the defects in which ophthalmoplegia or ptosis are a primary presenting symptom. This is merely a brief overview of the many distinct CMSs and should not be considered an exhaustive reference.

Clinical features. General features of congenital myasthenia in the newborn include respiratory insufficiency with ptosis, ophthalmoplegia, feeding difficulties or choking spells. In infants and children general signs and symptoms may include delayed acquisition of motor skills, speech problems, and difficulty coughing or swallowing in addition to ocular symptoms. Ptosis usually fluctuates depending on the infant's degree of fatigue; it may involve both eyes or just one. Ophthalmoplegia may fluctuate or present as a static deficit. Associated extraocular findings help narrow the genetic workup.

Approximately 50% of CMSs are due to postsynaptic deficits. Of these, the most common is acetylcholine receptor (AchR) deficiency, which may be due to pathogenic variants in the *CHRNA1*, *CHRNB1*, *CHRND*, or *CHRNE* genes. Phenotypes are variable but include early-onset ptosis, ophthalmoplegia, and bulbar and limb weakness ranging from mild to severe. Deficits in the AchR clustering pathway account for much of the remaining postsynaptic forms, which present with ptosis with or without associated ophthalmoplegia; associated weakness may be severe, and some affected infants experience acute respiratory failure which overshadows any ophthalmologic concerns.

Synaptic CMSs include endplate acetylcholinesterase deficiency due to pathogenic *COLQ* variants, which are often characterized by severe weakness, external ophthalmoplegia, and slowed pupillary light response.

Presynaptic CMSs are uncommon. Pathogenic *VAMP1* variants cause ophthalmoplegia, severe hypotonia, and feeding difficulty. *MYO9A* mutations cause ptosis, ophthalmoplegia, and weakness in addition to developmental delays or intellectual disability.[4]

Diagnosis. Suspect the diagnosis in any newborn with bilateral ptosis or limitation of eye movement, particularly if respiratory distress is also present. Repetitive nerve stimulation of the limbs at a frequency of 3 Hz may evoke a decremental response after 5–10 minutes of stimulation; single nerve testing is often helpful. If clinical suspicion is high, consider testing a nerve in the face if two limbs produce negative results. Multigene panels are available and are usually the most efficient route to diagnosis.

Management. Management depends, to some extent, on the underlying genetic deficit. Some CMSs respond to acetylcholinesterase inhibitors while others do not. All affected children require a developmental evaluation and implementation of therapies as indicated. Monitor feeding, nutrition, and pulmonary function. Assess periodically for joint contractures and consider involvement of orthopedics or physical medicine and rehabilitation.

Congenital Ptosis

Congenital drooping of one or both lids is relatively common, and the drooping is unilateral in 70% of cases. It is caused by dysgenesis of the levator palpebrae superioris muscle, which is the main elevator of the upper lid. It is usually idiopathic, but at times may be associated with an underlying genetic syndrome.

Clinical features. Congenital ptosis may be unnoticed until early childhood or even adult life and then misdiagnosed as an "acquired" ptosis. Miosis is sometimes an associated feature and suggests the possibility of Horner syndrome, except that the pupil responds normally to pharmacological agents. Some patients have synkinesis between the oculomotor and trigeminal nerves; jaw movements produce opening of the eye (*Marcus-Gunn phenomenon*).

Diagnosis. Box 15.1 lists the differential diagnosis of ptosis. Distinguishing congenital ptosis from acquired ptosis is essential. The examination of baby pictures is

BOX 15.1   Causes of Ptosis

Congenital
- Congenital fibrosis of extraocular muscles
- Horner syndrome[a]
- Myasthenia[a]
- Oculomotor nerve palsy[a]

Acquired
- Horner syndrome[a]
- Lid inflammation
- Mitochondrial myopathies (see Chapter 8)
- Myasthenia gravis[a]
- Oculomotor nerve palsy[a]
- Orbital cellulitis
- Recurrent painful optic neuropathy
- Trauma

[a]The most common conditions and the ones with disease modifying treatments.

more cost-effective than MRI to make the distinction. The presence of other eye abnormalities such as blepharophimosis or epicanthus inversus should prompt a genetic workup.

Management. If ptosis is severe enough to compromise vision, then early corrective surgery is essential to avoid the development of amblyopia. Otherwise, no treatment is required, although surgery is often pursued for cosmetic reasons.

Acute Unilateral Ophthalmoplegia

Box 15.2 summarizes the causes of acquired ophthalmoplegia. The discussion of many of these conditions is in other chapters.

In acute ophthalmoplegia symptoms peak within 1 week. The deficit may be partial or complete (Box 15.3). Generalized increased intracranial pressure is always an

BOX 15.2   Causes of Acquired Ophthalmoplegia

Brainstem
- Brainstem encephalitis[a] (see Chapter 10)
- Intoxication
- Multiple sclerosis[a] (see Chapter 10)
- Subacute necrotizing encephalopathy (see Chapter 10)
- Tumor
  - Brainstem glioma[a]
  - Craniopharyngioma (see Chapter 16)
  - Leukemia
  - Lymphoma
  - Metastases
  - Pineal region tumors
- Vascular
  - Arteriovenous malformation
  - Hemorrhage
  - Infarction
  - Migraine[a]
  - Vasculitis

Nerve
- Familial recurrent cranial neuropathies (see Chapter 17)
- Increased intracranial pressure (see Chapter 4)
- Infectious
  - Diphtheria
  - Gradenigo syndrome
  - Meningitis (see Chapter 4)
  - Orbital cellulitis
- Inflammatory
  - Miller Fisher syndrome[a] (see Chapter 10)

- Polyradiculoneuropathy (see Chapter 7)
- Sarcoid
- Postinfectious
- Trauma
  - Head
  - Orbital
- Tumor
  - Cavernous sinus hemangioma
  - Orbital tumors
  - Sellar and parasellar tumors (see Chapter 16)
  - Sphenoid sinus tumors
- Vascular
  - Aneurysm
  - Carotid-cavernous fistula
  - Cavernous sinus thrombosis
  - Migraine

Neuromuscular Transmission
- Botulism[a] (see Chapter 7)
- Myasthenia gravis[a]
- Tick paralysis

Myopathies
- Fiber-type disproportion myopathies (see Chapter 6)
- Kearns-Sayre syndrome
- Mitochondrial myopathies (see Chapter 8)
- Orbital inflammatory disease
- Thyroid disease
- Vitamin E deficiency

[a]The most common conditions and the ones with disease modifying treatments.

- Aneurysm[a,b]
- Brain tumors
  - Brainstem glioma
  - Parasellar tumors (see Chapter 16)
  - Tumors of pineal region (see Chapter 4)
- Brainstem stroke[a]
- Cavernous sinus fistula
- Cavernous sinus thrombosis
- Gradenigo syndrome
- Idiopathic ocular motor nerve palsy[a]
- Increased intracranial pressure (see Chapter 4)
- Multiple sclerosis[a] (see Chapter 10)
- Myasthenia gravis[a]
- Ophthalmoplegic migraine[a,b]
- Orbital inflammatory disease[a,b]
- Orbital tumor[b]
- Recurrent familial[a] (see Chapter 17)
- Trauma
  - Head
  - Orbital

[a]May be recurrent.
[b]May be associated with pain.

important consideration in patients with unilateral or bilateral abducens palsy (see Chapter 4).

Aneurysm

The full discussion of arterial aneurysms is in Chapter 4, because the important clinical feature in children is hemorrhage rather than nerve compression. This section deals only with possible ophthalmoplegic features.

Clinical features. Aneurysms at the junction of the internal carotid and posterior communicating arteries are an important cause of unilateral oculomotor palsy in adults; these are less frequent in children but remain an important consideration in any case of acquired cranial nerve III palsy. Compression of the nerve by expansion of the aneurysm causes the weakness. Intense pain in and around the eye is frequently experienced at the time of hemorrhage, but prior to rupture the symptoms are painless. Because the parasympathetic fibers are at the periphery of the nerve, mydriasis is an almost constant feature of ophthalmoplegia caused by aneurysms of the posterior communicating artery. However, pupillary involvement may develop several days after the onset of an incomplete external ophthalmoplegia. A normal

pupil with complete external ophthalmoplegia makes aneurysm very unlikely.

Sometimes, aneurysms affect the superior branch of the oculomotor nerve earlier and more severely than the inferior branch. Ptosis may precede the development of other signs by hours or days.

Diagnosis. Contrast-enhanced MRI and magnetic resonance angiography or computed tomography (CT) angiogram identify most aneurysms.

Management. Surgical intervention is the treatment of choice whenever technically feasible. Oculomotor function often returns to normal after the procedure.

Brainstem Glioma

Brainstem glioma is a general term that encompasses any tumor of glial origin arising in the brainstem, including diffuse intrinsic pontine glioma (DIPG) and pilocytic astrocytoma. DIPG is by far the most common form, comprising 75%–80% of childhood brainstem glioma. Onset is usually between 5 and 10 years of age. Symptoms progress rapidly and diagnosis is rarely delayed more than 6 months after onset; one exception is children with neurofibromatosis type I who may have slowly growing pilocytic astrocytomas discovered during routine screening studies.

Clinical features. Abducens palsy is one of the most common presenting signs, in addition to other cranial neuropathies, spasticity, and ataxia. DIPG can cause obstructive hydrocephalus and some children present primarily with symptoms of increased intracranial pressure such as positional headache, vomiting, and altered mental status. Intractable vomiting may also occur due to direct irritation of the brainstem emetic center.

Unfortunately, DIPG has a terrible prognosis due to its location, and survival is typically less than 1 year. Children with pilocytic astrocytoma have a much better outlook and 5-year survival is over 90%.[5]

Diagnosis. MRI delineates the tumor well and differentiates tumor from inflammatory and vascular disorders (Fig. 15.1). DIPG can often be diagnosed based on imaging findings alone. Biopsy is typically required for pilocytic astrocytomas.

Management. As with most childhood brain tumors, there are no clearly established treatment guidelines. Pilocytic astrocytomas can sometimes be resected but this is rarely the case for DIPG. Radiation treatment is often used with or without chemotherapy, although

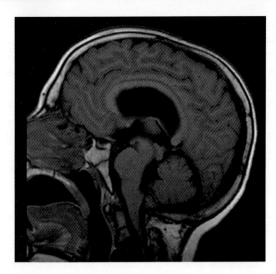

Fig. 15.1 Brainstem Glioma. T$_1$ sagittal magnetic resonance imaging shows a distorted and homogeneous pons.

evidence for the use of specific chemotherapeutic regimens is scarce. Increasing recognition of genetic markers may help guide treatment in the future.

Brainstem Stroke

Box 11.2 summarizes the causes of stroke in children. Small brainstem hemorrhages resulting from emboli, leukemia, or blood dyscrasias have the potential to cause isolated ocular motor palsies, but this is not the rule. Other cranial nerves are also involved, and hemiparesis, ataxia, and decreased consciousness are often associated features.

Carotid-Cavernous Sinus Fistula

Clinical features. Arteriovenous communications between the carotid artery and the cavernous sinus may be congenital, but trauma is more common in children. The carotid artery or one of its branches ruptures into the cavernous sinus, increasing pressure in the venous system. The results are a pulsating proptosis, redness and swelling of the conjunctiva, increased intraocular pressure, and ophthalmoplegia. If a bruit is present over the eye, compression of the ipsilateral carotid artery reduces the volume.

Diagnosis. Carotid arteriography reveals rapid cavernous sinus filling, poor filling of the distal intracranial branches, and engorgement of and retrograde flow within venous drainage pathways.

Management. Transarterial balloon embolization or coiling of the affected cavernous sinus is the mainstay of treatment.

Cavernous Sinus Thrombosis

Cavernous sinus thrombosis may produce either unilateral or bilateral ophthalmoplegia. The cause is usually the anterograde spread of infection from the mouth, face, nose, or paranasal sinuses.

Clinical features. Cavernous sinus thrombosis is a rare complication of otitis media, mastoiditis, or dental infections. The child develops fever, malaise, and frontal headache, followed by increasingly severe symptoms, including proptosis, orbital congestion, ptosis, external ophthalmoplegia, pupillary paralysis, and blindness. The infection begins in one cavernous sinus and may spread to the other. If untreated, it may extend to the meninges. Even with vigorous antibiotic treatment, the mortality rate is 8% and neurological morbidity approaches 25%.[6]

Diagnosis. The ocular signs may suggest orbital cellulitis or orbital pseudotumor. The cerebrospinal fluid is normal early in the course. A mixed leukocytosis develops, and the protein concentration is moderately elevated even in the absence of meningitis. Once the meninges are involved, the pressure becomes elevated, the leukocytosis increases, and the glucose concentration falls.

Cranial CT may show clouding of infected paranasal sinuses but fails to show the thrombus. Contrast-enhanced MRI or CT are the most sensitive diagnostic modalities.

Management. Intravenous antibiotic therapy similar to that used to treat meningitis. Surgical drainage of infected paranasal sinuses is sometimes necessary.

Gradenigo Syndrome

Clinical features. The abducens nerve lies adjacent to the medial aspect of the petrous bone before entering the cavernous sinus. Infections of the middle ear sometimes extend to the petrous bone and cause thrombophlebitis of the inferior petrosal sinus. The infection involves not only the abducens nerve but also the facial nerve and the trigeminal ganglion. The resulting syndrome consists of ipsilateral paralysis of abduction, facial palsy, and facial pain.

Diagnosis. The combination of unilateral abducens and facial palsy also occurs after closed head injuries. The diagnosis of Gradenigo syndrome requires the demonstration of middle ear infection. CT of the mastoid bone shows the infection. Lumbar puncture reveals a cellular response and an elevation of protein content.

Management. Prompt antibiotic therapy prevents permanent nerve damage.

Postviral Cranial Nerve VI Palsy

Isolated unilateral abducens nerve palsy can occur following viral infections, although it is a diagnosis of exclusion. Abducens palsy has been reported in the setting of otherwise asymptomatic SARS-CoV-2 infection.[7]

Myasthenia Gravis

The discussion of some neonatal forms of myasthenia is in Chapter 6; congenital myasthenia is included in the "Congenital Ophthalmoplegia" section earlier in this chapter, and limb-girdle myasthenia in Chapter 7. This section describes the immune-mediated form of myasthenia encountered from late infancy through adult life. The two clinical forms are *ocular myasthenia*, which primarily or exclusively affects the eye muscles, and *generalized myasthenia*, in which weakness of bulbar and limb muscles is moderate to severe. Autoantibodies against the nicotinic AchR cause 85% of cases. Most of the remainder are caused by antibodies against muscle-specific kinase (MuSK) or lipoprotein receptor–related protein 4 (LRP4). MuSK and LRP4 are both proteins involved in facilitating the clustering of AchRs, thus enabling muscle excitability.

Clinical features. The initial symptoms do not appear until after 6 months of age; 75% of children first have symptoms after age 10. Prepubertal onset is associated with a male predominance, only ocular symptoms, and seronegativity for AChR antibodies, whereas postpubertal onset is associated with a strong female preference, generalized myasthenia, and seropositivity. In general the disease is less severe in boys than in girls.

The initial features of both the ocular and the generalized form are usually ptosis, diplopia, or both. Myasthenia is the most common cause of acquired unilateral or bilateral ptosis. Pupillary function is normal. Between 40% and 50% of patients have weakness of other bulbar or limb muscles at the onset of ocular symptoms. Ocular motor weakness is generally not constant initially, and the specific muscles affected may change from examination to examination. Usually both eyes are affected, but one is more affected than the other.

Children with ocular myasthenia may have mild facial weakness and easy fatigability of the limbs. However, they do not have respiratory distress or difficulty speaking or swallowing. The subsequent courses of ocular myasthenia may be one of steady progression to complete ophthalmoplegia or by relapses and remissions. The relapses are of varying severity and last for weeks to years. At least 20% of patients have permanent remissions. Prepubertal onset is more commonly associated with spontaneous remission than postpubertal onset.

Children with generalized myasthenia have generalized weakness within 1 year of the initial ocular symptoms. The symptoms include dysarthria, dysphagia, difficulty chewing, and limb muscle fatigability. Spontaneous remissions are unusual. Respiratory insufficiency (*myasthenic crisis*) occurs in one-third of untreated children.

Children with generalized myasthenia, but not those with ocular myasthenia, have a higher than expected incidence of other autoimmune disorders, especially thyroiditis and collagen vascular diseases. Thymoma is present in 15% of adults with generalized myasthenia but occurs in less than 5% of children. When thymoma occurs in children, it is likely to be malignant.

Diagnosis. Ptosis worsens with fatigue. Ask the child to sustain upgaze for as long as possible; patients with untreated ocular myasthenia will develop ptosis relatively rapidly. Some physicians use the *ice-pack test*, which involves placing a very cold compress on the ptotic lid for 2 minutes. Partial opening of the lid suggests myasthenia. Five minutes of resting with the eye closed may accomplish the same result without the ice pack.

Repetitive nerve stimulation is useful for diagnosing generalized myasthenia but is less sensitive for ocular myasthenia. Single-fiber EMG is much more sensitive for ocular myasthenia and is the preferred electrophysiologic study.

Eighty-five percent of patients with generalized immune-mediated myasthenia have elevated serum concentrations of antibodies against the AChR. MuSK or LRP4 antibodies account for the remaining 15%; rarely other antibodies can be detected such as those against cortactin or agrin. Negative antibody tests should prompt consideration of genetic testing to rule out congenital myasthenia gravis, particularly if the child has other symptoms such as intellectual disability or a history of neonatal respiratory distress. Conversely, LARP4 and cortactin antibodies are not disease-specific and can be seen in other autoimmune conditions, so care must be taken in interpretation of positive results.[8]

Management. The basis for managing nongenetic myasthenia in children is experience and retrospective studies, primarily done in adults.[9] Children with ocular myasthenia, but not those with generalized myasthenia, have a reasonable hope of spontaneous remission. Anticholinesterase therapy is the treatment of choice for ocular myasthenia. The initial dose of neostigmine is 0.5 mg/kg every 4 hours in children younger than 5 years and 0.25 mg/kg in older children, not to exceed 15 mg per dose in any child. The equivalent dose of pyridostigmine is four times greater. After initiating treatment, the dose slowly increases as needed and tolerated. Diarrhea and gastrointestinal cramps are the usual limiting factors. In general pyridostigmine is more effective at treating ptosis than diplopia.

Several retrospective studies in adults suggest that early immunotherapy[10,11] and thymectomy reduce the conversion of ocular myasthenia to generalized myasthenia. Evidence for children is lacking.

Recurrent Painful Ophthalmoplegic Neuropathy

Recurrent painful ophthalmoplegic neuropathy (RPON), previously referred to as ophthalmoplegic migraine, is a rare entity that is poorly understood. The mechanism remains unknown, but there seems to be a genetic connection to migraine given the strong family history of migraine in affected patients.

Clinical features. RPON occurs most frequently in children under the age of 10, with a male preponderance. The child typically presents with a headache and unilateral cranial nerve III palsy, although there are reports of CN IV and CN VI involvement. Pupillary responses may be affected. The associated headache may or may not be migrainous. Photophobia, nausea, and vomiting are common. Headaches may be prolonged, lasting up to a week.

Ophthalmoplegia may not occur simultaneously to the headache and has been reported to start up to 14 days after a headache attack. Ophthalmoplegia self-resolves with time but may persist for weeks or even months.

Diagnosis. Cranial neuropathy in the setting of headache is always worrisome, and most patients will undergo contrasted MRI of the brain and orbits to rule out tumor, vascular abnormalities, or other pathologies. Diagnosis is based on the history of past and present attacks; formal criteria have been suggested by the International Headache Society.

Management. There are no evidence-based treatment guidelines for RPON. Because there have been some studies suggesting an inflammatory mechanism, steroids may be used, but there is limited evidence of efficacy. Pregabalin and indomethacin have been reported to be effective in some case reports.[12,13] Prophylaxis with calcium channel blockers, beta blockers, or topiramate is only indicated if the child also suffers from typical migraines.

Orbital Inflammatory Disease

The term *orbital inflammatory disease* encompasses a group of nonspecific inflammatory conditions involving the orbit. Inflammation may be diffuse or localized to specific tissues within the orbit. The differential diagnosis includes idiopathic inflammatory orbit disease, orbital myositis, dacryoadenitis, sarcoidosis, Graves disease, histiocytosis, orbital pseudotumor, lymphoproliferative disease, Wegener granulomatosis, rhabdomyosarcoma, retinoblastoma, and neuroblastoma.[14]

Clinical features. The disorder is unusual before the age of 20 years but may occur as early as 3 months of age. Males and females are equally affected. Acute and chronic forms exist. The main features are pain, ophthalmoplegia, proptosis, and lid edema evolving over several days or weeks. One or both eyes may be involved. Ocular motility is disturbed in part by proptosis but mainly by myositis. Some patients have only myositis, whereas others have inflammation in other orbital structures. Vision is initially preserved, but loss of vision is a threat if the condition remains untreated.

Diagnosis. The development of unilateral pain and proptosis in a child suggests an orbital tumor. Bilateral proptosis suggests thyroid myopathy. MRI shows a soft tissue mass without sinus involvement or bone erosion. Orbital involvement by lymphoma or leukemia produces a similar imaging appearance. The extraocular muscles may appear enlarged. Biopsy should be considered in cases where refractory or rebound inflammation is noted during or after steroid treatment.

Management. Orbital inflammatory disease has a self-limited course, but treatment is required to prevent vision loss or permanent ophthalmoplegia. Administer prednisone, 1 mg/kg/day, for at least 1 month before tapering. Reinitiate the full dose if the disorder recurs during the taper. Treatment of the underlying inflammatory disorder is required.

Orbital Tumors

Clinical features. The initial feature of intraorbital tumors is proptosis, ophthalmoplegia, or rarely ptosis. When the globe displaces forward, the palpebral fissure widens, and closing the eye fully may not be possible. The exposed portion of the eye becomes dry and erythematous and may develop exposure keratitis. The direction of displacement of the globe is the best clue to the tumor's position. Ophthalmoplegia may occur because of forward displacement of the globe, causing direct pressure on one or more ocular muscles.

Diagnosis. The differential diagnosis of proptosis in children includes infection and inflammation, hemorrhage and other vascular disorders, orbital tumors, hyperthyroidism and other metabolic disorders, developmental anomalies, and Hand-Schüller-Christian disease (a form of Langerhans cell histiocytosis) and related disorders; some are idiopathic. The most common orbital tumors are dermoid cyst, hemangioma, metastatic neuroblastoma, anterior visual pathway glioma, and rhabdomyosarcoma. Orbit CT and MRI, and biopsy are necessary for the diagnosis and selection of treatment.

Management. Treatment varies with the tumor type. Many require surgical resection.

Trauma

Trauma accounts for 40% of isolated acquired ocular motor nerve palsies and 55% of multiple nerve palsies in children. Hemorrhage and edema into the nerves or muscles may occur from closed head injuries even in the absence of direct orbital injury. In the presence of orbital fractures the nerves and muscles are vulnerable to laceration, avulsion, or entrapment by bone fragments.

Clinical features. Superior oblique palsy, caused by trochlear nerve damage, is a relatively common consequence of closed head injuries. Usually the trauma is severe, often causing loss of consciousness, but it may be mild. The palsy is more often unilateral than bilateral. Patients with unilateral superior oblique palsy have a marked hypertropia in the primary position and a compensatory head tilt to preserve fusion; 65% of cases resolve spontaneously. When bilateral involvement is present, the hypertropia is milder and alternates

between the two eyes; spontaneous recovery occurs in only 25% of cases.

Transient lateral rectus palsy is rare in newborns and is attributed to birth trauma. The palsy is unilateral and clears completely within 6 weeks.

Diagnosis. Direct injuries to the orbit with associated hemorrhage and swelling do not pose a diagnostic dilemma. CT of the head with orbital views shows the extent of fracture so that the need for surgical intervention can be determined. CT may also show a lateral midbrain hemorrhage as the cause of trochlear nerve palsy.

A delay between the time of injury and the onset of ophthalmoplegia makes diagnosis more problematic. The possible mechanisms of delayed ophthalmoplegia following trauma to the head include progressive local edema in the orbit; progressive brainstem edema; progressive increased intracranial pressure; development of meningitis, mastoiditis, or petrous osteomyelitis; venous sinus or carotid artery thrombosis; and carotid-cavernous fistula.

Management. Local trauma and fracture of the orbit may require surgical repair. Surgery directed at rebalancing the extraocular muscles sometimes improves vision after permanent paralysis of ocular motor nerves following head injury. Botulinum toxin is another treatment option for bilateral sixth nerve palsies.

Acute Bilateral Ophthalmoplegia

Many of the conditions that cause acute unilateral ophthalmoplegia (see Box 15.3) may also cause acute bilateral ophthalmoplegia. The conditions listed in Box 15.4

> **BOX 15.4   Causes of Acute Bilateral Ophthalmoplegia**
>
> - Basilar meningitis (see Chapter 4)
> - Brainstem encephalitis[a] (see Chapter 10)
> - Carotid-cavernous fistula
> - Cavernous sinus thrombosis
> - Diphtheria
> - Intoxication
> - Miller Fisher syndrome[a] (see Chapter 10)
> - Myasthenia gravis[a]
> - Polyradiculoneuropathy (see Chapter 7)
> - Subacute necrotizing encephalomyelopathy (see Chapter 5)
> - Tick paralysis (see Chapter 7)
>
> [a]The most common conditions and the ones with disease modifying treatments.

often have a high incidence of bilateral involvement. The discussion of thyroid ophthalmopathy occurs only with chronic conditions because progression of ophthalmoplegia usually occurs over a period greater than 1 week.

Botulism

Several strains of the bacterium *Clostridium botulinum* elaborate a toxin that disturbs neuromuscular transmission. The discussion of the infantile form of botulism, which causes ptosis but not ophthalmoplegia, is in Chapter 6. This section deals with late-onset cases.

Clinical features. The cause of botulism is most often the ingestion of a toxin in home-canned food. This is most likely when canning at high altitudes, where the boiling temperature is too low to destroy spores. Because *C. botulinum* spores are ubiquitous in soil, infection may also follow burns, wounds, and the sharing of needles among drug addicts. Blurred vision, diplopia, dizziness, dysarthria, and dysphagia begin 12–36 hours after ingestion of the toxin. The pupillary response is usually normal. An ascending paralysis similar to Guillain-Barré syndrome follows the early symptoms and may lead to death from respiratory paralysis. Patients remain conscious and alert throughout. Most patients make a complete recovery within 2–3 months, but those with severe involvement may not return to normal for a year.

Diagnosis. The presence of ophthalmoplegia, and the EMG findings, distinguishes botulism from Guillain-Barré syndrome. Motor and sensory nerve conduction velocities are normal, the amplitude of evoked muscle action potentials reduced, and a decremental response is not ordinarily present at low rates of stimulation, although facilitation may be present at high rates of stimulation. Showing the organism or the toxin in food, stool, or a wound establishes the diagnosis.

Management. Intravenous botulism immune globulin is the recommended treatment. Assure the availability of mechanical respiratory support when the diagnosis is suspect.

Intoxications

Clinical features. Anticonvulsants, tricyclic antidepressants, and many other psychoactive drugs selectively impair ocular motility at toxic blood concentrations. Overdose may be accidental or intentional. A child, found unconscious, arrives at the emergency department. The state of consciousness varies from obtundation to stupor, but the eyes do not move, either

by rapidly rotating the head laterally or with ice water irrigation of the ears. Complete ophthalmoplegia is expected in a comatose child if brainstem function is otherwise impaired (see Chapter 2), but in a noncomatose child with otherwise intact brainstem function, ingestion of a drug that selectively impairs ocular motility should be suspected.

Diagnosis. Question the family about drugs available in the household and screen the blood and urine for toxic substances.

Management. Specific treatment depends on the drug ingested; in most cases, supportive care is sufficient.

Chronic Bilateral Ophthalmoplegia

Box 15.5 lists the conditions responsible for bilateral ophthalmoplegia developing over a period longer than 1 week. The discussion of most conditions is in previous sections of this chapter or in other chapters.

Thyroid Ophthalmopathy

The association of ophthalmopathy with hyperthyroidism is not causal. The two conditions are associated autoimmune diseases. One hypothesis suggests the presence of a cross-reacting antigen in thyroid and orbital tissues. Myasthenia gravis may be associated as well.

BOX 15.5 Causes of Chronic Bilateral Ophthalmoplegia

- Brainstem glioma
- Chronic meningitis (see Chapter 4)
- Chronic orbital inflammation
- Kearns-Sayre syndrome
- Myasthenia gravis[a]
  - Thyroid orbitopathy[a]
  - Congenital
  - Juvenile
- Myopathies
  - Fiber-type disproportion myopathy (see Chapter 6)
  - Mitochondrial myopathies (see Chapter 8)
  - Myotubular myopathy (see Chapter 6)
  - Oculopharyngeal muscular dystrophy (see Chapter 17)
- Subacute necrotizing encephalomyelopathy (see Chapter 5)
- Thyroid disease[a]
- Vitamin E deficiency

[a]The most common conditions and the ones with disease modifying treatments.

Clinical features. Disorders of ocular motility are sometimes present in most patients with hyperthyroidism and may precede systemic features of nervousness, heat intolerance, diaphoresis, weight loss, tachycardia, tremulousness, and weakness. The main orbital pathology is a myopathy of the extraocular muscles. They become inflamed, swollen with interstitial edema, and finally fibrotic. If the two eyes are equally affected, the patient may not complain of diplopia despite considerable limitation of ocular motility. Staring or lid retraction occurs in more than 50% of cases, lid lag on downward gaze in 30%–50%, and proptosis (exophthalmos) in almost 90%. Severe exophthalmos is due to edema and infiltration of all orbital structures.

Diagnosis. Thyroid disease is a consideration in any child with evolving ophthalmoplegia. CT of the orbit shows enlargement of the extraocular muscles. Thyroid function tests are often normal, but a thyroid-releasing hormone stimulation test and a measure of the concentration of thyroid-stimulating immunoglobulin may confirm the diagnosis.

Management. Meticulous control of hyperthyroidism does not necessarily cure ophthalmopathy. While treating hyperthyroidism, avoid overtreatment causing hypothyroidism. If the exophthalmos progresses, even after the patient is euthyroid, corticosteroids may prevent further proptosis, but persistent optic nerve compression requires surgical decompression. Newer biologics such as teprotumumab (Tepezza) offer an additional treatment option specifically for thyroid ophthalmopathy.

Kearns-Sayre Syndrome

Nearly all cases of Kearns-Sayre syndrome (KSS) are sporadic and caused by a single large deletion or duplication of the mitochondrial DNA (mtDNA), arising either in the maternal oocyte or in early embryonic life.[15]

Clinical features. The triad of progressive external ophthalmoplegia, onset before age 20 years, and at least one of the following: short stature, pigmentary retinopathy, cerebellar ataxia, heart block, and elevated cerebrospinal fluid protein (>100 mg/dL) define KSS. The onset is so insidious that patients usually do not complain of diplopia. The clinical course is progressive, but life expectancy can be normal with appropriate support.

Diagnosis. The basis for diagnosis is the major clinical criteria. Electrocardiographic monitoring for cardiac arrhythmia and cerebrospinal fluid examination are essential.

Management. Treatment with vitamins or coenzyme Q, depending on the specific respiratory complex defect, is common but of uncertain benefit. This mitochondrial cocktail includes riboflavin 100 mg/day, pyridoxine 20 mg/kg/day, coenzyme Q 10–20 mg/kg/day, biotin 5–20 mg/day, and carnitine 50–100 mg/kg/day. Ongoing ophthalmologic, nutritional, and endocrinologic surveillance is recommended, and regular cardiac evaluations are vital. A cardiac pacemaker may be lifesaving.

Gaze Palsies

This section deals with supranuclear palsies. The examiner must show that the eyes move normally in response to brainstem gaze center reflexes (doll's head maneuver, caloric testing, and Bell phenomenon) to verify supranuclear palsy. Box 15.6 gives the differential diagnosis of gaze palsies.

Apraxia of Horizontal Gaze

Ocular motor apraxia is a deficiency in voluntary, horizontal, lateral, fast eye movements (saccades) with retention of slow pursuit movements. Bringing the eyes to a desired position requires jerking movements of the head. The rapid phases of optokinetic nystagmus are absent.

Congenital Ocular Motor Apraxia

Clinical features. Although ocular motor apraxia is present at birth, detection is not until late infancy. Failure of fixation raises questions concerning visual impairment. Refixation requires overshooting head thrusts, often accompanied by blinking of the eyes. With the head held immobile, the child makes no effort to initiate horizontal eye movements.

Many children with ocular motor apraxia have other signs of cerebral abnormality, such as psychomotor delays, learning disabilities, and clumsiness. When hypotonia is present, the child may have difficulty making the head movements needed for refixation. Agenesis of the corpus callosum and agenesis of the cerebellar vermis are comorbidities in some children. The association does not indicate that the malformations are responsible for ocular motor apraxia.

Diagnosis. Consider the possibility of ocular motor apraxia in any infant referred for evaluation of visual impairment. Children with ocular motor apraxia require brain MRI to search for other cerebral malformations,

BOX 15.6   Gaze Palsies

Apraxia of Horizontal Gaze
- Ataxia-telangiectasia (see Chapter 10)
- Ataxia-ocular motor apraxia (see Chapter 10)
- Brainstem glioma
- Congenital ocular motor apraxia
- Huntington disease (see Chapter 5)

Internuclear Ophthalmoplegia
- Brainstem stroke
- Brainstem tumor
- Exotropia (pseudointernuclear ophthalmoplegia [INO])
- Multiple sclerosis
- Myasthenia gravis (pseudo-INO)
- Toxic-metabolic

Vertical Gaze Palsy
- Aqueductal stenosis (see Chapter 18)
- Congenital vertical ocular motor apraxia
- Gaucher disease (see Chapter 5)

- Hydrocephalus (see Chapters 4 and 184, 18)
- Miller Fisher syndrome (see Chapter 10)
- Niemann-Pick disease type C (see Chapter 5)
- Tumor (see Chapter 4)
  - Midbrain
  - Pineal region
  - Third ventricle

Horizontal Gaze Palsy
- Adversive seizures (see Chapter 1)
- Brainstem tumors
- Destructive lesions of the frontal lobe (see Chapter 11)
- Familial horizontal gaze palsy

Convergence Paralysis
- Head trauma
- Idiopathic
- Multiple sclerosis (see Chapter 10)
- Pineal region tumors (see Chapter 4)

---

and tests for ataxia-telangiectasia (see Chapter 10) and lysosomal storage diseases (see Chapter 5).

Management. Management depends on the underlying condition. Reading is often difficult, even if the affected child has normal intelligence, and educational accommodations are required.

Internuclear Ophthalmoplegia

The medial longitudinal fasciculus (MLF) contains fibers that connect the abducens nucleus to the contralateral oculomotor nucleus to perform horizontal conjugate lateral gaze. Unilateral lesions in the MLF disconnect the two nuclei, so that, when the patient attempts a lateral gaze, the adducting eye ipsilateral to the abnormal MLF is unable to move medially but the abducting eye is able to move laterally. Nystagmus (actually *overshoot dysmetria*) is often present in the abducting eye. This symptom complex, which may be unilateral or bilateral, is called *internuclear ophthalmoplegia* (INO). The usual cause of unilateral INO is vascular occlusive disease, and the cause of bilateral INO is either demyelinating disease or, rarely, toxic-metabolic causes.

Patients with myasthenia gravis sometimes have ocular motility dysfunction that resembles an INO except that nystagmus is usually lacking. The disorder is a *pseudo-INO* because the MLF is intact. Exotropia is another cause of pseudo-INO. When the normal eye is fixating

in full abduction, there is no visual stimulus to bring the paretic eye into full adduction. Nystagmus is not present in the abducting eye.

The combination of an INO in one direction of lateral gaze and complete gaze palsy in the other is termed a *one-and-a-half syndrome.* The underlying pathology is a unilateral lesion in the dorsal pontine tegmentum that affects the pontine lateral gaze center and the adjacent MLF. Multiple sclerosis is the usual cause. Other causes include brainstem glioma, infraction, or myasthenia gravis.

Toxic-Metabolic Disorders

Clinical features. Toxic doses of several drugs may produce the clinical syndrome of INO. Usually, the patient is comatose and may have complete ophthalmoplegia that evolves into a bilateral INO. The drugs reported to produce INO include amitriptyline, barbiturates, carbamazepine, doxepin, phenothiazine, and phenytoin. INO may also occur during hepatic coma.

Diagnosis. Drug intoxication is always a consideration in children with decreased consciousness who were previously well. The presence of INO following drug ingestion suggests the possibility of anticonvulsant or psychotropic drug ingestion.

Management. The INO resolves as the blood concentration of the drug falls.

Vertical Gaze Palsy

Children with supranuclear vertical gaze palsies are unable to look upward or downward fully, but they retain reflex eye movements such as the doll's eye reflex and the Bell phenomenon. Disorders of upward gaze in children generally are due to damage to the dorsal midbrain; the usual cause is a tumor in the pineal region. *Parinaud syndrome* is the combination of paralysis of upgaze, a dilated pupil unresponsive to light but becoming smaller when focusing on a near object (light near dissociation or *Argyll Robertson pupil*), convergence retraction nystagmus (the eyes pull in and retract with attempt to look upward), eyelid retraction (*Collier's sign*), and a tendency to look down in primary gaze position. Isolated paralysis of upward gaze may be the initial feature of the Miller Fisher syndrome and of vitamin B_1 deficiency.

Bilateral lesions in the midbrain reticular formation cause isolated disturbances of downward gaze. They are rare in children but may occur in neurovisceral lipid storage disease.

Congenital vertical ocular motor apraxia.

Clinical features. Congenital vertical ocular motor apraxia is a rare syndrome similar to congenital horizontal ocular motor apraxia, except for the direction of gaze palsy. At rest, the eyes are fixated in either an upward or a downward position, with little random movement. Initially, the child uses head flexion or extension to fixate in the vertical plane; later, the child learns to use head thrusts. The Bell phenomenon is present.

Diagnosis. Vertical gaze palsy suggests an intracranial tumor, and a head MRI is required. However, gaze palsies present from birth without the later development of other neurological signs usually indicate a nonprogressive process. Bilateral restriction of upward eye movement resulting from muscle fibrosis is a consideration. In children with ocular motor apraxia the eyes can move upward reflexively or by forced ductions; in children with muscle fibrosis, the eyes will not move upward by any means.

Management. Specific treatment is not available.

Horizontal Gaze Palsy

The usual cause of inability to look to one side is a lesion in the contralateral frontal or ipsilateral pontine gaze center. Immediately after developing a frontal lobe lesion, the eyes are tonically deviated toward the side of the lesion and contralateral hemiplegia is often present. The eyes move horizontally reflexively by stimulation of the brainstem gaze center with ice water caloric techniques. In contrast an irritative frontal lobe lesion, such as one causing an epileptic seizure, generally causes the eyes to deviate in a direction opposite to the side with the seizure focus. When the focus is parietal, the eye deviation may be ipsilateral. Movements of the head and eyes during a seizure are called *adversive seizures* (see Chapter 1). The initial direction of eye deviation reliably predicts a contralateral focus, especially if the movement is forced and sustained in a unilateral direction. Later movements that are mild and transient are not predictive.

Convergence Paralysis

Convergence paralysis, inability to adduct the eyes to focus on a near object in the absence of medial rectus palsies, can be caused by a pineal region tumor; in such cases, however, other signs of midbrain compression are usually present. Convergence paralysis is sometimes factitious or due to lack of motivation or attention. The absence of pupillary constriction when convergence is attempted identifies factitious convergence paralysis.

Convergence insufficiency is common after closed head injuries. The head injury need not be severe. Patient complaints may include diplopia, headache, or eyestrain while reading or other close work. Convergence insufficiency also occurs in the absence of prior head injury. The onset often follows a change in study time or intensity, poor lighting in the workplace, or the use of new contact lenses or eyeglasses. Treatment consists of convergence exercises.

NYSTAGMUS

Nystagmus is an involuntary, rhythmic ocular oscillation in which at least one phase is slow. With *pendular nystagmus*, both phases are slow. The oscillations of congenital pendular nystagmus are in the horizontal plane, even with the eyes in vertical gaze. On lateral gaze, the oscillations may change to jerk nystagmus.

Movements of unequal speed characterize *jerk nystagmus*. Following an initial slow component in one direction is a fast component with saccadic velocity in the other direction. Oscillation may be horizontal or vertical. The direction of jerk nystagmus is named for the fast (saccadic) component. Nystagmus intensity increases in the horizontal plane when gaze is in the direction of the fast phase.

TABLE 15.2   Abnormal Eye Movements

Movement	Appearance	Pathology
Nystagmus	Rhythmic oscillation	Variable
Opsoclonus	Nonrhythmic, chaotic conjugate movements	Neuroblastoma
Ocular flutter	Intermittent bursts of rapid horizontal oscillations during fixation	Cerebellar/brainstem disease
Ocular dysmetria	Overshooting, undershooting, or oscillation on refixation	Cerebellar disease
Ocular bobbing	Intermittent, rapid downward movement	Pontine lesions
Periodic alternating gaze	Cyclic conjugate lateral eye deviations, alternating from side to side	Posterior fossa

BOX 15.7   Differential Diagnosis of Nystagmus

- Physiologic
- Vestibular
  - Migraine
  - Labyrinthine disorders
- Congenital
  - Albinism
  - Associated with blindness
  - Familial
  - Idiopathic
- Acquired
  - Spasmus nutans (often pendular or monocular)
  - Drug Induced
  - Ictal
  - Glioma
- Monocular
  - Spasmus nutans
  - Chiasmal tumors
- See-saw
  - Congenital
  - Tumors of the sella/parasellar region
- Downbeat
  - Abnormalities of cervicomedullary junction
- Upbeat
  - Vascular lesions
  - Brainstem tumor
  - Lesions of cerebellar vermis
- Divergence
  - Midline cerebellar or dorsal pontine lesions

Table 15.2 describes other eye movements that cannot be classified as nystagmus but that have diagnostic significance. *Opsoclonus* consists of conjugate, rapid, chaotic movements in all directions of gaze, often referred to as "dancing eyes." It occurs in infants with neuroblastoma (see Chapter 10) and children with opsoclonus-myoclonus-ataxia syndrome (see Chapter 14). *Ocular flutter* is a brief burst of conjugate horizontal saccadic eye movements that interrupt fixation. It occurs in the recovery phase of opsoclonus or in association with cerebellar disease. *Ocular dysmetria* is overshooting or undershooting of the eyes during refixation or an oscillation before the eyes come to rest on a new fixation target. *Ocular bobbing* is not downbeat nystagmus, but is a sudden downward movement of both eyes with a slow drift back to midposition. It most often occurs in comatose patients with pontine dysfunction. The discussions of congenital and acquired nystagmus are separate because their differential diagnoses are distinct (Box 15.7).

Physiological Nystagmus

A high frequency (1–3 Hz), low-amplitude oscillation of the eyes occurs normally when sustaining lateral gaze to the point of fatigue. A jerk nystagmus, present at the endpoint of lateral gaze, is also normal. A few beats are usual, but even sustained nystagmus occurring at the endpoint is normal unless associated with other signs of neurological dysfunction or distinctly asymmetric.

Congenital Nystagmus

To be termed congenital nystagmus must be present by 6 months of age. Nystagmus that develops after 6 months of age is considered acquired and requires neuroimaging. The distinction may be complicated by the fact that although congenital nystagmus is present at birth, it may be unnoticed until infancy or childhood and then misdiagnosed as acquired nystagmus. One reason that congenital nystagmus may remain unnoticed is that the *null point*, the angle of ocular movement at which the nystagmus is minimal, may be very wide. Often, nystagmus is mistaken for normal movement. There are two distinct types of congenital nystagmus: those with normal vision, and those with visual impairment. Congenital nystagmus associated with abnormal vision is termed *congenital sensory nystagmus*, because the child's sense of vision is deficient. Congenital nystagmus with normal vision typically is due to defective control of eye movements and may be termed *congenital motor nystagmus*.

Congenital sensory nystagmus may be caused by a variety of conditions including albinism, cataracts, optic nerve hypoplasia, choroidal coloboma, achromatopsia, and severe refractive errors. Congenital motor nystagmus often has no identified cause, but rare genetic etiologies have been discovered in families with multiple affected members.

Clinical features. Congenital nystagmus is usually horizontal in plane but may be either pendular or jerk in character. Convergence generally diminishes and fixation increases the intensity of nystagmus. Because a null zone often exists where nystagmus is minimal, the head may be held to one side, or tilted, or both, to improve vision. Periodic head turning may accompany periodic alternating nystagmus.

Two forms of head oscillation are associated with congenital nystagmus. One is involuntary and does not improve vision. The other, also seen in spasmus nutans, is opposite in direction to the nystagmus but not phase locked and improves vision. Many children have impaired vision from the nystagmus in the absence of a primary disturbance in visual acuity.

Diagnosis. Determination that the nystagmus was present at birth is important but not always possible. A formal dilated eye exam is needed to rule out other ocular conditions. MRI is typically unrevealing but is necessary if it is unclear whether nystagmus is congenital or acquired.

Management. Treatment depends on the underlying deficit. For example, children with congenital sensory nystagmus secondary to a severe refractive error will benefit from corrective lenses.

ACQUIRED NYSTAGMUS

Spasmus Nutans

Spasmus nutans is an acquired nystagmus with onset in early infancy characterized by the triad of nystagmus,

head nodding, and torticollis. The underlying pathology is unclear, but it may be that the main abnormality is nystagmus, and head bobbing and torticollis are compensatory mechanisms.

Clinical features. Onset typically occurs between 6 and 12 months of age. Nystagmus is characteristically binocular but may be monocular or asymmetric and is frequently described as "shimmering." Head tilt and movement may be more prominent than nystagmus, and torticollis is often the first complaint (see Chapter 14). Affected children are unlikely to have imaging abnormalities, although structural abnormalities have been reported in a small minority of cases.[16] There is a rare association with retinal dystrophy.

Previously, parents were counseled that spasmus nutans would persist for 1–2 years then spontaneously resolve. However, longitudinal follow-up studies demonstrate that nystagmus is persistent in many children, even if head nodding and torticollis resolve.[17]

Diagnosis. Diagnosis is based on clinical symptoms. Imaging studies are usually normal but are often performed to rule out structural abnormalities. The ophthalmologist may obtain an electroretinogram to rule out retinal dystrophy.

Management. There is no specific treatment for the disorder, but ongoing ophthalmologic follow-up is recommended due to the potential for persistent nystagmus and amblyopia.

Pendular Nystagmus

Pendular nystagmus may be either congenital or acquired. In adults the usual causes of acquired pendular nystagmus are brainstem infarction and multiple sclerosis. In children, pendular nystagmus in the absence of other neurological signs is either congenital or the first sign of spasmus nutans. However, the development of optic atrophy in a child with pendular nystagmus indicates a glioma of the anterior visual pathway.

Vertical pendular nystagmus is unusual and sometimes occurs in association with rhythmic vertical oscillations of the palate (*palatal myoclonus or tremor*). One encounters the syndrome of oculopalatal oscillation in some spinocerebellar degenerations and in ischemic disorders of the deep cerebellar nuclei and central tegmental tract.

Drug-Induced Nystagmus

Clinical features. Many psychoactive drugs, including tranquilizers, antidepressants, anticonvulsants, and alcohol, produce nystagmus at high therapeutic or toxic blood concentrations. The nystagmus evoked by lateral gaze is either horizontal or horizontal-rotary. Vertical nystagmus may be present on upward, but rarely on downward, gaze. Toxic dosages of most antiepileptic drugs and lithium produce primary-position downbeat nystagmus as well.

Diagnosis. Suspect drug overdose in patients with nystagmus and decreased consciousness. Request a quantitative and qualitative drug screen.

Management. Nystagmus resolves when the blood concentration of the drug falls.

Ictal Nystagmus

Clinical features. Nystagmus as a seizure manifestation is binocular. It may occur alone or in association with other ictal manifestations. Sometimes, pupillary oscillations synchronous with nystagmus are present. As a rule, concurrent epileptiform discharges are focal, contralateral to the fast phase of nystagmus in frontal foci (saccades center) and ipsilateral to the fast phase of nystagmus in parieto-occipital foci (pursuit center). However, individual cases exist of nystagmus accompanying generalized 3 Hz spike-wave discharges and periodic lateralized epileptiform discharges.

Diagnosis. Other seizure manifestations that identify the nature of the nystagmus are usually present. The electroencephalogram confirms the diagnosis by the presence of epileptiform activity concurrent with nystagmus.

Management. Ictal nystagmus responds to anticonvulsant drug therapy (see Chapter 1).

Vestibular Nystagmus

Vestibular nystagmus occurs with disorders of the labyrinth, vestibular nerve, vestibular nuclei of the brainstem, or vestibulocerebellum.

Clinical features. Labyrinthine disease (especially labyrinthitis) is usually associated with severe vertigo, nausea, vomiting, and autonomic features such as tachycardia and diaphoresis (see Chapter 17). Deafness, tinnitus, or both may be present as well. Movement of the head enhances the nystagmus and is more critical to the mechanism of nystagmus than the position obtained. Nystagmus is usually horizontal and torsional, with an initial slow phase followed by a rapid return. It is worse when gaze is in the direction of the fast phase. Fixation reduces nystagmus and vertigo.

Vertigo and nausea are mild when nystagmus is of central origin. Nystagmus is constantly present and not affected by head position. It may be horizontal or vertical and not affected by fixation. Other neurological disturbances referable to the brainstem or cerebellum are frequently associated features.

Diagnosis. Observation alone readily identifies vestibular nystagmus. It is identical to the nystagmus provoked by caloric stimulation or rotation. Labyrinthine disorders in children are usually infectious, sometimes viral, and sometimes a result of otitis media. Central causes of vestibular nystagmus include spinocerebellar degeneration, brainstem glioma or infarction, subacute necrotizing encephalomyelitis, periodic ataxias, and demyelinating disorders. Migraine with brainstem aura and vestibular migraine can produce nystagmus in the setting of vertigo and headache.

Management. Several different classes of drugs appreciably reduce the vertigo and nausea associated with labyrinthine disease. Diazepam is especially effective. Other useful drugs include meclizine, scopolamine, and other antihistamines. Venlafaxine is helpful for vestibular migraine.

Downbeat Nystagmus

Clinical features. In primary position the eyes drift slowly upward and then reflexively beat downward. The intensity of the nystagmus is usually greatest when directing the eyes slightly downward and laterally. Downbeat nystagmus is distinguishable from *downward-beating nystagmus*, in which the nystagmus is present only on downward gaze. The cause of downward-beating nystagmus is toxic doses of anticonvulsant and sedative drugs, whereas downbeat nystagmus often indicates a structural abnormality of the brainstem, especially the cervicomedullary junction or cerebellum. Patient complaints include dizziness, oscillopsia, blurred vision, and difficulty reading. Approximately one-third of patients are asymptomatic. Cerebellar ataxia is present in about half of patients and usually is the only associated neurological sign.

Diagnosis. Downbeat nystagmus is an unusual finding and is typically associated with abnormalities of the cervicomedullary junction. Nutritional deficiencies, gluten ataxia, paraneoplastic syndromes, and congenital or acquired cerebellar degeneration are other potential etiologies.

Management. In addition to disease-specific treatments, aminopyridines such as 4-AP are first-line therapy. Ophthalmology may pursue strabismus surgery or the use of prisms to broaden the null point.[18]

Upbeat Nystagmus

Clinical features. In primary position the eyes drift slowly downward and then spontaneously beat upward. Upward gaze accentuates the nystagmus. A large- and a small-amplitude type occur. Large-amplitude nystagmus increases in intensity during upward gaze and indicates a lesion in the anterior vermis of the cerebellum or an abnormality in the anterior visual pathway. Anterior visual pathway abnormalities include Leber congenital amaurosis, bilateral optic nerve hypoplasia, and congenital cataract (see Chapter 16). Small-amplitude nystagmus decreases in intensity during upward gaze and, when present, suggests an intrinsic lesion of the medulla.

Diagnosis. Upbeat nystagmus is usually an acquired disorder caused by vascular lesions or tumors of the brainstem or cerebellar vermis. Therefore every child with a normal anterior visual pathway requires a head MRI. Upbeat nystagmus also occurs with impairment of smooth pursuit movements in dominantly inherited cerebellar vermian atrophy.

Management. Specific treatment is not available. Sometimes, gabapentin or DAP are useful.

Dissociated Nystagmus

Divergence Nystagmus

Divergence nystagmus is a rare condition in which both eyes beat outward simultaneously. The mechanism, while poorly understood, can be seen with lesions in the midline cerebellum and dorsal pons.[19]

Monocular Nystagmus

Monocular nystagmus may be congenital or acquired. The most important diagnostic considerations in children are spasmus nutans and chiasmal tumors.

A coarse pendular vertical nystagmus may develop in an amblyopic eye years after the visual loss. The nystagmus occurs in the blind eye when attempting distance fixation with the sighted eye and is inhibited by convergence.

See-Saw Nystagmus

See-saw nystagmus is the result of two different oscillations. One is a pendular vertical oscillation. The other is a torsional movement in which one eye rises and intorts while the other falls and extorts. It may be congenital or acquired. The congenital form is sometimes associated with absence of the chiasm and a horizontal pendular nystagmus. Acquired cases are usually due to tumors of the sellar and parasellar regions and are associated with bitemporal hemianopia.

REFERENCES

1. Chung M, Stout JT, Borchert MS. Clinical diversity of hereditary Duane's retraction syndrome. *Ophthalmology*. 2000;107:500-503.
2. Verzijl HT, van der Zwaag B, Cruysberg JR, Padberg GW. Möbius syndrome redefined. A syndrome of rhombencephalic maldevelopment. *Neurology*. 2003;61:327-333.
3. Whitman M, Hunter DG, Engle EC. Congenital fibrosis of the extraocular muscles (April 27, 2004). In: Adam MP, Ardinger HH, Pagon RA, et al., eds. *GeneReviews®*. University of Washington; 1993–2018. https://www.ncbi.nlm.nih.gov/books/NBK1348/. Updated January 14, 2016.
4. Abicht A, Müller JS, Lochmüller H. Congenital myasthenic syndromes overview (May 9, 2003). In: Adam MP, Feldman J, Mirzaa GM, et al., eds. *GeneReviews®*. University of Washington; 1993–2023. https://www.ncbi.nlm.nih.gov/books/NBK1168/. Updated December 23, 2021.
5. PDQ Pediatric Treatment Editorial Board *Childhood Brain Stem Glioma Treatment (PDQ®): Health Professional Version. PDQ Cancer Information Summaries [Internet]*. National Cancer Institute (US); 2002. https://www.ncbi.nlm.nih.gov/books/NBK65812/.
6. Smith DM, Vossough A, Vorona GA, Beslow LA, Ichord RN, Licht DJ. Pediatric cavernous sinus thrombosis: a case series and review of the literature. *Neurology*. 2015;85(9):763-769. https://doi.org/10.1212/WNL.0000000000001886. Epub 2015 Jul 31. PMID: 26231260; PMCID: PMC4553026.
7. Anilkumar A, Tan E, Cleaver J, Morrison HD. Isolated abducens nerve palsy in a patient with asymptomatic SARS-CoV-2 infection. *Journal of Clinical Neuroscience*. 2021;89:65-67. https://doi.org/10.1016/j.jocn.2021.04.011. Epub 2021 Apr 19. PMID: 34119296; PMCID: PMC8055164.
8. Behbehani R. Ocular myasthenia gravis: a current overview. *Eye and Brain*. 2023;15:1-13. https://doi.org/10.2147/EB.S389629. PMID: 36778719; PMCID: PMC9911903.
9. Richman DP, Agius MA. Treatment of autoimmune myasthenia gravis. *Neurology*. 2003;61:1652-1661.
10. Kuppersmith MJ. Does early immunotherapy reduce the conversion of ocular myasthenia gravis to generalized

myasthenia gravis. *Journal of Neuro-Ophthalmology.* 2003;23:249-250.

11. Mee J, Paine M, Byrne E, et al. Immunotherapy of ocular myasthenia gravis reduces conversion to generalized myasthenia gravis. *Journal of Neuro-Ophthalmology.* 2003;23:251-255.

12. Zamproni LN, Ribeiro RT, Cardeal M. Treatment of recurrent painful ophthalmoplegic neuropathy: a case where pregabalin was successfully employed. *Case Reports in Neurological Medicine.* 2019;2019:1-5. https://doi.org/10.1155/2019/9185603.

13. Pareja J, Churruca J, de la Casa Fages B, de Silanes CL, Sanchez C, Barriga F. Ophthalmoplegic migraine. Two patients with an absolute response to indomethacin. *Cephalalgia.* 2010;30(6):757-760. https://doi.org/10.1111/j.1468-2982.2009.02003.x.

14. Belanger C, Zhang KS, Reddy AK, et al. Inflammatory disorders of the orbit in childhood: a case series. *American Journal of Ophthalmology.* 2010;150:460-463.

15. Goldstein A, Falk MJ, Mitochondrial DNA. Deletion Syndromes. In: Adam MP, Ardinger HH, Pagon RA, et al., eds. *GeneReviews®*. University of Washington; 1993–2019. https://www.ncbi.nlm.nih.gov/books/NBK1203.

16. Bowen M, Peragallo JH, Kralik SF, Poretti A, Huisman TAGM, Soares BP. Magnetic resonance imaging findings in children with spasmus nutans. *Journal of AAPOS.* 2017;21(2):127-130. https://doi.org/10.1016/j.jaapos.2017.03.001. Epub 2017 Mar 8. PMID: 28284856.

17. Parikh RN, Simon JW, Zobal-Ratner JL, Barry GP. Long-term follow-up of spasmus nutans. *Journal of Binocular Vision and Ocular Motility.* 2018;68(4):137-139. https://doi.org/10.1080/2576117X.2018.1527639. Epub 2018 Oct 17. PMID: 30332338.

18. Tran TM, Lee MS, McClelland CM. Downbeat nystagmus: a clinical review of diagnosis and management. *Current Opinion in Ophthalmology.* 2021;32(6):504-514. https://doi.org/10.1097/ICU.0000000000000802. PMID: 34456290.

19. Kwon E, Lee J-Y, Kim H-J, Choi J-Y, Kim J-S. Pearls & oy-sters: divergence nystagmus. *Neurology.* 2021;96(6):290-293. https://doi.org/10.1212/WNL.0000000000011273.

16

Disorders of the Visual System

OUTLINE

Assessment of Visual Acuity, 367
  Clinical Assessment, 367
  Visual Evoked Response, 368
Congenital Blindness, 368
  Congenital Cataract, 368
  Congenital Optic Nerve Hypoplasia, 369
  Coloboma, 370
Acute Monocular or Binocular Blindness, 371
  Cortical Blindness, 371
Posttraumatic Vision Loss, 372
  Optic Neuropathies, 372
  Pituitary Apoplexy, 374
  Retinal Disease, 374
Progressive Loss of Vision, 375
  Compressive Optic Neuropathy, 375
Hereditary Optic Neuropathy, 377

Leber Congenital Amaurosis/Early-Onset Severe
  Retinal Dystrophy, 377
Wfs1-Spectrum Disorder (Wolfram Syndrome), 377
Retinoblastoma, 378
Syndromes of Retinal Degeneration, 378
  Bardet-Biedl Syndrome, 378
  Laurence-Moon Syndrome, 378
  Cockayne Syndrome, 378
Disorders of the Pupil, 379
  Aniridia, 379
  Benign Essential Anisocoria, 379
  Fixed, Dilated Pupil, 379
  Horner Syndrome, 379
  Tonic Pupil Syndrome (Adie Syndrome), 380
References, 380

Both congenital and acquired visual impairments in children are often associated with neurological disorders. The most common visual disorders are uncorrected refractive errors, amblyopia, strabismus, cataracts, and genetic disorders.

ASSESSMENT OF VISUAL ACUITY

The assessment of visual acuity in preverbal children relies mainly on assessing fixation and tracking as the infant or young child interacts with the environment. Some pediatrician's offices have autorefractors that provide an estimate of refractive errors, but such devices are rare in the pediatric neurology clinic.

Clinical Assessment

The pupillary light reflex is a test of the functional integrity of the subcortical afferent and efferent pathways and is reliably present after 31 weeks' gestation. A blink response to light develops at about the same time, and the lid may remain closed for as long as the light is present (the dazzle reflex). The blink response to threat may not be present until 5 months of age. These responses are integrated into the brainstem and do not provide information on the cognitive (cortical) aspects of vision.

Observing fixation and following behavior is the principal means to assess visual function in newborns and infants. The human face, at a distance of approximately 30 cm, is the best target for fixation. Ninety percent of infants fixate on faces by 9 weeks of age. After obtaining fixation, the examiner slowly moves from side to side to test *tracking*. Visually directed grasping is present in normal children by 3 months of age but is difficult to test before 6 months of age. Absence of visually directed grasping may indicate a motor rather than a visual disturbance.

The *refixation reflex* evaluates the visual fields in infants and young children by moving an interesting stimulus in the peripheral field. Clues to visual impairment are structural abnormalities (e.g., microphthalmia, cloudy cornea), an absent or asymmetric pupillary response to light, dysconjugate gaze, nystagmus, and failure to fixate or track. Staring at a bright light source and oculodigital stimulation indicate severe visual impairment.

Visual Evoked Response

The visual evoked response to strobe light demonstrates the anatomical integrity of visual pathways without patient cooperation. At 30 weeks' gestation, a positive "cortical" wave with a peak latency of 300 ms is first demonstrable. The latency linearly declines at a rate of 10 ms each week throughout the last 10 weeks of gestation. In the newborn the morphology of the visual evoked response is variable during wakefulness and active sleep and easiest to obtain just after the child goes to sleep. By 3 months of age, the morphology and latency of the visual evoked response are mature.

CONGENITAL BLINDNESS

Cortical blindness is the most common cause of congenital visual impairment among children referred to a neurologist. Ophthalmologists are more likely to see ocular abnormalities. The causes of congenital visual impairment are numerous and include prenatal and perinatal disturbances. Optic nerve hypoplasia, with or without other ocular malformations, is the most common ocular abnormality, followed by congenital cataracts and corneal opacities. Corneal abnormalities usually do not cause visual loss unless clouding is extensive. Such extensive clouding may develop in the mucopolysaccharidoses and in Fabry disease. Box 16.1 lists conditions with corneal clouding present during childhood.

Congenital Cataract

For the purpose of this discussion, congenital cataract includes cataracts discovered within the first 3 months. Box 16.2 lists the differential diagnosis. Approximately one-third are hereditary, one-third are syndromic, and one-third are idiopathic.

In previous studies intrauterine infection accounted for one-third of congenital cataracts. That percentage has declined with the prevention of rubella embryopathy by immunization. Genetic and chromosomal disorders account for a significant number of cases, but in

BOX 16.1   Corneal Clouding in Childhood

- Cerebrohepatorenal syndrome (Zellweger syndrome)
- Congenital syphilis[a]
- Fabry disease (ceramide trihexosidosis)
- Familial high-density lipoprotein deficiency
- Fetal alcohol syndrome
- Glaucoma[a]
- Infantile GM_1 gangliosidosis
- Juvenile metachromatic dystrophy
- Marinesco-Sjögren disease
- Mucolipidosis
- Mucopolysaccharidoses
- Multiple sulfatase deficiency
- Pelizaeus-Merzbacher disease
- Trauma (forceps at birth)

[a]The most common conditions and the ones with disease modifying treatments.

a large minority, the cause is unknown. The mode of transmission of syndromic congenital cataracts varies. In many hereditary syndromes cataracts can be either congenital or delayed in appearance until infancy, childhood, or even adulthood. Several of these syndromes are associated with dermatoses: incontinentia pigmenti (irregular skin pigmentation), *Marshall syndrome* (anhidrotic ectodermal dysplasia), hereditary mucoepithelial dysplasia, and congenital ichthyosis.

Congenital cataracts occur in approximately 10% of children with trisomy 13 and trisomy 18 and many children with trisomy 21. The association of congenital cataract and lactic acidosis or cardiomyopathy suggests a mitochondrial disorder.

Clinical features. Small cataracts may impair vision and may be difficult to detect by direct ophthalmoscopy. Large cataracts appear as a white mass in the pupil and, if left in place, quickly cause deprivation amblyopia. The initial size of a cataract does not predict its course; congenital cataracts may remain stationary or increase in density but never improve spontaneously. Other congenital ocular abnormalities, aniridia, coloboma, and microphthalmos occur in 40%–50% of newborns with congenital cataracts.

Diagnosis. Large cataracts are obvious on inspection. Smaller cataracts distort the normal red reflex when the direct ophthalmoscope is at arm's length distance from the eye and a +12 to +20 lens is used.

Genetic disorders and maternal drug exposure are important considerations when cataracts are the only

BOX 16.2 Cataract Etiology

Congenital Cataract
- Chromosomal aberrations
  - Trisomy 13
  - Trisomy 18
  - Trisomy 21[a]
  - Turner syndrome[a]
- Drug exposure during pregnancy
  - Chlorpromazine
  - Corticosteroids
  - Sulfonamides
- Galactokinase deficiency
- Galactose-1-phosphate uridyltransferase deficiency
- Galactosemia
- Genetic
  - Hereditary spherocytosis[a]
  - Incontinentia pigmenti[a]
  - Marshall syndrome[a]
  - Myotonic dystrophy[a]
  - Schäfer syndrome[a]
  - Without other anomalies
- Autosomal dominant inheritance
- Autosomal recessive inheritance
  - Congenital ichthyosis[a]
  - Congenital stippled epiphyses (Conradi disease)
  - Marinesco-Sjögren syndrome[a]
  - Siemens syndrome[a]
  - Smith-Lemli-Opitz syndrome
  - X-linked inheritance (oculocerebrorenal syndrome)[a]
- Idiopathic
  - Intrauterine infection[a]
  - Mumps
  - Rubella
  - Syphilis
- Maternal factors
  - Diabetes

- Malnutrition
- Radiation
- Prematurity

Acquired Cataract
- Drug-induced
  - Corticosteroids
  - Long-acting miotics
- Genetic
  - Cockayne disease
  - Hepatolenticular degeneration (Wilson disease)
  - Rothmund-Thompson syndrome
  - Werner syndrome
  - Autosomal dominant inheritance (Alport syndrome)
  - Autosomal recessive inheritance
  - X-linked inheritance (pseudo-pseudohypoparathy-roidism)
- Chromosomal (Prader-Willi syndrome)
- Metabolic
  - Cretinism
  - Hypocalcemia
  - Hypoparathyroidism
  - Juvenile diabetes
  - Pseudohypoparathyroidism
- Trauma
- Varicella (postnatal)

Dislocated Lens
- Crouzon syndrome
- Ehlers-Danlos syndrome
- Homocystinuria
- Hyperlysinemia
- Marfan syndrome
- Sturge-Weber syndrome
- Sulfite oxidase deficiency

[a]Cataracts may not be noted until infancy or childhood

abnormality. Intrauterine disturbances, such as maternal illness and fetal infection, are usually associated with growth retardation and other malformations. Dysmorphic features are always an indication for ordering chromosome analysis. Galactosemia is suspected in children with hepatomegaly and milk intolerance (see Chapter 5), but cataracts may be present even before the development of systemic features.

Management. Developmental amblyopia is preventable by recognizing and removing cataracts before the age of 3 months. Urgent referral to a pediatric ophthalmologist is the standard of care.

Congenital Optic Nerve Hypoplasia

Optic nerve hypoplasia is a developmental defect in the number of optic nerve fibers and may result from excessive regression of retinal ganglion cell axons. Hypoplasia may be bilateral or unilateral and varies in severity. It may occur as an isolated defect or be associated with intracranial anomalies. The most common association is with midline defects of the septum pellucidum and hypothalamus (septo-optic dysplasia). The cause of septo-optic dysplasia is unknown in most cases, but some causative genetic mutations have been discovered.

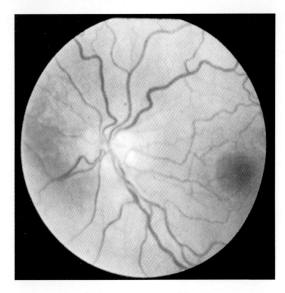

Fig. 16.1 Optic Nerve Hypoplasia. The optic nerve is small and pale, but the vessels are of normal size.

Clinical features. The phenotype is highly variable; 62% of affected children have isolated hypopituitarism and 30% have the complete phenotype of pituitary hypoplasia, optic nerve hypoplasia, and agenesis of midline structures.[1] In one study group of 55 patients with optic nerve hypoplasia,[2] 49% had an abnormal septum pellucidum on magnetic resonance imaging (MRI), and 64% had a hypothalamic-pituitary axis abnormality. Twenty-seven patients (49%) had endocrine dysfunction, and 23 of these had a hypothalamic-pituitary axis abnormality. The frequency of endocrinopathy was higher in patients with an abnormal septum pellucidum (56%) than a normal septum pellucidum (39%) and the appearance of the septum pellucidum predicts the likely spectrum of endocrinopathy.

When hypoplasia is severe, strabismus and nystagmus are present, indicating severe visual impairment. Ophthalmoscopic examination reveals a small, pale nerve head (Fig. 16.1). A pigmented area surrounded by a yellowish mottled halo is sometimes present at the edge of the disk margin, giving the appearance of a double ring. The degree of hypothalamic-pituitary involvement varies. Possible symptoms include neonatal hypoglycemia and seizures, recurrent hypoglycemia in childhood, growth retardation, diabetes insipidus, and disorders of sexual development, including premature or delayed puberty. Some combination of intellectual disability cerebral palsy, and epilepsy is often present and indicates malformations in other portions of the brain.

Diagnosis. All infants with ophthalmoscopic evidence of optic nerve hypoplasia require cranial MRI and an assessment of endocrine status. The common findings on MRI are cavum septum pellucidum, hypoplasia of the cerebellum, aplasia of the corpus callosum, aplasia of the fornix, and an empty sella. Absence of the pituitary infundibulum with posterior pituitary ectopia indicates congenital hypopituitarism. Endocrine studies should include assays of growth hormone, antidiuretic hormone, and the integrity of hypothalamic-pituitary control of the thyroid, adrenal, and gonadal systems. Infants with hypoglycemia usually have growth hormone deficiency.

Superior segmental optic nerve hypoplasia is associated with congenital inferior visual field defects and occurs in children born to mothers with insulin-dependent diabetes.

Management. No treatment is available for optic nerve hypoplasia, but endocrine abnormalities respond to replacement therapy. Children with corticotrophin deficiency are at risk for sudden death and require appropriate emergency steroid administration during times of stress or illness. Children with visual impairment may benefit from visual aids. Almost all affected children require educational accommodations including those specific to those with visual disabilities.

Coloboma

Coloboma is a defect in embryogenesis that may affect only the disk or may include the retina, iris, ciliary body, and choroid. Colobomas isolated to the nerve head appear as deep excavations, deeper inferiorly. They may be unilateral or bilateral. The causes of congenital coloboma are genetic (monogenic and chromosomal) and intrauterine disease (toxic and infectious). Retinochoroidal colobomas are glistening white or yellow defects inferior or inferior nasal to the disk. The margins are distinct and surrounded by pigment. *Morning glory disk* is not a form of coloboma; it is an enlarged dysplastic disk with a white excavated center surrounded by an elevated annulus of pigmentary change. Retinal vessels enter and leave at the margin of the disk, giving the appearance of a morning glory flower. The morning glory syndrome is associated with transsphenoidal encephaloceles. Affected children are dysmorphic with midline facial anomalies.

ACUTE MONOCULAR OR BINOCULAR BLINDNESS

The differential diagnoses of acute and progressive blindness show considerable overlap. Although older children recognize sudden visual loss, slowly progressive ocular disturbances may produce an asymptomatic decline until vision is severely disturbed, especially if unilateral. When finally noticed, the child's loss of visual acuity seems acute. Teachers or parents are often the first to recognize a slowly progressive visual disturbance. Box 16.3 lists conditions in which visual acuity is normal and then suddenly lost. Box 16.4 lists disorders in which the underlying pathological process is progressive. Consult both lists in the differential diagnosis of acute blindness. The duration of a transitory monocular visual loss suggests the underlying cause: seconds indicate optic disk disorders such as papilledema or drusen, minutes indicate emboli, hours indicate migraine, and days indicate optic neuropathy, most commonly optic neuritis.

Cortical Blindness

Cortical blindness in children may be permanent or transitory, depending on the cause. The causes of transitory cortical blindness in childhood include migraine (see Chapter 3), mild head trauma, brief episodes of hypoglycemia or hypotension, and benign occipital

---

BOX 16.3   Causes of Acute Loss of Vision

- Carotid dissection[a] (see Chapter 11)
- Cortical blindness
  - Demyelinating
  - Ischemic
  - Toxic
  - Traumatic
- Anoxic encephalopathy (see Chapter 2)
- Benign occipital epilepsy[a] (see Chapter 1)
- Hydrocephalus[a]
- Hypoglycemia[a]
- Hypertension[a] (malignant or accelerated)
- Hyperviscosity
- Hypotension
- Migraine[a] (see Chapter 3)
- Occipital metastatic disease
- Posttraumatic transient cerebral blindness
- Systemic lupus erythematosus
- Toxic[a] (cyclosporine, etc.)
- Trauma
- Disorders affecting the optic nerves
- Optic neuropathy[a]
  - Idiopathic optic neuritis
  - Multiple sclerosis (see Chapter 10)
  - Neuromyelitis optica (see Chapter 12)
- Pituitary apoplexy
- Pseudotumor cerebri[a] (see Chapter 4)
- Retinal disease
  - Central retinal artery occlusion
  - Migraine
  - Trauma

[a]The most common conditions and the ones with disease modifying treatments.

BOX 16.4   Causes of Progressive Loss of Vision

- Compressive optic neuropathies
  - Aneurysm[a] (see Chapters 4 and 15)
  - Arteriovenous malformations[a] (see Chapters 4, 10, and 11)
  - Craniopharyngioma[a]
  - Hypothalamic and optic tumors
  - Pituitary adenoma[a]
  - Pseudotumor cerebri[a] (see Chapter 4)
- Disorders of the lens (see Box 16.3)
  - Cataract
  - Dislocation of the lens
- Hereditary optic atrophy
  - Leber hereditary optic neuropathy
  - Wolfram syndrome
- Intraocular tumors
- Retinal degenerations
  - Mucopolysaccharidosis (see Chapter 5)
  - Primary hyperoxaluria
- Abnormal carbohydrate metabolism
- Abnormal lipid metabolism
  - Abetalipoproteinemia (see Chapter 10)
  - Hypobetalipoproteinemia (see Chapter 10)
  - Multiple sulfatase deficiency (see Chapter 5)
  - Neuronal ceroid lipofuscinosis (see Chapter 5)
  - Niemann-Pick disease (see Chapter 5)
  - Refsum disease (see Chapter 7)
- Other syndromes
  - Bardet-Biedl syndrome
  - Cockayne syndrome
  - Laurence-Moon syndrome
- Refsum disease (see Chapter 7)

[a]The most common conditions and the ones with disease modifying treatments.

epilepsy (see Chapter 1). Acute and sometimes permanent blindness may occur following anoxia; secondary to massive infarction of, or hemorrhage into, the visual cortex; and when multifocal metastatic tumors or abscesses are located in the occipital lobes. The main feature of cortical blindness is loss of vision with preservation of the pupillary light reflex. Fundoscopic examination is normal.

Hypoglycemia

Repeated episodes of acute cortical blindness may occur at the time of mild hypoglycemia in children with glycogen storage diseases and following insulin overdose in diabetic children.

Clinical features. Sudden blindness is associated with clinical evidence of hypoglycemia (sweating and confusion). Ophthalmoscopic and neurological findings are normal. Recovery is usually complete in minutes to hours provided the underlying hypoglycemia is treated.

Diagnosis. During an episode of cortical blindness caused by hypoglycemia, electroencephalography (EEG) shows high-voltage slowing over both occipital lobes. Afterward the EEG returns to normal. Brain MRI shows diffuse edema in the occipital lobes.

Management. Recovery occurs when blood glucose concentration normalizes; however, permanent damage may occur with prolonged hypoglycemia.

POSTTRAUMATIC VISION LOSS

There are multiple potential etiologies of posttraumatic vision loss, and prognosis varies depending on the cause. The optic nerve is vulnerable to shear injury, stretch injury, and ischemia, as well as avulsion or direct injury from penetrating eye trauma or intraorbital foreign bodies. Chiasmatic injury or compression, anoxic, ischemic, or hemorrhagic brain injuries can all cause visual disturbance.

The diagnosis of posttraumatic visual loss may be delayed if other injuries are severe or if the child is unable to communicate their symptoms. Some forms of posttraumatic vision loss are temporary, but others result in permanent deficits.

Clinical features. Orbital injuries in the setting of clinical trauma are often clinically evident on inspection. Lid laceration, pupillary irregularity, hyphema, collapsed globe, subconjunctival hemorrhage, or corneal laceration should prompt emergent ophthalmologic consultation.

The neurologist is more likely to be consulted in cases of traumatic optic neuropathy, which may be direct or indirect. Direct neuropathy results from direct trauma to the nerve such as shear injury, avulsion, or acute compression due to hemorrhage. Indirect neuropathy is caused by the concussive effects of energy absorbed by the nerve within the bony confines of the optic nerve canal; this is often seen following blunt injury to the forehead.[3] Indirect optic neuropathy may occur even with mild head trauma and is the likely cause of most transient postconcussive visual loss. In both cases the patient experiences partial or complete visual loss which may be immediate (as in nerve avulsion) or delayed (as in gradual compression from swelling or hemorrhage). Associated symptoms depend on the nature of the injury.

Other causes of traumatic visual loss include traumatic carotid cavernous fistula (see Chapter 15) and cerebral injuries anywhere along the course of the visual pathway.

Diagnosis. Neuroimaging studies and ophthalmologic evaluation are almost always required in cases of posttraumatic vision loss.

Management. Treatment depends on the underlying etiology. Direct optic neuropathy may improve with decompressive surgery if acute compression is the cause. Indirect optic neuropathy historically has been treated with high-dose steroids or optic canal decompression; however, there is no evidence that either of these treatment modalities is efficacious.[4]

Optic Neuropathies
Demyelinating Optic Neuropathy

Demyelination of the optic nerve (optic neuritis) may occur as an isolated finding affecting one or both eyes, or it may be associated with demyelination in other portions of the nervous system. Discussion of neuromyelitis optica (*Devic syndrome*), the syndrome combining optic neuritis and transverse myelitis, is in Chapter 12, and multiple sclerosis in Chapter 10. MRI is a useful technique for surveying the central nervous system for demyelinating lesions (see Fig. 10.1). The incidence of later multiple sclerosis among children with optic neuritis is 15% or less if the child has no evidence of more diffuse involvement when brought to medical attention. The incidence is much higher when diffuse involvement is present or when optic neuritis recurs within 1 year.

Unilateral optic neuritis, and retrobulbar as opposed to papillitis, has a higher incidence of later multiple sclerosis than bilateral optic neuritis.

Clinical features. Monocular involvement is characteristic of optic neuritis in adults, but binocular involvement occurs in more than half of children. Binocular involvement may be concurrent or sequential, sometimes occurring over a period of weeks. The initial feature in some children is pain in the eye, but for most it is blurred vision, progressing within hours or days to partial or complete blindness. Visual acuity reduces to less than 20/200 in almost all affected children within 1 week. A history of a preceding "viral" infection or immunization is common, but a cause-and-effect relationship between optic neuritis and these events is not established.

Results of ophthalmoscopic examination may be normal at the onset of symptoms if neuritis is primarily retrobulbar. Visual loss readily distinguishes papillitis from papilledema. In optic neuritis visual loss occurs early; in papilledema, visual loss is a late feature.

Neuroretinitis is the association of swelling of the optic nerve head with macular edema or a macular star. Ophthalmoscopic examination shows disk swelling, peripapillary retinal detachment, and a macular star (Fig. 16.2). Neuroretinitis suggests the possibility of conditions other than idiopathic optic neuritis.

Diagnosis. Optic neuritis is a consideration whenever monocular or binocular blindness develops suddenly in a child. Ophthalmoscopic or slit-lamp examination confirms the diagnosis. Visual evoked response testing further confirms the diagnosis. MRI of the orbit may reveal swelling and demyelination of the optic nerve. Perform a lumbar puncture to assess cerebrospinal fluid for markers of demyelinating disease, such as oligoclonal bands, IgG index, and aquaporin-4 antibodies. Such examination sometimes shows a leukocytosis and an increased concentration of protein. Accelerated hypertension causes bilateral swelling of the optic nerves and recording blood pressure is an essential part of the evaluation.

Management. Treatment is detailed in Chapter 10.

Ischemic Optic Neuropathy

Infarction of the anterior portion of the optic nerve is rare in children and is usually associated with systemic vascular disease or hypotension.

Clinical features. Ischemic optic neuropathy usually occurs as a sudden segmental loss of vision in one eye, but slow or stepwise progression over several days

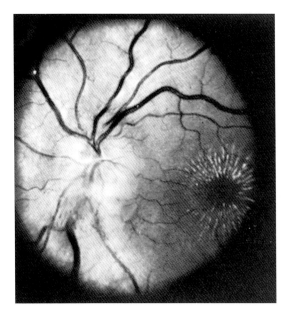

Fig. 16.2 Neuroretinitis. The optic disk is swollen and the peripapillary nerve fiber layer opacified. Exudates surround the macula in a star pattern. (Courtesy Patrick Lavin, MD.)

is possible. Recurrent episodes are unusual except with migraine and some idiopathic cases.

Diagnosis. Altitudinal visual field defects are present in 70%–80% of patients. Color vision loss is roughly equivalent in severity to visual acuity loss, whereas in demyelinating optic neuritis the disturbance of color vision is greater than that of visual acuity. Ophthalmoscopic examination reveals diffuse or partial swelling of the optic disk. When swelling is diffuse, it gives the appearance of papilledema and flame-shaped hemorrhages appear adjacent to the disk margin. After acute swelling subsides, optic atrophy follows.

Management. Treatment depends on the underlying cause of ischemia.

Toxic-Nutritional Optic Neuropathies

Drugs, toxins, and nutritional deficiencies alone or in combination may cause an acute or progressive optic neuropathy. These factors may cause optic neuropathy by inducing mitochondrial changes, perhaps in susceptible populations with mitochondrial DNA (mtDNA) mutations.

Clinical features. Implicated drugs include barbiturates, antibiotics (chloramphenicol, isoniazid, streptomycin, and sulfonamides), chemotherapeutic agents, chlorpropamide, digitalis, ergot, halogenated hydroxy-quinolines, penicillamine, and quinine. Nutritional deficiencies that may cause such optic neuropathies include folic acid and vitamins B_1, B_2, B_6, and B_{12}.

Symptoms vary with the specific drug, but progressive loss of central vision is typical. In some cases visual loss is rapid and develops as acute binocular blindness that may be asymmetric at onset, suggesting monocular involvement. Many of the drugs produce optic neuropathy by interfering with the action of folic acid or vitamin B_{12} and thereby causing a nutritional deficiency.

Diagnosis. Suspect drug toxicity whenever central and paracentral scotomas develop during the course of drug treatment. Optic nerve hyperemia with small paracentral hemorrhages may be an early feature. Later the disk becomes pale.

Management. Drug-induced optic neuropathy is dose-related. Dosage reduction may be satisfactory in some cases, especially if concurrent treatment with folic acid or vitamin B_{12} reverses the process. Some drugs require complete cessation of therapy.

Pituitary Apoplexy

Pituitary apoplexy in children is a very rare, life-threatening condition caused by hemorrhagic infarction of the pituitary gland.

Clinical features. Pituitary infarction occurs most often when there is a preexisting pituitary tumor but may also occur in the absence of a tumor. Several different clinical features are possible, depending on the structures affected by the swollen gland, including monocular or binocular blindness, visual field defects, ophthalmoplegia, chemical meningitis, cerebrospinal fluid rhinorrhea, and shock from hypopituitarism. Leakage of blood and necrotic material into the subarachnoid space causes chemical meningitis associated with headache, meningismus, and loss of consciousness.

Diagnosis. An MRI of the head with views of the pituitary gland establishes the diagnosis. Endocrine testing may show a deficiency of all pituitary hormones.

Management. Patients deteriorate rapidly and may die within a few days without prompt administration of corticosteroids. Replacement of other hormones is required but is not lifesaving. In patients who continue to do poorly, as evidenced by loss of consciousness, hypothalamic instability, or loss of vision, urgent surgical decompression of the expanding pituitary mass is required. In patients who develop acute secondary adrenal crisis, intravenous hydrocortisone at 1–1.5 mg/kg followed by 1.5–2.5 mg/kg over 24 hours and continuous infusion of intravenous fluids with continuous cardiovascular monitoring is required to decrease fatalities.[5]

Retinal Disease
Central Retinal Artery Occlusion
The most common risk factors for central retinal artery occlusion are congenital heart disease, mitral valve prolapse, sickle cell disease, migraine, vasculitis, and pregnancy.

Clinical features. Most affected children have an abrupt loss of monocular vision of variable intensity without premonitory symptoms. Some describe spots, a shadow, or a descending veil before the loss of vision. Bilateral retinal artery occlusion is very rare in children.

Diagnosis. The clinical history and ophthalmoscopic examination are the basis for the diagnosis of retinal artery obstruction. The posterior pole of the retina becomes opacified except in the foveal region, which contains a cherry-red spot. The peripheral retina appears normal. Visual field examination and angiography help confirm the diagnosis in some cases. One must seek the underlying cause once the diagnosis is established. Evaluation should include a cranial MRI and MR angiography or CT angiography, auscultation of the heart, radiographs of the chest, echocardiography in selected cases, complete blood cell count with sedimentation rate, cholesterol and triglyceride screening, coagulation studies, hemoglobin electrophoresis, and lupus anticoagulant and antiphospholipid antibodies.

Management. Acute treatment requires immediate ophthalmological consultation. The management of idiopathic occlusion of the retinal artery in adults is controversial, with growing evidence to suggest that early systemic fibrinolytic therapy may be beneficial.[6]

In children, systemic fibrinolysis is not routinely used, and steroids should be considered only in suspected vasculitis. Visual acuity is more likely to improve when the obstruction is in a branch artery rather than in the central retinal artery.

Retinal ischemia lasting longer than 240 minutes may lead to irreversible loss of vision. Restoration of blood flow within 100 minutes may preserve vision, so timely therapy is critical. Spontaneous recovery is rare. Visual acuity at presentation is a predictive of eventual acuity after the event. Although several treatment modalities are available, none has been prospectively shown to have more than a limited or marginal benefit. Traditional therapies include ocular massage to dislodge the embolus, decreasing intraocular pressure through anterior chamber paracentesis or administering intravenous diuretics. The use of vasodilators or inhaling carbogen (95% oxygen and 5% carbon dioxide) has also been tried. A more aggressive approach involves using thrombolytics similar to their use in acute myocardial infarction and ischemic stroke. For patients with sickle cell disease, exchange transfusion, used similarly in other vaso-occlusive crises, may be employed but the evidence is unclear.[6]

Retinal Migraine (Ocular Migraine or Ophthalmic Migraine)

Clinical features. Visual symptoms are relatively common during an attack of migraine with aura (see Chapter 3). Scintillating scotomas, or "fortification spectra," are field defects caused by altered neuronal function in the occipital cortex. The affected field is usually contralateral to the headache. Visual symptoms associated with migraine aura are *homonymous*; they occur in one visual field but are present in both eyes. Retinal migraine is distinguished from migraine aura by its clear *monocular* presentation.

The International Classification of Headache Disorders defines retinal migraine as reversible "repeated attacks of monocular visual disturbance, including scintillation, scotoma or blindness, associated with migraine headache."[7] The visual loss is sudden in most cases, may be partial or complete, and often precedes and is ipsilateral to the headache. Recurrences are usually in the same eye, and attacks may occur without headache. Family history is often positive for migraine in one or both parents.

Diagnosis. Retinal migraine with typical monocular scintillating scotoma and migrainous head pain rarely requires diagnostic evaluation beyond a thorough history and physical examination, but an episode of true monocular blindness demands further workup with MRI/MRA of the brain and orbits as well as a formal ophthalmologic examination. Consider EEG to rule out occipital seizures if the history is unclear.

Management. Treatment is often similar to that used for other types of migraine, but specific evidence-based treatment protocols are lacking.

Retinal Trauma

Direct blunt injury to the orbit causes visual impairment by retinal contusion, tear, or detachment. A diminished pupillary response characterizes all three. Contusion is associated with retinal edema. Although visual loss is immediate, the retina appears normal for the first few hours and only later becomes white and opaque. The severity of visual loss varies, but complete recovery is the rule.

A retinal tear is often associated with vitreous hemorrhage. Visual loss is usually immediate and easily diagnosed by its ophthalmoscopic appearance. Recovery is spontaneous unless there is detachment, for which cryotherapy is required.

PROGRESSIVE LOSS OF VISION

Compressive Optic Neuropathy

Compression of one or both optic nerves often occurs in the region of the chiasm. The visual loss may involve one eye or one visual field. In children with tumors in and around the diencephalon, the most constant feature is growth failure, which may be unrecognized until other symptoms develop.

Craniopharyngioma

Clinical features. Craniopharyngiomas are the most common nonglial tumors in children. The peak age range for diagnosis of this tumor is 6–14 years. The typical onset is insidious, and a 1- to 2-year history of slowly progressive symptoms is common. These symptoms may include progressive visual loss, delayed sexual maturation, growth failure, weight gain, and diabetes insipidus. Field defects are frequently asymmetric or unilateral. Bitemporal hemianopia is present in 50% of children with craniopharyngioma, and homonymous hemianopia in 10%–20%. Diminished visual acuity in one or both eyes and optic atrophy are constant features.

Approximately 25% of children have hydrocephalus that causes headache and papilledema. Hypothalamic involvement may produce diabetes insipidus or the hypodipsia-hyponatremia syndrome, characterized by lethargy, confusion, and hypotension. Other features depend on the direction of tumor growth. Anterior extension may compress the olfactory tract, causing anosmia, whereas lateral extension may compress the third and fifth nerves.

Diagnosis. MRI is diagnostic. The important feature is a multicystic and solid enhancing suprasellar mass, which causes hydrocephalus and stretches the optic nerves and chiasm.[8]

Management. Surgical removal of the tumor is the most effective treatment. Recurrences occur in 30% of cases after "complete" resection, 57% after incomplete resection, and 30% when radiation follows subtotal resection. The 5- and 10-year survival rates after post-operative radiotherapy are over 90%; however, most long-term survivors experience panhypopituitarism, cognitive impairment, and obesity.[9]

Optic Pathway and Diencephalic Gliomas

Sixty percent of optic pathway gliomas are pilocytic astrocytomas and the remaining 40% are fibrillary astrocytomas. Optic gliomas represent 3%–5% of childhood brain tumors. They may involve any part of the optic pathway from the optic nerves to the optic radiations. They also infiltrate the adjacent hypothalamus and temporal lobes. More than 50% of children with optic gliomas have neurofibromatosis type 1 (NF1) and often present with precocious puberty. Children with NF1 have a greater incidence of optic pathway gliomas but experience slower tumor growth, and some exhibit static lesions or even regression in tumor volume over time.

Clinical features. Initial symptoms depend on the location, but hypothalamic tumors eventually affect the optic chiasm and optic chiasm tumors affect the hypothalamus. In children younger than 3 years, tumors of the hypothalamus may produce *diencephalic syndrome,* characterized by marked loss of subcutaneous fat and total body weight with maintenance or acceleration of long bone growth. Despite the appearance of cachexia, the infant is mentally alert and does not seem as sick as the appearance suggests. Pendular or see-saw nystagmus may be associated. The precise endocrine mechanism that leads to diencephalic syndrome is unknown. Hamartomas of the tuber cinereum, optic pathway gliomas that compress the hypothalamus, and craniopharyngiomas are also associated with the syndrome. Precocious puberty, rather than diencephalic syndrome, can be the initial feature of hypothalamic tumors in infants and children.

Age is an important prognostic factor for optic gliomas. Children less than 5 years have a more aggressive course. The presenting features of unilateral optic nerve gliomas are visual loss, proptosis, and optic atrophy. Chiasmatic tumors in infants present as large suprasellar masses that may also extend into the hypothalamus and third ventricle, producing hydrocephalus and endocrine abnormalities. Binocular involvement suggests involvement of the optic chiasm or tract. Visual field deficits vary. Increased intracranial pressure suggests extension of the tumor from the chiasm to the hypothalamus.

Although the tumor is usually benign, its location results in serious morbidity. Children with NF1 have a better progression-free survival, while an age of less than 1 year is associated with a higher risk of tumor progression.[10]

Diagnosis. MRI of the hypothalamus identifies gliomas as high-density signals on T_2-weighted studies. MRI permits visualization of the hypothalamus in several different planes and identification of brainstem extension of the tumor (Fig. 16.3).

MRI with enhancement identifies optic pathway gliomas as an enlarged tubular appearance of the nerve and chiasm. Examine the entire visual pathway in all children with optic nerve gliomas because many tumors involve retrochiasmal pathways in addition to the chiasm. Routine MRI screening for optic pathway gliomas in asymptomatic children with NF1 does not affect the outcome.[11] Regular ophthalmological examinations are the preferred method for surveillance.

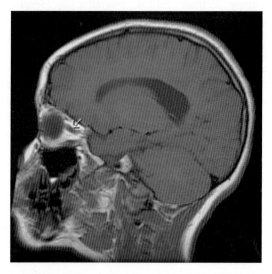

Fig. 16.3 Optic Nerve Glioma. Sagittal T_1 magnetic resonance imaging shows an enlarged optic nerve in a patient with neurofibromatosis.

Management. Several factors influence management decisions. The indications for early intervention are younger age, progressive symptoms, and extensive central nervous system involvement. Chemotherapy, the initial treatment, may provide stabilization or regression.[12] Older children and those who fail chemotherapy receive radiation therapy, which provides 5-year survival rates up to 90%. Biologics are increasingly used depending on specific tumor markers. Stereotaxic-guided biopsy should be considered when feasible as it may provide genetic information that assists with formulating a treatment plan.

Optic pathway gliomas associated with NF1 rarely progress significantly after the time of diagnosis. Biopsy or removal of tumor from a sighted eye is only a consideration when the tumor is malignant, progressively enlarging or causing severe proptosis, and likely to cause blindness or death.

Pituitary Adenoma

Pituitary adenomas represent only 1%–2% of intracranial tumors of childhood. Visual field defects may be unilateral temporal, bitemporal, or occasionally homonymous. Optic atrophy is present in 10%–20% of cases.

Clinical features. The onset of symptoms is usually during adolescence. The presenting features relate to the hormone secreted by the tumor. Approximately one-third of adenomas secrete prolactin, one-third are nonfunctioning, and many of the rest secrete growth hormone or adrenocorticotropic hormone (ACTH). Amenorrhea is usually the first symptom in girls with prolactin-secreting tumors. Galactorrhea may also be present. In boys the initial features are growth retardation, delayed puberty, and headache.

Gigantism results when increased concentrations of growth hormone circulate before the epiphyses close. After closure, growth hormone causes acromegaly. Increased concentrations of ACTH cause Cushing syndrome.

Diagnosis. MRI provides excellent visualization of the tumor and identification of its extrasellar extent. Measurement of hormone production is useful in distinguishing the tumor type.

Management. Surgical resection is the preferred treatment for tumors that compress the optic pathways. Medical treatment may suffice for small tumors. Perform an endocrine evaluation, as hormone replacement may be needed.

HEREDITARY OPTIC NEUROPATHY

Hereditary optic neuropathies may affect only the visual system, or the visual system and central nervous system, or multiple systems. The underlying abnormality may lie in nuclear or mitochondrial DNA. These disorders can cause acute, subacute, or chronic visual decline.

Leber Congenital Amaurosis/Early-Onset Severe Retinal Dystrophy

Leber congenital amaurosis and early-onset severe retinal dystrophy (LCA/EOSRD), a group of inherited retinal dystrophies, is the most common genetic cause of congenital visual impairment. Multiple different genes are implicated in pathogenesis, usually inherited in an autosomal recessive manner; rare autosomal dominant or de novo mutations have been reported. The common feature is disturbance of the retinal pigmentary epithelium.

Clinical features. The clinical characteristics of LCA are moderate to severe visual impairment at or within a few months of birth, nystagmus, keratoconus, and sluggish pupillary responses. EOSRD may have a later onset but always begins prior to age 5. Additional features include nystagmus and hypermetropic refractive errors. While substantial variation between families exists, the phenotype is relatively constant within families. Ophthalmoscopy of the retina shows progressive retinal stippling and pallor of the disk. Visual acuity is rarely better than 20/400. A characteristic finding is *oculodigital sign*, comprising eye poking, pressing, and rubbing. Several mutations are associated with kidney disease.[13]

Diagnosis. The retinal appearance and abnormal electroretinogram suggest the diagnosis in infants. Confirmatory genetic testing is available. Other disorders that may be mistaken for LCA are peroxisomal disorders and several varieties of infantile-onset progressive retinal degeneration.

Management. Gene therapy for the treatment of LCA/EOSRD is under active investigation.

Wfs1-Spectrum Disorder (Wolfram Syndrome)

There are two types of *WFS1*-spectrum disorders: classic and nonclassic. The nonclassic phenotype tends to be milder than the classic. Classic *WFS1*-SD is caused by biallelic pathogenic variants in the *WFS1* gene while nonclassic forms are caused by heterozygous pathogenic variants.[14]

Clinical features. Wolfram syndrome is a progressive neurodegenerative disorder characterized by diabetes mellitus, optic atrophy, hearing loss, dementia, ataxia, and neuropathy. Onset in the classic form is before age 16 with onset of diabetes in the first decade. Insulin therapy is required soon after diagnosis. Visual loss progresses rapidly in the second decade but does not lead to complete blindness. Diabetes does not cause optic atrophy, rather all clinical features result from a progressive neurodegenerative process. Sensorineural hearing loss affects high frequencies first. The hearing loss is progressive but rarely leads to severe hearing loss. Features reported in some patients include anosmia, autonomic dysfunction, ptosis, external ophthalmoplegia, tremor, ataxia, nystagmus, seizures, central diabetes insipidus, and other endocrinopathies. Psychiatric illness occurs in most classic cases, and patients affected with the nonclassic form have a predisposition for psychiatric disorders.

Diagnosis. Genetic testing is available.

Management. Symptomatic treatment is required for each of the clinical features. Multiple different treatments are currently under investigation, including gene therapy, but none are yet widely available.[15]

Retinoblastoma

Although retro-orbital tumors generally cause strabismus and proptosis, intraocular tumors always diminish vision. Retinoblastoma is the only malignant intraocular tumor of childhood. Its prompt recognition can be lifesaving.

The typical features of retinoblastoma in a young child are an abnormal appearance of the eye, loss of vision, and strabismus. Monocular blindness is usually unrecognized by parents. Older children may complain of visual blurring and floaters. Ocular pain is uncommon.

Leukocoria, a white pupillary reflex, is the initial feature in most children with retinoblastoma. In bright sunlight or in a flash photograph, the pupil does not constrict and has a white color. Strabismus occurs when visual acuity is impaired. The sighted eye fixates and the other remains deviated outward in all directions of gaze.

Refer all children with intraocular tumors to an ophthalmologist. A neurologist may be the primary consulting physician when the tumor is part of a larger syndrome that includes intellectual disability. Such syndromes include retinoblastoma associated with deletion of the long arm of chromosome 13, retinal astrocytoma associated with tuberous sclerosis, choroidal hemangioma associated with Sturge-Weber disease, and optic nerve glioma in children with neurofibromatosis.

SYNDROMES OF RETINAL DEGENERATION

Bardet-Biedl Syndrome

Bardet-Biedl syndrome is a genetic cone-rod dystrophy best characterized as a multisystem nonmotile ciliopathy. Several genes have been implicated.

Clinical features. Both major and minor clinical criteria exist. The most common symptoms are retinal cone-rod dystrophy, obesity, polydactyly, cognitive impairment, genitourinary or renal malformations, hypogonadotropic hypogonadism, and renal disease. Other features may include olfactory dysfunction, gastrointestinal disorders such as celiac or Hirschsprung's disease, epilepsy, ataxia, or psychiatric problems.[16]

Diagnosis. Diagnosis depends on recognition of the clinical constellation of symptoms and signs. There is significant clinical and genetic overlap with other ciliopathies. Genetic testing is available, but in approximately 25% of cases no genetic mutation is identified.

Management. Treatment is symptomatic.

Laurence-Moon Syndrome

Laurence-Moon syndrome is similar to Bardet-Biedl syndrome but represents a genetically distinct disorder with intellectual disability, pigmentary retinopathy, obesity, and postaxial polydactyly. Some authors consider the two syndromes to be part of the same spectrum of disease due to their phenotypic similarities.

Cockayne Syndrome

Cockayne syndrome (CS), like xeroderma pigmentosum (see Chapter 5), is a disorder of DNA repair. It has several types: CS types I, II, III, and a severe fetal form called COFS. Inheritance is autosomal recessive.

Clinical features. In CS type I prenatal growth is normal. Growth and developmental failure begin in the first 2 years with height, weight, and head circumference all below the 5th percentile. Progressive impairment of vision, hearing, and central and peripheral nervous system function lead to severe disability. Death typically occurs in the first or second decade.

CS type II is characterized by growth failure at birth with virtually no postnatal neurological development. Congenital cataracts or other structural anomalies of the eye may be present. Kyphosis, scoliosis, and joint contractures develop early, and death occurs by age 5.

CS type III is rare and has a later onset (after age 2). Growth and development are better than that seen in CS type I, but severe disability is still the rule.

COFS is characterized by very severe fetal anomalies including arthrogryposis and microphthalmia.

Diagnosis. The diagnosis is by the clinical features and by molecular genetic testing, which demonstrates biallelic pathogenic variants in the *ERCC6* or *ERCC8* genes.[17]

Management. Treatment is symptomatic and focuses on nutrition and feeding, management of spasticity and joint contractures, and behavioral and developmental support. Patients should wear sunglasses to protect the lens and retina. There is no cure for the underlying syndrome.

DISORDERS OF THE PUPIL

When the person is awake, the size of the pupil is constantly changing in response to light and autonomic input. This pupillary unrest is *hippus*. An isolated disturbance of pupillary size is not evidence of intracranial disease.

Aniridia

Hypoplasia of the iris may occur as a solitary abnormality or may be associated with intellectual disability, genitourinary abnormalities, and Wilms tumor. About two-thirds of cases are genetic and transmitted as an autosomal dominant trait. One-third of sporadic cases are associated with Wilms tumor. In some cases the short arm of chromosome 11 is abnormal.

Benign Essential Anisocoria

Between 20% and 30% of healthy people have an observable difference in pupillary size. Like congenital ptosis, it may go unnoticed until late childhood or adult life and is then thought to be a new finding. The size difference is constant at all levels of illumination but may be greater in darkness. The absence of other pupillary dysfunction or disturbed ocular motility suggests essential anisocoria, but old photographs are invaluable to confirm the diagnosis.

Fixed, Dilated Pupil

Clinical features. A fixed, dilated pupil is an ominous sign in unconscious patients because it suggests transtentorial herniation (see Chapter 4). However, a dilated pupil that does not respond to light or accommodation in a child who is otherwise well and has no evidence of ocular motor dysfunction or ptosis can result only from the application of a pharmacological agent or from a damaged iris sphincter. The application may be accidental, as when inadvertently wiping a drug or chemical from the hand to the eye, or when a droplet from a nebulized or aerosolized breathing treatment lands in the eye. Albuterol can produce mydriasis, as can some cosmetics or hair sprays. A careful history is essential for diagnosis.

Diagnosis. Instill 1% pilocarpine in both eyes using the normal eye as a control. Parasympathetic denervation produces prompt constriction. A slow or incomplete response indicates pharmacological dilation.

Management. Pharmacologically induced mydriasis is often long lasting, but eventually resolves.

Horner Syndrome

Horner syndrome results from sympathetic denervation; it may be congenital or acquired. When acquired, it may occur at birth as part of a brachial plexus injury, during infancy from neuroblastoma, or in childhood from tumors or injuries affecting the superior cervical ganglion or the carotid artery.

Clinical features. Unilateral Horner syndrome consists of the following ipsilateral features: mild to moderate ptosis (ptosis of the lower lid in one-third); miosis, which is best appreciated in dim light so that the normal pupil dilates; and anhidrosis of the face, heterochromia, and apparent enophthalmos when the syndrome is congenital.

Diagnosis. Disruption of the sympathetic system, anywhere from the hypothalamus to the eye, causes Horner syndrome. Brainstem disturbances from stroke are common in adults, but peripheral lesions are more common in children. Topical instillation of 1% hydroxyamphetamine usually produces pupillary dilation after 30 minutes when postganglionic denervation is present. However, false-negative results can occur during the first week after injury.[18] Ten percent cocaine solution produces little or no dilation, regardless of the site of abnormality, but the compound is difficult to obtain and cocaine metabolites can be detected in urine which limits the utility of the test.

Management. Treatment depends on the underlying cause.

Tonic Pupil Syndrome (Adie Syndrome)

Clinical features. The cause of tonic pupil syndrome is a defect in the orbital ciliary ganglion. The onset usually occurs after childhood but may occur as early as 5 years of age. Women are more often affected than men.

The defect is usually monocular and manifests as anisocoria or photophobia. The abnormal pupil is slightly larger in bright light but changes little, if at all, with alteration in illumination. In a dark room the normal pupil dilates and becomes larger than the tonic pupil. With attempted accommodation, which may also be affected, the pupil constricts slowly and incompletely and redilates slowly afterward. Binocular tonic pupils occur in children with dysautonomia and in association with diminished tendon reflexes (Holmes-Adie syndrome).

Diagnosis. The tonic pupil is supersensitive to parasympathomimetic agents; 0.125% pilocarpine achieves constriction.

Management. The condition is benign and seldom needs treatment.

REFERENCES

1. Thomas PQ, Dattani MT, Brickman JM, et al. Heterozygous HESX1 mutations associated with isolated congenital pituitary hypoplasia and septo-optic dysplasia. *Human Molecular Genetics.* 2001;10:39-45.
2. Birkebaek NH, Patel L, Wright NB, et al. Endocrine status in patients with optic nerve hypoplasia: relationship to midline central nervous system abnormalities and appearance of the hypothalamic-pituitary axis on magnetic resonance imaging. *The Journal of Clinical Endocrinology and Metabolism.* 2003;88:5281-5286.
3. Atkins EJ, Newman NJ, Biousse V. Post-traumatic visual loss. *Reviews in Neurological Diseases.* 2008;5(2):73-81. PMID: 18660739; PMCID: PMC2998754.
4. Wladis EJ, Aakalu VK, Sobel RK, et al. Interventions for indirect traumatic optic neuropathy: a report by the American Academy of Ophthalmology. *Ophthalmology.* 2021;128(6):928-937. https://doi.org/10.1016/j.ophtha.2020.10.038.
5. Arlt W, Alloli B. Adrenal insufficiency. *Lancet.* 2003;361:1881-1893.
6. Grory BM, Schrag M, Biousse V, et al. Management of central retinal artery occlusion: a scientific statement from the American Heart Association. *Stroke.* 2021;52(6):e282-e294. https://doi.org/10.1161/STR.0000000000000366.
7. Chong YJ, Mollan SP, Logeswaran A, Sinclair AB, Wakerley BR. Current perspective on retinal migraine. *Vision (Basel).* 2021;5(3):38. https://doi.org/10.3390/vision5030038. PMID: 34449754; PMCID: PMC8396291.
8. Brunel H, Raybaud C, Peretti-Viton P, et al. Craniopharyngioma in children: MRI study of 43 cases. *Neurochirurgie.* 2002;48:309-318.
9. Muller HL. Craniopharyngioma. *Endocrine Reviews.* 2014;35(3):513-543.
10. Opocher E, Kremer LCM, Da Dalt L, et al. Prognostic factors for progression of childhood optic pathway glioma: a systematic review. *European Journal of Cancer.* 2006;42:1807-1816.
11. Listernick R, Louis DN, Packer RJ, et al. Optic pathway gliomas in children with neurofibromatosis 1: consensus statement from the NF1 optic pathway glioma task force. *Annals of Neurology.* 1997;41:143-149.
12. Silva MM, Goldman S, Keating G, et al. Optic pathway hypothalamic gliomas in children under three years of age: the role of chemotherapy. *Pediatric Neurosurgery.* 2000;33(3):151-158.
13. Kumaran N, Pennesi ME, Yang P, et al. Leber congenital amaurosis/early-onset severe retinal dystrophy overview (October 4, 2018). In: Adam MP, Feldman J, Mirzaa GM, et al., eds. *GeneReviews®.* University of Washington; 1993–2023. https://www.ncbi.nlm.nih.gov/books/NBK531510/. Updated March 23, 2023.
14. Barrett T, Tranebjærg L, Gupta R, et al. WFS1 spectrum disorder (February 24, 2009). In: Adam MP, Feldman J, Mirzaa GM, et al., eds. *GeneReviews®.* University of Washington; 1993–2023. https://www.ncbi.nlm.nih.gov/books/NBK4144/. Updated December 1, 2022.
15. Mishra R, Chen BS, Richa P, Yu-Wai-Man P. Wolfram syndrome: new pathophysiological insights and therapeutic strategies. *Therapeutic Advances in Rare Disease.* 2021;2:26330040211039518. PMID: 37181110; PMCID: PMC10032446. https://doi.org/10.1177/26330040211039518.
16. Forsyth RL, Gunay-Aygun M. Bardet-Biedl syndrome overview (July 14, 2003). In: Adam MP, Feldman J, Mirzaa GM, et al., eds. *GeneReviews®.* University of Washington; 1993–2023. https://www.ncbi.nlm.nih.gov/books/NBK1363/. Updated March 23, 2023.
17. Laugel V. Cockayne syndrome (December 28, 2000). In: Adam MP, Feldman J, Mirzaa GM, et al., eds. *GeneReviews®.* University of Washington; 1993–2023. https://www.ncbi.nlm.nih.gov/books/NBK1342/. Updated August 29, 2019.
18. Donahue SP, Lavin PJM, Digre K. False-negative hydroxyamphetamine (Paredrine) test in acute Horner's syndrome. *American Journal of Ophthalmology.* 1996;122:900-901.

17

Lower Brainstem and Cranial Nerve Dysfunction

OUTLINE

Facial Weakness and Dysphagia, 381
  Anatomical Considerations, 381
  Approach to Diagnosis, 382
  Congenital Syndromes, 384
  Immune-Mediated and Infectious Disorders, 386
  Genetic Disorders, 387
  Hypertension, 389
  Infection, 389
  Metabolic Disorders, 390
  Syringobulbia, 390
  Toxins, 390
  Trauma, 391
  Tumors, 391

Hearing Impairment and Deafness, 391
  Anatomical Considerations, 391
  Symptoms of Auditory Dysfunction, 391
  Tests of Hearing, 392
  Congenital Deafness, 393
  Later-Onset Genetic Disorders, 395
  Acquired Hearing Impairment, 396
Vertigo, 397
  Anatomical Considerations, 397
  Approach to Vertigo, 398
  Causes of Vertigo, 399
References, 401

This chapter will review disorders causing dysfunction of cranial nerves VII through IX. Many such disorders also disturb ocular motility and the discussion of those is in Chapter 15. The basis for chapter assignment is by the most usual initial clinical feature. For example, the discussion of myasthenia gravis is in Chapter 15 because diplopia is a more common initial complaint than dysphagia.

An acute isolated cranial neuropathy, such as facial palsy, is usually a less ominous sign than multiple cranial neuropathies and is likely to have a self-limited course. However, an isolated cranial neuropathy may be the first sign of progressive cranial nerve dysfunction. Therefore the discussion of conditions causing isolated and multiple cranial neuropathies are together because they may not be separable at onset.

FACIAL WEAKNESS AND DYSPHAGIA

Anatomical Considerations
Facial Movement

The motor nucleus of the facial nerve is a column of cells in the ventrolateral tegmentum of the pons. Nerve fibers leaving the nucleus take a circuitous path in the brainstem before emerging close to the pontomedullary junction. The fibers then enter the internal auditory meatus with the acoustic nerve. Fibers for voluntary and reflexive facial movements separate rostral to the lower pons. After bending forward and downward around the inner ear, the facial nerve traverses the temporal bone in the facial canal and exits the skull at the stylomastoid foramen. Extracranially, the facial nerve passes into the parotid gland where it divides into several branches that innervate all muscles of facial expression except the levator palpebrae superioris, which is innervated by cranial nerve III.

Sucking and Swallowing
The sucking reflex requires the integrity of the trigeminal, facial, and hypoglossal nerves. Stimulation of the lips produces coordinated movements of the face, jaw, and tongue. The automatic aspect of the reflex disappears after infancy but may return with bilateral dysfunction of the cerebral hemispheres.

Fibers of the trigeminal and glossopharyngeal nerves ending in the nucleus solitarius form the afferent arc of the swallowing reflex. The motor roots of the trigeminal nerve, the glossopharyngeal and vagus fibers from the nucleus ambiguous, and the hypoglossal nerves form the efferent arc. A swallowing center that coordinates the reflex is located in the lower pons and upper medulla. A bolus of food stimulates the pharyngeal wall or back of the tongue, and the combined action of the tongue, palatine arches, soft palate, and pharynx move the food into the esophagus.

Approach to Diagnosis

The causes of facial muscle weakness may be supranuclear palsy (pseudobulbar palsy), intrinsic brainstem disease, or disorders of the motor unit: facial nerve, neuromuscular junction, and facial muscles (Boxes 17.1 and 17.2). The differential diagnosis of dysphagia is similar (Box 17.3), except that isolated dysfunction of the nerves that enable swallowing is very uncommon.

Pseudobulbar Palsy

Because the corticobulbar innervation of most cranial nerves is bilateral, pseudobulbar palsy occurs only when the hemispheric disease is bilateral. Many children with pseudobulbar palsy have a progressive degenerative disorder of gray or white matter. The discussion of most of these disorders is in Chapter 5 because dementia is usually the initial feature. Bilateral strokes, simultaneous or in sequence, cause pseudobulbar palsy in children; the usual causes are coagulation defects, leukemia, and trauma (see Chapter 11). Pseudobulbar palsy is the main feature of congenital bilateral perisylvian syndrome, discussed in this chapter. Episodic pseudobulbar palsy (oral apraxia, dysarthria, and drooling) may indicate acquired epileptiform opercular syndrome (see Chapter 1).

BOX 17.2   Causes of Postnatal Facial Weakness

- Autoimmune and postinfectious
  - Bell palsy[a]
  - Miller Fisher syndrome[a] (see Chapter 10)
  - Myasthenia gravis[a] (see Chapter 15)
- Genetic
  - Riboflavin transporter deficiency
  - Muscular disorders
  - Facioscapulohumeral syndrome (see Chapter 7)
  - Facioscapulohumeral syndrome, infantile form
  - Fiber-type disproportion myopathies (see Chapter 6)
  - Melkersson-Rosenthal syndrome
  - Myotonic dystrophy (see Chapter 7)
  - Myasthenic syndromes[a]
  - Congenital myasthenia[a] (see Chapter 15)
  - Familial infantile myasthenia[a] (see Chapter 6)
  - Osteopetrosis
  - Recurrent facial palsy
- Hypertension
- Infectious
  - Diphtheria
  - Herpes zoster oticus[a]
  - Infectious mononucleosis
  - Lyme disease[a] (see Chapter 2)
  - Otitis media[a]
  - Sarcoidosis[a]
  - Tuberculosis[a]
- Metabolic disorders
  - Hyperparathyroidism[a]
  - Hypothyroidism[a]
- Multiple sclerosis (see Chapter 10)
- Syringobulbia[a]
- Toxins
- Trauma
  - Delayed
  - Immediate
- Tumor
  - Glioma of brainstem (see Chapter 15)
  - Leukemia
  - Meningeal carcinoma
  - Neurofibromatosis

[a]The most common conditions and the ones with disease-modifying treatments.

BOX 17.1   Causes of Congenital Facial Weakness

- Aplasia of facial muscles
- Birth injury
- Congenital myotonic dystrophy (see Chapter 6)
- Congenital bilateral perisylvian syndrome
- Fiber-type disproportion myopathies (see Chapter 6)
- Myasthenic syndromes[a]
  - Congenital myasthenia (see Chapter 15)
  - Familial infantile myasthenia (see Chapter 6)
  - Transitory neonatal myasthenia (see Chapter 6)

[a]The most common conditions and the ones with disease-modifying treatments.

BOX 17.3 Neurological Causes of Dysphagia

- Autoimmune/postinfectious
  - Dermatomyositis (see Chapter 7)
  - Guillain-Barré syndrome (see Chapter 7)
  - Myasthenia gravis[a] (see Chapter 15)
  - Transitory neonatal myasthenia gravis[a] (see Chapter 6)
- Congenital or perinatal
  - Aplasia of brainstem nuclei
  - Cerebral palsy (see Chapter 5)
  - Chiari malformation[a] (see Chapter 10)
  - Congenital bilateral perisylvian syndrome
  - Syringobulbia[a]
- Genetic
  - Degenerative disorders (see Chapter 5)
  - Familial dysautonomia (see Chapter 6)
  - Familial infantile myasthenia (see Chapter 6)
  - Fiber-type disproportion myopathies (see Chapter 6)
  - Myotonic dystrophy (see Chapters 6 and 7)
- Glioma of brainstem
- Infectious
  - Botulism[a] (see Chapters 6 and 7)
  - Diphtheria
  - Poliomyelitis (see Chapter 7)
- Riboflavin transporter deficiency

[a]The most common conditions and the ones with disease-modifying treatments.

BOX 17.4 Causes of Recurrent Cranial Neuropathies/Palsies

- Familial
  - Isolated facial palsy
  - Melkersson-Rosenthal syndrome
- Hypertensive facial palsy[a]
- Myasthenia gravis[a]
- Sporadic multiple cranial neuropathies
- Toxins

[a]The most common conditions and the ones with disease-modifying treatments.

Motor Unit Disorders

Disorders of the facial nuclei and nerves always cause ipsilateral facial weakness and atrophy, but associated features vary with the site of abnormality:

1. *Motor nucleus*: Hyperacusis is present, but taste, lacrimation, and salivation are normal.
2. *Facial nerve between the pons and the internal auditory meatus*: Taste sensation is spared, but lacrimation and salivation are impaired, and hyperacusis is present.
3. *Geniculate ganglion*: Taste, lacrimation, and salivation are impaired, and hyperacusis is present.
4. *Facial nerve from the geniculate ganglion to the stapedius nerve*: Taste and salivation are impaired, and hyperacusis is present, but lacrimation is normal.
5. *Facial nerve from the stapedius nerve to the chorda tympani*: Taste and salivation are impaired, hyperacusis is not present, and lacrimation is normal.
6. *Facial nerve below the exit of the chorda tympani nerve*: Only facial weakness is present.

Disturbances of cranial nerve nuclei seldom occur in isolation; they are often associated with other features of brainstem dysfunction (bulbar palsy). Usually some combination of dysarthria, dysphagia, and diplopia is present. Examination may show strabismus, facial diplegia, loss of the gag reflex, atrophy of bulbar muscles, and fasciculations of the tongue.

The facial weakness associated with myasthenia gravis and facial myopathies is usually bilateral. In contrast, brainstem disorders usually begin on one side and eventually progress to bilateral impairment. Facial nerve palsies are usually unilateral. The differential diagnosis of recurrent facial palsy or dysphagia is limited to disorders of the facial nerve and neuromuscular junction (Box 17.4).

The characteristic feature of pseudobulbar palsy is an inability to use bulbar muscles in voluntary effort, while reflex movements, initiated at a brainstem level, are normal. Extraocular motility is unaffected. The child can suck, chew, and swallow but cannot coordinate these reflexes for eating; movement of a food bolus from the front of the mouth to the back has a volitional component. Emotionally derived facial expressions occur, but voluntary facial movements do not. Severe dysarthria is often present. Affected muscles do not show atrophy or fasciculations. The gag reflex and jaw jerk are usually exaggerated, and emotional volatility is often an associated feature.

Newborns with familial dysautonomia have difficulty feeding, despite normal sucking and swallowing, because they fail to coordinate the two reflexes (see Chapter 6). Box 6.7 summarizes the differential diagnosis of feeding difficulty in an alert newborn. Children with cerebral palsy often have a similar disturbance in the coordination of chewing and swallowing that impairs feeding.

Congenital Syndromes

Congenital Bilateral Perisylvian Syndrome

This syndrome results from a disturbance in neuronal migration that results in pachygyria of the Sylvian and Rolandic regions. Most cases are sporadic. The transmission of familial cases is by X-linked inheritance; such cases are more severe in males than in females.[1]

Clinical features. All affected children have a pseudobulbar palsy that causes failure of speech development (apraxia) and dysphagia. Cognitive impairment and seizures are present in approximately 85% of cases. The cognitive deficit varies from mild to severe, and the seizures, which begin between 4 and 12 years, may be atypical absence, atonic/tonic, focal, or generalized tonic-clonic.

Diagnosis. Magnetic resonance imaging (MRI) shows bilateral perisylvian gyral dysgenesis including pachygyria and polymicrogyria (Fig. 17.1). Postmortem studies have confirmed the MRI impression.

Management. The seizures are usually difficult to control, and palliative corpus callosotomy has been useful in some cases with intractable drop attacks. Speech therapy does not overcome the speech disorder, and instruction in sign language is the better alternative for children of near-normal intelligence. Drooling is very

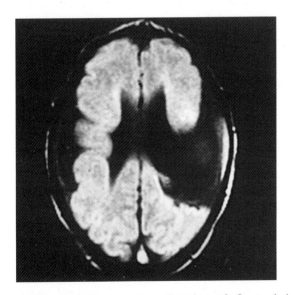

Fig. 17.1 Magnetic Resonance Imaging of Congenital Bilateral Perisylvian Syndrome. This child has lissencephaly and schizencephaly. Bilateral disturbances in the perisylvian region caused a pseudobulbar palsy.

disruptive and may benefit from the use of glycopyrrolate, excision of the submandibular glands, ligation of parotid gland ducts, or botulinum toxin injections to the parotid glands.

Congenital Dysphagia

Congenital dysphagia is usually associated with infantile hypotonia and therefore discussed in Chapter 6. Because the neuroanatomical substrates of swallowing and breathing are contiguous, congenital dysphagia and dyspnea are often concurrent. Isolated aplasia of the cranial nerve nuclei subserving swallowing is not established.

Congenital Facial Asymmetry

The cause of most facial asymmetries at birth is congenital aplasia of muscle and not trauma to the facial nerve. Facial diplegia, whether complete or incomplete, suggests Möbius syndrome or other congenital muscle aplasia. Complete unilateral palsies are likely to be traumatic in origin, whereas partial unilateral palsies may be either traumatic or aplastic. The term *neonatal facial asymmetry* is probably more accurate than facial nerve palsy to denote partial or complete unilateral facial weakness in the newborn and emphasizes the difficulty in differentiating traumatic nerve palsies from congenital aplasias. A common cause of asymmetry of the lower face/mouth is the unilateral absence of the depressor anguli oris.

Aplasia of facial muscles

Clinical features. Möbius syndrome is the best-known congenital aplasia of facial nerve nuclei and facial muscles. The site of pathology is usually the facial nerve nuclei and their internuclear connections. Facial diplegia may occur alone, with bilateral abducens palsies, or with the involvement of several cranial nerves.[2] Many children with the syndrome have micrognathia and microstomia and may have cleft palate and dental anomalies, which contribute to speech delays. Congenital malformations elsewhere in the body (dextrocardia, talipes equinovarus, absent pectoral muscles, and limb deformities) are sometimes associated features. Although affected children may have intellectual impairment and speech delays, use caution in diagnosing autism spectrum disorders as the syndrome can cause difficulty with normal expression and eye contact that can be misleading. Most cases are sporadic, but familial recurrence with autosomal dominant inheritance has been reported in a very small number of cases.

Other developmental causes of unilateral facial palsy are *Goldenhar syndrome*, the *Poland anomaly*, *DiGeorge syndrome*, osteopetrosis, and trisomy 13 and 18.

Diagnosis. Congenital facial diplegia is, by definition, Möbius syndrome. All such cases require MRI of the brain to determine if other cerebral malformations are present. Causes other than primary malformations include intrauterine toxins (e.g., thalidomide), vascular malformations, or infarction.

Electromyography (EMG) can help determine the timing of injury. Denervation potentials are only present if injury to the facial nuclei or nerve occurred 2–6 weeks before the study. Facial muscles that are aplastic, as in Möbius syndrome, or nerve injury occurring early in gestation, do not show active denervation.

Management. Surgical procedures may provide partial facial movement.

Depressor anguli oris aplasia ("Asymmetric crying facies")

Clinical features. Isolated unilateral weakness of the depressor anguli oris muscle (DAOM) is the most common cause of facial asymmetry at birth. One corner of the mouth fails to move downward when the child cries. All other facial movements are symmetrical. The lower lip on the paralyzed side feels thinner to palpation, even at birth, suggesting antepartum hypoplasia.

Diagnosis. Traumatic lesions of the facial nerve would not selectively injure nerve fibers to the DAOM and spare all other facial muscles. Electrodiagnostic studies are typically not needed but may aid in differentiating aplasia of the DAOM from traumatic injury. In aplasia, the conduction velocity and latency of the facial nerve are normal. Fibrillations are not present at the site of the DAOM. Instead, motor unit potentials are absent or decreased in number. The pulling of the mouth in the direction of the healthy DAOM when crying often causes the referring physician to believe that this is the abnormal side. While the anomaly itself is relatively mild, approximately 10% of cases are associated with other, more significant congenital abnormalities, most notably of the cardiovascular system.[3]

Management. No treatment is available or needed. The DAOM is not a significant component of facial expression in older children and adults, and absence of the muscle is often unnoticed. The child should be carefully examined for evidence of other malformations.

Birth injury. Perinatal traumatic facial palsy is a disorder of large-term newborns delivered vaginally after prolonged labor. Nerve compression against the sacrum during labor is more often the cause than is the misapplication of forceps. Children with forceps injuries, an unusual event, have forceps marks on the cheeks.

Clinical features. The clinical expression of complete unilateral facial palsy in the newborn can be subtle and may not be apparent immediately after birth. Failure of eye closure on the affected side is the first noticeable evidence of weakness. Only when the child cries does the flaccid paralysis of all facial muscles become obvious. The eyeball rolls up behind the open lid, the nasolabial fold remains flat, and the corner of the mouth droops during crying. The normal side appears paralyzed because it pulls and distorts the face; the paralyzed side appears to be normal. When paralysis of the facial nerve is partial, the orbicularis oculi is the muscle most frequently spared. In these injuries the compression site is usually over the parotid gland, with sparing of nerve fibers that course upward just after leaving the stylomastoid foramen.

Facial nerve palsies can be graded according to several scales. The most widely accepted is the House-Brackmann scale, which is useful to provide consistency among treating physicians although it does not provide details regarding the specific muscle deficits:

- Grade I: Symmetric at rest and with movement, with no abnormalities.
- Grade II: Mild weakness, symmetric at rest, minimal asymmetry with movement, complete eye closure with gentle effort, possible mild synkinesis.
- Grade III: Moderate weakness, symmetric at rest, moderate asymmetry with movement, complete eye closure only with full effort, possible moderate synkinesis.
- Grade IV: Moderate-to-severe weakness, symmetric at rest, moderate asymmetry with movement, incomplete eye closure.
- Grade V: Severe weakness, grossly asymmetric at rest, significant asymmetry with movement, incomplete eye closure.
- Grade VI: No visible movement, grossly asymmetric at rest ("facial droop").

Diagnosis. The diagnosis of facial asymmetry is by observing the face of the crying newborn. Carefully examine the facial skin for lacerations. Otoscopic examination is useful to establish the presence of hemotympanum. EMG does not alter the management of the palsy.

Management. The majority of cases of perinatal facial nerve injuries spontaneously recover within 4 months, although recovery may be incomplete. As expected, grade I and II injuries have the best prognosis, while grades V and VI usually cause permanent deficits.

Most newborns are not candidates for surgical intervention unless the nerve laceration occurs at delivery. In that event the best response is to reconstitute the nerve if possible or at least to allow the proximal stump a clear pathway toward regeneration by debridement of the wound. Surgical repairs are sometimes attempted in less severe cases after age 4 months if recovery is incomplete, but the outcomes are uncertain and published clinical trials are scarce.

Immune-Mediated and Infectious Disorders

Postinfectious demyelination of the VII nerve is the cause of most cases of acute unilateral facial neuritis (Bell palsy) or bilateral facial neuritis. The basis for distinguishing bilateral Bell palsy from Guillain-Barré syndrome (acute inflammatory demyelinating polyneuropathy) is the preservation of limb tendon reflexes in Bell palsy. Discussion of Guillain-Barré syndrome is in Chapter 7.

Bell Palsy

Bell palsy is an acute, idiopathic, self-limited, typically monophasic, paralysis of the face caused by dysfunction of the facial nerve. The pathogenesis is believed to be viral (most often herpes simplex) but may also be postviral, immune-mediated, or demyelinating. The annual incidence is approximately 3/100,000 in the first decade, 10/100,000 in the second decade, and 25/100,000 in adults. Only 1% of cases have clinical evidence of bilateral involvement, but many have electrophysiological abnormalities on the unaffected side. Bilateral or recurrent Bell palsy should prompt consideration of neurosarcoidosis (see section later in this chapter).

Clinical features. A history of viral infection, usually upper respiratory, is recorded in many cases, but the frequency is not significantly greater than expected by chance. The initial feature of neuritis is often pain or tingling in the ear canal ipsilateral to the subsequent facial palsy. Pain accompanies facial weakness in 60%, impaired lacrimation in 60%, taste changes in 30%–50%, and hyperacusis in 15%–30% of patients.

Ipsilateral facial sensory symptoms are usually mild and explained by extension of inflammation from the facial nerve to the trigeminal nerve via the greater superficial petrosal nerve.[4] The palsy has an explosive onset and becomes maximal within hours. Either the child or the parents may first notice the palsy, which affects all muscles on one side of the face. Half of the face sags, enlarging the palpebral fissure. Weakness of the orbicularis muscle prevents closure of the lid. Efforts to use muscles of expression cause the face to pull to the normal side. Eating and drinking become difficult and dribbling of liquids from the weak corner of the mouth causes embarrassment.

The most commonly affected portion of the nerve is within the temporal bone; taste, lacrimation, and salivation are impaired, and hyperacusis is present. However, examination of all facial nerve functions in small children is difficult, and precise localization is not critical to diagnosis or prognosis.

Children generally exhibit good recovery although outcomes are variable among studies. However, prognosis depends largely on the House-Brackmann scale at the time of presentation, and those who present with weakness grade V or VI typically experience residual deficits regardless of treatment.[5]

Diagnosis. Complete neurological examination is required in every child with acute unilateral facial weakness to determine whether the palsy is an isolated abnormality. Mild facial weakness on the other side or the absence of tendon reflexes in the limbs suggests the possibility of Guillain-Barré syndrome. Such children require observation for the development of progressive limb weakness.

Exclude possible underlying causes (e.g., hypertension, infection, trauma) of facial nerve palsy before considering the diagnosis of Bell palsy. Examine the ear ipsilateral to the facial palsy for herpetic lesions (see the "Herpes Zoster Oticus [Ramsay-Hunt Syndrome]" section). MRI shows contrast enhancement of the involved nerve, but acute, isolated facial palsy is not an indication for MRI in every child. A more reasonable approach is to watch the child and recommend an imaging study if other neurological disturbances develop or if the palsy does not begin to resolve within 1 month.

Management. Always protect the cornea if the blink reflex is absent and especially if the palpebral fissure remains open while sleeping. This may result in corneal ulcers due to prolonged ocular exposure and dryness. Ophthalmological ointments are needed to prevent this complication. Patch the eye when the child is outside the home or at play and apply artificial tears several times a day to keep the cornea moist. The use of steroids and an antiviral agent such as acyclovir is standard if the patient presents early in the course, but there is no evidence of efficacy in long-standing or severe cases.

Polyneuritis Cranialis

Polyneuritis cranialis is extremely rare in the pediatric population. The presumed mechanism is postinfectious, and many consider it a variant of Guillain-Barré syndrome.

Clinical features. Onset is usually in adults, and most childhood cases occur in adolescence. Similar cases described in infants subsequently developed limb weakness, and infantile botulism was the more likely diagnosis (see Chapter 6).

Constant, aching facial pain usually precedes weakness by hours or days. The pain is often localized to the temple or frontal region but can be anywhere in the face. Weakness may develop within 1 day or may evolve over several weeks. Extraocular motility is usually affected. Facial and trigeminal nerve disturbances occur in half of cases, but lower cranial nerve involvement is uncommon. Occasional patients have transitory visual disturbances, ptosis, pupillary abnormalities, and tinnitus. Tendon reflexes in the limbs remain active. Recurrent idiopathic cranial neuropathies occur as sporadic cases in adults but usually occur on a familial basis in children.

Diagnosis. The differential diagnosis includes Guillain-Barré syndrome, infant and childhood forms of botulism, brainstem glioma, juvenile progressive bulbar palsy, pontobulbar palsy with deafness, and Tolosa-Hunt syndrome. Preservation of tendon reflexes in polyneuritis cranialis is the main feature distinguishing it from Guillain-Barré syndrome. Prominent autonomic dysfunction and limb weakness separate it from botulism (see Chapters 6 and 7). Cranial nerve dysfunction in patients with brainstem glioma, juvenile progressive bulbar palsy, and pontobulbar palsy with deafness usually evolves over a longer period. Tolosa-Hunt syndrome of painful ophthalmoplegia and idiopathic cranial polyneuropathy share many features, and they may be a variant of the same disease process (see Chapter 15).

All laboratory findings are normal. The possibility of a brainstem glioma requires MRI of the brainstem in all cases. Examination of the cerebrospinal fluid occasionally reveals a mild elevation of protein concentration and a lymphocyte count of 5–6/mm^3.

Management. The disease is self-limited, and full recovery is the expected outcome 2–4 months after onset. The use of corticosteroids is routine and believed to ease facial pain and shorten the course. The relief of pain may be dramatic, but evidence documenting a shortened course is lacking.

Genetic Disorders
Facioscapulohumeral Dystrophy

Facioscapulohumeral dystrophy (FSHD) sometimes begins during infancy as bilateral facial weakness (facial diplegia). Two types exist: FSHD1 and FSHD2, which are clinically indistinguishable but genetically distinct. Inheritance of FSHD1 is by autosomal dominant transmission; FSHD2 is inherited in a digenic pattern, meaning two separate genetic changes are needed to cause the condition.[6] The majority of individuals with FSHD1 inherited the disease-causing deletion from a parent, and the rest are de novo deletions. There is evidence that having both *FSHD1* and *FSHD2* mutations causes more severe and rapidly progressive disease. Prenatal testing is available.

Clinical features. The onset of infantile FSHD is usually no later than age 5 years. Facial diplegia is the initial feature. When onset is early in infancy, the common misdiagnosis is congenital aplasia of facial muscles. Later, nasal speech and sometimes ptosis develop. Progressive proximal weakness begins 1–2 years after onset, first affecting the shoulders and then the pelvis. Scapular winging is often seen, and the child may have difficulty combing their hair or throwing a ball. Pseudohypertrophy of the calves may be present. Tendon reflexes are depressed and then absent in weak muscle. Typical features are a striking asymmetry of muscle involvement from side to side and sparing of bulbar extraocular and respiratory muscles. The weakness may also stabilize for long intervals and not cause severe disability until adult life. Approximately 20% of patients eventually become nonambulatory.

Retinal telangiectasia and high-frequency hearing loss occur in about half of affected families.[7] Both conditions are progressive and may not be symptomatic in early childhood.

Diagnosis. The diagnosis of FSHD is a possibility in every child with progressive facial diplegia. A family history of FSHD syndrome is not always obtainable because the affected parent may show only minimal expression of the phenotype. Molecular-based testing is reliable for diagnosis.

Myasthenia gravis and brainstem glioma are a consideration in infants with progressive facial diplegia. The serum concentration of creatine kinase is helpful in differentiating these disorders. It is usually elevated in the infantile FSHD syndrome and normal in myasthenia gravis and brainstem glioma. Electrophysiological studies show brief, small-amplitude polyphasic potentials in weak muscles, and a normal response to repetitive nerve stimulation.

Management. Treatment is supportive.

Riboflavin Transporter Deficiency

Riboflavin transporter deficiency encompasses a spectrum of disorders including juvenile progressive bulbar palsy (previously known as *Fazio-Londe disease*) and pontobulbar palsy with deafness (*Brown-Vialetto-Van Laere syndrome*).

Clinical features. The phenotype is variable but includes progressive peripheral and cranial neuropathies leading to weakness, sensorineural hearing loss, vision loss, and sensory ataxia. The initial symptom is often rapidly progressive deafness with other symptoms beginning within 1–2 years. Optic nerve atrophy and pallor occur and are associated with vision loss and nystagmus. Involvement of cranial nerves IX, X, and XII results in bulbar palsy and tongue fasciculations. Cranial nerve III and VII palsies are less common but may occur, causing ptosis and facial weakness. Peripheral neuropathy leads to muscle weakness and can cause respiratory compromise; the arms are more affected than the legs, and tendon reflexes are absent. Cognition usually remains normal.

Diagnosis. The major diagnostic considerations are myasthenia gravis and brainstem glioma. MRI excludes brainstem tumors. EMG shows chronic partial denervation and nerve conduction studies demonstrate sensory more than motor axonal neuropathies. Visual evoked potentials are usually abnormal. Molecular genetic testing reveals biallelic pathogenic variants in either the *SLC52A2* or *SLC52A3* genes.[8]

Management. Treatment is high-dose oral riboflavin (vitamin B_2) supplementation between 10 and 50 mg/kg/day. Begin supplemental riboflavin immediately if the diagnosis is suspected; do not wait for the results of confirmatory genetic testing. Prompt treatment can be lifesaving, and outcomes are better when treatment is started early in the disease before neuronal damage.

CLCN7-Related Osteopetrosis

There are three distinct phenotypes: infantile malignant *CLCN7*–related autosomal recessive osteopetrosis (ARO); intermediate autosomal osteopetrosis (IAO), and autosomal dominant osteopetrosis type II (also known as Albers-Schönberg disease). Cranial nerve compression and cranial neuropathies can occur in any of the three but are most common in ARO.

Clinical features. ARO onset is at birth. Sclerosis of the skull base produces multiple compressive cranial neuropathies, including visual impairment, sensorineural hearing loss, and facial weakness. The bone marrow cavity is significantly reduced or absent leading to severe anemia and thrombocytopenia. Fractures, hyperparathyroidism, and hypocalcemia with tetany and seizures are possible. Life expectancy without treatment is less than 10 years. IAO begins in childhood with increased incidence of fractures, mild anemia, and occasional optic nerve compression with normal life expectancy. AOII begins in adolescence and is the mildest phenotype; optic nerve compression is unusual.[9]

Diagnosis. Molecular genetic testing demonstrates biallelic or pathogenic heterozygous mutations in the *CLCN7* gene.

Management. ARO should be treated with hematopoietic stem cell transplantation, which can be curative. Unfortunately, the cranial neuropathies usually result in permanent deficits even after stem cell transplant.

Melkersson-Rosenthal Syndrome

Melkersson-Rosenthal syndrome is a rare disorder of unknown cause resulting in recurrent attacks of facial palsy and oro-facial edema. Rare familial cases have been reported but the vast majority are of unknown cause.

Clinical features. Melkersson-Rosenthal syndrome is a rare disorder characterized by the triad of recurrent facial palsy, lingua plicata, and facial edema. Attacks of facial palsy usually begin in the second decade, but 20%–40% have a deeply furrowed tongue that is present from birth.

The first attack of facial weakness is indistinguishable from Bell palsy except that a migraine-like headache may precede the attack. Subsequent attacks are associated with eyelid edema, which is soft, painless, nonerythematous, and nonpruritic. The edema is most often asymmetric, involving only the upper lip on the paralyzed side, but it may affect the cheek and eyelid on one or both sides. Cold weather or emotional stress may precipitate an attack of facial swelling. Lingua plicata is present in 30%–50% of cases. Furrowing and deep grooving on the dorsal surface of the tongue may lead to infection or loss of taste. Often, family members have similar tongue findings. Nonneurologic complications include allergy tendency and immune dysfunction including ulcerative colitis and uveitis.[10]

Diagnosis. The diagnosis of Melkersson-Rosenthal syndrome is established when two features of the triad are present. It is a consideration in any child with a personal or family history of recurrent facial palsy or recurrent facial edema. The presence of lingua plicata in any member of the kindred confirms the diagnosis. Histopathology of the affected eyelid reveals a granulomatous lymphangitis unique to the disease.[11]

Management. Due to the allergy and immune comorbidities, corticosteroids are often used although evidence-based treatment protocols are lacking.

Hypertension

Unilateral facial palsy may be a feature of malignant hypertension in children. The cause of the palsy is swelling and hemorrhage into the facial canal.

Clinical features. The course of facial paralysis is indistinguishable from that in Bell palsy. Nerve compression occurs in its proximal segment, impairing lacrimation, salivation, and taste. The onset coincides with a rise in diastolic blood pressure to greater than 120 mm Hg, and recovery begins when the pressure reduces. The duration of palsy varies from days to weeks. Recurrences are associated with repeated episodes of hypertension.

Diagnosis. The occurrence of facial palsy in a child with known hypertension suggests that the hypertension is out of control.

Management. Control of hypertension is the only effective treatment.

Infection

The facial nerve is sometimes involved when bacterial infection spreads from the middle ear to the mastoid. External otitis may lead to facial nerve involvement by the spread of infection from the tympanic membrane to the chorda tympani.

Diphtheria may cause single or multiple cranial neuropathies from a direct effect of its toxin. Facial palsy, dysarthria, and dysphagia are potential complications. Basilar meningitis, from tuberculosis or other bacterial

infections, causes inflammation of cranial nerves as they leave the brain and enter the skull. Multiple and bilateral cranial nerve involvement is usually progressive.

Herpes Zoster Oticus (Ramsay-Hunt Syndrome)

Herpes zoster infection of the geniculate ganglion causes herpes zoster oticus.

Clinical features. The initial feature is pain in and behind the ear. This pain is often more severe and persistent than that expected with other causes of Bell palsy. Unilateral facial palsy, indistinguishable from Bell palsy by appearance, follows. However, examination of the ipsilateral ear, especially in the fossa of the helix and behind the lobule, shows a vesicular eruption characteristic of herpes zoster. Hearing loss is associated in 25% of cases.

Diagnosis. The only historical feature distinguishing herpes zoster oticus from Bell palsy is the severity of ear pain. Examination of the ear for vesicles is critical to the diagnosis.

Management. Herpes zoster infections are usually self-limited but painful. A combination of oral acyclovir and oral prednisone improves the outcome of facial nerve function in people 15 years and older.[12] Complete recovery occurs in 75% of those treated within 7 days of onset and in 30% treated after 7 days. The varicella vaccine may reduce the incidence of new cases and decrease the severity of symptoms.[13]

Sarcoidosis

Cranial nerve dysfunction is the most common neurological complication of sarcoidosis. Basilar granulomatous meningitis is the usual cause (Fig. 17.2), but the facial nerve may also be involved when parotitis is present.

Clinical features. Onset is usually in the third decade but may be as early as adolescence. Neurological complications occur in only 5% of patients with sarcoidosis but, when present, they are often an early feature of the disease. Facial nerve palsy, unilateral or bilateral, is the single most common feature. Visual impairment or deafness is next in frequency. Single cranial neuropathies are present in 73% and multiple cranial neuropathies in 58%. Any cranial nerve except the accessory nerve may be involved. Systemic features of sarcoidosis occur in almost every case: intrathoracic involvement is present in 81% and ocular involvement in 50%. Uveoparotitis is an uncommon manifestation

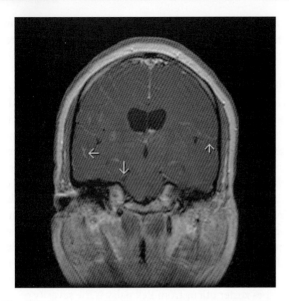

Fig. 17.2 Neurosarcoidosis. T_1 coronal magnetic resonance imaging with contrast shows enhancing leptomeninges (*arrows*).

of sarcoidosis. The patient ordinarily comes to medical attention because of visual impairment and a painful eye. The mouth is dry and the parotid gland is swollen. Facial nerve compression and palsy are present in 40% of cases.

Diagnosis. Sarcoidosis is a consideration in any patient with single or multiple cranial neuropathies. Documentation of multisystem disease confirms the diagnosis. Radiographs of the chest either establish or are compatible with the diagnosis in almost all patients with neurological manifestations. Contrast-enhanced MRI demonstrates cranial neuropathies and may show other evidence of neurosarcoidosis such as periventricular white matter lesions or enhancing parenchymal lesions.

Increased serum concentrations of angiotensin-converting enzyme (ACE) are detectable in 75% of patients with active pulmonary disease, and patients with neurosarcoidosis may have elevated cerebrospinal fluid concentrations of ACE. Biopsy of lymph nodes or other affected tissues provides histological confirmation.

Management. Treatment of neurosarcoidosis depends on symptom severity. Steroids are the mainstay of therapy for facial palsies. Prednisone therapy, 0.5–1 mg/kg/day, is maintained until a clinical response is evident and then slowly tapered at a rate that prevents relapse. Cranial neuropathies associated with other manifestations require more aggressive management with methotrexate, mycophenolate mofetil, or TNF-α inhibitors.[14]

Metabolic Disorders
Hyperparathyroidism

The most common neurological features of primary hyperparathyroidism are headache and confusion (see Chapter 2). Occasionally, hyperparathyroidism is associated with a syndrome that is similar to amyotrophic lateral sclerosis and includes ataxia and internuclear ophthalmoplegia. Dysarthria and dysphagia are prominent features.

Hypothyroidism

Cranial nerve abnormalities are unusual in hypothyroidism. Deafness is the most common feature, but acute facial nerve palsy resembling Bell palsy also occurs.

Syringobulbia

Syringobulbia is usually the medullary extension of a cervical syrinx (see Chapter 12) but may also originate in the medulla. The syrinx usually involves the nucleus ambiguous and the spinal tract and motor nucleus of the trigeminal nerve. Symptoms in order of frequency are headache, vertigo, dysarthria, facial paresthesias, dysphagia, diplopia, tinnitus, and palatal palsy.

Toxins

Most neurotoxins produce either diffuse encephalopathy or peripheral neuropathy. Only ethylene glycol, trichloroethylene, and chlorocresol exposure cause selective cranial nerve toxicity. Ethylene glycol is antifreeze. Ingestion causes facial diplegia, hearing impairment, and dysphagia. Trichloroethylene intoxication can cause multiple cranial neuropathies but has a predilection for the trigeminal nerve. It was once a treatment for tic douloureux. Chlorocresol, a compound used in the industrial production of heparin, caused recurrent unilateral facial palsy in one exposed worker. Inhalation of the compound caused tingling of one side of the face followed by weakness of the muscles. The neurological disturbance was brief, relieved by exposure to fresh air, and could be reproduced experimentally.

Trauma

Facial palsy following closed head injury is usually associated with bleeding from the ear and fracture of the petrous bone.

Clinical features. The onset of palsy may be immediate or delayed for as long as 3 weeks after injury. In most cases the interval is between 2 and 7 days. Delays may be due to late effects of swelling or axonal degeneration following shear injury.

Diagnosis. Electrophysiological studies are helpful in prognosis. If the nerve is intact but shows a conduction block, recovery usually begins within 5 days and is complete. Most patients with partial denervation recover full facial movement but have evidence of aberrant reinnervation. Full recovery is not an expected outcome when denervation is complete.

Management. The management of traumatic facial palsy is controversial and depends on the severity of the injury and resultant deficits. Corticosteroids followed by surgical decompression are common, but management varies greatly depending on the specific type and location of the injury. Surgical options include direct coaptation in cases of complete transection, nerve grafting, or nerve transfer.[15]

Tumors

Tumors of the facial nerve are rare in children. The major neoplastic cause of facial palsy is brainstem glioma (see Chapter 15), followed by tumors that infiltrate the meninges, such as leukemia, meningeal carcinoma, and eosinophilic granuloma. Acoustic neuromas are unusual in childhood and are limited to children with neurofibromatosis type 2 (NF2). These neuromas cause hearing impairment before facial palsy and are discussed in the following section.

HEARING IMPAIRMENT AND DEAFNESS

Anatomical Considerations

Sound, mechanically funneled through the external auditory canal, causes the tympanic membrane to vibrate. Ossicles transmit the vibrations to the oval window of the cochlea, the sensory organ of hearing. The air-filled space extending from the tympanic membrane to the cochlea comprises *the middle ear*. The membranous labyrinth within the osseous labyrinth is the principal structure of *the inner ear*. It contains the cochlea, the semicircular canals, and the vestibule. The semicircular canals and vestibule are the sensory organs of vestibular function. The cochlea consists of three fluid-filled canals wound into a snail-like configuration.

The organ of Corti is the transducer within the cochlea that converts mechanical to electrical energy. The auditory portion of the eighth nerve transmits impulses to the ipsilateral cochlear nuclei of the medulla. The transmission of information from the cochlear nuclei on each side is to both superior olivary nuclei, causing a bilateral representation of hearing throughout the remainder of the central pathways. From the superior olivary nuclei, transmission is by the lateral lemniscus to the inferior colliculus. Further cross-connections occur in collicular synapses. Rostrally directed fibers from the inferior colliculi ascend to the medial geniculate and auditory cortex of the temporal lobe.

Symptoms of Auditory Dysfunction

The major symptoms of disturbance in the auditory pathways are hearing impairment, tinnitus, and hyperacusis. The characteristic feature of hearing impairment in infants is failure to develop speech (see Chapter 5) and in older children inattentiveness and poor school performance. Fifty percent of infants use words with meaning by 12 months and join words into sentences by 24 months. Failure to accomplish these tasks by 21 months and 3 years, respectively, is always abnormal. A hearing loss of 25–30 dB is sufficient to interfere with normal acquisition of speech.

Hearing Impairment

Hearing impairment is classified as conductive, sensorineural (perceptive), or central. The cause of conductive hearing impairment is a disturbance in the external or middle ear. Faithful delivery of the mechanical vibrations that make up the sensory input of hearing to the inner ear does not occur because the external canal is blocked or the tympanic membrane or ossicles are abnormal. The major defect in conductive hearing loss is sound amplification. Patients with conductive hearing impairment are better able to hear loud speech in a noisy background than soft speech in a quiet background. Tinnitus may be associated.

Sensorineural hearing impairment may be congenital or acquired and is caused by a disturbance of the cochlea or auditory nerve. The frequency content of sound is improperly analyzed and transduced. High frequencies may be selectively lost. Individuals with sensorineural hearing impairment have difficulty discriminating speech when there is background noise. Central hearing impairment results from disturbance of the cochlear nuclei or their projections to the cortex. Brainstem lesions usually cause bilateral hearing impairment. Cortical lesions lead to difficulty in processing information. Pure-tone audiometry is normal, but background noise or competing messages impair speech discrimination. The cause of approximately one-third of childhood deafness is genetic, one-third acquired, and one-third idiopathic. Many of the idiopathic cases are probably genetic as well.

Tinnitus

Tinnitus is the illusion of noise in the ear. The noise is usually high-pitched and constant. In most cases the cause of tinnitus is a disturbance of the auditory nerve, but it may also occur as a simple partial seizure originating from the primary auditory cortex. Sounds generated by the cardiovascular system (heartbeat and bruit) are sometimes audible, especially while a person is lying down but should not be confused with tinnitus.

Hyperacusis

The cause of hyperacusis is failure of the stapedius muscle to dampen sound by its effect on the ossicles. This occurs with damage to the chorda tympani branch of the facial nerve (see the discussion of "Bell Palsy" section). Transient hypersensitivity to sound is relatively common during migraine attacks but should not be confused with true hyperacusis.

Tests of Hearing
Office Testing

Hearing assessment in the office is satisfactory for severe hearing impairment but is unsatisfactory for detecting loss of specific frequency bands. The speech and hearing disability generated by a high-frequency hearing impairment should not be underestimated. When testing an infant, the physician should stand behind the patient and provide interesting sounds to each ear. Bells, chimes, rattles, or a tuning fork are useful for that purpose. Dropping a large object and watching the infant and parents startle from the noise is not a test of hearing. Once the infant sees the source of the interesting sound or hears it several times, interest is lost. Therefore the use of different high- and low-frequency sounds is

required for each ear. The normal responses of the infant are to become alert and to attempt to localize the source of the sound.

In older children observing their response to spoken words at different intensities and with tuning forks that provide pure tones of different frequencies tests hearing. The *Rinne test* compares air conduction (conductive plus sensorineural hearing) with bone conduction (sensorineural hearing). Hold a tuning fork against the mastoid process until the sound fades and is then held 1 inch from the ear. Normal children hear the vibration produced by air conduction twice as long as that produced by bone conduction. Impaired air conduction with normal bone conduction indicates a conductive hearing loss.

The *Weber test* compares bone conduction in the two ears. Localization of the signals transmitted by bone conduction is to the better-hearing ear or the ear with the greater conductive deficit. With a tuning fork placed at the center of the forehead, inquire whether the perception of sound is equal in both ears. A normal response is to hear the sound in the center of the head. If bone conduction is normal in both ears, sound localization is to the ear with impaired air conduction because the normal blocking response of air conduction is lacking. If a sensorineural hearing impairment is present in one ear, the perception of bone conduction is in the good ear. Otoscopic examination is imperative in every child with hearing problems or tinnitus. The cause seen through the speculum may be impacted wax, otitis media, perforated tympanic membrane, or cholesteatoma.

Specialized Testing

The usual battery of auditory tests includes pure-tone air and bone conduction testing, and measures of speech threshold and word discrimination.

Pure-tone audiometry. With selected frequencies presented by earphones (air conduction) or by vibration applied to the mastoid (bone conduction), the minimum level perceived for each frequency is determined. International standards define normal hearing levels. The test can be performed adequately only in children old enough to cooperate. With conductive hearing impairment, air conduction is abnormal and bone conduction is normal; with sensorineural hearing impairment, both are abnormal; and with central hearing impairment, both are normal.

Speech tests. The speech reception threshold measures the intensity at which a subject can repeat 50% of presented words. The speech discrimination test measures the subject's ability to understand speech at normal conversational levels. Both tests are abnormal out of proportion to pure-tone loss with auditory nerve disease, abnormal in proportion to pure-tone loss with cochlear disease, and normal with conductive and central hearing loss.

Special tests. Cochlear lesions may cause diplacusis and recruitment. Auditory nerve lesions produce tone decay. Diplacusis is a distortion of pure tones so that the subject perceives a mixture of tones. With recruitment, the sensation of loudness increases at an abnormally rapid rate as the intensity of sound is increased. Tone decay is diminished perception of a suprathreshold tone with time.

Brainstem Auditory Evoked Response

The brainstem auditory evoked response (BAER) is a useful test of hearing and the integrity of the brainstem auditory pathways in infants and small children. No cooperation is required, and sedation improves the accuracy of results.

When each ear is stimulated with repetitive clicks, an electrode over the ipsilateral mastoid referenced to the forehead records five waves. Wave I is generated by the acoustic nerve, wave II by the cochlear nerve, wave III by the superior olivary complex, wave IV by the lateral lemniscus, and wave V by the inferior colliculus. The BAER first appears at a conceptional age of 26–27 weeks. The absolute latencies of waves I and V and the V–I interpeak interval decline progressively with advancing conceptional age. The latency of wave V bears an inverse relationship to the intensity of the stimulus and tests hearing.

An initial test uses a stimulus intensity of 70 dB. Failure to produce wave V indicates a hearing impairment. Repeated tests at higher intensities find the response threshold. If wave V is present, the repeated tests at sequential reductions of 10 dB establish the lowest intensity capable of producing wave V, the *hearing threshold*. Because the latency of wave V is proportional to the intensity of the stimulus, a latency-intensity curve is drawn. In normal newborns the latency of wave V will decrease by 0.24–0.44 ms for each 10 dB in sound intensity between 70 and 110 dB.

In children with conductive hearing impairment prolonged time is required to transmit sound across the middle ear and activate the cochlea. This reduces the total amount of sound energy, prolongs the latency of wave I, and shifts the latency-intensity curve of wave V to the right. The amount of shift is equivalent to the hearing impairment, without altering the slope of the curve.

In children with sensorineural hearing impairment the latency-intensity curve of wave V shifts to the right because of the hearing impairment. In addition, the slope of the curve becomes steeper, exceeding 0.55 ms/dB.

Zellweger spectrum disorders. Newborns with severe Zellweger spectrum disorder (ZSD) have multiple congenital malformations and a leukodystrophy phenotype; they typically die within the first year of life. Those with intermediate ZSD do not have congenital malformations, but rather present with progressive sensorineural hearing loss and retinal dystrophy in addition to hypotonia and developmental delays. Sensory loss is due to the underlying peroxisome dysfunction. While cognitive dysfunction is the rule, intellect can be normal in some cases.

Clinical features. Features include early-onset cognitive impairment, dysmorphisms, hypotonia, retinitis pigmentosa, sensorineural hearing deficit, hepatomegaly, osteoporosis, failure to thrive, and renal stones.

Diagnosis. The concentration of protein in the spinal fluid is elevated, and electroencephalography (EEG) may show epileptiform activity. Liver transaminase levels are elevated, as is the plasma concentration of very long-chain fatty acids. Molecular genetic testing reveals biallelic pathogenic variants in one of the multiple implicated *PEX* genes. Multigene panels are available.[16]

Management. No curative therapy is presently available for ZSD. Symptomatic therapy includes evaluation of feeding, hearing, vision, liver function, and endocrine evaluation (including bone density scan) in addition to an evaluation of neurological function and treatment of seizures if needed. All affected children benefit from appropriate educational placement and the use of hearing aids.

Congenital Deafness

The diagnosis of congenital deafness in newborns is rarely entertained in the absence of an external ear deformity or a family history of genetic hearing loss. Congenital ear malformations are present in approximately 2% of newborns with congenital deafness.

Pediatric hearing loss can be classified as congenital (present at birth), prelingual (starting before speech is acquired), or postlingual (occurring after speech has been acquired). Hearing loss may be syndromic or non-syndromic. Eighty percent of prelingual hearing loss is genetic. More than 120 genes have been identified causing nonsyndromic hearing loss, and over 600 genes are associated with syndromic hearing loss. Inheritance can be autosomal dominant, autosomal recessive, X-linked, or mitochondrial.[17]

Maternal use of heparin during pregnancy produces an embryopathy characterized by skeletal deformities, flattening of the nose, cerebral dysgenesis, and deafness.

In the absence of an external malformation or family history deafness often goes unnoticed until the infant fails to develop speech. Intrauterine infection with cytomegalovirus is an important cause of congenital deafness (see Chapter 5). Ten percent of newborns infected in utero with cytomegalovirus develop sensorineural hearing loss. Mass immunization has now almost eliminated rubella embryopathy, once a significant cause of childhood deafness in the United States.

Aplasia of the Inner Ear

Inner ear aplasia is always associated with auditory nerve abnormalities. The three main types are the *Michel defect*, complete absence of the otic capsule and eighth cranial nerve; the *Mondini defect*, incomplete development of the bony and membranous labyrinths and dysgenesis of the spiral ganglion; and the *Scheibe defect*, dysplasia of the membranous labyrinth and atrophy of the eighth nerve.

Waardenburg syndrome. Waardenburg syndrome (WS) is a group of autosomal dominant disorders that cause similar clinical phenotypes. It is the most common cause of autosomal dominant syndromic hearing loss. Four distinct types are recognized, with types 1 and 2 being the most common. Both WS1 and WS2 involve abnormal distribution of melanocytes, resulting in depigmentation of the hair (white forelock), skin, and eyes (heterochromia iridia). Loss of pigmentary cells in the stria vascularis of the cochlea results in sensorineural hearing loss. WS1 is caused by pathogenic heterozygous mutations in the *PAX3* gene. Heterozygous pathogenic mutations in the *MITF* gene cause most cases of WS2.

Clinical features. WS is relatively easy to recognize because of its cutaneous features: a white forelock, eyes of different colors (usually different shades of blue, or one blue and one brown), and depigmented dermal patches. Hearing loss is not a constant feature but occurs in approximately 50% of WS1 and 70%–80% of WS2.

The presence of other abnormalities differentiates four subtypes. Patients with WS1 have hypertelorism and a broad nasal bridge due to the lateral displacement of the inner canthus of the eyes. These features are not present in WS II. In WS III upper limb abnormalities are present, and Hirschsprung disease is part of WS IV.

Diagnosis. The family history and the cutaneous features suggest the diagnosis. Single gene testing is available but because multiple genes can cause similar symptoms, a multigene panel or comprehensive genomic testing is more useful.[18]

Management. Treatment is symptomatic.

Usher syndrome. Usher syndrome is a group of autosomal recessive conditions and the most common cause of deaf-blindness, accounting for approximately 50% of cases. All affected individuals have profound sensorineural hearing loss followed by the development of retinitis pigmentosa and vision loss. Vestibular function is impaired in some patients. There are several different subtypes caused by distinct genetic mutations.

Clinical features. Three main types of Usher syndrome are recognized, which have been further subdivided as additional genetic information comes to light. Severe-to-profound congenital or prelingual sensorineural hearing loss and abnormal vestibular dysfunction characterize type 1. The vestibular deficit delays developmental motor milestones for sitting and walking. Mild-to-severe prelingual sensorineural hearing loss and normal or only mildly impaired vestibular function characterize type 2. Hearing aids provide effective amplification and oral communication is possible. Characteristic features of type 3 are progressive postlingual hearing loss, late-onset retinitis pigmentosa, and progressive deterioration of vestibular function. Most children are otherwise healthy with normal or near-normal intellectual function.

Diagnosis. Multigene panels are available. Single gene testing is usually not helpful due to the wide variety of potential causative mutations.[19,20]

Management. Evaluate all affected children for hearing aids or cochlear implants as soon as possible. There is currently no treatment for the visual loss caused by retinitis pigmentosa, but multiple clinical trials are in progress. Some patients benefit from vestibular rehabilitation.

Pendred syndrome. Pendred syndrome is an auto-somal recessive defect in thyroxine synthesis that accounts for up to 10% of cases of congenital syndromic hearing loss, caused by biallelic pathogenic variants in the *SLC26A4* gene. Goiter and sensorineural hearing impairment are the characteristic features. The hearing impairment is profound. Goiter is not present at birth and develops in early puberty (40%) or adulthood (60%).

Clinical features. Sensorineural hearing impairment is congenital and often severe. Milder hearing impairment may not be detectable until the child is 2 years of age. Vestibular function may also be impaired. A diffuse goiter becomes apparent during the first decade and is typically euthyroid and nonnodular. Growth and intelligence are usually normal.

Diagnosis. Thin-cut CT with detailed cochlear anatomy demonstrates abnormalities in the temporal bones.

Thin-section high-resolution MRI in the axial and sag-ittal planes shows enlargement of the endolymphatic sac and duct in association with a large vestibular aqueduct.[21]

Management. Affected children should be evaluated for hearing aids or cochlear implants. The goiter is usu-ally euthyroid but patients must be monitored for the development of hypothyroidism or nodules.

Later-Onset Genetic Disorders

The discussion of several of the disorders listed in Box 17.5 is in other chapters. Sensorineural hearing impairment occurs as part of several spinocerebellar degenerations, hereditary motor sensory neuropathies, and sensory autonomic neuropathies. It is a major feature of Refsum disease (hereditary motor sensory neuropathy type IV), the treatment of which is dietary measures to reduce serum concentrations of phytanic acid.

BOX 17.5 Hearing Impairment and Deafness

- Congenital
  - Aplasia of inner ear
  - Michel defect
  - Mondini defect
  - Scheibe defect
- Chromosome disorders
  - Trisomy 13
  - Trisomy 18
- Genetic disorders
  - Pendred syndrome
  - Usher syndrome
  - Waardenburg syndrome
- Intrauterine viral infection (see Chapter 5)
- Maternal drug use
  - Drugs
  - Antibiotics
  - β-Blockers
  - Chemotherapy
- Genetic neurological disorders
  - Familial spastic paraplegia (see Chapter 12)
  - Hereditary motor sensory neuropathies (see Chapter 7)
  - Hereditary sensory autonomic neuropathies (see Chapter 9)
  - Infantile Refsum disease (Zellweger spectrum disorders)
  - Neurofibromatosis type 2 (see the "Acoustic Neuroma" section)
- Riboflavin transporter deficiency
- Mitochondrial disorders (see Chapter 8)
- Spinocerebellar degenerations (see Chapter 10)
- Wolfram syndrome (see Chapter 16)
- Xeroderma pigmentosum (see Chapter 5)
- Infectious diseases
  - Bacterial meningitis[a]
  - Otitis media[a] (see the "Vertigo" section)
  - Viral encephalitis (see Chapter 2)
  - Viral exanthemas
- Metabolic disorders
  - Hypothyroidism[a]
  - Ménière disease (see the "Vertigo" section)
- Skeletal disorders
  - Apert acrocephalosyndactyly
  - Cleidocranial dysostosis
  - Craniofacial dysostosis (Crouzon disease)
  - Craniometaphyseal dysplasia (Pyle disease)
  - Klippel-Feil syndrome
  - Mandibulofacial dysostosis (Treacher-Collins syndrome)
  - Osteogenesis imperfecta
  - Osteopetrosis (Albers-Schönberg disease)
- Susac syndrome
- Trauma (see the "Vertigo" section)
- Tumor
  - Acoustic neuroma[a]
  - Cholesteatoma[a] (see the "Vertigo" section)

[a]The most common conditions and the ones with disease-modifying treatments.

Deafness-Dystonia-Optic Neuronopathy Syndrome

Inheritance of this disorder is as an X-linked trait involving the *TIMM8A* gene. Carrier females are unaffected.[22]

Clinical features. Progressive deafness begins before the age of 2 and progresses to profound hearing loss by age 10. Dystonia and/or ataxia develop in the second decade followed by decreased vision from optic neuropathy in the third decade, and dementia at age 40.

Diagnosis. The clinical features are diagnostic. The serum IgG is <200 mg/dL and the IgM and IgA are <20 mg/dL. Molecular genetic testing is available.

Management. Treatment is symptomatic.

Acquired Hearing Impairment

Drug-Induced Impairment

Antibiotics are the most commonly used class of drugs with potential ototoxicity in children. The incidence of toxic reactions is greatest with amikacin, furosemide, and vancomycin and only a little less with kanamycin and neomycin. Permanent damage is unusual with any of these drugs. The characteristic syndrome consists of tinnitus and high-frequency hearing impairment. Vancomycin produces hearing loss only when blood concentrations exceed 45 µg/mL. By contrast, aminoglycosides may cause irreversible cochlear toxicity, which begins as tinnitus, progresses to vertigo and high-frequency hearing impairment, and finally impairs all frequencies. This is of special concern in sick preterm newborns given aminoglycosides for periods of 15 days or longer.

β-Adrenoceptor blocking drugs are a rare cause of hearing impairment and tinnitus. Cessation of therapy reverses symptoms. Cisplatin, an anticancer drug, has ototoxic effects in 30% of recipients. Tinnitus is the major feature. The hearing impairment is at frequencies above those used for speech.

Salicylates tend to concentrate in the perilymph of the labyrinth and are ototoxic. Tinnitus and high-frequency hearing impairment result from long-term exposure to high doses.

Infectious Diseases

Otitis media is a common cause of reversible conductive hearing impairment in children, but only rarely does infection spread to the inner ear (see the "Vertigo" section). Hearing impairment is a relatively common symptom of viral encephalitis (see Chapter 2) and may be an early feature. Sudden hearing loss may also accompany childhood exanthemas (chickenpox, mumps, and measles), and in such cases viruses can be isolated from the cochlear and auditory nerves.

The overall incidence of persistent unilateral or bilateral hearing loss in children with acute bacterial meningitis is 10%. Early treatment with dexamethasone reduces the risk (see Chapter 4). *Streptococcus pneumoniae* meningitis is also associated with a 20% incidence of persistent dizziness, gait ataxia, and other neurological deficits.

The site of disease is probably the inner ear or auditory nerve. Organisms may gain access to the inner ear from the subarachnoid space. Otitis media is the source of meningitis in many children and produces transient conductive hearing loss but does not cause a permanent sensorineural hearing loss. It is common in many centers to screen all children hospitalized for treatment of acute bacterial meningitis with BAER audiometry prior to discharge.

Metabolic Disorders

Tinnitus and decreased hearing are common features of hypothyroidism and are reversible by thyroid replacement therapy.

Skeletal Disorders

The combination of hearing impairment and skeletal deformities almost always indicates a genetic disease. Skeletal disorders may be limited, usually to the face and digits, or generalized. The partial list in Box 17.5 highlights the more common syndromes. Genetic transmission is variable and may be autosomal dominant or recessive.

Trauma

Acute auditory and vestibular injuries occur with fractures of the petrous portion of the temporal bone. Vestibular function is more likely to be impaired than auditory function (see the "Vertigo" section).

Tumor

Acoustic neuroma and cholesteatoma are the tumors most likely to impair children's hearing. Other cerebellopontine angle tumors are extremely rare before the third or fourth decade. The discussion of cholesteatoma is in the "Vertigo" section.

Acoustic neuroma. Acoustic neuromas are actually schwannomas of the eighth nerve. Only 6% of acoustic neuromas come to medical attention in the second decade, and even fewer in the first decade. Children with acoustic neuroma usually have NF2, a genetic disease distinct from neurofibromatosis type 1 (see Chapter 5). Genetic transmission of NF2 is by autosomal dominant inheritance, with the *NF2* gene locus on chromosome 22. Acoustic neuromas are the most constant feature of the phenotype. Later, other cerebral tumors such as meningioma, glioma, schwannoma, and juvenile posterior subcapsular lenticular opacity may develop. Café au lait spots may be present on the skin but are fewer than five in number.

Clinical features. Deafness or tinnitus is the usual initial complaint. Approximately one-third of patients have nonaudiological symptoms, such as facial numbness or paresthesia, vertigo, headache, and ataxia. Hearing impairment is present in almost every patient; ipsilateral diminished corneal reflex occurs in half; and ataxia, facial hypoesthesia or weakness, and nystagmus in 30%–40%. Large tumors cause obstructive hydrocephalus with symptoms of increased intracranial pressure and brainstem compression.

Diagnosis. Molecular genetic testing demonstrates pathogenic heterozygous mutations in the *NF2* gene. Exploration of the family history for acoustic neuroma or other neurological disturbance is also required.

Abnormalities in pure-tone audiometry and the BAER are present in almost every patient but are not necessary for diagnosis. Gadolinium-enhanced MRI is the test of choice to visualize tumors in the cerebellopontine angle (Fig. 17.3).

Management. MRI surveillance is required annually. If negative for tumor, it can be spaced to every 2 years. However, if a tumor is seen, the MRI should be repeated in 6 months. Return to annual surveillance if tumor size is stable.

Surgery is the treatment of choice for symptomatic acoustic neuromas or meningiomas. There is emerging evidence regarding the use of disease-specific treatments; however, none are yet standard of case.

VERTIGO

Vertigo is the sensation of rotation or spinning. It terrifies small children. Balance is lost and posture is difficult to maintain, giving the appearance of ataxia (see

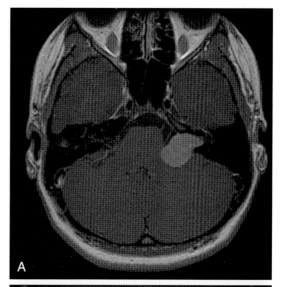

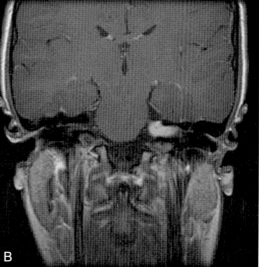

Fig. 17.3 Acoustic Neuroma. (A) T_1 coronal and (B) axial magnetic resonance imaging of a left acoustic neuroma.

Chapter 10). Nausea and nystagmus are often associated features. When nystagmus is present, the fast phase is in the same direction as the perceived rotation. Movement of the head exacerbates all symptoms.

Anatomical Considerations

The semicircular canals and the vestibule, within the labyrinth, are the sensory organs of the vestibular system. The stimulus for excitation of the semicircular canals is rotary motion of the head; for the vestibule, it is gravity. The vestibular portion of the VIII cranial nerve transmits information from the sensory organs to the vestibular nuclei in the brainstem and the cerebellum. The vestibular nuclei have extensive connections with the cerebellum and medial longitudinal fasciculus. Cortical projections terminate in the superior temporal gyrus and frontal lobe.

Approach to Vertigo
History and Physical Examination
Children often complain of dizziness or lightheadedness but rarely complain of vertigo. Carefully question those who complain of dizziness or lightheadedness about the sensation of spinning. Whether the subject or the environment rotates is irrelevant. The illusion of rotation separates vertigo from presyncope, ataxia, and other disturbances of balance, and localizes the disturbance to the vestibular system. Vertigo implies dysfunction of the labyrinth or vestibular nerve (peripheral vertigo) or the brainstem or temporal lobe (central vertigo).

Important historical points to document include the course of vertigo (acute, recurrent, or chronic), precipitating events (trauma, infection, or position change), association of hearing impairment and tinnitus, drug exposure, cardiovascular disease, and family history of migraine. Migraine and epilepsy are the usual causes of acute, episodic attacks of vertigo, not induced by motion, with migraine as the more common of the two. The usual cause of a single, prolonged attack of vertigo,

especially in combination with nausea and vomiting, is infection of the labyrinth or vestibular nerve. Chronic vertigo often waxes and wanes and may seem intermittent rather than chronic. Both central and peripheral causes of vertigo are considerations (Box 17.6), but the clinical and laboratory features readily distinguish central from peripheral vertigo (Table 17.1).

BOX 17.6   Causes of Vertigo
- Drugs and toxins
- Epilepsy
  - Complex partial seizures
  - Simple partial seizures
- Infections
  - Otitis media
  - Vestibular neuronitis
- Ménière disease
  - Migraine
  - Migraine with brainstem aura (see Chapter 10)
  - Benign paroxysmal vertigo (see Chapter 10)
- Motion sickness
- Multiple sclerosis (see Chapter 10)
- Psychogenic
  - Hyperventilation syndrome (see Chapter 1)
  - Panic attacks
- Trauma
  - Temporal bone fracture
  - Vestibular concussion
  - Whiplash injury

TABLE 17.1   Distinguishing Peripheral and Central Vertigo

	Clinical Features	Laboratory Features
Peripheral vertigo	Hearing loss, tinnitus, and otalgia may be associated features Past pointing and falling in the direction of unilateral disease occur Ataxia occurs with the eyes closed in bilateral disease Vestibular and positional nystagmus is present	Caloric testing reveals vestibular paresis, directional preponderance, or both Pure-tone audiometry reveals sensorineural hearing loss Recruitment is present with end-organ disease and tone decay with nerve disease
Central vertigo	Cerebellar and cranial nerve dysfunction are frequently associated Hearing is intact Loss of consciousness may be associated	Pure-tone audiometry and speech discrimination are normal Comprehension of competing messages is impaired Caloric testing may reveal directional preponderance but not vestibular paresis Brainstem evoked response, EEG, CT, or MRI may be abnormal

CT, Computed tomography; EEG, electroencephalography; MRI, magnetic resonance imaging.

Special Tests

Not every child who complains of dizziness requires caloric and audiometric testing.[23] A description of caloric testing is in this section and audiometric testing is in the "Hearing Impairment and Deafness" section. The Dix-Hallpike test is useful to define position-induced vertigo. Electronystagmography (ENG) is often helpful for lateralizing which side is affected and localizing the lesion.

Caloric testing. The simplest method of caloric testing is to instill small quantities of cool water into the external auditory canal with a rubber-tipped syringe. Before instilling the water, inspect the canal to determine whether there is a clear passage to an intact tympanic membrane. Use a sufficient quantity of water, depending on the child's size, to keep the tympanic membrane cooled for 20 seconds. A normal response is slow deviation of the eyes to the side stimulated, followed by a fast component to the opposite side. If stimulation with cool water fails to produce a response, repeat the procedure with ice water. Absence of nystagmus indicates absence of peripheral vestibular function. Partial dysfunction of one vestibular apparatus results in asymmetry of response (directional preponderance).

Dix-Hallpike test. The Dix-Hallpike test requires tilting the patient backward from the sitting position to the supine position so that the head hangs down below the level of the examining table. Observe the eyes for position-induced nystagmus after turning the head 45 degrees to the right and then to the left.

Causes of Vertigo

Drugs

Many drugs that disturb vestibular function also disturb auditory function. This section deals only with drugs affecting vestibular function more than auditory function. Toxic doses of anticonvulsant and neuroleptic medications produce ataxia, incoordination, and measurable disturbances of vestibular function, but patients do not ordinarily complain of vertigo.

Antibiotics are the main class of drugs with vestibular toxicity. Streptomycin, minocycline, and aminoglycosides have a high incidence of toxic reactions, and sulfonamides have a low incidence.

Streptomycin disturbs vestibular function but has little effect on hearing. Variation in individual susceptibility prevents the establishment of a toxic milligram-per-kilogram dose. However, the vestibular toxicity of streptomycin is so predictable that high dosages of the drug are therapeutic to destroy vestibular function in patients with severe Ménière disease.

Minocycline produces nausea, vomiting, dizziness, and ataxia at standard therapeutic doses. Symptoms begin 2–3 days after starting treatment and cease 2 days after cessation. Gentamicin and other aminoglycosides have an adverse effect on both vestibular and auditory function. Some disturbance occurs in 2% of patients treated with gentamicin. Vestibular dysfunction, either alone or in combination with auditory dysfunction, occurs in 84% of cases, whereas auditory dysfunction alone occurs in only 16%. Ototoxic effects develop when the total dose exceeds 17.5 mg/kg.

Epilepsy

Vertigo can be the only feature of a simple partial seizure or the initial feature of a complex partial seizure. The experience of vertigo is an aura in 10%–20% of patients with complex partial seizures.

Clinical features. The recognition of vertigo as an aura is straightforward when a complex partial seizure follows. Diagnosis is more problematic when vertigo is the only feature of a simple partial seizure. The child ceases activity, becomes pale, appears frightened, and then recovers. Unsteadiness and nausea may be associated features.

Diagnosis. All children with unexplained brief attacks of vertigo, especially when vestibular and auditory function is normal between attacks, require EEG. Ambulatory EEG or 24-hour video monitoring is required to capture an attack if interictal EEG is normal.

Management. Discussion of the management of simple and complex partial seizures is in Chapter 1.

Infections

Bacterial infection. Otitis media and meningitis are leading causes of vestibular and auditory impairment in children. Acute suppurative labyrinthitis resulting from extension of bacterial infection from the middle ear has become uncommon since the introduction of antibiotics. However, even without direct bacterial invasion, bacterial toxins may cause serous labyrinthitis.

Chronic otic infections cause labyrinthine damage by the development of cholesteatoma. A cholesteatoma is a sac containing keratin, silvery-white debris shed by squamous epithelial cells. Such cells are not normal constituents of the middle ear but gain access from the external canal after infection repeatedly perforates the eardrum. Cholesteatomas erode surrounding tissues, including bone, and produce a fistula between the peri-lymph and the middle ear.

Clinical features. The characteristics of acute sup-purative or serous labyrinthitis are the sudden onset of severe vertigo, nausea, vomiting, and unilateral hearing loss. Meningismus may also be present. Chronic otitis causes similar symptoms. Severe vertigo that is pro-voked by sneezing, coughing, or merely applying pres-sure on the external canal indicates fistula formation. Otoscopic examination reveals evidence of otitis media and tympanic membrane perforation and allows visual-ization of cholesteatoma.

Diagnosis. When vestibular dysfunction develops in children with otitis media, order radiographs or CT of the skull to visualize erosion of bone or mastoiditis. The presence of meningismus or increased intracranial pres-sure (see Chapter 4) necessitates CT or MRI to exclude the possibility of abscess and then examination of cere-brospinal fluid to exclude meningitis.

Management. Vigorous antibiotic therapy and drainage of the infected area are required in every case. Myringotomy and mastoidectomy provide drain-age when needed. Cholesteatomas are progressive and require surgical excision.

Viral Infections. Viral infections may affect the lab-yrinth or vestibular nerve. The two are difficult to dif-ferentiate by clinical features, and the terms *vestibular neuritis* or *neuronitis* describe acute peripheral vestibu-lopathies. Vestibular neuritis may be part of a systemic viral infection, such as mumps, measles, and infectious mononucleosis, or it may occur in epidemics without an identifiable viral agent, or as part of a postinfectious cranial polyneuritis. The incidence in children is low, accounting for less than 7% of all cases.

Clinical features. The main feature is the acute onset of vertigo. Any attempt to move the head results in a severe exacerbation of vertigo, nausea, and vom-iting. Nystagmus is present on fixation and increased by head movement. The patient is unable to maintain posture and lies motionless in bed. Recovery begins during the first 48 hours. Spontaneous nausea dimin-ishes, and nystagmus on fixation ceases. With each day, vertigo decreases in severity, but positional nystagmus is still present. Recovery is usually complete within 3 weeks.

Diagnosis. The clinical features are the basis for establishing the diagnosis. Brain imaging is unneces-sary when acute-onset vertigo is an isolated symptom and begins improving within 48 hours.[24]

Management. Consider antiviral medications on a case-by-case basis. During the acute phase, keep the child in bed and encourage hydration. Diazepam or lorazepam are very effective in dampening the labyrinth and relieving the symptoms. As recovery progresses, gradually increase activity.

Ménière Disease

Ménière disease is uncommon in children. An overac-cumulation of endolymph that results in rupture of the labyrinth is the mechanism of disease.

Clinical features. Rupture of the labyrinth causes the clinical features, hearing impairment, tinnitus, and vertigo. Hearing impairment fluctuates and may tempo-rarily return to normal when the rupture heals. Tinnitus is ignorable, but vertigo demands attention and is often the complaint that brings the disorder to attention. A typical attack consists of disabling vertigo and tinnitus lasting for 1–3 hours. Tinnitus, fullness in the ear, or increased loss of hearing may precede vertigo. Tinnitus becomes worse during the attack. Pallor, sweating, nausea, and vomiting are often associated features. Afterward, the patient is tired and sleeps. Attacks occur at unpredictable intervals for years and then subside, leaving the patient with permanent hearing loss. Bilateral involvement is present in 20% of cases. Nystagmus is present during an attack. At first, the fast component is toward the abnor-mal ear (irritative); later, as the attack subsides, the fast component is away (paralytic). Between attacks, the results of examination are normal, with the exception of unilateral hearing impairment.

Diagnosis. Pure-tone audiometry shows threshold fluctuation. Speech discrimination is preserved, and recruitment is present on the abnormal side. Caloric stimulation demonstrates unilateral vestibular paresis or directional preponderance.

Management. The underlying disease is not revers-ible. Management of the acute attack and increasing the interval between attacks is the goal of therapy. Bed rest, sedation, and antiemetic drugs are the treatment of acute attacks. Maintenance therapy usually consists of a low-salt diet and diuretics. Surgery and intratympanic injection of ototoxic medications are reserved for severe, intractable cases.

Migraine

Seventeen percent of migraineurs report vertigo at the time of an attack. Such individuals have no difficulty in recognizing vertigo as a symptom of migraine. Another 10% experience vertigo in the interval between attacks and may have difficulty relating vertigo to migraine. Brief (minutes), recurrent episodes of vertigo in infants and small children are usually a migraine equivalent, despite the absence of headache. The attacks later evolve into classic migraine. Affected children appear ataxic; discussion of the syndrome is therefore in Chapter 10 (see the "Benign Paroxysmal Vertigo" section).

Motion Sickness

Unfamiliar body accelerations or a mismatch in information provided to the brain by the visual and vestibular systems during acceleration of the body induces motion sickness. Motion in the visual field opposed to actual body movement induces motion sickness. Therefore allowing a child to look out of the window while riding in a car reduces the incidence of motion sickness. Small children in the back seat, where the only visual input is the car interior, are at the greatest risk for motion sickness.

The prevalence of motion sickness depends on how violent the movement is and approaches 100% in the worst case. Twenty-five percent of a ship's passengers become sick during a 2- to 3-day Atlantic crossing, and 0.5% of commercial airline passengers are affected. The first symptom is pallor, which is followed by nausea and vomiting. Because nausea usually precedes vomiting, there is time to prevent vomiting in some situations. Stopping the motion is the best way to abort an attack. Watching the environment move opposite the direction of body movement may inhibit early attacks. Individuals with known susceptibility to motion sickness should take an antihistamine, diazepam, or scopolamine before travel.

Trauma

Fifty percent of children complain of dizziness and headache during the first 3 days after a closed head injury, with or without loss of consciousness. One-third have persistent vertigo without hearing loss. This group is separable into patients with direct trauma to the labyrinth (vestibular concussion) and those in whom the vestibular apparatus is not injured.

Vestibular concussion

Clinical features. Vestibular concussion usually follows blows to the parieto-occipital or temporoparietal region of the skull. Severe vertigo is present immediately after injury. The child is unsteady and sways toward the affected side. Symptoms persist for several days and then improve, but specific movements of the head (paroxysmal positional vertigo) precipitate recurrent episodes of vertigo and nausea lasting for 5–10 seconds. Such lingering symptoms may persist for months after the initial injury.

Diagnosis. All children with vertigo following a head injury require a head CT. Fractures through the petrous pyramid require special attention. Bleeding from the ear or a facial palsy should raise suspicion of such a skull fracture. Moving the injured ear downward induces positional nystagmus by the Dix-Hallpike technique. Caloric testing or ENG shows a reduced response from the injured ear.

Management. Immediately after injury, treat with an antihistamine and diazepam until the acute phase is over. Vestibular rehabilitation is useful for children with prolonged symptoms.

Whiplash injury. Whiplash injuries are frequently associated with vestibular and auditory dysfunction. The mechanism depends on the specific mechanical forces involved. Significant controversy remains regarding the incidence and nature of vertigo in the setting of whiplash.

Clinical features. Vertigo may be present immediately after injury and usually subsides within a few days. Brief attacks of vertigo and tinnitus, sometimes associated with headache or nausea, may develop months later in children who appear fully recovered from the injury. Many features of the attacks suggest posttraumatic migraine.

Diagnosis. During the acute phase, the Dix-Hallpike technique induces vertigo and caloric testing documents unilateral dysfunction. Vestibular evoked potentials and other types of vestibular testing are often obtained.

Management. Treatment is symptomatic and usually consists of vestibular rehabilitation.

REFERENCES

1. Villard L, Nguyen K, Cardoso C, et al. A locus for bilateral perisylvian polymicrogyria maps to Xq28. *American Journal of Human Genetics.* 2002;70:1003-1008.
2. Harriette TFM, van der Zwaag B, Cruysberg JRM, et al. Mobius syndrome redefined. A syndrome of rhombencephalic maldevelopment. *Neurology.* 2003;61:327-333.

3. Lahat E, Heyman E, Barkay A, et al. Asymmetric crying facies and associated congenital anomalies: prospective study and review of the literature. *Journal of Child Neurology*. 2000;15(12):808-810.

4. Vanopdenbosch LJ, Verhoeven K, Casselman JW. Bell's palsy with ipsilateral numbness. *Journal of Neurology, Neurosurgery, and Psychiatry*. 2005;76:1017-1018.

5. Yoo MC, Park DC, Byun JY, Yeo SG. Clinical prognostic factors associated with good outcomes in pediatric Bell's palsy. *Journal of Clinical Medicine*. 2021;10(19):4368. https://doi.org/10.3390/jcm10194368. PMID: 34640384; PMCID: PMC8509832.

6. Lemmers RJLF, Tawil R, Petek L, et al. Digenic inheritance of an SMCHD1 mutation and an FSHD-permissive D4Z4 allele causes facioscapulohumeral muscular dystrophy type 2. *Nature Genetics*. 2012;44(12):1370-1374.

7. Padberg GW, Brouwer OF, de Keizer RJW, et al. On the significance of retinal vascular disease and hearing loss in facioscapulohumeral muscular dystrophy. *Muscle & Nerve*. 1995;2(suppl):S73-S80.

8. Cali E, Dominik N, Manole A, et al. Riboflavin transporter deficiency (June 11, 2015). In: Adam MP, Feldman J, Mirzaa GM, et al., eds. *GeneReviews®*. University of Washington; 1993–2023. https://www.ncbi.nlm.nih.gov/books/NBK299312/. Updated April 8, 2021.

9. Sobacchi C, Villa A, Schulz A, et al. CLCN7-related osteopetrosis (February 12, 2007). In: Adam MP, Feldman J, Mirzaa GM, et al., eds. *GeneReviews®*. University of Washington; 1993–2023. https://www.ncbi.nlm.nih.gov/books/NBK1127/. Updated January 20, 2022.

10. Dhawan SR, Saini AG, Singhi PD. Management strategies of Melkersson-Rosenthal syndrome: a review. *International Journal of General Medicine*. 2020;13:61-65. https://doi.org/10.2147/IJGM.S186315. PMID: 32161488; PMCID: PMC7049838.

11. Cockerham KP, Hidayat AA, Cockerham GC, et al. Melkersson-Rosenthal syndrome: new clinicopathologic findings in 4 cases. *Archives of Ophthalmology*. 2000;118:227-232.

12. Murakami S, Hato N, Horiuchi J, et al. Treatment of Ramsay Hunt syndrome with acyclovir-prednisone: significance of early diagnosis and treatment. *Annals of Neurology*. 1997;41:353-357.

13. Hato N, Kisaki H, Honda N, et al. Ramsay-Hunt syndrome in children. *Archives of Neurology*. 2000;48:254-256.

14. Voortman M, Drent M, Baughman RP. Management of neurosarcoidosis: a clinical challenge. *Current Opinion in Neurology*. 2019;32(3):475-483. https://doi.org/10.1097/WCO.0000000000000684. PMID: 30865007; PMCID: PMC6522203.

15. Gordin E, Lee TS, Ducic Y, Arnaoutakis D. Facial nerve trauma: evaluation and considerations in management. *Craniomaxillofacial Trauma & Reconstruction*. 2015;8(1):1-13. https://doi.org/10.1055/s-0034-1372522. PMID: 25709748; PMCID: PMC4329040.

16. Steinberg SJ, Raymond GV, Braverman NE, et al. Zellweger spectrum disorder (December 12, 2003). In: Adam MP, Feldman J, Mirzaa GM, et al., eds. *GeneReviews®*. University of Washington; 1993–2023. https://www.ncbi.nlm.nih.gov/books/NBK1448/. Updated October 29, 2020.

17. Shearer AE, Hildebrand MS, Schaefer AM, et al. Genetic hearing loss overview (February 14, 1999). In: Adam MP, Feldman J, Mirzaa GM, et al., eds. *GeneReviews®*. University of Washington; 1993–2023. https://www.ncbi.nlm.nih.gov/books/NBK1434/. Updated September 28, 2023.

18. Milunsky JM. Waardenburg syndrome type I (July 30, 2001). In: Adam MP, Feldman J, Mirzaa GM, et al., eds. *GeneReviews®*. University of Washington; 1993–2023. https://www.ncbi.nlm.nih.gov/books/NBK1531/. Updated October 20, 2022.

19. Koenekoop RK, Arriaga MA, Trzupek KM, et al. Usher syndrome type I (December 10, 1999). In: Adam MP, Feldman J, Mirzaa GM, et al., eds. *GeneReviews®*. University of Washington; 1993–2023. https://www.ncbi.nlm.nih.gov/books/NBK1265/. Updated October 8, 2020.

20. Koenekoop R, Arriaga M, Trzupek KM, et al. Usher syndrome type II (December 10, 1999). In: Adam MP, Feldman J, Mirzaa GM, et al., eds. *GeneReviews®*. University of Washington; 1993–2023. https://www.ncbi.nlm.nih.gov/books/NBK1341/. Updated March 23, 2023.

21. Phelps PD, Coffey RA, Trembath RC, et al. Radiological malformations of the ear in Pendred syndrome. *Clinical Radiology*. 1998;53:268-273.

22. Tranebjærg L. Deafness-dystonia-optic neuronopathy syndrome (February 6, 2003). In: Adam MP, Feldman J, Mirzaa GM, et al., eds. *GeneReviews®*. University of Washington; 1993–2023. https://www.ncbi.nlm.nih.gov/books/NBK1216/. Updated November 21, 2019.

23. Fife TD, Tusa RJ, Furman JM, et al. Assessment: vestibular testing techniques in adults and children. Report of the Therapeutics and Technology Assessment Subcommittee of the American Academy of Neurology. *Neurology*. 2000;55:1431-1441.

24. Hotson JR, Baloh RW. Acute vestibular syndrome. *The New England Journal of Medicine*. 1998;333:680-686.

18

Disorders of Cranial Volume and Shape

OUTLINE

Measuring Head Size, 403
Macrocephaly, 403
    Communicating Hydrocephalus, 404
    Noncommunicating Hydrocephalus, 407
    Megalencephaly (*PIK3CA*-Related Overgrowth
      Spectrum), 412
    Metabolic Megalencephaly, 414
Microcephaly, 415
    Primary Microcephaly, 415

Anencephaly, 416
Encephalocele, 416
Defective Prosencephalization, 417
Secondary Microcephaly, 419
Abnormal Head Shape, 420
    Intracranial Forces, 420
    Extracranial Forces, 420
    Craniosynostosis, 420
References, 422

The brain, cerebrospinal fluid (CSF), and blood are the three intracranial compartments that determine the size of the skull during infancy. Expansion of one compartment comes at the expense of another in order to maintain volume and pressure (see Chapter 4). The epidural, subdural, and subarachnoid spaces may expand with blood or CSF fluid and significantly affect cranial volume and the other intracranial compartments. Less important factors contributing to head size are the thickness of the skull bones and the rate of their fusion.

The intracranial content, the fusion of the sutures, and external forces on the skull determine its shape. Infants left supine all the time tend to develop flat occiputs (plagiocephaly). Premature infants resting on one side of the head all the time develop heads with large frontooccipital diameter (dolichocephaly).

MEASURING HEAD SIZE

Head circumference is determined by measuring the greatest frontooccipital circumference. Influencing the accuracy of the measurement is the head shape and fluid in and beneath the scalp. Following a prolonged and difficult delivery, edema or blood may thicken the scalp and a cephalohematoma may be present as well. Fluid that infiltrates from a scalp infusion can markedly increase head circumference.

A round head has a larger intracranial volume than an oval head of equal circumference. A head with a relatively large frontooccipital diameter has a larger volume than a head with a relatively large biparietal diameter.

Head circumference measurements are most informative when plotted over time (head growth). The head sizes of male and female infants are different, and one should not rely on head growth charts that provide median values for both sexes. The rate of head growth in premature infants is considerably faster than in full-term newborns (Fig. 18.1). For this reason, the charting of head circumference is always by conceptional age and not by postnatal age.

MACROCEPHALY

Macrocephaly means a large head, larger than two standard deviations (SD) from the normal distribution. Thus 2% of the "normal" population has macrocephaly. Investigation of such individuals may show an abnormality causing macrocephaly, but many are normal, often with a familial tendency for a large head. When

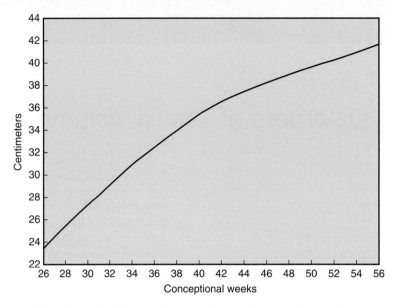

Fig. 18.1 Normal Growth of Head Circumference in Boys. The rate of growth in premature infants is greater than in full-term infants.

asked to evaluate a large head in an otherwise normal child, first measure and plot the parents' heads.

The causes of a large head include hydrocephalus (an excessive volume of CSF intracranially), megalencephaly (enlargement of the brain), thickening of the skull, and hemorrhage into the subdural or epidural spaces. Hydrocephalus is traditionally communicating (nonobstructive) or noncommunicating (obstructive), depending on whether or not there is CSF communication between the ventricles and subarachnoid space (Box 18.1). Hydrocephalus is the main cause of macrocephaly at birth in which intracranial pressure (ICP) is increased.

The causes of megalencephaly are anatomical and metabolic. The anatomical disorders are primary megalencephaly and neurocutaneous disorders (Box 18.2). Children with anatomical megalencephaly are often macrocephalic at birth but have normal ICP. Children with metabolic megalencephaly are usually normocephalic at birth and develop megalencephaly from cerebral edema, and often elevated ICP, during the neonatal period.

Increased thickness of the skull bones does not cause macrocephaly at birth or in the newborn period. Macrocephaly develops during infancy. Box 18.3 lists the conditions associated with increased skull growth.

The text does not contain a separate discussion. The discussion of intracranial hemorrhage in the newborn is in Chapter 1, and intracranial hemorrhage in older children is in Chapter 2.

Communicating Hydrocephalus

This is a condition caused by functional obstruction of CSF leading to ventricular dilation. The usual cause of communicating hydrocephalus is impaired absorption of CSF secondary to meningitis or subarachnoid hemorrhage. Meningeal malignancy, usually by leukemia or primary brain tumor, is a less common cause. Any of these processes may cause arachnoiditis or arachnoid infiltration and decrease reabsorption of CSF by the arachnoid villi. The excessive production of CSF by a choroid plexus papilloma rarely causes communicating hydrocephalus because the potential rate of CSF reabsorption far exceeds the productive capacity of the choroid plexus (see Chapter 4). Such tumors more commonly cause hydrocephalus by obstructing one or more ventricles.

Benign Enlargement of Subarachnoid Space

The terms used to describe benign enlargement of the subarachnoid space include *external hydrocephalus, extraventricular hydrocephalus, benign subdural*

BOX 18.1   Causes of Hydrocephalus

Communicating
- Achondroplasia
- Basilar impression (see Chapter 10)
- Choroid plexus papilloma[a] (see Chapter 4)
- Meningeal malignancy
- Meningitis[a] (see Chapter 4)
- Posthemorrhagic (see Chapter 4)

Noncommunicating
- Abscess[a] (see Chapter 4)
- Aqueductal stenosis[a]
- Chiari malformation (see Chapter 10)
- Dandy-Walker malformation
- Hematoma[a] (see Chapters 1 and 2)
- Infectious[a]
- Klippel-Feil syndrome
- Mass lesions[a]
- Tumors and neurocutaneous disorders
- Vein of Galen malformation[a]
- Walker-Warburg syndrome
- X-linked

Other Causes of Increased Intracranial Cerebrospinal Fluid
- Benign enlargement of subarachnoid space
- Holoprosencephaly
- Hydranencephaly
- Porencephaly

[a]The most common conditions and the ones with disease modifying treatments.

BOX 18.2   Causes of Megalencephaly

Genetic Megalencephaly
- Megalencephaly with *PIK3CA*-related overgrowth spectrum disorders
- Megalencephaly with achondroplasia
- Megalencephaly with gigantism (Sotos syndrome)
- Neurocutaneous disorders
  - Epidermal nevus syndromes
  - Schimmelpenning syndrome
  - Hypomelanosis of Ito
  - Incontinentia pigmenti (see Chapter 1)
  - Neurofibromatosis (see Chapter 5)
  - Tuberous sclerosis (see Chapter 5)

Metabolic Megalencephaly
- Alexander disease (see Chapter 5)
- Canavan disease (see Chapter 5)
- Galactosemia: transferase deficiency (see Chapter 5)
- Gangliosidosis (see Chapter 5)
- Globoid leukodystrophy (see Chapter 5)
- Glutaric aciduria type I (see Chapter 14)
- Maple syrup urine disease[a] (see Chapter 1)
- Megalencephalic leukoencephalopathy with subcortical cysts
- Metachromatic leukodystrophy (see Chapter 5)
- Mucopolysaccharidoses (see Chapter 5)

[a]The most common conditions and the ones with disease modifying treatments.

BOX 18.3   Conditions With a Thickened Skull Causing Macrocephaly

- Anemia[a]
- Cleidocranial dysostosis
- Craniometaphyseal dysplasia of Pyle
- Epiphyseal dysplasia
- Hyperphosphatemia
- Leontiasis ossea
- Orodigitofacial dysostosis
- Osteogenesis imperfecta
- Osteopetrosis
- Pyknodysostosis
- Rickets[a]
- Russell-Silver syndrome

[a]The most common conditions and the ones with disease modifying treatments.

effusions, and *benign extracerebral fluid collections*. It is a relatively common cause of macrocephaly in infants, a fact not fully appreciated before the widespread use of computed tomography (CT) to investigate large head size. A genetic cause is likely in some cases, with the infant's father often having a large head.

Clinical features. The condition occurs more commonly in males than females. A large head circumference is the only feature. An otherwise normal infant is brought to medical attention because serial head circumference measurements show an enlarging head size. The circumference is usually above the 90th percentile at birth, grows to exceed the 98th percentile, and then parallels the normal curve (Fig. 18.2). The anterior fontanelle is large but soft. Neurological findings are normal, but motor development is often slower. Head control is one of the earliest achievements in motor development

for an infant. Macrocephalic infants take longer to control their heads and this delays other milestones such as sitting and standing; however, the ultimate development is normal in these children.

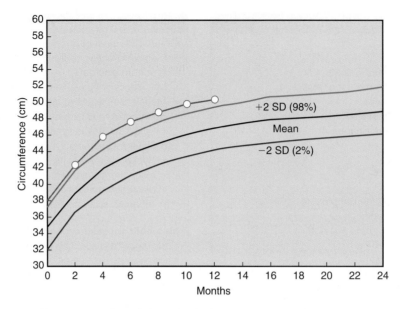

Fig. 18.2 Benign Enlargement of the Subarachnoid Space. Head circumference is already large at birth, grows to exceed the 98th percentile, and then parallels the curve.

Diagnosis. Magnetic resonance imaging (MRI) of the head shows an enlarged frontal subarachnoid space, widening of the sylvian fissures and other sulci, and normal or minimally enlarged ventricular size (Fig. 18.3). Normal ventricular size and large head circumference distinguish this condition from cerebral atrophy. In infants the upper limit of normal size for the frontal subarachnoid space is 5.7 mm and for the sylvian fissure 7.6 mm. The MRI of the head often is read as brain atrophy as the brain looks smaller than the container; however, both the brain and the cranium are large.

Management. Most affected infants develop normally and do not require ventricular shunts. Plot head circumference measurements monthly until the head growth is paralleling the normal curve. Repeat imaging is often unnecessary unless head growth continues to deviate from the normal curve 6 months after the onset of abnormal enlargement, neurological examination is abnormal, or social and language development is slow or regressing.

Meningeal Malignancy

Tumors that infiltrate the meninges and subarachnoid space impair the reabsorption of CSF and cause communicating hydrocephalus. Meningeal spread usually occurs from a known primary tumor site. Diffuse

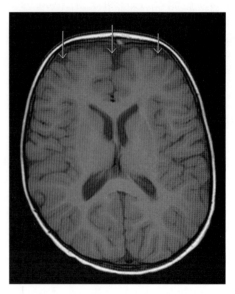

Fig. 18.3 Benign Enlargement of the Subarachnoid Space. T_1 axial magnetic resonance imaging showing enlargement of the subarachnoid space (*arrows*) in a child with macrocephaly and normal development.

meningeal gliomatosis is the exception where the initial feature may be hydrocephalus.

Clinical features. Tumors that infiltrate the meninges are usually aggressive and cause rapid progression of symptoms. Headache and vomiting are the initial features and lethargy and personality change follow. Meningismus and papilledema are common features and may suggest bacterial meningitis. Multifocal neurological disturbances may be present.

Diagnosis. MRI shows dilatation of the entire ventricular system but not of the subarachnoid space, which may appear obliterated except for a layer of enhancement. The pressure of the CSF and its protein concentration are increased. The glucose concentration may be decreased or normal. Tumor cell identification in the CSF is rarely successful and meningeal biopsy is usually required for tissue diagnosis.

Management. Ventricular shunt relieves symptoms of increased ICP. Radiation therapy and chemotherapy provide palliation and extend life in some cases, but the outcome is generally poor.

Noncommunicating Hydrocephalus

Complete obstruction of the flow of CSF from the ventricles to the subarachnoid space causes increased pressure and dilation of all ventricles proximal to the obstruction. The incidence of congenital hydrocephalus is 1 in 1000 live births. The best estimate is that 40% of the cases of congenital hydrocephalus have a genetic basis. X-linked hydrocephalus associated with stenosis of the aqueduct of Sylvius (HSAS) accounts for 10% of cases in males with idiopathic hydrocephalus and is part of the spectrum of L1 disorders described later.[1] The responsible gene is at Xq28 encoding for L1CAM. Other environmental factors that may lead to congenital hydrocephalus are exposure to radiation, alcohol, or infections in utero.[2]

Noncommunicating hydrocephalus is the most common form of hydrocephalus in fetuses. Aqueductal stenosis is the usual cause of congenital hydrocephalus in the absence of other associated cerebral malformations. Aqueductal stenosis is less common during infancy but its frequency increases during childhood. Mass lesions are the most common cause of aqueductal obstruction during childhood. Children with congenital hydrocephalus who have seizures usually have other cerebral malformations. Such children have a higher incidence of cognitive impairment.

Congenital Aqueductal Stenosis

At birth, the mean length of the cerebral aqueduct is 12.8 mm and its smallest cross-sectional diameter is usually 0.5 mm. The small lumen of the cerebral aqueduct, in relation to its length, makes it especially vulnerable to internal compromise from infection and hemorrhage, and to external compression by tumors and venous malformations. Congenital atresia or stenosis of the cerebral aqueduct can occur as a solitary malformation or can occur as part of a spectrum of abnormalities associated with the L1 spectrum.

Clinical features. Hydrocephalus is present at birth. Head circumference ranges from 40 to 50 cm and may cause cephalopelvic disproportion and poor progress of labor requiring cesarean section. The forehead is bowed, the scalp veins are dilated, the skull sutures are widely separated, and the fontanelles are large and tense. These signs exaggerate when the child cries, but they are also present in a quiet state. The eyes deviate downward so that the sclera shows above the iris (*setting-sun sign*), and abducens palsies may be present.

Diagnosis. Intrauterine sonography is diagnostic after 20 weeks when the ventricles expand. Sonograms performed earlier are misleading. When macrocephaly is present in the fetus, amniotic fluid assay of α-fetoprotein is useful for the detection of neural tube defects (see Chapter 12). Chromosomal analysis provides further information concerning the integrity of the fetal nervous system to develop a management plan.

CT or MRI readily provides the postpartum diagnosis of aqueductal stenosis. Marked enlargement of the lateral ventricle, the third ventricle, and the cephalic end of the cerebral aqueduct is easily visualized. The remainder of the cerebral aqueduct and the fourth ventricle cannot be seen (Fig. 18.4).

Management. Congenital hydrocephalus caused by aqueductal stenosis is severe, does not respond to medical therapy directed at decreasing the volume of CSF, and progresses to a stage that harms the brain. Diversion of the CSF from the ventricular system to an extracranial site is the only effective method of management.

VP shunt is the procedure of choice for newborns and small infants with aqueductal stenosis. It is easier to revise and is better tolerated than a ventriculoatrial shunt. Mechanical obstruction and infection are the most common complications of shunt placement in infancy (see Chapter 4).

The relief of hydrocephalus increases the potential for normal development, even when the cerebral mantle

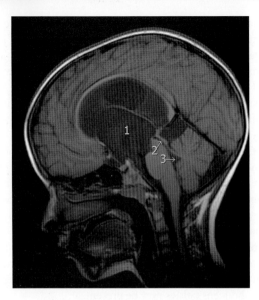

Fig. 18.4 Aqueduct Stenosis. T_1 sagittal magnetic resonance imaging shows *(1)* dilated third ventricle; *(2)* stenosis of aqueduct; and *(3)* normal size fourth ventricle.

appears very thin preoperatively, but does not necessarily result in a normal child. The growth of intelligence is often uneven, with better development of verbal skills than of nonverbal skills. Associated anomalies may cause motor deficits and seizures.

X-Linked Hydrocephalus (L1 Syndrome)

The L1CAM syndrome encompasses HSAS syndrome (X-linked hydrocephalus with stenosis of the aqueduct of Sylvius), MASA syndrome (mental retardation [intellectual disability], aphasia, spastic paraplegia, and adducted thumbs), X-linked complicated hereditary spastic paraplegia type 1, and X-linked complicated corpus callosum agenesis.[1,3]

Clinical features. Hydrocephalus, cognitive impairment, spasticity of the legs, and adducted thumbs are possible characteristic features in affected males. The spectrum of severity is wide depending on the nature of the mutation. Cognitive impairment ranges from mild to severe, and gait abnormalities range from shuffling gait to spastic paraplegia. Adducted thumbs are characteristic of several phenotypes.

Diagnosis. Molecular genetic testing is commercially available.

Management. Most affected infants require early ventriculoperitoneal (VP) shunt placement.

Fibroblast Growth Factor Receptor–Associated Craniosynostosis Syndromes and Hydrocephalus

Pathogenic mutations in the fibroblast growth factor receptor (*FGFR*) gene cause several forms of craniosynostosis, many but not all of which are associated with hydrocephalus. Specific disorders in which hydrocephalus is a concern include Apert syndrome, Pfeiffer syndrome, Crouzon syndrome, and Beare-Stevenson cutis gyrata syndrome.

Clinical features. Features that are common to all syndromes include craniosynostosis, Chiari I malformation, and midface retrusion, which may be associated with proptosis if severe. Children with Beare-Stevenson cutis gyrate syndrome, Pfeiffer syndrome, and Apert syndrome usually have some degree of intellectual disability. Conversely, intellectual disability is uncommon in Crouzon syndrome. Digital abnormalities occur in Apert and Pfeiffer syndromes, and children with Pfeiffer syndrome may develop epilepsy.

Diagnosis. Molecular genetic testing is available and reveals pathogenic mutations in the *FGFR* gene.

Management. Most affected children require multiple surgeries for cranial reconstruction. Stable ventriculomegaly can be monitored, but progressive hydrocephalus requires placement of a ventriculoperitoneal shunt.[4]

Dandy-Walker Malformation

The Dandy-Walker malformation consists of a ballooning of the posterior half of the fourth ventricle, often associated with failure of the foramen of Magendie to open, aplasia of the posterior cerebellar vermis, heterotopia of the inferior olivary nuclei, pachygyria of the cerebral cortex, and other cerebral and sometimes visceral anomalies. Hydrocephalus may not be present at birth but develops during childhood or later. The size of the lateral ventricles does not correlate with the size of the fourth ventricle. Other malformations are present in two-thirds of children. The most common associated malformation is agenesis of the corpus callosum. Other malformations include heterotopia, abnormal gyrus formation, dysraphic states, aqueductal stenosis, and congenital tumors.[5]

A wide variety of etiologies exist, including congenital infections, chromosomal disorders, and specific gene mutations.

Clinical features. Many infants are diagnosed based on prenatal ultrasound. Postnatal diagnosis often does not occur until the child is several months old and presents with macrocephaly. Bulging of the skull, when present, is more prominent in the occipital than in the frontal region. The speed of head growth is considerably slower than with aqueductal stenosis. Compression of posterior fossa structures leads to neurological dysfunction, including apneic spells, nystagmus, truncal ataxia, cranial nerve palsies, and hyperreflexia in the legs.

Diagnosis. Macrocephaly or ataxia is the indication for head imaging, which shows cystic dilatation of the posterior fossa and partial or complete agenesis of the cerebellar vermis (Fig. 18.5). MRI is more useful because it also identifies other cerebral abnormalities such as heterotopia. Incomplete vermian agenesis may be difficult to differentiate from an enlarged cisterna magna.

Management. Decompression of the cyst alone provides immediate relief of symptoms; however, hydrocephalus recurs and ventricular shunting or endoscopic third ventriculostomy (ETV) is required in two-thirds of affected children. Shunting of the lateral ventricle or ETV alone provides immediate relief of hydrocephalus but fails to relieve brainstem compression. The procedure of choice is a dural shunt of both the lateral ventricle and the posterior fossa cyst.

Even after successful shunt placement, some children have transitory episodes of lethargy, personality change, and vomiting that falsely suggest shunt failure. The mechanism of such episodes, which in rare cases may prove fatal, is unknown but some authors have suggested vascular compromise as a potential etiology.[6]

Klippel-Feil Syndrome

Klippel-Feil syndrome is a malformation of the craniocervical skeleton that may be associated with Chiari I malformation and basilar impression. It involves the congenital fusion of at least two cervical vertebrae. The incidence is about 1 in 40,000–42,000 live births. Obstruction of the flow of CSF from the fourth ventricle to the subarachnoid space causes hydrocephalus. Several different entities comprise the syndrome, which may be autosomal recessive, autosomal dominant, or have no known genetic basis. There are three types of Klippel-Feil syndrome: type I is the single fusion of two cervical vertebrae; type II is the fusion of multiple noncontiguous cervical vertebrae; and type III is the fusion of multiple contiguous cervical vertebrae. Scoliosis occurs in about 50% of the cases and occurs more often with involvement of the lower cervical vertebrae, with multiple fusions, and with hemivertebrae.[7]

Clinical features. The essential features of the Klippel-Feil syndrome are a low posterior hairline, a short neck, and limitation of neck movement. Head asymmetry, facial asymmetry, scoliosis, and mirror movements of the hands are common. Unilateral or bilateral failure of downward migration of the scapula (*Sprengel deformity*) is present in 25%–35% of patients. Malformations of the genitourinary system and deafness are associated features. Deafness may be of the sensorineural, conductive, or mixed type. Hydrocephalus affects the fourth ventricle first and then the lateral ventricles. The resulting symptoms are those of posterior fossa compression: ataxia, apnea, and cranial nerve dysfunction.

Diagnosis. Radiographs of the spine reveal the characteristic fusion and malformations of vertebrae. MRI may show an associated Chiari malformation and dilatation of the ventricles.

Management. Children with unstable cervical vertebrae require cervical fusion to prevent myelopathy. Those with symptoms of obstructive hydrocephalus require a VP shunt or ETV to relieve pressure in the posterior fossa.

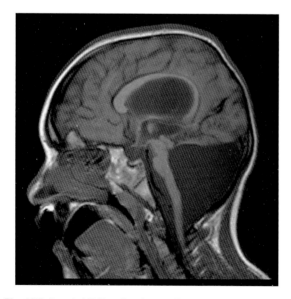

Fig. 18.5 Dandy-Walker Syndrome. T_1 sagittal magnetic resonance imaging shows a large cystic area in the posterior fossa with narrowing and elongation of the brainstem.

Congenital Brain Tumors

Congenital brain tumors and congenital brain malformations are both disorders of cellular proliferation. A noxious agent active during early embryogenesis might stimulate either or both abnormalities. The relative oncogenicity or teratogenicity depends on the virulence of the agent, the timing of the insult, the duration of exposure, and the genetic background and health of the fetus. The most common tumors of infancy are astrocytoma, medulloblastoma, teratoma, and choroid plexus papilloma.

Clinical features. Congenital tumors are more often supratentorial than infratentorial and more often in the midline than situated laterally. Newborns with hemispheric gliomas and teratomas may develop hydrocephalus in utero or in the first days or weeks postpartum. The point of obstruction is usually at the cerebral aqueduct (see Chapter 4). Choroid plexus papillomas are usually located in one lateral ventricle and become symptomatic during infancy rather than in the perinatal period. They produce hydrocephalus either by obstruction of the foramen of Monro or less likely by excessive production of CSF (see Chapter 4). Medulloblastomas are located in the posterior fossa and obstruct the fourth ventricle and cerebral aqueduct (see Chapter 10).

The clinical features of all congenital tumors are those of increasing ICP: enlarging head size, separation of the sutures, lethargy, irritability, difficult feeding, and vomiting. Seizures are unusual. Because of its posterior fossa location, medulloblastoma also produces nystagmus, downward deviation of the eyes, opisthotonos, and apnea. Large tumors may hemorrhage due to birth trauma; although rare, such neonates may present with shock and symptoms of disseminated intravascular coagulation.

Diagnosis. MRI, performed to investigate hydrocephalus, readily visualizes all congenital tumors. CT identifies most tumors and head ultrasound identifies some tumors.

Management. Complete resection of congenital brain tumors is unusual, with the exception of choroid plexus papilloma. Discussion of individual tumor management is in Chapters 4 and 10.

Vein of Galen Malformation

Arteriovenous malformations (AVMs) of the cerebral circulation may become symptomatic during infancy and childhood (see Chapters 4 and 10), but the malformation associated with congenital hydrocephalus is the vein of Galen malformation. Vein of Galen vascular malformations are not aneurysms and do not involve the vein of Galen. Instead, the normal vein of Galen does not develop and the median prosencephalic vein of Markowski persists, dilates, and drains to the superior sagittal sinus. Multiple arteriovenous fistulas are associated. Vein of Galen aneurysms account for 1% of all AVMs and 30% of all pediatric vascular malformations.[8]

Clinical features. Eighty percent of newborns with vein of Galen malformations are male. The usual initial feature is either enlargement of jugular veins with high-output cardiac failure or an enlarging head size. Hydrops fetalis is also possible. Hemorrhage almost never occurs early in the course. A cranial bruit is invariably present. Some affected children experience unexplained persistent hypoglycemia.

Large midline AVMs produce a hemodynamic stress in the newborn because of the large quantities of blood shunted from the arterial to the venous system. The heart enlarges in an effort to keep up with the demands of the shunt, but high-output cardiac failure ensues. Affected newborns often come first to the attention of a pediatric cardiologist because of the suspicion of congenital heart disease, and the initial diagnosis may be made during cardiac catheterization. Always auscultate the head of a newborn, infant, or toddler with macrocephaly or heart failure.

When hemodynamic stress is not severe and cardiac compensation is possible, the initial symptoms are in infancy or early childhood. In such a case obstructive hydrocephalus results from compression of the tegmentum and aqueduct. Symptoms usually begin before the age of 5 and always before the age of 10. The lateral ventricles enlarge, causing headache, lethargy, and vomiting. In infants the head enlarges and the fontanelle feels full.

Diagnosis. Contrast-enhanced CT (Fig. 18.6) or MRI readily visualizes the vein of Galen malformation. The lateral and third ventricles dilate behind the compressed cerebral aqueduct. MRI may provide additional information regarding prognosis. Injury to the cerebral gray and white matter is called "melting brain," and it is secondary to chronic hypoxia and venous stasis. The injury may be partially hemorrhagic and better seen on T_1-weighted images.[8] Radiographs of the chest in newborns with high-output cardiac failure show an enlarged heart with a normal shape.

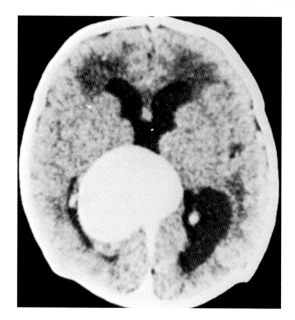

Fig. 18.6 Vein of Galen Malformation. The malformation is visible on contrast-enhanced computed tomography as a large aneurysmal sac compressing the midbrain and producing obstructive hydrocephalus.

Management. The overall results of direct surgical approaches are poor; the mortality rate and neurological morbidity in survivors are high. Endovascular embolization is the standard of care at most institutions.

Walker-Warburg Syndrome

Walker-Warburg syndrome (WWS) is the most severe of the alpha-dystroglycanopathies (other types include Fukuyama congenital muscular dystrophy and muscle-eye-brain disease). Multiple causative genetic mutations have been identified. It is often lethal within the first few months of life.

Clinical features. Hydrocephalus, severe ocular and brain malformations, and profound intellectual disability constitute the main clinical findings. Hydrocephalus is usually present at birth. The cause may be aqueductal stenosis or the Dandy-Walker malformation. Most children with both a Dandy-Walker malformation and ocular abnormalities have the WWS. Some children are born with microcephaly yet have enlarged ventricles. Severe neurological abnormalities are caused by partial or total agyria (lissencephaly) resulting from failure of neuronal migration. Both the brainstem and cerebellum are very small, the brainstem is often kinked, and

cerebral cysts are present.[9] The pattern of architectural abnormalities throughout the neuraxis suggests a disruption of cerebral maturation in the fourth conceptional month.

Several ocular abnormalities may be present, usually in combination: hypoplasia of the iris, abnormal anterior chamber, microphthalmos, cataracts, persistence of primary vitreous, optic disk coloboma, retinal detachment, retinal dystrophy, hypoplasia of the optic nerve, glaucoma, or buphthalmos.

Muscular dystrophy is present but relatively mild, but affected infants are hypotonic and have difficulty feeding. Seizures are uncommon. Most affected children die before the age of 3.

Diagnosis. MRI of the brain and orbits delineates the abnormalities. Multigene panels are the most useful tool to identify the specific genetic defect. Clinically, the features suggest the diagnosis, but can overlap significantly with other alpha-dystroglycanopathies such as muscle-eye-brain disease.

Management. The management of hydrocephalus is by ventriculoperitoneal shunt or ETV, but the outcome is poor because of concomitant severe cerebral malformations.

Hydranencephaly

The term *hydranencephaly* encompasses several conditions that result in the extensive replacement of the brain by CSF. The cause of hydranencephaly may be failure of normal brain development or an intrauterine disorder that destroys brain parenchyma. Progressive obstructive hydrocephalus, if left untreated, may cause a clinical picture very similar to hydranencephaly. Excessive pressure within the lateral ventricles destroys the midline structures and reduces the cerebral mantle to a thin membrane. However, pure hydranencephaly lacks any cerebral mantle.

Head circumference at birth is large in cases of severe hydrocephalus. Hydranencephaly is associated with microcephaly when the condition is due to intrauterine diseases and may be associated with any head size when caused by primary malformations.

Porencephaly

Porencephaly is a term used loosely in the literature. Originally, the term described hemispheric cysts that communicated with both the subarachnoid space and the lateral ventricle secondary to defects in the final stages of prosencephalization. The present use of the term is broader and includes any hemispheric cyst; the usual causes are intrauterine or perinatal infarct or trauma. The injured immature brain loses neurons, glia, and supporting structures. A fluid-filled cyst is formed in the injured area and may not communicate with either the ventricular system or the subarachnoid space. Pressure within the cyst often becomes excessive, causing compression of adjacent structures and macrocephaly.

Megalencephaly (*PIK3CA*-Related Overgrowth Spectrum)

Megalencephaly includes conditions in which the brain enlarges because the number or size of cells increases. Unlike other conditions causing macrocephaly discussed earlier, in this condition the actual size of the brain is enlarged.

Clinical features. The clinical symptom of megalencephaly was previously a feature of several different disorders, but since the discovery of the causative *PIK3CA* mutation they have been reorganized as a spectrum of a single underlying condition termed *PIK3CA*-related overgrowth spectrum (PROS).

PROS is a general or segmental overgrowth syndrome that may involve multiple body parts in addition to the brain. Various phenotypes exist including megalencephaly-capillary malformation syndrome, dysplastic megalencephaly, hemimegalencephaly, and Klippel-Trenaunay syndrome. In general any overgrowth syndrome involving the brain should raise suspicion of PROS. The most commonly affected tissues include the brain and vasculature. Other manifestations include abnormalities of muscle and adipose tissue, syndactyly or polydactyly, lymphatic malformations, and kidney malformations.

Affected children often present with increased head circumference, developmental delays, and seizures that may be resistant to treatment. Brain overgrowth can lead to progressive hydrocephalus or development of a Chiari I malformation, with associated symptoms of increased ICP. Skin manifestations may include café au lait spots or other findings suggestive of a neurocutaneous disorder.

Diagnosis. Brain MRI demonstrates dysplastic megalencephaly, hemimegalencephaly, or focal cortical dysplasias. Genetic testing reveals a pathogenic, usually mosaic variant in *PIK3CA*. The mutation is usually de novo, and risk to siblings is no greater than the general population.[10]

Management. Apelisib (Vijoice) 50 mg with food once daily is recommended for those between 2 and 18 years of age. After age 6, the dose can be increased to 125 mg daily, provided the child has been taking it for at least 6 months prior. Apelisib has been shown to reduce functional overgrowth and vascular lesions, but it is not known if it has any effect on the neurologic complications.

Epilepsy requires treatment with anticonvulsants. Patients with hemimegalencephaly often benefit from hemispherectomy early in the course of the disease to prevent permanent sequelae from uncontrolled seizures. Serial MRI of the brain is recommended for those with neurologic manifestations; perform imaging every 6 months until age 8, then annually thereafter to monitor for the development of progressive hydrocephalus and Chiari malformation.

Achondroplasia

Achondroplasia is a genetic disorder, transmitted as an autosomal dominant trait via heterozygous pathogenic variants in the *FGFR3* gene. De novo mutations account for more than 80% of cases. It is the most frequent form of short-limbed dwarfism.[11] It is the result of mutations that exaggerate the signal output of FGFR3, a receptotyrosine kinase that negatively regulates growth plate activity and linear bone growth.[12]

Clinical features. The main features are short stature caused by rhizomelic shortening of the limbs (the proximal portion of the limbs is shorter than the distal portion), large head with frontal bossing and midface hypoplasia, lumbar lordosis, and limitation of elbow extension. Stunted formation of enchondral bone causes the typical recessed facial appearance.

Affected newborns have true megalencephaly. Increased ICP occurs at times secondary to stenosis of the sigmoid sinus at the level of the jugular foramina. Despite considerable, and sometimes alarming, enlargement of head circumference, individuals with achondroplasia seldom show clinical evidence of increased ICP or progressive dementia. However, respiratory disturbances are common. Dyspnea, hyperreflexia, spasticity, and sensory disturbances of the limbs may result from cervicomedullary compression.

Diagnosis. Clinical examination and radiological features establish the diagnosis. Accurate molecular diagnosis is available. MRI shows a small posterior fossa and enlargement of the sphenoid sinuses. Basilar impression is sometimes present. Ventricular size varies from normal in newborns and young infants to moderate or severe dilatation in older children and adults.

Management. Ventricular size, after initial dilatation, usually remains stable but occasionally ventriculoperitoneal shunting is needed. Decompressive surgery is required in children with evidence of progressive cervicomedullary compromise or hydrocephalus. Vosoritide is a C-type natriuretic peptide analog approved to increase height; it has no effect on potential neurologic complications.[13]

Benign Familial Macrocephaly

Clinical features. The term describes a familial condition in which neurological and mental function are normal, but head circumference is larger than the 98th percentile. The suspected mechanism of transmission is autosomal dominant inheritance, but the genetic basis for nonsyndromic macrocephaly is probably multifactorial, with a polymorphic genetic basis. Head circumference may not be large at birth but increases during infancy, usually to between 2 and 4 cm above the 98th percentile. Body size is normal, and no physical deformities are present.

Diagnosis. The enlargement is indistinguishable by physical examination from benign enlargement of the subarachnoid space, but imaging distinguishes the two. MRI or CT are normal in benign familial macrocephaly.

Management. Treatment is not required.

Megalencephaly With Gigantism

Megalencephaly with gigantism, termed *cerebral gigantism* or *Sotos syndrome*, is a haploinsufficiency of the *NSD1* (nuclear receptor binding SET domain protein 1) gene. Ninety percent of cases are due to mutations or microdeletions of the *NSD1* gene[14].

Clinical features. Affected children are in the 75th–90th percentile at birth and grow at an excessive rate in height, weight, head circumference, and bone age up to the age of 3. Afterward, the rate of growth is normal. A prominent forehead, high-arched palate, and hypertelorism are present in almost every case. All have overgrowth with advanced bone age, macrocephaly, and the majority have intellectual disabilities or autism.[15]

Diagnosis. Head MRI or CT are usually normal except for mild ventricular widening. Extensive studies of endocrine function have failed to show a consistent abnormality other than glucose intolerance. Plasma somatomedin levels are elevated during the first year in some infants and fall below normal during early childhood.

Management. Treatment is symptomatic and based on the phenotype.

Neurocutaneous Disorders

Neurocutaneous syndromes are often associated with seizures (see Box 1.8) and cognitive impairment (see Chapter 5). The skin manifestations may be present at birth (incontinentia pigmenti) or during infancy (neurofibromatosis, tuberous sclerosis). The cause of macrocephaly is either hydrocephalus or megalencephaly. PROS (discussed earlier in this chapter) causes hemimegalencephaly, hemihypertrophy of the body, or hypertrophy of a single limb as well as characteristic skin manifestations, and should be considered in the differential if megalencephaly is present.

Hypomelanosis of Ito. Hypomelanosis of Ito, also called *incontinentia pigmenti achromians*, is a mosaic syndrome and the third most common neurocutaneous disorder after neurofibromatosis 1 and tuberous sclerosis. The etiology remains unclear, and there is no definite evidence of genetic transmission.

Clinical features. The cutaneous feature is a large, hypopigmented area that has a whorled or streaked appearance following the lines of Blashko (migratory routes for fetal epidermal cells). It appears in the first year and is a negative image of the hyperpigmented lesions of incontinentia pigmenti (see Chapter 1). Other cutaneous features are café au lait spots, angiomatous nevi, heterochromia of the iris or hair, and other nevi. Seizures and cognitive impairment are the most common neurological abnormalities. Intelligent quotient (IQ) scores are below 70 in more than half of patients, but approximately 20% have IQ scores above 90. Approximately half of patients have seizures, usually with onset in the first year. Focal seizures are most common, although occasional patients have infantile spasms and epilepsies refractory to treatment evolving into the spectrum of epileptic encephalopathy/Lennox-Gastaut syndrome. Spastic diplegia may also be present. Disturbances of neuronal migration cause these symptoms. Megalencephaly occurs in approximately 25% of cases.

One-third of patients have skeletal and eye anomalies, including limb hypertrophy or atrophy, facial hemiatrophy, poorly formed ears, dysplastic teeth, hypertelorism, strabismus, and corneal opacities.

Diagnosis. The characteristic skin lesions are critical to the diagnosis. Use a Wood's lamp to emphasize hypomelanotic areas and fully define the lesion. MRI may show generalized cerebral or cerebellar hypoplasia, severe cortical neuronal migration anomalies, and hemimegalencephaly and lissencephaly. Hemimegalencephaly may be ipsilateral or contralateral to the cutaneous hypopigmentation.

Management. Treatment is symptom directed. Educational accommodations and anticonvulsants are often necessary.

Epidermal nevus syndromes. Epidermal nevus syndromes (ENS) refer to several disorders that have in common an epidermal nevus, neurological manifestations such as seizures or hemimegalencephaly, endocrine dysfunction, and often skeletal or ocular abnormalities. These disorders are clinically similar in certain ways but are not genetically related. It is likely that this group of disorders will be reclassified in the future based on the causative genetic mutation.

Clinical features. Signs and symptoms are highly variable between disorders, but in general all affected children have an epidermal nevus or nevi that may be linear, sebaceous, or large. Nevi on the face and head are more often associated with brain malformations, while nevi on the trunk are more likely to be associated with scoliosis and other skeletal abnormalities.

Schimmelpenning Syndrome. In the past authors frequently referred to Schimmelpenning syndrome as "epidermal nevus syndrome" and many times it is the disorder that is actually being discussed in the literature when speaking of the ENS. It is the most common ENS and is characterized by multiple congenital sebaceous nevi that become more noticeable as the child ages. Sebaceous nevi are smooth, hairless, yellow- or salmon-colored patches that may become warty or thickened after puberty. Neurologic symptoms include epilepsy, developmental delays, intellectual disability, and cerebral malformations. Many children have ocular abnormalities, including coloboma or retinal abnormalities. Some children have epibulbar lipodermoid tumors, which are benign, yellowish tumors of the outer portion of the eye. Skeletal abnormalities are common.

Diagnosis. Diagnosis relies on recognition of the nevus with associated extra-cutaneous signs. MRI of the brain frequently reveals various types of cerebral malformations. Most ENS are thought to be due to postzygotic mutations; causative mutations have been identified in a few specific syndromes, but in many the genetic defect remains unknown.

Management. Seizures may respond to standard anticonvulsant therapy (see Chapter 1), but treatment is not available for the underlying cerebral malformation.

Metabolic Megalencephaly

Several inborn errors of metabolism produce megalencephaly by storage of abnormal substances or by producing cerebral edema (see Box 18.2). Their discussion is elsewhere in the text because the initial features are usually developmental regression (see Chapter 5) or seizures (see Chapter 1). Two exceptions are glutaric aciduria type I (see Chapter 14) and metabolic leukoencephalopathy with subcortical cysts. Infants with glutaric aciduria type I are normal up to 3 years, except for macrocephaly, and then develop an acute illness that resembles encephalitis. Most infants with metabolic megalencephaly have a normal head circumference at birth. Head enlargement parallels neurological regression and clinical evidence of increased ICP. The ventricles are often small.

Megalencephalic Leukoencephalopathy With Subcortical Cysts

The metabolic defect in megalencephalic leukoencephalopathy with subcortical cysts (MLC) is a mutation in the *MLC1* gene, which encodes a protein expressed in brain astrocytes. The presence in affected sibling pairs and in instances of parental consanguinity establish autosomal recessive inheritance.[16]

Clinical features. Early-onset macrocephaly combined with mild developmental delay and seizures are characteristic. The gradual development of ataxia and spasticity follows. Extrapyramidal findings may develop, and mild mental deterioration occurs late in life. The degree of macrocephaly is variable and can be as much as 4–6 SD above the mean in some individuals. After the first year of life, head growth rate normalizes and growth follows a line several centimeters above the 98th percentile. Mental deterioration is late and mild. Motor impairment ranges from independent walking only during early childhood to independent walking in the fifth decade. Some individuals have died in their teens or twenties; others are alive in their forties. Exacerbation of symptoms after minor head injury or infection is common.[17]

Diagnosis. MRI shows severe leukoencephalopathy that suggests a demyelinating white matter disorder. The hemispheres appear swollen, with cyst-like spaces in the frontoparietal and anterior temporal areas, but with relative sparing of the occipital white matter. Sequence analysis, available commercially, reveals mutations in *MLC1* in approximately 60%–70% of affected individuals.

Management. Treatment is symptomatic.

MICROCEPHALY

Microcephaly means a head circumference that is smaller than two SD below the normal distribution of the mean. A small head circumference indicates a small brain. Most full-term newborns whose head circumferences are smaller than two SD, but who are neurologically normal, will have normal intelligence at age 7, but a head circumference smaller than three SD usually indicates later cognitive impairment.

A small head circumference at birth suggests a prenatal brain insult but does not distinguish primary from secondary microcephaly (Box 18.4). Primary microcephaly encompasses conditions in which the brain is small and has never formed properly because of genetic or chromosomal abnormalities. Secondary microcephaly implies that the brain was forming normally but a disease process impaired further growth. Normal head circumference at birth, followed by failure of normal head growth, usually indicates a secondary microcephaly. Chromosomal disorders are an exception to that rule unless they cause defective prosencephalization or cellular migration.

Perinatal brain insult does not cause a recognizable decrease of head circumference until 3–6 months postpartum. Failure of normal brain growth removes the force keeping the cranial bones separated, and they fuse prematurely. A primary disorder of the skull (craniosynostosis) may cause premature closure of the cranial sutures even though the brain is attempting to grow normally. The distinction between the two is relatively simple: craniosynostosis is always associated with an abnormal skull shape and heaping up of bone along the cranial sutures; failure of brain growth produces a relatively normal-shaped skull with some overlapping of skull bones.

MRI may be informative in distinguishing primary from secondary microcephaly. In most children with primary microcephaly MRI results are normal, or a recognizable pattern of cerebral malformation is present. In those with secondary microcephaly imaging is usually abnormal, characterized by one or more of the

BOX 18.4 Conditions Causing Microcephaly

Primary Microcephaly
- Chromosomal disorders
- Defective neurulation
  - Anencephaly
  - Encephalocele
- Defective prosencephalization
  - Agenesis of the corpus callosum
  - Holoprosencephaly (arrhinencephaly)
- Defective cellular migration
- Microcephaly vera (genetic)

Secondary Microcephaly
- Intrauterine disorders
  - Infection
  - Toxins
  - Vascular
- Perinatal brain injuries
  - Hypoxic-ischemic encephalopathy[a]
  - Intracranial hemorrhage
  - Meningitis and encephalitis[a]
  - Stroke
- Postnatal systemic diseases
  - Chronic cardiopulmonary disease
  - Chronic renal disease
  - Malnutrition

[a]The most common conditions and the ones with disease modifying treatments.

following features: ventricular enlargement, cerebral atrophy, and porencephaly.

Primary Microcephaly

Many cerebral malformations are of uncertain cause, and classification as primary or secondary is not possible. Morphogenetic errors, although lacking in the traditional stigmata of tissue injury, could result from exposure of the embryo to a noxious agent during the first weeks after conception. At this early stage, disorganization of the delicate sequencing of neuronal development could occur when the brain is incapable of generating a cellular response.

Microcephaly Vera (Microcephaly Primary Hereditary)

The term *microcephaly vera* encompasses various disorders that decrease bulk growth of the brain. Multiple causative genetic defects have been identified.

Clinical features. Children with microcephaly vera have a characteristic disproportion in size between the face and the skull. The forehead slants backward, and the reduced size of the skull causes the scalp to wrinkle in the occipital region. The chin is small, and the ears and nose are prominent. In a study of children at 7 years old, of those with a head circumference 2–3 SD below the mean, 10% had an IQ < 70 while only 14% had an IQ > 100. With head circumferences greater than 3 SD below the mean, 51% had IQ < 70 while none were above average.[18]

Diagnosis. Results of brain imaging are normal other than the size.

Management. Treatment is symptomatic, and most children require educational accommodations. Treat seizures if they occur.

Chromosomal Disorders

Chromosomal disorders are not usually a cause of microcephaly at birth unless cerebral aplasia, such as holoprosencephaly (HPE), is part of the syndrome. Hypotonia and dysmorphism are the prominent features of chromosomal disorders in the newborn (see Chapter 5), and microcephaly becomes evident during infancy.

Defective Neurulation

At the end of the first week, a rostrocaudal axis appears on the dorsal aspect of the embryo. This axis is responsible for the subsequent induction of a neural plate, which is the rudimentary basis of the nervous system. The neural plate evolves into a closed neural tube during the third and fourth weeks. Defects in closure are *dysraphic states.* The most rostral portion of the neural tube, the anterior neuropore, closes at about the 24th day.

Anencephaly

Anencephaly is the result of defective closure of the anterior neuropore and is distinct from hydranencephaly in that it is a dysraphic state rather than the result of failure of brain growth, brain destruction, or catastrophic hydrocephalus. Myelomeningocele is the result of defective closure of the posterior neuropore (see Chapter 12). The rate of each is declining. Folic acid supplementation from 400 µg to 4 mg a day has reduced the incidence of spinal dysraphism; however, in 2012, nutritional fortification was only preventing 25% of preventable cases of spinal bifida and anencephaly.[19]

Clinical features. Less than half of anencephalic children are born alive, and those who are rarely survive the first month. The scalp is absent, and the skull is open from the vertex to the foramen magnum. The exposed brain appears hemorrhagic and fibrotic. It consists mainly of the hindbrain and parts of the diencephalon; the forebrain is completely lacking. The orbits are shallow, and the eyes protrude. The neck is in retroflexion, and the proximal portions of the arms seem overgrown compared with the legs.

Diagnosis. Following the birth of a child with a neural tube defect, the chance of anencephaly or myelomeningocele in subsequent pregnancies increases two- to fivefold. After two affected children have been born, the chance of having another affected child doubles again. The section on myelomeningocele (Chapter 12) contains the discussion of prenatal diagnosis of dysraphic states.

Management. The condition is universally fatal, although affected infants may survive for a brief period of time depending on the functionality of the brainstem. Provide support to the family and palliative or comfort care for the infant. Do not recommend interventions that prolong life; such interventions are medically futile.

Encephalocele

An encephalocele is a protrusion of brain and meninges, covered by skin, through a defect in the skull. An encephalocele may occur in any location; however, most are midline-occipital, except in Asians, in whom the defects are usually midline-frontal.

Clinical features. The size of the encephalocele may range from a small protrusion to a cyst as big as the skull. When the protrusion is large, the skull is likely to be microcephalic. The size of the mass does not predict its contents, but an encephalocele with a sessile base is more likely to contain cerebral tissue than one with a pedunculated base. Encephaloceles rarely occur as a solitary cerebral malformation and are usually associated with abnormalities of the cerebral hemispheres, cerebellum, and midbrain.

Diagnosis. MRI is reasonably accurate in defining the contents of the encephalocele. Despite its midline location, the derivation of the protruded material is usually from the smaller hemisphere that is displaced across the midline by the larger hemisphere.

Management. The surgical treatment of meningoceles has an excellent prognosis as the protrusion includes only meninges and CSF. The prognosis for surgical resection of encephalocele depends on the size and the location of the protruding brain. The extent of comorbid malformations should also influence any decision to remove or repair the encephalocele surgically. Children with protruded brain material and associated malformations usually die during infancy.

Defective Prosencephalization

The forebrain develops between 25 and 30 days' gestation from a midline vesicle generated from the closed anterior neuropore. Between 30 and 40 days' gestation, bilateral cerebral vesicles are formed by the cleavage and outpouching of the midline vesicle. The midline vesicle is the primordium of the third ventricle, and the bilateral cerebral vesicles are the primordia of the lateral ventricles.

Holoprosencephaly

Defective cleavage of the embryonic forebrain leads to a spectrum of malformations subdivided into three main types: alobar, semilobar, and lobar in which alobar is the most severe form and lobar the mildest.

Total failure of cleavage produces a small brain with a midline vesicle covered by a horseshoe of limbic cortex (lobar HPE). With less severe defects, the third ventricle and diencephalon differentiate, and partial cleavage of the occipital hemispheres occurs. The corpus callosum is hypoplastic or absent (semilobar HPE). The minimal defect (lobar HPE or arrhinencephaly) is the unilateral or bilateral absence of the olfactory bulbs and tracts associated with some degree of rhinic lobe aplasia. Hemispheric cleavage is complete, the ventricles are normal, and the corpus callosum is present in part or in total.

Almost half of patients with HPE have an abnormal numerical or structural chromosomal abnormality. Trisomy 13 is the most common cause. Multiple other triploidy and aneuploidy conditions have been associated as well as various chromosome deletion or duplication syndromes. Single-gene disorders occur in a minority of cases.

Clinical features. Craniofacial dysplasia is usually associated, and malformations in other organs are common. The facial deformities are primarily in the midline (cyclopia or ocular hypotelorism, flat nose, cleft lip, and cleft palate), and their severity is often predictive of the severity of the brain malformation. Associated malformations include congenital heart defects, clubbing of the hands or feet, polydactyly and syndactyly, hypoplasia of the genitourinary system, an accessory spleen and liver, and malrotation of the intestine.

Many children with severe defects in cleavage of the forebrain are stillborn or die in the neonatal period. Microcephaly, hypotonia, apnea, and seizures are prominent features. Hypotonia is especially severe when the defect is associated with a chromosomal abnormality. Infants who survive have severe intellectual, motor, and sensory impairment. Conversely, children with lobar HPE may appear physically normal and may display minor disturbances in neurological function such as learning disabilities and seizures.

Diagnosis. Suspect HPE in every child with midline facial deformities, especially when malformations are present in other organs. MRI provides excellent visualization of the malformation. Chromosomal analysis and molecular genetic testing should be considered.

Management. The management is symptomatic. The appearance of the ventricles is often confused with hydrocephalus but the pathogenesis is different and shunting is not usually needed. The extent of supportive care depends on the severity of the defect. In cases of alobar HPE palliative care should be an option for families.

Agenesis of the Corpus Callosum

Anomalous development of the three telencephalic commissures (the corpus callosum and the anterior and hippocampal commissures) is an almost constant feature of defective prosencephalization. The incidence of callosal abnormalities (complete or partial agenesis or hypoplasia of corpus callosum) detected by MRI obtained for all reasons was reported to be about 0.25%.[20] However, a study population in Hungary found the prevalence in newborns to be about 0.018% in a group of subjects with agenesis of corpus callosum as an isolated finding.[21] Agenesis also occurs in association with other prosencephalic dysplasias and with some metabolic defects (see the "Glycine Encephalopathy" section in Chapter 1) and as a solitary genetic defect. When only the corpus callosum is absent, the anterior and hippocampal commissures may be normal or enlarged. Callosal agenesis is part of the Aicardi syndrome (see Chapter 1), the Andermann syndrome (autosomal recessive callosal agenesis, intellectual disability, and peripheral neuropathy), and trisomies 8, 11, and 13.

Clinical features. Solitary agenesis of the corpus callosum is clinically silent except for subtle disturbances in the interhemispheric transfer of information, for which special testing is needed. Cognitive impairment or learning disabilities occur in some cases, and epilepsy usually indicates concurrent additional brain dysgenesis (focal heterotopias, cortical dysplasia, etc.). Agenesis of the corpus callosum is a congenital condition in which the corpus callosum fails to develop (about 200 million axons); such individuals may exhibit deficits in non-literal language comprehension, humor, theory of mind, and social reasoning. These findings together with parent reports suggest a phenotype within the autism spectrum, particularly in social interaction and communication.[22]

Diagnosis. Neuroimaging shows lateral displacement of the lateral ventricles and upward displacement of the third ventricle. Intraventricular pressure is normal.

Management. Treatment is symptomatic.

Defective Cellular Migration

Lissencephaly is a failure of cerebral cortical development because of defective neuroblast migration.[23] When neurons that should form the superficial layers of the cerebral cortex are unable to pass through the already established deeper layers of neurons, the cortical convolution pattern is lacking (agyria) and neurons accumulate in the white matter (*heterotopia*). Complete absence of gyri causes a smooth cerebral surface (*lissencephaly-1*), whereas incomplete gyral formation reduces the number and enlarges the size of the existing convolutions (*pachygyria*). Neurons that come close to their cortical position form a subcortical band (*band heterotopia*).

The migrations of the cerebellum and the brainstem also are usually involved, but the embryonic corpus ganglio-thalamic pathway is not disturbed, so the thalamus and basal ganglia form properly. Structural and metabolic abnormalities of the fetal ependyma may be important factors in disturbing the normal development of radial glial cells. Decreased brain size leads to microcephaly, with widened ventricles representing a fetal stage rather than pressure from hydrocephalus and an uncovered sylvian fossa representing lack of operculation.

The second form of cortical architectural abnormality in lissencephaly is disorganized clusters of neurons with haphazard orientation, forming no definite layers or predictable pattern (*lissencephaly-2*). Lissencephaly-2 is associated with several closely related genetic syndromes: WWS, Fukuyama muscular dystrophy, muscle-eye-brain disease of Santavuori, and Meckel-Gruber syndrome. Microcephaly and characteristic facies that includes micrognathia, high forehead, thin upper lip, short nose with anteverted nares, and low-set ears characterize *Miller-Dieker syndrome*. A microdeletion at the 17p13.3 locus occurs in most patients with Miller-Dieker syndrome, and deletions on chromosome 17 occur in many other lissencephaly syndromes.

Genetic transmission of lissencephaly also occurs as an X-linked dominant trait with two different phenotypes; males show classical lissencephaly, while females show bilateral periventricular nodular heterotopia (BPNH) (Fig. 18.7).

Clinical features. Referral of most children with lissencephaly is for evaluation of developmental delay or intractable myoclonic seizures. Many initially exhibit muscular hypotonia that later evolves into spasticity and opisthotonus. Microcephaly is not always present, but all children have severe cognitive impairment, epilepsy, and cerebral palsy. BPNH usually presents with sporadic or familial epilepsy and normal intelligence. Small, isolated heterotopic cortical nodules are an important

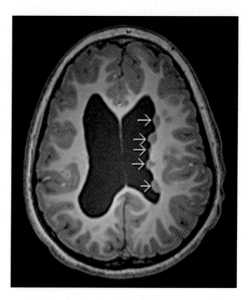

Fig. 18.7 Nodular Heterotopias. T$_1$ axial MRI shows (*arrows*) multiple nodular heterotopias protruding into a dilated ventricular system.

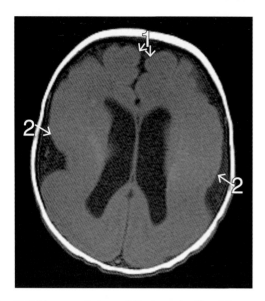

Fig. 18.8 Lissencephaly and Pachygyria. T_1 axial magnetic resonance imaging shows *(1)* frontal pachygyria and *(2)* posterior lissencephaly.

cause of intractable epilepsy in an otherwise normal child (see Chapter 1).

Diagnosis. MRI abnormalities establish the diagnosis. A smooth cortical surface except for rudimentary sulci (agyria) may be limited to the parietal or frontal regions or encompass the whole brain (Fig. 18.8). The sylvian fissure is broad and triangular, the interhemispheric fissure is widened, and nests of gray matter are present within the white matter. The ventricles may be enlarged, and the corpus callosum may be absent. Molecular genetic testing is available for several specific syndromes.

Management. Seizures are usually intractable, but standard drugs for the management of infantile spasms or myoclonic seizures may provide partial relief (see Chapter 1). Focal defects may respond to surgery. Prognosis depends largely on the extent of the malformation and the severity of seizures.

Secondary Microcephaly
Intrauterine Disorders

Intrauterine infection is an established cause of microcephaly. Cytomegalovirus infection (see Chapter 5) can manifest as microcephaly, without any features of systemic disease. Because maternal infection is asymptomatic, such cases are difficult to identify as caused by

cytomegalovirus disease. However, surveys of cytomegalovirus antibody demonstrate a higher rate of seropositive individuals among microcephalic than normocephalic children. This suggests that such cases do exist.

Efforts to identify environmental toxins that produce cerebral malformation have had only limited success. Drugs of abuse and several pharmaceutical agents are suspects, but the evidence is rarely compelling. The only absolute conclusion derived from an abundance of studies is that a negative impact occurs on fetuses of women whose lifestyle includes some combination of heavy alcohol or drug use, poor nutrition, and inadequate health care. The expression of the negative impact includes intrauterine growth restriction, dysmorphic features, and microcephaly.

Aplasia of major cerebral vessels is a rare malformation of unknown cause. Brain tissue that the aplastic vessels should have supplied with blood either never forms or is infarcted and replaced by calcified cystic cavities. The cavities are present at birth, and the CT appearance suggests an intrauterine infection except that the cysts conform to a vascular distribution.

Zika Virus

Zika virus was first identified in a rhesus monkey in Uganda in 1947. Sporadic human cases were reported in southeast Asia and sub-Saharan Africa, spread to Yap Island Micronesia in 2007, and then French Polynesia, New Caledonia, the Cook Islands, and Easter Island in 2013 and 2014. The outbreak in Brazil in 2015 caused worldwide alarm and led to the recognition of Zika as a global health threat.

Clinical features. Clinical manifestations in a healthy, nonpregnant person are usually mild and include malaise, fever, headache, arthralgia, and rash; occasionally, children or adults develop acute inflammatory demyelinating polyradiculoneuropathy (Guillain-Barré syndrome).[24] Effects on the fetus are potentially devastating and include severe microcephaly with lifelong neurological deficits.

Diagnosis. Zika virus RNA is detected in serum or amniotic fluid using reverse transcription polymerase chain reaction, or the presence of anti-Zika IgM antibodies confirms the diagnosis.

Management. The only effective management is preventing pregnant women from exposure, either by limiting traveling to endemic areas or by effective control of the Aedes mosquito population.

Perinatal Brain Injuries

Perinatal brain injuries are an important cause of failure of brain growth during infancy when head circumference is normal at birth. The initial features of this group of disorders are neonatal encephalopathy and seizures (see Chapter 1). Children with microcephaly and cognitive impairment from perinatal brain injuries virtually always have cerebral palsy and often have epilepsy. Microcephaly and cognitive impairment in the absence of motor impairment suggest a prenatal origin.

Postnatal Systemic Disease

Infants who are chronically ill and malnourished fail to thrive. All growth is slowed, but usually head growth maintains itself better than length and weight. If body size is below the 3rd percentile, head circumference might be at the 5th or 10th percentile. Failure to correct the systemic disturbance usually causes brain injury, brain growth slows, and head circumference falls into the microcephalic range.

ABNORMAL HEAD SHAPE

Whereas skull content almost exclusively determines skull size, skull shape results from forces acting from within and without, and of the time of closure of the cranial sutures.

Intracranial Forces

The shape of the brain contributes to the shape of the skull by influencing the time of closure of cranial sutures. Temporal lobe agenesis results in a narrower calvarium, and cerebellar agenesis results in a small posterior fossa. Hydrocephalus produces characteristic changes in skull shape. Large lateral ventricles cause bowing of the forehead, and the Dandy-Walker malformation causes bowing of the occiput. In infants with subdural hematomas separation of the sagittal suture may cause bitemporal widening.

Extracranial Forces

Constricting forces in utero, such as a bicornuate uterus or multiple fetuses, may influence head shape. Physical constraint of the skull in utero may contribute to premature closure of a cranial suture, but perinatal and postnatal constraints do not. Molding of the skull is common during a prolonged vaginal delivery, but the closure of

TABLE 18.1   Terms That Describe Head Shapes

Term	Description
Acrocephaly	High, tower-like head with vertical forehead
Brachycephaly	Broad head with recessed lower forehead
Oxycephaly	Pointed head
Plagiocephaly	Flattening of one side of head
Scaphocephaly (dolichocephaly)	Abnormally long, narrow head
Trigonocephaly	Triangular head with prominent vertical ridge in the midforehead

cranial sutures is unaffected. Molding does not influence eventual head shape.

In premature infants, *scaphocephaly* (Table 18.1) often develops because the poorly mineralized skull flattens on one side and then the other with turning of the child from side to side. The shape of the skull becomes normal with maturity.

Plagiocephaly or occipital flattening is the rule in normal infants who always sleep on their backs, and is especially frequent in hypotonic infants who constantly lay in the same position. The hair over the flattened portion of skull is usually sparse from rubbing against the bed surface. A normal head shape resumes by changing the infant's position or through the use of helmet therapy.

Craniosynostosis

Craniosynostosis is the premature closure of one or more cranial sutures; the result is always an abnormal skull shape. The term is only applicable to infants in whom the sutures close while the brain is growing. Early closure of sutures in infants with microcephaly is not premature because the ICP required to keep sutures apart is lacking.

Most cases of craniosynostosis are sporadic and of uncertain etiology. Autosomal dominant and recessive forms of single-suture closure occur. Autosomal dominant inheritance is more common than autosomal recessive inheritance but is also more easily identifiable as hereditary. Many sporadic cases could represent autosomal recessive inheritance.

TABLE 18.2   Distinguishing Clinical Features in the Fibroblast Growth Factor Receptor –Related Craniosynostosis Syndromes

Disorder	Thumbs	Hands	Great toes	Feet
Muenke syndrome	Normal	± Carpal fusion	± Broad	± Tarsal fusion
Crouzon syndrome	Normal	Normal	Normal	Normal
Crouzon syndrome with acanthosis nigricans	Normal	Normal	Normal	Normal
Jackson-Weiss syndrome	Normal	Variable	Broad, medially deviated	Abnormal tarsals
Apert syndrome	Occasionally fused to fingers	Bone syndactyly	Occasionally fused to toes	Bone syndactyly
Pfeiffer syndrome	Broad, medially deviated	Variable brachydactyly	Broad, medially deviated	Variable brachydactyly
Beare-Stevenson syndrome	Normal	Normal	Normal	Normal
FGFR2-related isolated coronal synostosis	Normal	Normal	Normal	Normal

(Data from Robin NH, Falk MJ, Haldeman-Englert CR. FGFR-related craniosynostosis syndromes. In: *GeneClinics: Medical Genetic Knowledge Base [database online]*. University of Washington. http://www.geneclinics.org.)

Craniosynostosis may be one feature of a larger recognized syndrome of chromosomal or genetic abnormality. Many of the genetic disorders are secondary to mutations of *FGFR* (see Fibroblast Growth Factor Receptor-Associated Craniosynostosis Syndromes and Hydrocephalus section earlier in this chapter). Table 18.2 summarizes these disorders.[25]

Craniosynostosis is also associated with other disorders. Some of these associations are coincidental, but a cause-and-effect relationship probably does exist with metabolic disorders of bone.

Clinical features. In nonsyndromic craniosynostosis the only clinical feature is an abnormal head shape. Normal bone growth is impaired in a plane perpendicular to the fused sutures but is able to occur in a parallel plane. The cause of scaphocephaly is premature fusion of the sagittal suture, brachycephaly is premature fusion of both coronal sutures, plagiocephaly is premature fusion of one coronal or one lambdoid suture, trigonocephaly is premature fusion of the metopic suture, and oxycephaly is premature fusion of all sutures. When several sutures close prematurely, the growing brain is constricted and symptoms of increased ICP develop. Communicating and noncommunicating hydrocephalus occur more frequently in children with craniosynostosis than in normal children. It is more likely that a common underlying factor causes both rather than one causing the other. Two-suture craniosynostosis is common. The sagittal suture is usually involved, in combination with either the metopic or the coronal suture.

Diagnosis. Visual inspection of the skull and palpation of the sutures are sufficient for diagnosis in most cases of one- or two-suture craniosynostosis, and three-dimensional cranial CT scans confirm the diagnosis. Plain films of the skull show a band of increased density at the site of the prematurely closed sutures. All children with craniosynostosis of multiple sutures and children with craniosynostosis of a single-suture and suspected hydrocephalus require an imaging study of the head.

Management. The two indications for surgery to correct craniosynostosis are to improve the appearance of the head and to relieve increased ICP. The cosmetic indication should be used sparingly and only to make severe deformities less noticeable. The early use of a helmet may be beneficial in reshaping the head in early cases of partial craniosynostosis.

422   **CHAPTER 18**   Disorders of Cranial Volume and Shape

REFERENCES

1. Tully HM, Dobyns WB. Infantile hydrocephalus: a review of epidemiology, classification and causes. *European Journal of Medical Genetics*. 2014;57(8):359-368.
2. Zhang J, Williams MA, Rigamonti D. Genetics of human hydrocephalus. *Journal of Neurology*. 2006;253:1255-1266.
3. Stumpel C, Vos YJ. L1 syndrome. In: Adam MP, Ardinger HH, Pagon RA, et al., eds. *GeneReviews*. University of Washington; 1993–2019. https://www.ncbi.nlm.nih.gov/books/NBK1484.
4. Wenger T, Miller D, Evans K. FGFR craniosynostosis syndromes overview (1998). In: Adam MP, Feldman J, Mirzaa GM, et al., eds. *GeneReviews®*. University of Washington; 1993–2023. https://www.ncbi.nlm.nih.gov/books/NBK1455/. Updated April 30, 2020.
5. Grinberg I, Northrup H, Ardinger H, et al. Heterozygous deletion of the linked genes ZIC1 and ZIC4 is involved in Dandy-Walker malformation. *Nature Genetics*. 2004;36:1053-1055.
6. Elterman RD, Bodensteiner JB, Barnard JJ. Sudden unexpected death in patients with Dandy-Walker malformation. *Journal of Child Neurology*. 1995;10(5):382-384. https://doi.org/10.1177/088307389501000508. PMID: 7499758.
7. Samartzis D, Kalluri P, Herman J, et al. Cervical scoliosis in the Klippel-Feil patient. *Spine*. 2011;36:E1501-E1508.
8. Wagner MW, Vaught AJ, Poretti A, et al. Vein of Galen aneurysmal malformation: prognostic markers depicted on fetal MRI. *The Neuroradiology Journal*. 2015;28(1):72-75.
9. Saito K. Fukuyama congenital muscular dystrophy (2006). In: Adam MP, Feldman J, Mirzaa GM, et al., eds. *GeneReviews®*. University of Washington; 1993–2023. https://www.ncbi.nlm.nih.gov/books/NBK1206/. Updated July 3, 2019.
10. Mirzaa G, Graham Jr JM, Keppler-Noreuil K. PIK3CA-related overgrowth spectrum (August 15, 2013). In: Adam MP, Feldman J, Mirzaa GM, et al., eds. *GeneReviews®*. University of Washington; 1993–2023. https://www.ncbi.nlm.nih.gov/books/NBK153722/. Updated April 6, 2023..
11. Pauli RM, Legare JM. Achondroplasia. In: Adam MP, Ardinger HH, Pagon RA, et al., eds. *GeneReviews®*. University of Washington; 1993–2019. https://www.ncbi.nlm.nih.gov/books/NBK1152.
12. Klag KA, Horton WA. Advances in the treatment of achondroplasia and osteoarthritis. *Human Molecular Genetics*. 2016;25(R1):R2-R8.
13. Legare JM. Achondroplasia (October 12, 1998). In: Adam MP, Feldman J, Mirzaa GM, et al., eds. *GeneReviews®*. University of Washington; 1993–2023. https://www.ncbi.nlm.nih.gov/books/NBK1152/. Updated May 11, 2023.
14. Tatton-Brown K, Cole TRP, Rahman N. Sotos syndrome. In: Adam MP, Ardinger HH, Pagon RA, et al., eds. *GeneReviews®*. University of Washington; 1993–2019. https://www.ncbi.nlm.nih.gov/books/NBK1479.
15. Lane C, et al. Characteristics of autism spectrum disorder in Sotos syndrome. *Journal of Autism and Developmental Disorders*. 2017;47(1):135-143.
16. van der Knaap MS, Abbink TE, Min R. Megancephalic leukoencephalopathy with subcortical cysts. In: Adam MP, Ardinger HH, Pagon RA, et al., eds. *GeneReviews®*. University of Washington; 1993–2019. https://www.ncbi.nlm.nih.gov/books/NBK1535.
17. Lanciotti A, et al. Megalencephalic leukoencephalopathy with subcortical cysts protein-1 regulates epidermal growth factor receptor signaling in astrocytes. *Human Molecular Genetics*. 2016;25(8):1543-1558.
18. Gilmore EC, et al. Genetic causes of microcephaly and lessons for neuronal development. *Wiley Interdisciplinary Reviews: Developmental Biology*. 2013;2(4):461-478.
19. Youngblood ME, et al. 2012 Update on global prevention of folic acid–preventable spina bifida and anencephaly. *Birth Defects Research*. 2013;(97):658-663.
20. Hetts SW, Sherr EH, Chao S, et al. Anomalies of the corpus callosum: an MR analysis of the phenotypic spectrum of associated malformations. *American Journal of Roentgenology*. 2006;187:1343-1348.
21. Szabó N, Gergev G, Kóbor J, et al. Corpus callosum anomalies: birth prevalence and clinical spectrum in Hungary. *Pediatric Neurology*. 2011;44:420-426.
22. Paul LK, et al. Agenesis of corpus callosum and autism: a comprehensive comparison. *Brain*. 2014;137:1813-1829.
23. Hehr U, Uyanik G, Aigner L, et al. DCX-related disorders. In: Adam MP, Ardinger HH, Pagon RA, et al., eds. *GeneReviews®*. University of Washington; 1993–2019. https://www.ncbi.nlm.nih.gov/books/NBK1185.
24. Mlakar J, et al. Zika virus associated with microcephaly. *New England Journal of Medicine*. 2016;374:951-958.
25. Robin NH, Falk MJ, Haldeman-Englert CR. FGFR-related craniosynostosis syndromes. In: Adam MP, Ardinger HH, Pagon RA, et al., eds. *GeneReviews®*. University of Washington; 1993–2019. https://www.ncbi.nlm.nih.gov/books/NBK1455.

Behavioral Neurology

OUTLINE

Depression and Suicidality, 423
Anxiety Disorders, 425
Obsessive-Compulsive Disorder, 426
  Autism Spectrum Disorder, 428
  Conduct Disorder and Oppositional Defiant
    Disorder, 430
  Treatment Options, 431
Psychogenic Disorders, 431
  Psychogenic Nonepileptic Spells, 431

Psychogenic (Functional) Movement Disorders, 433
Common Medications Used in the Treatment of
  Neurobehavioral Disorders, 433
  Selective Serotonin Reuptake Inhibitors, 433
  Selective Serotonin and Norepinephrine Reuptake
    Inhibitors, 434
  Stimulant Medications, 434
  Nonstimulant Medications, 435
References, 435

Behavioral conditions and psychiatric comorbidities are frequently seen in the practice of neurology. Psychiatric conditions land in our practice for many reasons. They are common comorbidities in patients with neurological diseases such as migraines, epilepsy, developmental delay, and neurogenetic disorders. Conversely, primary psychiatric disorders may present with neurologic symptoms such as dizziness, headache, spells, or paresthesias. At other times parents or psychiatrists want to rule out an underlying "neurologic" cause for behavioral symptoms. This can be a tricky question to address since both normative and pathological behaviors always have a neurologic cause (the brain being the source of all behaviors); however, it is extremely rare for typical childhood behavior problems to be secondary to structural brain disease or have an autoimmune or metabolic basis. Those patients often exhibit systemic symptomatology and frequently have encephalopathy, seizures, abnormal neurologic examination, or signs of other organ involvement in addition to the behavioral or psychiatric symptoms.

According to epidemiological studies, up to 25% of youth (defined as people aged 15–24 years) have experienced a mental disorder as defined by the Diagnostic and Statistical Manual of Mental Disorders (*DSM*) within the past year, and 33% will experience one within their lifetimes. The most common disorders encountered in a pediatric neurology practice are major depressive disorder (MDD), obsessive-compulsive disorder (OCD), generalized anxiety disorder (GAD), social anxiety disorder (SAD), panic disorder (PD), attention deficit disorder with or without hyperactivity (ADD/ADHD), autism spectrum disorder (ASD), and psychogenic symptoms. Not surprisingly, the American Board of Neurology and Psychiatry oversees our training and certification. Neurologic and psychiatric symptoms are abnormal manifestations of the same organ, the brain.

DEPRESSION AND SUICIDALITY

MDD is estimated to occur in about 4% of the population. The percentage is much higher when including minor depression or depression not otherwise specified. Peak onset in adolescence is ages 11–14.[1] Many of these patients present to the neurology clinic for headaches, cognitive complaints, decreased school performance, and generalized pain and fatigue. Depression is most likely a complex polygenetic disease and often runs in families; unfortunately, no objective biomarkers have yet been discovered.

Clinical features. Depression may manifest differently in children than in adults. Common features in all age groups include sleep disruption, changes in appetite, feeling of fogginess or general fatigue, and trouble concentrating. Both young children and adolescents may "act out" more during episodes of depression, and depression should be considered in any child with aggression or defiance (*externalizing behaviors*). *Somatization* is another common symptom. Many children are unable to articulate the vague feelings of sadness or hopelessness that characterize a depressive illness and may instead focus on concrete physical complaints such as head pain or nausea.

Suicidal ideation is common in children and adolescents with depression. In such cases it is critical to determine if the child is thinking about suicide in a general sense versus formulating a definite plan. Screening tools assume great importance in this regard because evidence shows that most pediatric patients with suicidal ideation will not disclose their symptoms to their parents or health care provider spontaneously but may do so when specifically asked. Adolescents are at particular risk for suicide but death by suicide has been reported in children as young as 7 years old, and the numbers have drastically increased in recent years.[2] The natural impulsivity of children is a significant danger when combined with suicidal thoughts or actions.

Diagnosis. A brief depression assessment should be performed on all children and adolescents at every clinic visit. The patient health questionnaire-9 (PHQ-9) is a free, widely available screening tool for depression (Box 19.1). The final score represents the probability of minimal, mild, moderate, or severe depression. The PHQ-2 is a shorter version but may fail to identify patients with clinically significant suicide risk. Every patient should be screened, but especially those exhibiting clinical signs of depression such as monotonous, slow speech or a flat affect. Prompt diagnosis and treatment of depression can be lifesaving.

Management. Selective serotonin reuptake inhibitors (SSRIs) and serotonin-norepinephrine reuptake inhibitors (SNRIs) are the mainstay of treatment. Specific medications and doses are listed later in this chapter. Cognitive behavioral therapy (CBT), behavioral modification, and interpersonal psychotherapy are often used concurrently. Avoid tricyclic antidepressants such as amitriptyline, clomipramine, and imipramine since their benefit is questionable and their cardiotoxicity can be fatal if taken in overdose during a suicide attempt. We do not use monoaminoxidase inhibitors due to lack

---

BOX 19.1 The Patient Health Questionnaire-9 (PHQ-9) Patient Screening Tool

Name _____ Date _____

Over the *last 2 weeks*, how often have you been bothered by any of the following problems?	Not at all	Several days	More than half the days	Nearly every day
1. Little interest or pleasure in doing things	0	1	2	3
2. Feeling down, depressed, or hopeless	0	1	2	3
3. Trouble falling or staying asleep, or sleeping too much	0	1	2	3
4. Feeling tired or having little energy	0	1	2	3
5. Poor appetite or overeating	0	1	2	3
6. Feeling bad about yourself—or that you are a failure or have let yourself or your family down	0	1	2	3
7. Trouble concentrating on things, such as reading the newspaper or watching television	0	1	2	3
8. Moving or speaking so slowly that other people could have noticed? Or the opposite—being so fidgety or restless that you have been moving around a lot more than usual	0	1	2	3
9. Thoughts that you would be better off dead or of hurting yourself in some way	0	1	2	3

(For office coding: Total Score ____ = ____ + ____ + ____)

of supportive evidence and likelihood of side effects.[3] Pharmacotherapy and psychotherapy are more effective when used in combination rather than individually.

Children with acute suicidality require urgent evaluation in the emergency department by a mental health crisis intervention team.

ANXIETY DISORDERS

According to the Centers for Disease Control and Prevention, 9.4% of children aged 3–17 years were diagnosed with anxiety between 2016 and 2019. The incidence is undoubtedly higher when we consider those who suffer from anxiety disorders but remain undiagnosed. The most common subtypes are GAD and SAD. Separation anxiety, panic attacks or PD, overanxious disorder (OAD), and specific phobias are also common. The prevalence is higher in females with a 2–3:1 female-to-male ratio by adolescence.[1,4]

Functional MRI demonstrates hyperactivation of the amygdala, the ventrolateral prefrontal cortex (VLPFC), and other pathways. The VLPFC functions to reduce feelings of anxiety and likely becomes hyperactive as a compensatory mechanism. Interestingly, fluoxetine and CBT also increase VLPFC activity. We note that while such studies elucidate the neurobiology of anxiety, imaging studies are rarely required or helpful in diagnosis or treatment.[4]

Clinical features. Patients with anxiety disorders present with a variety of symptoms. Children and adolescents with panic attacks or PD (which is simply the experience of recurrent panic attacks) often present with fainting, dizziness, shortness of breath, blurred or darkened vision, chest pain, tachycardia, and paresthesias of the hands, feet, and perioral region. Intense or prolonged hyperventilation results in generalized high amplitude slowing on the electroencephalogram (EEG) due to hypocapnia and hypoperfusion of the brain, sometimes with clinically evident encephalopathy such as decreased responsiveness or confusion. Hyperventilation also causes *carpopedal spasm*, in which the limbs stiffen, arms flex, and the hands assume a dystonic, clawed position. Carpopedal spasm can be misinterpreted as seizure, particularly in a patient who is poorly responsive due to panic or hyperventilation-induced encephalopathy.

Younger children may present with tantrums, meltdowns, irritability, or crying when trying to avoid the anxiety-provoking situation. Caregivers often misinterpret these behaviors as oppositional or disobedient. Many children and adolescents present with nausea which may evolve into recurrent vomiting; in severe cases this can lead to food refusal, weight loss, and dehydration. It is not unusual for a child to undergo multiple invasive gastrointestinal evaluations for undiagnosed anxiety-induced vomiting.

Most patients with anxiety experience disrupted sleep. Older children who can verbalize their feelings will tell you that their mind "never shuts down" and may endorse racing or unpleasant thoughts that prevent them from falling asleep. Younger children may appear unable to "settle" and repeatedly cry or get out of bed. Such symptoms must be differentiated from sleep disruption secondary to hyperactivity, restless legs syndrome, or other sleep disorders.

Anxiety disorders in children and adolescents are potentially fatal and increase the risk of suicide attempts and illicit substance use and dependence.[5–8]

Diagnosis. The GAD-7 is a validated tool for the diagnosis of anxiety in pediatric patients ages 11–17; however, we also find it helpful to detect traits in younger children (Box 19.2). The final score provides the probability of minimal, mild, moderate, or severe anxiety.[9] Other tools such as the multidimensional anxiety scale for children, the screen for child anxiety and related emotional disorders, and the Spence children's anxiety scale are also available.

Management. SSRIs and SNRIs are the medications used most frequently. Buspirone, an azapirone drug, has become increasingly popular due to its efficacy and relatively low side effect profile. Its mechanism of action is not fully known but appears to be related to its strong affinity for serotonin 5HT1a receptors, as well as weak affinity for 5HT2 receptors and weak antagonism against dopaminergic D2 receptors. Unlike benzodiazepines, it has no effect on gamma-aminobutyric acid. We do not recommend the long-term use of benzodiazepines due to the possibility of tolerance and dependence, but the short-term use is sometimes helpful for situational anxiety such as phlebotomy or during dental work.

CBT with systematic exposure to triggers, gradual desensitization, and habituation is often favored by parents who may themselves have anxiety traits and an aversion to medications. Large, controlled trials are scarce, but available evidence shows that CBT probably has some effect.[12] As in depression, the combination of

---

BOX 19.2   The GAD-7 Patient Screening Tool

Generalized Anxiety Disorder 7-item (GAD-7)

Over the last 2 weeks, how often have you been bothered by the following problems	Not at all	Several days	More than half the days	Nearly every day
1. Feeling nervous, anxious or on edge	0	1	2	3
2. Not being able to stop or control worrying	0	1	2	3
3. Worrying too much about different things	0	1	2	3
4. Trouble relaxing	0	1	2	3
5. Being so restless that it is hard to sit still	0	1	2	3
6. Becoming easily annoyed or irritable	0	1	2	3
7. Feeling afraid as if something awful might happen	0	1	2	3

GAD-7 score obtained by adding score for each question (total points).

A score of 8 points or higher is a reasonable and is the cut-off for needing further identifying evaluation to determine presence and type of anxiety disorder[10,11]

The following cutoffs correlate with level of anxiety severity:

Score 0–4	: Minimal Anxiety
Score 5–9	: Mild Anxiety
Score 10–14	: Moderate Anxiety
Score of 15 or greater	: Severe Anxiety

---

medication and CBT has significantly better efficacy when compared with either therapy alone. A list of SSRIs and SNRIs with dosages can be found later in this chapter.

OBSESSIVE-COMPULSIVE DISORDER

The prevalence of OCD is about 0.25%–4% depending on the study, and the disorder probably represents the extreme end of a spectrum of behaviors and personalities. A degree of obsessive-compulsiveness may be viewed as a positive attribute, in that people who have mild obsessive-compulsive traits are often organized, meticulous, and highly productive with a strong desire to perform tasks correctly and thoroughly. Such traits are often seen in the parents of affected children. Obsessive-compulsiveness becomes a disorder when it leads to an overwhelming degree of rigidity, intrusive thoughts, lack of flexibility, unusually intense fixations, and compulsions or rituals. OCD has a polygenic inheritance with many genes influencing the final phenotype, and a wide spectrum of the disorder may be seen within the same family.

When evaluating children with OCD, it is common to have both parents present; parents of affected children are often highly organized and want to be sure everything is fully addressed and understood. This experience is also common when evaluating conditions that have obsessive-compulsive behaviors such as parents of children with Tourette syndrome and autism.

Serotonergic, dopaminergic, and glutamatergic systems are affected. Functional neuroimaging studies show hyperactivation of the medial and lateral parts of the orbitofrontal cortex in OCD with decreased activity after CBT.[8] Currently, diagnostic genetics cannot identify OCD, and functional neuroimaging is not helpful in clinical practice.

Clinical features. Children with OCD often come to medical attention due to comorbid disorders such as anxiety or tics. Affected children are usually intelligent, but school performance may suffer when obsessions or compulsions (OC) prevent the child from focusing on their studies. Conversely, some children suffer from compulsive perfectionism. Such children are excellent students and intolerant of any perceived imperfections in their work. One revealing question to ask is if, when drawing or writing out an assignment, the child feels they must discard the entire paper and start again if any mistake is made, rather than simply correcting the mistake and moving on. We find that a surprisingly high number of children answer in the affirmative when asked this question.

Some obsessions and compulsions may not be apparent to family members, who often dismiss the child's behavior as "pickiness" or "fussiness." For example, a child with OCD may have a messy room with no apparent interest in cleanliness; however, the same child melts down if made to wear shoes with shoelaces, because they cannot rest unless the laces on each side are exactly even. Such children prefer shoes with Velcro closures long after they have learned to tie their laces. Many patients are extraordinarily sensitive to textures, preferring to wear sweatpants or leggings rather than jeans. Others insist on absolute separation of all foods and demand that parents discard their plate and make a new one if, for example, any of their carrots touch the rice. Likewise, some compulsive behaviors may be misdiagnosed as "complex tics" (e.g., needing to spin around three times upon entering a room).

Classic obsessions and compulsions are easier to identify, and include counting, ordering, cleaning, listing, and checking (e.g., repeatedly checking the door to make sure it is locked). Hoarding and trichotillomania are classified in a similar category. Sexual and religious obsessions are seen in adults but are less common in children. Deviation from a compulsive behavior causes such disruption and emotional distress that many families choose to accommodate the behavior rather than challenging it. In severe cases the child's OCD essentially kidnaps the entire family because restrictions on their activities are so extreme.

An explosive onset of OCD can be seen with pediatric autoimmune neuropsychiatric disorder associated with streptococcus and pediatric acute-onset neuropsychiatric disorder (PANS), which are described elsewhere and will not be addressed here.

Diagnosis. In order to meet diagnostic criteria OC must be present for more than 2 weeks. Patients are aware that OC originate in their own brain. OC are repetitive and distressing, and at least one is excessive. At least one OC is unsuccessfully resisted. Completion of OC may provide relief but is not a pleasurable experience. The symptoms are disabling.[13]

Management. Children usually respond to treatment. In our experience untreated OCD tends to become stronger over time and evolves into a chronic condition.

The treatment for OCD includes the use of SSRIs or SNRIs, clomipramine, and CBT. CBT consists of 12–20 sessions with the strategy to expose the patient to an obsession such as contamination by experiencing the feared situation (e.g., touching a door handle), and then trying to refrain from the immediate compulsion (e.g., washing hands). The intent is to desensitize the child from the feared situation and habituate to a better response.

The pathophysiological contribution of dopaminergic and glutaminergic mechanisms has been poorly investigated. Medications that work on these neurotransmitters may have a role in patients resistant to current treatments, but further research is needed.

Attention Deficit Disorder With or Without Hyperactivity

ADD/ADHD are controversial. They are some of the most prevalent disorders of childhood, occurring in approximately 5% of the pediatric population. However, diagnostic criteria are subjective, and there are no biological markers or consistent imaging findings to support the diagnosis, which is heavily dependent on the expertise and opinions of the treating physician. Concern has grown in recent years that ADD/ADHD is overdiagnosed and children medicated in order to promote conformity to certain societal expectations, rather than out of a true regard for the child's welfare. We wholeheartedly agree that, in general, children are not meant to sit still and be quiet for multiple hours each day, and that some cases of supposed "ADHD" are due to inappropriate expectations on the part of the teacher or parent. Nevertheless, it is clear that ADD and ADHD are real disorders that can cause significant distress, disability, and even physical harm in the children they afflict, and those cases require appropriate diagnosis and treatment.

Clinical features. Suspect the diagnosis when the triad of inattention, hyperactivity, and impulsiveness is present. The diagnosis of ADHD requires symptoms to be present before the age of 12 and noticed in at least two settings (such as school and home). Importantly, there must be evidence that symptoms are reducing the quality of social, school, or work functioning and do not have another explanation such as anxiety or a mood disorder. Males are diagnosed more often than females; this may be due to a genuine predilection for males to have the disorder or may reflect the fact that fewer females display hyperactivity and thus are less likely to draw the attention of exasperated teachers or parents. Children with ADHD often cause disruptions at home and at school and are more prone to accidental injuries due to risky behavior and poor decision-making.

Inattentiveness symptoms include:

- Often fails to give close attention to details or makes careless mistakes in schoolwork, at work, or with other activities.
- Often has trouble holding attention on tasks or play activities.
- Often does not seem to listen when spoken to directly.
- Often does not follow through on instructions and fails to finish schoolwork, chores, or duties in the workplace (e.g., loses focus, side-tracked).
- Often has trouble organizing tasks and activities.
- Often avoids, dislikes, or is reluctant to do tasks that require mental effort over a long period of time (such as schoolwork or homework).
- Often loses things necessary for tasks and activities (e.g., school materials, pencils, books, tools, wallets, keys, paperwork, eyeglasses, mobile telephones).
- Is often easily distracted.
- Is often forgetful in daily activities.
  Hyperactivity/impulsiveness symptoms include:
- Often fidgets with or taps hands or feet, or squirms in seat.
- Often leaves seat in situations when remaining seated is expected.
- Often runs about or climbs in situations where it is not appropriate (adolescents or adults may be limited to feeling restless).
- Often unable to play or take part in leisure activities quietly.
- Is often "on the go" acting as if "driven by a motor."
- Often talks excessively.
- Often blurts out an answer before a question has been completed.
- Often has trouble waiting their turn.
- Often interrupts or intrudes on others (e.g., butts into conversations or games).[14]

Diagnosis. The *DSM* criteria require six or more symptoms of inattention or hyperactivity/impulsiveness for children up to age 16, or five or more for adolescents aged 17 years and older and adults; symptoms for at least 6 months, and symptoms that are inappropriate for developmental level.[15]

Management. Educational accommodations are the first-line treatments in mild cases, in which school concerns virtually always overshadow any concerns that parents have for behavior in the home. Seat the child at the front of the room near the teacher and allow frequent breaks for movement. "Wobble chairs" are helpful for some children because they allow a certain amount of movement while still remaining seated; likewise, "fidget toys" offer an outlet for excessive hand movement. Specialized chairs and toys should not be used if they only serve to distract the child further. If the teacher allows, it is often helpful to allow the child to perform self-directed individual activities in the location and position of their choice within the classroom (e.g., some classrooms have a dedicated corner with bean bags and a rug to allow children to lie in various positions while reading).

In cases that are not adequately controlled with conservative measures, both stimulant and nonstimulant drugs are used for treatment. In general stimulants are more efficacious than nonstimulants. A list of these medications can be found later in this chapter. Sometimes treatment is delayed based on the family's fears of changing the child's personality or "making him a zombie." We must convey to the family that we understand their concerns and that such side effects will not be tolerated. The goals of treatment include better academic performance, fewer accidental injuries, greater acceptance among peers, and less stress overall for the patient and family. Environmental adaptations should continue; there is evidence that stimulant medications plus environmental accommodations allow adequate symptom control at lower doses than stimulants used without accommodations.[15]

Autism Spectrum Disorder

Autism is a neurodevelopmental disorder characterized by deficits in social communication, restricted interests, and repetitive behaviors. A separate category of social pragmatic communication disorder exists for those with impaired social communications without repetitive or restrictive behaviors. The World Health Organization estimates ASD prevalence at 0.76%, and the Centers for Disease Control and Prevention estimates the prevalence of ASD in the United States at 1.68%. The number of children diagnosed with ASDs has grown steadily over the last few decades. Many factors likely contribute to the increased incidence, including changing definitions and *DSM* diagnostic criteria, public awareness campaigns, increased childhood access to health care, evolving health care regulations, and reimbursements.[16] ASD is more common in males with a 3:1 male-to-female ratio.

ASD is a syndrome with multiple etiologies; it may be monogenetic, polygenetic, chromosomal, or of unknown cause. A meta-analysis of all published twin studies demonstrates strong heritability ranging from 64% to 91%.[17] Another study combining twin and family data across five (largely White European) countries found a heritability rate of 80.8%.[18] Autism is most properly conceived as a spectrum, and relatives of affected patients have higher rates of autism-like features such as abnormal social interactions and unusual personality traits. Other influences include advanced maternal or paternal age; older paternal age is particularly associated with an increased incidence of rare de novo mutations. The importance of genetic contributions appears to be similar for both mild and severe autism phenotypes, but some studies suggest a component of genetic loading.

To date, inherited or de novo mutations in more than 700 genes have been associated with ASD. Many of these genes exhibit pleiotropy and are implicated in other neurodevelopmental or psychiatric disorders. The strongest associations are between autism and ADHD and depression, but links exist to schizophrenia, Tourette syndrome, and OCD.[19]

Although autism is highly heritable, significant clinical variability exists even between monozygotic twins. This suggests that while genetic predisposition is strong, the specific phenotype is heavily influenced by environmental factors. The nature of such factors remains unclear.

Clinical features. Typically developing toddlers have an intense desire to communicate with their caregivers. They make eye contact, smile socially, recognize their own names, babble, and point. Slightly older children will excitedly share new discoveries and experiences with parents. In contrast early signs of autism include decreased eye contact, unresponsiveness to name, and a lack of showing and sharing, which evolves into rigidity, excessive fixation on certain interests, and a lack of pretend play. More subtle findings include concrete or literal thinking beyond that which is normal for age, and impaired language and social skills. Many children engage in "stimming," which involves producing repetitive movements or sounds. This may be a self-soothing mechanism and can also be a way of expressing excitement or other strong emotions. A small minority of people with autism display extraordinary cognitive abilities in certain subjects ("savants").

Children with ASD often have comorbid ADHD, OCD, insomnia, depression, anxiety, pathological shyness, and other treatable symptoms. In many cases the

child's distress is caused by associated disorders rather than autism itself. When evaluating a child with autism, it is vital to assess for the related disorders mentioned earlier.

Autistic children have higher rates of epilepsy than the general population, and any reported "spells" should be taken seriously. However, children with autism are more prone to staring with apparent unresponsiveness due to decreased social interaction at baseline, and often display abnormal repetitive movements, which may represent stimming rather than epileptic automatisms or clonic movements. Parental recordings of the spells and EEG are critical for diagnosis.

Diagnosis. Formal testing comprises extensive evaluations such as the Autism Diagnostic Observation Schedule (ADOS) and other validated tools. These are particularly useful when the child has some autistic features, but it is unclear if he meets criteria for a formal diagnosis. Assessments like ADOS are considered the gold standard of diagnosis but are time consuming and difficult to obtain, leading to diagnostic delay in many cases. In our opinion a child with obvious autism should not have their treatment delayed in order to administer a lengthy test, the outcome of which is already known. Nevertheless, some states, school districts, or insurance companies may require such testing to consider the diagnosis valid.

All children with autism deserve a genetic workup. Given the significant genetic heterogeneity of the disorder, whole exome sequencing or autism multigene panels are the most practical approach to diagnosis. Other tests include chromosome microarray, Fragile X for males, and specific gene testing in patients with unique symptoms suggestive of a specific disorder. Children with autism and epilepsy should undergo brain imaging with MRI. Prolonged EEG monitoring, including during sleep, is helpful to evaluate for the rare possibility of Landau-Kleffner syndrome (acquired epileptic aphasia) or other epileptic encephalopathies. However, EEG is not required unless there are specific concerns for epilepsy, and a routine EEG may suffice in cases in which acquired epileptic aphasia is not suspected.

Management. Applied behavioral analysis (ABA) is generally accepted as standard of care for children with autism. The therapy is intensive, up to 40 hours per week, and focuses on breaking desired behaviors down into manageable steps, with the child rewarded for achieving each step. Although ABA early in life is considered the gold standard for treatment of behavioral symptoms associated with ASD, high-quality objective evidence is limited due to the variability of symptoms and the lack of long-term studies. ABA has also become increasingly controversial as some older, verbal patients with autism reported that participating in ABA harmed their self-esteem and made them feel that they must hide their true natures in order to fit into society (this has been covered in multiple stories in the lay press, for example, "Is the Most Common Therapy for Autism Cruel?" published in *The Atlantic* in 2016). Our approach is that parents should pursue ABA therapy but should also feel free to discontinue it if they feel it is not helpful for their child or produces an undue amount of distress.

We mainly focus on managing the common comorbidities associated with autism. We have personally treated patients with severe, nonverbal autism who began speaking and interacting after only 2–3 weeks of treatment with an SSRI. Although this evidence is anecdotal and the number small, the life-altering nature of the response convinced us that every child with autism should receive a trial of SSRIs or SNRIs if there is any indication of underlying anxiety, depression, or OCD. ADHD is another common, highly treatable comorbidity. We treat ADHD in autism similarly to ADHD in nonautistic children (see the section on "Attention Deficit Disorder With or Without Hyperactivity" earlier in this chapter). Treat epilepsy with standard anticonvulsant therapy (see Chapter 1).

Children with autism may have drastically negative responses to stimuli they find unpleasant. At times, this interferes with standard caretaking and hygiene such as haircuts and fingernail trims. In those cases a small dose of an antipsychotic such as olanzapine (Zyprexa) or a short-acting benzodiazepine like alprazolam (Xanax) can make the experience less stressful and less likely to result in injury to the child or caregiver. Risperidone (Risperdal) and aripiprazole (Abilify) are specifically approved by the FDA for the treatment of tantrums, irritability, aggression, and self-injurious behaviors in ASD, and many other drugs are used off-label.

Sleep is a major concern for most parents of autistic children. Children with autism are highly routine-oriented, and the early establishment of a consistent bedtime routine is critical. However, many patients will continue to experience sleep disruptions even when a good routine is in place. We typically use clonidine or gabapentin to treat insomnia. Disrupted sleep in the setting of new developmental regression should prompt an overnight EEG to rule out nocturnal seizures.

Conduct Disorder and Oppositional Defiant Disorder

Conduct disorder (CD) is the presence of repetitive violation of the basic rights of others and of major age-appropriate rules or norms. The subcategories of CD include aggression to people and animals, destruction of property, deceitfulness or theft and serious violations of rules. It requires presence of symptoms for more than a year and for the behavior to cause academic or social dysfunction. CD is more common in males than females and is associated with the development of antisocial personality disorder later in life.[20,21]

Suspect oppositional defiant disorder (ODD) in children with anger, loss of temper, and bullying. The diagnosis is used for children with negativistic, defiant, and hostile behaviors. Children with ADHD often exhibit mild to moderate ODD symptoms; however, children with CD often exhibit intense or severe ODD symptoms.[20] CD and ODD are grouped together in the *DSM-5* under the heading of "Disruptive, Impulse Control, and Conduct Disorders." These disorders account for a significant portion of mental health costs and are considered strongly predictive of mental health disorders in adulthood, including anxiety, depression, suicidality, and substance abuse disorders. Children with CD and ODD are at increased risk of contact with law enforcement and involvement in the juvenile justice system.

Clinical features. Children with CD and ODD may show a high level of impulsivity and poor emotional regulation, and may display *callous-unemotional* traits, described as lack of empathy, deficient guilt/remorse, lack of concern over performance of important activities, and constricted displays of emotion. Patients with increased callous-unemotional traits, and those who become symptomatic in childhood rather than adolescence, are more likely to have persistent symptoms into adulthood.[22]

Diagnosis. Diagnostic criteria are defined by the *DSM-5.* Like many other psychiatric and neurobehavioral disorders, CD and ODD exist on a spectrum with no clear cutoffs. Typically developing toddlers often display aggression and oppositional behaviors, and some degree of rule-breaking is present in almost all children. It is therefore important to account for normative age-related behaviors when considering the diagnosis. The imprecise nature of the diagnostic tools increases the risk of inappropriate or biased results, especially in children of color or low socioeconomic status.[23] Perhaps more than in any other disorder, the treating physician must keep their own implicit biases in mind when evaluating a child for CD or ODD.

Treatment Options

The complexity and variability of CD manifestations and their overlapping comorbidities have limited the availability of good evidence-based treatments. Therapies are considered the standard of care, but there are few high-quality studies to support their efficacy. Such therapies focus on improving parenting skills to prevent or modify dysfunctional behaviors as well as CBT for the patient. Parental skill training is preferred for parents of younger children and consists of a group of parents who participate in 10–16 sessions lasting 90–120 minutes, during which the child's behavior is demonstrated and parents practice their response with feedback from the therapist. CBT for older children and adolescents consists of 10–18 weekly 2-hour sessions with similar role playing by peers and rehearsal of new skills with feedback from therapists.[10]

Pharmacologically, there is no specific treatment target for CD and ODD, but mood stabilizers, atypical antipsychotics (risperidone, aripiprazole, others), antiseizure medications used as mood stabilizers (valproic acid, lamotrigine, oxcarbazepine), psychostimulants, SSRIs, and SNRIs may decrease the impact of comorbid conditions.[20]

PSYCHOGENIC DISORDERS

Psychogenic Nonepileptic Spells

Pyschogenic nonepileptic spells (PNES) are episodes of altered behavior or responsiveness that may resemble epileptic seizures but are not. Such episodes are also called pseudoseizures, functional seizures, or nonepileptic seizures. We prefer to avoid the use of the word "seizure" in any of the descriptors, as it can confuse patients and caregivers who need to understand that the events in question are not, in fact, seizures. We also tend to avoid use of the term "functional seizure" as the presence of PNES indicates significant dysfunction despite a structurally and electrically normal brain. We note, however, that PNES are classified under "Functional Neurological Symptoms Disorders," formerly known as conversion disorders. PNES can also be conceived as a dissociative disorder, and spells are sometimes called "dissociative seizures."

PNES is a common problem representing between 3.5% and 20% of all admissions for EEG monitoring and 11%–38% of all children with nonepileptic spells.[11,24,25] The precise pathophysiology of PNES remains unknown, but recent studies have increased our understanding of the disorder. Many adults with PNES have a history of trauma such as prior physical or sexual abuse, posttraumatic stress disorder (PTSD), or other mood disorders. The same does not apply to children and adolescents, who are much more likely to report that their main stressors center around school and home life rather than a specific traumatic experience. While some pediatric patients have an obvious history of psychosocial stressors or psychiatric disease, these are not prerequisites for diagnosis. The theory that specific personality types are more vulnerable to PNES has gained traction in recent years, as well as the notion that certain cognitive traits are associated with the disorder, in particular *alexithymia* (difficulty of verbal expression of affect leading to an inner expression of psychic distress in the form of physical complaints) and a tendency toward dissociation.[26]

Small studies have demonstrated physical changes in the brains of PNES patients, such as increased limbic and paralimbic activity, increased sensitization of the amygdala, and increased functional connectivity between the amygdala and motor planning circuits in the those with PNES and other motor-based functional neurological disorders. This implies increased limbic control of motor outputs, but the results are preliminary. Functional connectivity studies have demonstrated increased connectivity between emotional (insula, cingulate) and motor control centers in patients with PNES. More research is needed to confirm and interpret these findings.[27]

Clinical features. As with epileptic seizures, PNES can present with a wide variety of symptoms. Certain findings or behaviors should raise concern for PNES, including multiple distinct spells, spells with inconsistent semiology, spells that only occur in specific locations (e.g., a certain classroom at school), spells that only occur around certain people (parents, significant others, specific friends), and spells that rapidly increase in frequency to the point that the patient is completely unable to participate in normal daily activities such as school, sports, or other hobbies. Clinically, PNES may have a stop-and-go quality as the patient pauses to rest before resuming movement. Episodes are often prolonged, lasting minutes to hours. Certain types of movements are more common in PNES, including side-to-side head or body shaking, pelvic thrusting, asynchronous or irregular jerking, back arching, and eye closure. Patients may whimper or cry during events. Of note, it is possible for patients to urinate, injure themselves, or bite their tongues during PNES. Exertion causes the patient to breathe rapidly once the spell is over, in contrast to postictal breathing following an epileptic seizure, which is slow and sonorous. Later, patients may have intact recall and report that they could hear but not see or speak during the event.

A significant minority of patients with PNES have comorbid epilepsy requiring anticonvulsant treatment. Other common comorbidities include anxiety, depression, perfectionism, obsessive-compulsive tendencies, and a tendency toward dissociation. Females outnumber males. *La belle indifference* may be seen, in which the patient insists that she is neither anxious nor sad despite the fact that she is utterly debilitated by her spells.

Diagnosis. A good history is usually enough to diagnose PNES; however, in the presence of frequent events (daily or near daily), the diagnosis can be confirmed by long-term video EEG. Imaging studies and laboratory investigations are not useful. Prolactin is elevated for about 20 minutes following a convulsive seizure but normalizes rapidly, rendering it essentially useless as a biomarker. Furthermore, prolactin may remain normal following focal seizures.

It is important to note that any highly stereotyped spell, no matter how bizarre, deserves thorough evaluation. There are endless anecdotes and case studies demonstrating the various unusual ways that epileptic seizures can present, and most practicing epileptologists can vividly recall cases in which they were convinced that spells were psychogenic when in fact they were epileptic. In cases in which the diagnosis is uncertain, always obtain prolonged EEG monitoring.

Treatment Options

In general children and adolescents with PNES have better outcomes than adults, with up to 89% either fully in remission or with significant decrease in spells 1 year after being treated in a pediatric PNES clinic. Interestingly, capturing episodes on video EEG did not correlate significantly with acceptance of the diagnosis or outcomes.[28]

The physician must deliver the diagnosis clearly and with compassion. Such conversations are time consuming, and the physician should set aside sufficient time for discussion. Outcomes are significantly better when patients and parents fully accept the diagnosis rather than continuing to seek additional testing. Many patients improve following diagnosis, even without specific treatment. The physician's explanation should help the patient and family understand that pediatric PNES often occurs in highly driven and caring individuals who tend to resist asking for help. Reassure them that PNES is a common problem in childhood and adolescence. It is not a sign of weakness, and the diagnosis is private health information that the patient is not obligated to share with anyone.

Treatment is focused on identifying and reducing stressors and addressing issues at home, in interpersonal relationships, and with the school (including allowing a brief period of reduced attendance or homebound schooling in certain cases). When speaking to patients, we emphasize that we want to help them regain control over their bodies and their lives. Therapy is needed to develop improved coping mechanisms. Anecdotally, we find that meditation techniques and grounding exercises used successfully in other dissociative disorders are often helpful in PNES. If patients have anxiety or depression, start treatment with SSRIs or SNRIs. Close follow-up with a therapist or physician is extraordinarily helpful, although sometimes difficult to achieve. Patients who fail to improve after diagnosis often report feelings of abandonment or a sense that they were "dumped" by their physician. Ongoing therapeutic support helps avoid such sentiments. Once therapy is established, gradual reintroduction of activities should be attempted.

During treatment, some patients will continue to have occasional spells, and parents often ask for direction in terms of acute management. Provided that the spell in question is the patient's typical nonepileptic spell, we advise the following: first, obtain some privacy for the patient if possible. Crowds tend to increase patient anxiety levels and intrude upon patient privacy and dignity. Second, reduce stimulation by dimming the lights and eliminating sources of noise. The caregiver must remain calm and supportive. Quietly talk to and reassure the patient. Do not escalate by becoming panicked or calling emergency services. Although such spells may be distressing to witness, they are not dangerous, and utilizing emergency services increases the risk of inappropriate use of potentially dangerous medications, as well as unnecessary testing and hospitalization.

Psychogenic (Functional) Movement Disorders

Psychogenic movement disorders comprise a large portion of functional neurologic disease. As with psychogenic nonepileptic seizures, our understanding has evolved into a biopsychosocial model that includes objective changes in brain connectivity as well as associated personality traits and the presence of underlying stressors. In the pediatric population tics are the most common functional movement disorder.

Patients and parents may worry that the explosive onset of apparent tics signals a serious underlying disorder such as PANS. The critical distinction is that the movement disorder in PANS is a true movement disorder accompanied by psychiatric symptoms; in contrast, functional movement disorders are due to an entirely different pathological process.

Clinical features. Tic disorders usually begin in early childhood. The onset of motor and vocal tics in adolescence is unusual, although not impossible, and should raise concern for a functional movement disorder. Functional tics are often varied and change rapidly; they tend to be large amplitude, obvious movements, or noises and have more complexity than typical simple tics. Patients often deny a premonitory urge and may report that they are unable to suppress tics at all, even for short periods of time.[29] Coprolalia (vocal tics characterized by cursing) is more common in patients with psychogenic tics. Parents may report that movements persist during sleep, which indicates that the movement is either not a tic or that the patient is not actually sleeping (*pseudosleep*). It is possible for certain movement disorders to persist during sleep, but this phenomenon is extremely uncommon (see Chapter 14).

Diagnosis. As with other psychogenic disorders, diagnosis can usually be made on the basis of a thorough history and physical examination. Unlike PNES, there is no objective device like EEG that we may use to confirm our suspicions, and no biomarkers for the disorder have yet been discovered. Therefore the diagnosis is entirely clinical.

Management. Management is largely the same as that for PNES and depends on the degree of disability. Treat comorbid anxiety, depression, ADHD, or OCD. CBT and counseling to address coping mechanisms are recommended.

COMMON MEDICATIONS USED IN THE TREATMENT OF NEUROBEHAVIORAL DISORDERS

Selective Serotonin Reuptake Inhibitors

SSRIs are used in the treatments of MDD, OCD, GAD, SAD, PD, PTSD, and premenstrual dysphoric disorder (PDD).

Currently, fluoxetine has the most evidence showing that benefits outweigh the risk for children and adolescents aged 8–18 years. Other SSRIs should be selected over SNRIs when pharmacogenomic testing supports that option. All antidepressants list suicidal ideation as a treatment-emergent adverse event. Studies report approximately 2 people of every 100 treated with an SSRI will have a "suicide-related" event compared to 1 person of every 100 treated with placebo. Suicidal-related events include short-term suicidal ideation, persistent suicidal ideation self-harm without suicide intent, and self-harm with suicide intent. One and two percent are very low numbers that suggest an underdetection of suicidal ideation in clinical trials as the prevalence of suicidal ideation is much higher in patients with depression. It may also suggest that patients with improvement are more likely to share these feelings than more severely depressed and withdrawn patients.

The main warnings and precautions for SSRIs include clinical worsening and suicidal ideation, serotonin syndrome, elevation of blood pressure, abnormal bleeding, angle closure glaucoma, and activation of hypomania or mania in patients with latent bipolar disorder.

Fluoxetine (Prozac) is approved for MDD and OCD in children with a start dose of 10 mg/day and may be increased to 20 mg daily after a week. Doses were increased up to 60 mg daily in adolescents with OCD. The maximum recommended dose for adults is 80 mg/day. The medication is indicated for adults with bulimia, PD, and depressive episodes associated with bipolar disease. Its half-life is 8.6 days; the metabolite half-life is longer.

Sertraline (Zoloft) is approved for the treatment of OCD in pediatrics. Doses used in pediatric patients 6–17 years were 50–200 mg daily. Sertraline is also indicated for adults with MDD, OCD, PTSD, SAD, and PDD. The initial dose recommended for adults is 25–50 mg daily and the maximum dose is 200 mg daily. The half-life is 26 hours.

Fluvoxamine (Luvox) is approved for the treatment of OCD in patients older than 8 years. The recommended starting dose is 25 mg nightly and can be titrated up to 200 mg if needed and tolerated. Adolescents could be adjusted up to 300 mg daily as adults. Doses higher than 50 mg are divided bid and titration can be up to 25 mg weekly. The half-life is 15 hours.

Citalopram (Celexa) is indicated for the treatment of MDD in adults with doses between 20 and 40 mg daily. The half-life is 35 hours.

Escitalopram (Lexapro) is indicated for the treatment of adults with MDD and GAD. The recommended dose is between 10 and 20 mg daily. The half-life is 27–32 hours.

Paroxetine (Paxil) is indicated for the treatment of adults with MDD, OCD, PD, SAD, GAD, and PTSD. The recommended doses are between 20 and 60 mg daily. The half-life is 21 hours.

Selective Serotonin and Norepinephrine Reuptake Inhibitors

SSNRIs are usually a second choice for patients that fail SSRIs and have pharmacogenomic profiles that show likely unresponsiveness to SSRI and better potential for SNRI.

Venlafaxine (Effexor) is indicated for the treatment of MDD, GAD, SAD, and PD. The starting dose is 37.5–75 mg daily, and the maximum dose is 225 mg daily. The half-life is 5.5 hours for immediate release and 11.5 hours for extended-release formulations.

Desvenlafaxine (Pristiq) is indicated for the treatment of MDD. The starting dose is 50 mg daily, and the maximum dose is 100 mg daily. The half-life is 11 hours.

Stimulant Medications

This class of medications is very effective at controlling ADHD symptoms; however, they have some obstacles when compared with the nonstimulant group. They are controlled substances and come with limitations regarding the amount to be dispensed (no more than 1 month) and require frequent visits to evaluate and document safety and the need for refills. They are also associated with the development of tolerance when used daily. In our practice we prefer to skip 1 or 2 days a week (usually weekends), to maintain the responsiveness when attending school. The main class warnings include serious cardiovascular reactions (avoid use in patients with cardiac abnormalities, cardiomyopathy,

coronary disease, and arrhythmias), increase in heart rate or blood pressure, potential psychosis or mania, priapism, Raynaud phenomena, and suppression of growth.

Methylphenidate (Generic, Ritalin, Aptensio XR, Azstarys, Concerta, Cotempla XR-ODT, Daytrana, Focalin, Jornay PM, Metadate, Methylin, Ritalin LA, Ritalin SR, and Quillivant XR) presumably activates the brainstem arousal system and cortex to produce a stimulant effect. Methylphenidate actions include dopamine and norepinephrine transporter inhibition, agonist activity at the serotonin type 1A receptor, and redistribution of the vesicular monoamine transporter 2. This translates into increased prefrontal efficiency with better attentional and executive functions. The starting dose is 5 mg bid with increments of 5–10 mg weekly up to 60 mg daily. Azstarys comprises serdexmethylphenidate (SDX), a prodrug of D-methylphenidate (D-MPH), coformulated with immediate-release D-MPH. Jornay PM capsules are filled with microbeads, each with a delayed release and extended-release layer. This prevents the medication from becoming active for the first 10–12 hours—meaning that, when taken in the evening before bedtime, the effects are felt when a child wakes up. The medication is then released into the body in steady amounts throughout the day. Potentially this may control the symptoms from awakening instead of waiting for absorption and onset of action after a morning dose.

D-**Amphetamines+ amphetamine** (Adderall, Adderall XR, Mydayis). The molecule peaks 3 hours postdose and has a half-life of 9.7–11 hours and 11.5–13.8 hours for the isomer. Amphetamine actions include the inhibition of dopamine and norepinephrine transporter, vesicular monoamine transporter 2, and monoamine oxidase activity. This translates into increased prefrontal efficiency with better attentional and executive functions. The recommended starting dose is 2.5 or 5 mg daily. It is rare for patients to require more than 40 mg/day. Increase the dose at 5 mg increments weekly if needed and tolerated.

Lisdexamfetamine (Vyvanse) is indicated for the treatment of ADHD and for adults with severe binge-eating disorder. The initial dose is 30 mg daily and can be titrating upward at increments of 10–20 mg weekly if needed. The maximum dose is 70 mg/day. The levels peak between 1 and 4 hours and the half-life is about 12 hours.

Nonstimulant Medications

Atomoxetine (Strattera) is a norepinephrine reuptake inhibitor that works by binding to the norepinephrine transporter, resulting in an increase in synaptic noradrenaline and dopamine in the prefrontal cortex. The medication is available in 10, 18, 25, 40, 60, 80, and 100 mg capsules. The maximum dose is 1.4 mg/kg or 100 mg daily. The most common side effects are nausea, vomiting, fatigue, decreased appetite, abdominal pain, and somnolence.

Clonidine and guanfacine are alpha-2 adrenaline receptor agonists. In the brainstem this reduces peripheral blood resistance and explains its use in hypertension. As with stimulants and atomoxetine, these drugs result in a higher noradrenergic effect in the prefrontal cortex with better attention and executive functions. Clonidine is about ten times more potent than guanfacine. The recommended starting dose is 0.1 mg of clonidine or 1 mg of guanfacine nightly with a maximum dose of 0.4 mg for clonidine and 4 mg for guanfacine. The most common limiting side effect is sedation. We often use a sedating dose for those children with comorbid insomnia, with the idea that the long half-life may provide nonsedating but still therapeutic levels during the daytime.

Viloxazine (Qelbree) is a norepinephrine reuptake inhibitor and as with the other medications mentioned earlier, it results in a higher noradrenergic effect in the prefrontal cortex with improved attention and executive functions. It also affects the serotonin system, which may partly explain why studies have shown an improvement in peer relations and social activities with this medication. It is indicated for the treatment of ADHD in children 6 years and older. The starting dose is 100 mg daily, which may be increased by 100 mg weekly up to 400 mg/day. The most common side effects are somnolence, decreased appetite, fatigue, nausea, emesis, insomnia, and irritability, similar to the other medications used in the treatment of ADHD.

REFERENCES

1. Merikangas KR, et al. Epidemiology of mental disorders in children and adolescents. *Dialogues in Clinical Neuroscience.* 2009;11:7-20.
2. Cwik MF, O'Keefe VM, Haroz EE. Suicide in the pediatric population: screening, risk assessment and treatment. *International Review of Psychiatry.* 2020;32(3):254-264.
   https://doi.org/10.1080/09540261.2019.1693351. Epub 2020 Jan 10. PMID: 31922455; PMCID: PMC7190447.
3. Bernaras E, et al. Child and adolescent depression: a review of theories, evaluation instruments, prevention programs, and treatments. *Frontiers in Psychology.* 2019;10:543. https://doi.org/10.3389/fpsyg.2019.00543.
4. Wehry, et al. Assessment and treatment of anxiety disorders in children and adolescents. *Current Psychiatry Reports.* 2015;17:52. https://doi.org/10.1007/s11920-015-0591-z.
5. Foley DL, Goldston DB, Costello EJ, Angold A. Proximal psychiatric risk factors for suicidality in youth: the Great Smoky Mountains study. *Archives of General Psychiatry.* 2006;63:1017-1024.
6. Jacobson CM, Muehlenkamp JJ, Miller AL, Turner JB. Psychiatric impairment among adolescents engaging in different types of deliberate self-harm. *Journal of Clinical Child & Adolescent Psychology.* 2008;37(2):363-375.
7. Beesdo-Baum K, Pine DS, Lieb R, Wittchen J. Mental disorders in adolescence and young adulthood: homotypic and heterotypic longitudinal associations. In: *American College of Neuropsychopharmacology 51st Annual Meeting*, Hollywood, Florida; 2012.
8. Pine DS, Cohen P, Gurley D, Brook J, Ma Y. The risk for early adulthood anxiety and depressive disorders in adolescents with anxiety and depressive disorders. *Archives of General Psychiatry.* 1998;55(1):56-64.
9. PHQ9 and GAD-7 Copyright © Pfizer Inc. PRIME-MD® is a trademark of Pfizer Inc.
10. Ghosh A, et al. Oppositional defiant disorder: current insight. *Psychology Research and Behavior Management.* 2017;10:353-367.
11. Kutluay E, Selwa L, Minecan D, Edwards J, Beydoun A. Nonepileptic paroxysmal events in a pediatric population. *Epilepsy & Behavior.* 2010;17:272-275.
12. James AC, Reardon T, Soler A, James G, Creswell C. Cognitive behavioural therapy for anxiety disorders in children and adolescents. *Cochrane Database of Systematic Reviews.* 2020;11(11):CD013162. https://doi.org/10.1002/14651858.CD013162.pub2. PMID: 33196111; PMCID: PMC8092480.
13. Krebs G, et al. Obsessive-compulsive disorder in children and adolescents. *Archives of Disease in Childhood.* 2015;100:495-499. https://doi.org/10.1136/archdischild-2014-306934.
14. American Psychiatric Association. *Diagnostic and Statistical Manual of Mental Disorders.* 5th ed. American Psychiatric Association; 2013.
15. Drechsler R, Brem S, Brandeis D, Grünblatt E, Berger G, Walitza S. ADHD: current concepts and treatments in children and adolescents. *Neuropediatrics.* 2020;51(5):315–335. https://doi.org/10.1055/s-

0040-1701658. Epub 2020 Jun 19. PMID: 32559806; PMCID: PMC7508636.

16. Masi A, et al. An overview of autism spectrum disorder, heterogeneity and treatment options. *Neuroscience Bulletin*. 2017;33(2):183-193. https://doi.org/10.1007/s12264-017-0100-y.

17. Tick B, Bolton P, Happé F, Rutter M, Rijsdijk F. Heritability of autism spectrum disorders: a meta-analysis of twin studies. *Journal of Child Psychology and Psychiatry and Allied Disciplines*. 2016;57(5):585-595. https://doi.org/10.1111/jcpp.12499.

18. Bai D, Yip BHK, Windham GC, et al. Association of genetic and environmental factors with autism in a 5-country cohort. *JAMA Psychiatry*. 2019;76(10).

19. Lee PH, Anttila V, Won H, et al. Genomic relationships, novel loci, and pleiotropic mechanisms across eight psychiatric disorders. *Cell*. 2019;179(7):1469-1482.e11. https://doi.org/10.1016/j.cell.2019.11.020.

20. Ghanizadeh A. Conduct behaviors and oppositional defiant behaviors in children and adolescents with ADHD. *Postgraduate Medicine*. 2015;127(3):289-294. https://doi.org/10.1080/00325481.2015.996434.

21. Bakker MJ, et al. Practitioner review: psychological treatments for children and adolescents with conduct disorder problems – a systematic review and meta-analysis. *Journal of Child Psychology and Psychiatry*. 2017;58(1):4-18.

22. Frick PJ, Kemp EC. Conduct disorders and empathy development. *Annual Review of Clinical Psychology*. 2021;17:391-416. https://doi.org/10.1146/annurev-clinpsy-081219-105809. Epub 2020 Dec 8. PMID: 33290109.

23. Cameron M, Guterman NB. Diagnosing conduct problems of children and adolescents in residential treatment. *Child & Youth Care Forum*. 2007;36:1-10. https://doi.org/10.1007/s10566-006-9027-6.

24. Kim SH, Kim H, Lim BC, et al. Paroxysmal nonepileptic events in pediatric patients confirmed by long-term video-EEG monitoring—single tertiary center review of 143 patients. *Epilepsy & Behavior*. 2012;24:336-340.

25. Jane Garland E. Update on the use of SSRIs and SNRIs with children and adolescents in clinical practice. *Journal of the Canadian Academy of Child and Adolescent*. 2016;25:4-10.

26. Albert DV. Psychogenic nonepileptic seizures in children and adolescents. *Seminars in Pediatric Neurology*. 2022;41:100949. https://doi.org/10.1016/j.spen.2021.100949. Epub 2021 Dec 16. PMID: 35450667.

27. Perez DL, Nicholson TR, Asadi-Pooya AA, et al. Neuroimaging in functional neurological disorder: state of the field and research agenda. *Neuroimage: Clinical*. 2021;30:102623. https://doi.org/10.1016/j.nicl.2021.102623. Epub 2021 Mar 11. PMID: 34215138; PMCID: PMC8111317.

28. Fredwall M, Terry D, Enciso L, Burch MM, Trott K, Albert DVF. Outcomes of children and adolescents 1 year after being seen in a multidisciplinary psychogenic nonepileptic seizures clinic. *Epilepsia*. 2021;62(10): 2528-2538. https://doi.org/10.1111/epi.17031. Epub 2021 Aug 2. PMID: 34339046.

29. Kola S, LaFaver K. Updates in functional movement disorders: from pathophysiology to treatment advances. *Current Neurology and Neuroscience Reports*. 2022;22(5):305-311. https://doi.org/10.1007/s11910-022-01192-9. Epub 2022 Apr 19. PMID: 35441333; PMCID: PMC9017419.

Note: Page numbers followed by *f* indicate figures, *t* indicate tables, and *b* indicate boxes.

A

Abducens nerve palsy/VI cranial nerve, 350

Abetalipoproteinemia, 275

Abnormal head shape, 420–422, 420*t*
  craniosynostosis causing, 420–422, 421*t*
  extracranial forces causing, 420
  intracranial forces causing, 420

Abscess, brain, in bacterial meningitis, 134–135

Absence epilepsy, 30–31, 34*f*, 43

Acanthocytosis, 275

Accommodative esotropia, 349

Acetazolamide
  ataxia responsive to, 260–261
  idiopathic intracranial hypertension, 139

Acetylcholine receptor (AChR), 198

Acetyl-coenzyme-A (acetyl-CoA), 240–241

Achondroplasia, 412–413

Acid maltase deficiency (Pompe disease), 204–205
  hypotonia, 184–185

Acidemia
  isovaleric, 12
  methylmalonic, 12–13
  propionic, 13–14

Acinetobacter baumanii, 130

Acoustic neuroma, 397, 397*f*

Acquired epileptiform aphasia, 37

Acquired epileptiform opercular syndrome, 37

Acquired hearing impairment, 396–397

Acquired immune-mediated myasthenia, 212

Acquired immunodeficiency syndrome (AIDS), 217
  encephalopathy, 152–153
  inflammatory myopathies, 217–219

Acquired nystagmus, 363–365

Acquired ophthalmoplegia, causes of, 352*b*

ACTH. *See* Adrenocorticotropic hormone

Action tremor, 344

Acute ataxic neuropathy, 264

Acute bilateral ophthalmoplegia, 357–358
  botulism, 358
  causes of, 357*b*
  intoxications, 358

Acute cerebellar ataxia, 264

Acute confusional migraine, 86

Acute disseminated encephalomyelitis (ADEM), 76–80, 77*f*
  ataxia, 265
  mimicking childhood ataxia with CNS hypomyelination/ vanishing white matter, 267
  transverse myelitis and, 309

Acute flaccid myelitis, 229

Acute generalized weakness, 227–231, 227*b*

Acute idiopathic brachial neuritis, 250

Acute idiopathic plexitis, 318–319

Acute infectious myositis, 217

Acute inflammatory demyelinating polyradiculoneuropathy (AIDP), 220, 249

Acute intermittent porphyria, 254–255

Acute motor axonal neuropathy (AMAN), 228

Acute reactions, in dystonia, 333–334

Acute stroke, 285

Acute symptomatic plexitis, 319–322
  asthmatic amyotrophy (Hopkins syndrome), 319
  neonatal traumatic brachial neuropathy, 320–321
  osteomyelitis-neuritis, 321
  postnatal injuries, 321–322

Acute unilateral ophthalmoplegia, 352–355
  causes of, 353*b*

Acute uremic encephalopathy, 84

Acyclovir, 72

ADCY5 dyskinesia, 27, 344

Addison disease, 239

ADEM. *See* Acute disseminated encephalomyelitis

Adenosine diphosphate (ADP), 240

Adenosine monophosphate (AMP) deaminase deficiency, 244

Adenosine triphosphatase (ATPase), 194, 286

Adenosine triphosphate (ATP), 240

ADHD. *See* Attention deficit hyperactivity disorder

Adie (tonic pupil) syndrome, 380

ADP. *See* Adenosine diphosphate

Adrenal disorders, 82

Adrenocorticotropic hormone (ACTH), 24–25

Adrenoleukodystrophy, 308
  X-linked, 278

Adrenomyeloneuropathy (AMN), 306, 308

Adverse reactions, antiepileptics
  brivaracetam, 45–46
  cannabidiol, 46
  carbamazepine, 46
  cenobamate, 46–47
  clobazam, 47
  clonazepam, 47
  ethosuximide, 47
  felbamate, 47
  felnfluramine, 47–48
  gabapentin, 48
  lacosamide, 48
  lamotrigine, 48
  levetiracetam, 48–49
  oxcarbazepine, 49
  perampanel, 49

Adverse reactions, antiepileptics
        (Continued)
    phenobarbital, 49
    phenytoin, 17
    pregabalin, 50
    primidone, 50
    rufinamide, 50
    stiripentol, 50
    tiagabine, 50
    topiramate, 50–51
    valproate, 51
    vigabatrin, 51
    zonisamide, 51
Adversive seizures, 361
Agenesis of corpus callosum, 417–418
Agitation, causes, 62b
Agyria, 418
Aicardi syndrome, 23, 145
AIDP. See Acute inflammatory
        demyelinating
        polyradiculoneuropathy
AIDS. See Acquired immunodeficiency
        syndrome
Akathisia, 328–329
Albers-Schönberg disease, 388
Albuterol, 213
Alcohol intake, maternal, 4–5
Alexander disease, 162
Alexithymia, 431
Alpers Huttenlocher syndrome, 163
Alpha-thalassemia X-linked disability
        syndrome, 150
Alprazolam (xanax), 430
Altered mental status, 64
Alternating esotropia, 348–349
AMAN. See Acute motor axonal
        Neuropathy
American Academy of Pediatrics, 141
Amino acid metabolism disorders,
        153–156
    homocystinuria, 153–154, 154f
    maple syrup urine disease, 154–155
    phenylketonuria, 155–156, 155f
Aminoacidopathies, 10–16
Aminoaciduria, for Hartnup disease, 262
Aminoglycosides, vertigo and, 399
Amitriptyline, migraine, 101
AMN. See Adrenomyeloneuropathy

Amphetamine abuse, 89
Amplitude EEG (aEEG), 2–3
Analgesic rebound headache, 105
Anaplastic astrocytoma, 122
Andersen-Tawil syndrome, 232–233
Anencephaly, 416
Aneurysms, 108
    in ophthalmoplegia, 353
Angelman syndrome, 149
Aniridia, 379
Anisocoria, benign essential, 379
Anoxia, acute, 67
Anterior fontanelle, palpation of, 115
Antibiotic therapy
    aseptic meningitis, 76
    cat-scratch disease, 68–69
    for cervical infections, 285
    gram-negative sepsis, 69
    Lyme disease, 70–71
    toxic shock syndrome, 71
    vertigo and, 400
Antibodies
    antithyroid, 77–78
    Lyme disease, 70
Anticoagulants, 15
Anticonvulsants
    anoxia and ischemia, 67–68
    autosomal dominant nocturnal
        frontal lobe epilepsy, 38
    benign childhood epilepsy with
        centrotemporal spikes, 40
    neonatal seizures, 16
    principles of therapy, 43
    subarachnoid hemorrhage, primary,
        16
Antiemetics, 331
Antiepileptic drugs, 17, 43–51
    administration
        brivaracetam, 45–46
        cannabidiol, 46
        carbamazepine (Tegretol/
            Tegreton-XR), 46
        cenobamate (Xcopri, SK Life
            Sciences), 46–47
        clobazam, 47
        clonazepam, 47
        ethosuximide, 47
        felbamate, 47

Antiepileptic drugs (Continued)
    felnfluramine, 47–48
    gabapentin, 48
    lacosamide, 48
    lamotrigine, 48
    levetiracetam, 48–49
    oxcarbazepine, 49
    perampanel, 49
    phenobarbital, 49
    phenytoin, 49–50
    pregabalin, 50
    primidone, 50
    rufinamide, 50
    stiripentol, 50
    tiagabine, 50
    topiramate, 50–51
    valproate, 51
    vigabatrin, 51
    zonisamide, 51
    adverse reactions, 45
    blood concentrations, 43–45
    for children, 44t
    discontinuing therapy, 43
    half-lives, 44–45
    idiosyncratic reactions, 45
    indications for starting, 43
    principles of therapy, 43–45
    selection, 45–51
Antihistamines, 49–50
Anti-N-methyl-D-aspartate receptor
        antibody encephalopathy,
        78–79
Antinuclear antibodies (ANAs),
        in systemic lupus
        erythematosus, 294
Antipsychotics, 87
Anxiety, autism/autistic spectrum
        disorders, 142
Anxiety disorders
    clinical features, 425
    diagnosis, 425
    management, 425–426
    VLPFC functions, 425
Apelisib, 412
Aplasia
    depressor anguli oris, 385
    of facial muscles, 384–385
    of inner ear, 394–395

Apnea
  in children under two, 18–19
  in newborn, 4
Apneic seizures, 18
Apneustic breathing, 65
Applied behavioral analysis (ABA),
    429–430
Apraxia
  of horizontal gaze, 359
  oculomotor apraxia type 2, with
    ataxia, 276
Aqueductal stenosis, congenital, 407–
    408, 408f
Arachnoid cysts, congenital
    malformations and, 301
Arbovirus-associated encephalitis,
    73–75
Arginase deficiency, 308
Aripiprazole (abilify), 430
Armodafinil, 28
Arrhythmias, 29
Arterial aneurysms, 128–129
Arterial oxygen pressure (P_2O_2), 66
Arteriosclerosis, 291
Arteriovenous malformations,
    129–130
  of childhood stroke, 285
  congenital malformations and, 301
Artery of Adamkiewicz, 308–309
Arthrogryposis, 184
  congenital myasthenic syndromes,
    198–199
  differential diagnosis of, 185b
  neurogenic, 196
ASD. See Autistic spectrum disorder
Aseptic meningitis, 75–76
  clinical features, 75
  description, 75
  diagnosis, 75–76
  versus encephalitis, 70
  management, 76
Aspartoacylase deficiency (Canavan
    disease), 169–170
Aspirin, for moyamoya disease, 292
Asthmatic amyotrophy (Hopkins
    syndrome), 319
Astrocytoma, 122–124, 123f
  cerebellar, 269–270

Astrocytoma (Continued)
  of cervical cord, 312f
  as spinal cord tumors, 312–313
Asymmetric crying facies, 385
Ataxia
  abetalipoproteinemia, 275
  acetazolamide-responsive, 260–261
  acute cerebellar, 264
  acute/recurrent, 258–269, 259b
  autosomal dominant inheritance,
    274–275
  autosomal recessive inheritance, 275
  brain tumor, 259, 269–272
  cerebellar, 331
  childhood, with CNS
    hypomyelination/ vanishing
    white matter, 267
  chronic/progressive, 259b, 269–278
  congenital malformations, 272–273
  conversion reaction, 259–260
  defined, 258
  dominant recurrent, 260–261
  drug ingestion, 261
  encephalitis, 261–262
  episodic type 1 (paroxysmal ataxia
    and myokymia), 260
  episodic type 2 (acetazolamide
    responsive ataxia), 260–261
  Friedreich ataxia, 276–277
  Hartnup disease, 262, 278
  hypobetalipoproteinemia, 275
  inborn errors of metabolism,
    262–263
  juvenile sulfatide lipidosis, 277
  maple syrup urine disease, 262, 278
  Marinesco-Sjögren syndrome, 277
  migraine, 263–264
  Miller Fisher syndrome, 264–265
  in motor development, delayed, 143
  multiple sclerosis, 265–266
  myoclonic encephalopathy/
    neuroblastoma syndrome,
    266–267, 266f
  with oculomotor apraxia type 1, 276
  with oculomotor apraxia type 2, 276
  other episodic, 261
  postinfectious/immune-mediated
    disorders, 264–267

Ataxia (Continued)
  progressive
    hereditary, 274–275
    metabolic screening in, 278t
  pseudoataxia, 267
  pyruvate dehydrogenase deficiency,
    262–263
  spinocerebellar degenerations,
    274–275
  trauma, 267
  vascular disorders, 268
  viral infections, 264
  X-linked inheritance, 278
Ataxia telangiectasia (AT), 275, 331
Ataxic breathing, 65
Athetosis, in chorea, 329
Atomoxetine (strattera), 435
ATP. See Adenosine triphosphate
ATP7A-related copper transport
    disorders, 173
Attention deficit disorder (ADD/
    ADHD)
  clinical features, 427–428
  diagnosis, 428
  inattentiveness symptoms, 428
  management, 428
  overview, 427
Attention deficit hyperactivity disorder
    (ADHD), in tics and Tourette
    syndrome, 326
Atypical/teratoid/rhabdoid tumors,
    124
Audiometry, pure-tone, 392
Auditory dysfunction, symptoms of,
    391–392
Auditory hallucinations, 64
Aura, 32
  migraine with, 99
  migraine without, 99
Autism. See Autistic spectrum disorder
Autism Diagnostic Observation
    Schedule (ADOS), 429
Autism spectrum disorder (ASD), 142
  clinical features, 429
  diagnosis, 429
  management, 429–430
  multiple etiologies, 428–429
Autoimmune encephalopathies, 76

Automatisms, complex partial seizures, 32

Autoregulation, cerebral blood flow of, 114

Autosomal dominant ataxia, 274–275

Autosomal dominant cerebellar ataxias, 274t

Autosomal dominant dystonias, 336

Autosomal dominant intellectual disability syndromes, 150–151
Coffin-Siris syndrome, 151
GRIN2B-related neurodevelopmental disorder, 150–151
SLC6A1-related neurodevelopmental disabilities, 151
SYNGAP1-related intellectual disability, 150

Autosomal dominant osteopetrosis type II (Albers-Schönberg disease), 388

Autosomal dominant sleep-related hypermotor epilepsy, 37–38

Autosomal recessive chorea-acanthocytosis, 332

Autosomal recessive distal myopathy, 225–227
dysferlinopathies, 225–226
emery-dreifuss muscular dystrophy, 226–227
myotonic dystrophy, 226
nebulin myopathy, 226

Autosomal recessive distal (dysferlin) myopathy, 225–227

Autosomal recessive inheritance, 275

Autosomal recessive intellectual disabilities, 151–152

B

Bacterial infections
altered states of consciousness, 68–76
arbovirus-Associated Encephalitis, 73–75
aseptic meningitis, 75–76
cat-scratch disease, 68–69
COVID-19 encephalitis, 75
enterovirus encephalitis, 73
gram-negative sepsis, 69
herpes simplex virus encephalitis, 72

Bacterial infections (Continued)
human parechovirus encephalitis, 72–73
meningitis. See Bacterial meningitis
rabies encephalitis, 73
Rickettsial, 70–71
toxic shock syndrome, 71
vaccine-preventable encephalitis, 75
viral encephalitis, 71–72

Bacterial meningitis, 130–135
acquired hearing impairment from, 396
brain abscess, 134–135
in infants and young children, 131–133
meningococcus, 133
in newborns, 130–131
pneumococcus, 133
in school-age children, 133
subdural and epidural empyema, 135
tuberculous meningitis, 133–134

Ballismus, in chorea, 329
Band heterotopia, 418
Barbiturate coma, 67–68, 120
Bardet-Biedl syndrome, 378
Bartonella (Rochalimaea) henselae, 68–69
Basilar impression, 272–273
Basilar meningitis, 389
Basilar skull fracture, 92
Bassen-Kornzweig syndrome, 275
Batten disease, 166–167, 175–176
BCAA. See Branched-chain amino acids
Becker disease, 238
Becker muscular dystrophy, 214–216
Becker muscular dystrophy (BMD), 213
BECTS. See Benign childhood epilepsy with centrotemporal spikes

Behavioral neurology
anxiety disorders, 425–426
clinical features, 425
diagnosis, 425
management, 425–426
VLPFC functions, 425
autism spectrum disorder (ASD), 428–430
clinical features, 429
diagnosis, 429

Behavioral neurology (Continued)
management, 429–430
multiple etiologies, 428–429
depression and suicidality, 423–425
clinical features, 424
diagnosis, 424
management, 424–425
nonstimulant medications, 435
atomoxetine (strattera), 435
clonidine and guanfacine, 435
viloxazine (qelbree), 435
obsessive-compulsive disorder (OCD), 426–431
clinical features, 426–427
diagnosis, 427
management, 427
obsessions and compulsions, 427
prevalence of, 426
treatment, 431–433
psychogenic (functional) movement disorders, 433
biopsychosocial model, 433
clinical features, 433
diagnosis, 433
management, 433
pseudosleep, 433
pyschogenic nonepileptic spells (PNES), 431–433
clinical features, 431–432
diagnosis, 432
overview, 431
treatment, 432–433
selective serotonin and norepinephrine reuptake inhibitors (SSNRIs), 434
selective serotonin reuptake inhibitors (SSRIs), 433–434
citalopram (celexa), 434
escitalopram (lexapro), 434
fluoxetine (prozac), 433
fluvoxamine (luvox), 434
paroxetine (paxil), 434
sertraline (zoloft), 433
stimulant medications, 434
D-Amphetamines+ amphetamine, 434
lisdexamfetamine (vyvanse), 434
methylphenidate, 434

Bell palsy, 386–387

Benign childhood epilepsy with centrotemporal spikes (BECTS), 36

Benign enlargement of subarachnoid space, 404–406, 406f

Benign essential anisocoria, 379

Benign exertional headache, 104

Benign familial neonatal seizures, 7

Benign infantile myoclonus, 4

Benign myoclonic epilepsy, 25

Benign nocturnal myoclonus, newborns, 4

Benign occipital epilepsy, of childhood, 26

Benign paroxysmal torticollis, 335

Benign paroxysmal vertigo, 26, 263–264

Benign spasms of infancy, 25

Benzodiazepines, 53, 65

Bethlem myopathy, 213–214

Bickerstaff encephalitis, 76

Bielschowsky test, 350

Bilateral ophthalmoplegia
    acute, 357–358, 357b
    chronic, 358–359, 358b

Bilateral periventricular nodular heterotopia, 418, 418f

Bilateral striatal necrosis (BSN), 338–339

Bilateral (central) transtentorial herniation, 118

Bilirubin encephalopathy, 7–8

Biotinidase deficiency, infants and young children, 25–26

Birth injury, 385–386

Bleeding diathesis, 290–295

Blepharospasm, in dystonia, 334

Blindness
    acute monocular or binocular, 371–372, 371b
    cerebral, 98
    congenital, 368–371
    cortical, 371–372
    hypoglycemia and, 372
    optic neuropathies and, 372–374
        demyelinating, 372–373
        ischemic, 373
        toxic-nutritional, 373–374

Blindness (Continued)
    traumatic, 373–374
    from pituitary apoplexy, 374
    retinal disease and, 374–375

Blink response, 367

Bloch–Sulzberger syndrome, 16. See also Incontinentia pigmenti

Borrelia burgdorferi, 70, 328

Botox, 103

Botulinum toxin, 103

Botulism, 230
    in acute bilateral ophthalmoplegia, 358
    infantile, 198

Brachial monoplegia, chronic progressive, 317

Brachial neuritis, 318

Brachial plexitis, 250, 318–319

Brachial plexus, 321–322

Bradycardia, apnea with, 4

Brain abscess, in bacterial meningitis, 134–135

Brain death, 68, 68b

Brain injury, 190, 300

Brain tumors
    anaplastic, 122
    astrocytoma, 122–124, 123f, 269–270
    ataxia and, 259, 269–272
    atypical/teratoid/rhabdoid tumors, 124
    cerebellar astrocytoma, 269–270
    cerebellar hemangioblastoma, 270
    of cerebrovascular disease, 287
    in children, 121b
    choroid plexus tumors, 121–122
    ependymoma, 124, 270
    germ cell, 125–126
    glial, glianeuronal, and neuronal tumors, 122–124
    medulloblastoma, 271–272
    meningioma, 126
    metastases, 125–126
    pineal region tumors, 125
    primitive neuroectodermal tumors, 124, 269–270
    supratentorial, 120–121

Brainstem auditory evoked response, 393

Brainstem glioma, in ophthalmoplegia, 353–354, 354f

Brainstem stroke, in ophthalmoplegia, 354

Branched-chain amino acids (BCAA), 10–12
    maple syrup urine disease, 11–12

Branched-chain ketoacid (BCKA) dehydrogenase, 11f

Breath-holding spells, 18–19

Breech presentation, in spinal cord injury, 192

Brief, small-amplitude, polyphasic potentials, 193

Brivaracetam (antiepileptic)
    administration, 45
    adverse effects, 45
    indications for, 45

Brody myopathy, 245

Brown syndrome, 350

Brown-Vialetto-Van Laere syndrome, 388

BSN. See Bilateral striatal necrosis

Burn encephalopathy, 85–86

C

Caffeine headache, 105

Caffeine ingestion, 327

Calcineurin inhibitor encephalopathy, 87–88

Calcinosis universalis, 218

Calcitonin gene-related peptide (CGRP), 100, 102

Calcitonin gene-related peptide receptor antagonists, 102

Calcium channel blockers, 103

Caloric testing, for vertigo, 399

Candidal meningoencephalitis, 136

Cannabidiol (Epidiolex, Greenwich)
    administration, 46
    adverse effects, 46
    indications for, 46

Capillary necrosis, 218

Carbamazepine (Tegretol/Tegreton-XR), 342
    administration, 46
    adverse effects, 46
    indications for, 46

Carbamazepine (Tegretol/Tegreton-XR) *(Continued)*
    oxcarbazepine replacing, 46
Carbohydrate utilization defects, 241–242
Carbohydrate-deficient glycoprotein syndromes, 161
Cardiac arrest, 67
Cardiac disorders
    arrhythmia, 29
    physical examination, 64–65
Cardiopulmonary bypass surgery, in chorea, 330
Carnitine
    consciousness, altered states, 83
    deficiency, 82–83, 83*b*, 219–220
    paroxysmal disorders, 12
Carnitine palmitoyl transferase (CPT) 2 deficiency, 242
Carotid and vertebral artery disorders, 285–286
    trauma to carotid artery, 285–286
    trauma to vertebral artery, 286
Carotid-cavernous sinus fistula, in ophthalmoplegia, 354
Carpopedal spasm, 425
Cataract, congenital, 368–369, 369*b*
CATCH acronym, hypocalcemia, 8
Cat-scratch disease, 68–69
Cauda equina tumors, 313
Caudal regression syndrome, congenital malformations and, 302
Caveolinopathies, 247
Cavernous sinus thrombosis, in ophthalmoplegia, 354
CCAD. *See* Cervicocephalic arterial dissection
CDKL5 deficiency disorder, 168–169
Ceftriaxone, 70
Cenobamate (Xcopri, SK Life Sciences), 46–47
Centers for Disease Control and Prevention, 230, 307–308
Central congenital insensitivity to pain, 252–255
Central core disease, 200, 200*f*
Central hearing impairment, 391–392

Central nervous system (CNS)
    hypomyelination, childhood ataxia with, 267
    isolated angiitis, 293–294
    systemic lupus erythematosus and, 294
Central retinal artery occlusion, 374–375
Centronuclear myopathies, 201–202
Cephalic presentation, in spinal cord injury, 192–193
Cerebellar astrocytoma, 269–270
Cerebellar ataxia, 331
Cerebellar hemangioblastoma (Von Hippel- Lindau disease), 270
Cerebellar hemorrhage, 268
Cerebellar herniation, 118
Cerebellar malformations, 272–273
    congenital hemisphere hypoplasia, 272–273
    vermal aplasia, 272–273
    X-linked cerebellar hypoplasia, 273
Cerebellum, aplasia of, 272*f*
Cerebral blindness, transitory, 98
Cerebral blood flow, in increased intracranial pressure, 114
Cerebral cysticercosis, 37
Cerebral dysgenesis, 189–190
Cerebral edema, 80
    diabetic ketoacidosis, 80
    hypernatremia, 81
    increased intracranial pressure in, 115
Cerebral hypotonia, 183, 188–192
    benign congenital hypotonia, 188
    chromosomal disorders, 188–189
    clues to the diagnosis of, 187, 187*b*
    genetic disorders, 190–192
    and motor unit hypotonia, 186*b*
Cerebral infarction
    evaluation of, 290*t*
    focal clonic seizures, 3
    inherited states promoting, 284*b*
Cerebral malformations, 145
Cerebral palsy (CP)
    disorders mistaken as, 314*t*
    hemiplegic, 281–283
    in motor development, delayed, 143
    quadriplegia and, 313–315

Cerebral paraplegia, 313–315
Cerebral perfusion, 114
Cerebral quadriplegia, 313–315
Cerebral venous sinus thrombosis (CVST), 288
Cerebrospinal fluid (CSF)
    aseptic meningitis, 75
    in bacterial meningitis, 130–135
    in cerebral edema, 115
    in choroid plexus tumors, 121–122
    in coccidioidomycosis, 136–137
    in cryptococcal meningitis, 137
    in herpes zoster myelitis, 307
    in hydrocephalus, 120–126
    increased intracranial pressure in, 114
    lymphocytosis in, 69
    in primary arachnoid cysts, 126
    in tuberculous meningitis, 133
    in tuberculous osteomyelitis, 307
Cerebrotendinous xanthomatosis, 178–179
Cerebrovascular accidents (CVAs), in systemic lupus erythematosus, 294
Cerebrovascular disease, 290. *See also* Strokes
    brain tumors, 287
    carotid and vertebral artery disorders, 285–286
Cervical cord, astrocytoma of, 312*f*
Cervical roots, pain from, 96
Cervicocephalic arterial dissection (CCAD), 286
CFEOM. *See* Congenital fibrosis of extraocular muscles
Cheyne-Stokes respiration, 65
Chiari malformations, congenital, 273, 274*f*, 302–303
Childhood
    alternating hemiplegia, 286–287
    benign paroxysmal vertigo, 263–264
    early-onset childhood occipital epilepsy, 38–39
    late-onset/idiopathic childhood occipital epilepsy, 38–39
    myocerebrohepatopathy spectrum, 163
    stroke, 284–287

Childhood and Adolescent Migraine Prevention (CHAMP) study, 101
Childhood stroke, 284–287
  arteriovenous malformations, 285
Children
  absence epilepsy, 30–31, 34f
  acquired epileptiform aphasia, 37
  acquired epileptiform opercular syndrome, 37
  ADCY5 dyskinesia, 27
  antiepileptic drugs for, 44t
  autosomal dominant sleep-related hypermotor epilepsy, 37–38
  brain tumors in, 121b
  electrical status epilepticus during slow wave sleep, 40
  epilepsy
    absence, 30–31, 34f, 43
    autosomal dominant sleep-related hypermotor epilepsy, 37–38
    electrical status epilepticus during slow wave sleep, 40
    epilepsia partialis continuans, 40
    with generalized tonic-clonic seizures on awakening, 42, 42b
    hemiplegia and, 287–288
    juvenile myoclonic, 33–34, 54f, 89–90
    with occipital paroxysms, 38–39
    reading, 41
    surgical approaches, 55–56
    temporal lobe, 41
  eyelid myoclonia with/without absences, 31–33
  familial paroxysmal nonkinesiogenic dyskinesia, 27
  generalized seizures, 41–43
  hemiconvulsions-hemiplegia syndrome, 40–41
  hyperventilation syndrome, 29
  increased intracranial pressure in, 115–117
  juvenile myoclonic epilepsy, 33–34, 54f
  Lafora disease, 35–36
  Lennox-Gastaut syndrome, 34–35

Children (*Continued*)
  Panayiotopoulos syndrome, 39
  paroxysmal disorders, 26–43
  paroxysmal dyskinesias, 26–27
  paroxysmal exertion-induced dyskinesia, 27
  paroxysmal kinesiogenic dyskinesia, 26–27
  PRICKLE1-related disorders, 36
  progressive myoclonic epilepsy type 1, 36
  progressive myoclonus epilepsies, 35–36, 35b
  pseudoseizures, 42
  reading epilepsy, 41
  seizures
    consciousness, altered states, 67
    generalized, 75
    inborn errors of metabolism, 83–84
Chlorocresol, 390
Cholesteatoma, 396–397, 399–400
Chorea, 328–333
  akathisia in, 328–329
  athetosis in, 329
  ballismus in, 329
  cardiopulmonary bypass surgery in, 330
  choreoacanthocytosis, 332–333
  definition of, 328–329
  differential diagnosis of, as an initial or prominent symptom, 330b
  drug-induced, 330–331
  emergent withdrawal syndrome in, 331
  Fahr disease in, 332
  genetic disorders and, 331–333
  hyperthyroidism in, 333
  idiopathic basal ganglia calcification in, 332
  lupus erythematosus in, 333
  myoclonus and, 340
  NKX2.1-related choreiform disorders, 331–332
  in pregnancy (chorea gravidarum), 333
  primary familial brain calcification in, 332

Chorea (*Continued*)
  Sydenham (rheumatic), 329–330
  systemic disorders in, 333
  tardive dyskinesia in, 331
  VPS13A disease, 332–333
Chorea gravidarum, 333
Choreoacanthocytosis, 332–333
Choreoathetoid cerebral palsy, 329–330
Choroid plexus tumors, 121–122
Chromosomal disorders, microcephaly and, 416
Chromosomal disturbances
  cerebral hypotonia, 188–189
  MECP2 duplication syndrome, 188
  Prader-Willi syndrome, 188–189, 189b
Chromosome 5q13, spinal muscular atrophies, 211
Chromosome 5q33.1, carnitine deficiency, 220
Chromosomes, gene mutations
  chromosome 5p15, Hartnup disease, 262
  chromosome 17, hereditary brachial plexopathy, 319
Chronic bilateral ophthalmoplegia, 358–359
  causes of, 358b
  Kearns-Sayre syndrome, 359
  thyroid ophthalmopathy, 358–359
Chronic inflammatory demyelinating polyradiculoneuropathy, 228–229
Chronic nonprogressive encephalopathy, 189–190
Chronic paroxysmal hemicrania, 104
  versus cluster headache, 103
Chronic posthypoxic myoclonus, 342
Chronic progressive headache, 108
Chronic uremic encephalopathy, 84–85
Citalopram (celexa), 434
Citrobacter diversus, 130
Classic Leigh syndrome, 163
CLCN1 gene, 239
CLCN7-related osteopetrosis, 388
Clonazepam (Klonapin), 20
  administration, 47
  adverse effects, 47

Clonazepam (Klonapin) *(Continued)*
  benign nocturnal myoclonus, 4
  indications for, 47
  infantile spasm, 24, 47
  stiff infant syndrome, 20
Clonidine, 435
Closed head injuries, 91–92
Clostridium botulinum, 198, 358
Cluster headache, 103–104
CMS. *See* Congenital myasthenic
      syndrome
CMUA. *See* Continuous motor unit
      activity
CNTNAP1 gene, 197
Coagulation factor deficiencies,
      hypocoagulable states, 290
COASY protein-associated
      neurodegeneration, 339
Cocaine abuse
  cerebral malformations in, 145
  in intracranial hemorrhage, 130
Coccidioidomycosis, 136–137, 138b
Cochlear lesions, special tests for, 393
Cockayne syndrome, 378–379
Coenzyme Q10, 101
Coffin-Siris syndrome, 151
Collagen type VI-related dystrophy, 203
Coloboma, 370
Coma
  barbiturate, 67–68, 120
  diagnostic approach to, 63b–64b,
      65–66
  hepatic, 83
  high road to, 62–63
  low road to, 63
  migraine, 86
  ocular motility assessment, 66
  pentobarbital, 120
  pupillary reflex, absent in comatose
      patient, 66
Communicating hydrocephalus,
      404–407
  benign enlargement of subarachnoid
      space in, 404–406, 406f
  meningeal malignancy as, 406–407
Complex regional pain syndrome
      (CRPS), 250–251. *See also*
      Reflex sympathetic dystrophy

Comprehensive behavioral intervention
      for tics (CBIT), 327
Compressed vertebral body fractures,
      310–312
Compressive optic neuropathy, 375–377
Computed tomography (CT)
  in arteriovenous malformations, 285
  in atlantoaxial dislocation, 302
  cat-scratch disease, 69
  in Chiari malformations, 303
  concussion, 90
  in congenital heart disease, 288
  consciousness, altered states, 65, 69,
      90
  focal clonic seizures, 3
  gram-negative sepsis, 69
  head injuries, severe, 90
  headache, 95
  in neonatal hemorrhage, 283
  of postconcussion syndrome, 268
  shaking injuries, 90
  single-photon emission, 55
  sinusitis, 109–110
  in spinal paraplegia, 300
  subarachnoid hemorrhage, primary,
      16
  in Takayasu arteritis, 294–295
Concussion, 90
Conduct disorder (CD)
  clinical features, 430
  diagnosis, 430–431
  overview, 430
  treatment, 431
Congenital aqueductal stenosis, 407–
      408, 408f
Congenital bilateral Perisylvian
      syndrome, 384, 384f
Congenital blindness, 368–371
Congenital brain tumors, 410
Congenital cataract, 368–369, 369b
Congenital cervical spinal muscular
      atrophy, 196
Congenital deafness, 393–395
  from aplasia of inner ear, 394–395
  from later-onset genetic disorders,
      395–396
Congenital disorders of glycosylation,
      161

Congenital dysphagia, 384
Congenital dystrophinopathy, 202
Congenital facial asymmetry, 384–386
Congenital fiber-type disproportion
      myopathy, 201
Congenital fibrosis of extraocular
      muscles (CFEOM), 350
Congenital heart disease, 288–289
Congenital hemisphere hypoplasia,
      272–273
Congenital hypomyelinating
      neuropathy, 197–198
Congenital lymphocytic
      choriomeningitis, 147
Congenital malformations
  arachnoid cysts, 301
  arteriovenous malformations, 301
  ataxia and, 272–273
  atlantoaxial dislocation, 301–302
  basilar impression, 272–273
  caudal regression syndrome, 302
  cerebellar, 272–273
  Chiari, 273, 274f, 302–303
  hemiplegic cerebral palsy, 282–283,
      282f
  myelomeningocele, 303–304
  perinatal stroke, 282–283
  of spinal paraplegia, 300–305
  tethered spinal cord, 304–305
Congenital mirror movements, 340
Congenital muscular dystrophy, 202
Congenital myasthenia gravis, 351
Congenital myasthenic syndrome
      (CMS), 198–199, 351
Congenital myopathies, 199–202
  central core disease, 200
  congenital fiber-type disproportion
      myopathy, 201
  multi-minicore disease, 200–201, 246
  myotubular (centronuclear)
      myopathy, 201–202
  nemaline (rod) myopathy, 199–200,
      200f
Congenital myotonic dystrophy, 185–
      186, 204, 204f
Congenital nystagmus, 362–363
Congenital ocular motor apraxia,
      359–360

Congenital ophthalmoplegia, 349–352

Congenital optic nerve hypoplasia, 369–370, 370f

Congenital ptosis, 351–352

Congenital superior oblique palsy, 350

Congenital syphilis, 146

Congenital vertical ocular motor apraxia, 361

Connective tissue disorders, headache associated with, 108–109

Consciousness, altered states, 61–94
  acute disseminated encephalomyelitis, 76–80, 77f
  agitation, causes, 62b
  anoxia, acute, 67
  brain death, 68
  concussion, 90
  delirium, diagnostic approach to, 64–65
  endocrine causes of encephalopathy, 82
  fever illness refractory epileptic syndrome, 78–79
  generalized seizures, 41–43
  head injuries, severe, 90–92
  hepatic encephalopathy, 82–83
  history, 64–65
  hypoxia, prolonged, 66
  inborn errors of metabolism, 83–84
    in newborns, 6b, 83–84
  ischemia, acute, 67
  laboratory investigations, 65
  lethargy and coma, diagnostic approach to, 65–66
  locked-in syndrome, 62
  metabolic and systemic disorders, 80–86
  metabolic encephalopathies, 85–86
  osmolality disorders, 80–82
  persistent vegetative state, 68
  physical examination, 64–65
  postimmunization encephalopathy, 80
  psychological disorders, 86–87
  renal disorders, 84–85
  responsiveness, lack of, 62
  Reye syndrome, 79–80, 120
  syncope, 29

Consciousness, altered states (Continued)
  systemic lupus erythematosus, 78
  trauma, 89–92

Continuous motor unit activity (CMUA), 237–238

Contralateral homonymous hemianopia, 118

Convergence insufficiency, 361

Convergence paralysis, 361

Conversion reaction, of ataxia, 259–260

Corneal clouding, 368, 368b

Cortical blindness, 371–372

Cortical thumb, 187

Corticosteroid psychosis, 87

Corticosteroid-induced quadriplegia, 230

Corticosteroids
  Hashimoto encephalopathy, 77–78
  for herpes zoster myelitis, 307
  infantile spasms, 24
  systemic lupus erythematosus, 78
  for X-linked inheritance, 278

COVID-19 (SARS-CoV-2), 148

COVID-19 encephalitis, 75

CP. See Cerebral palsy

Cramps
  definition of cramp, 236
  and familial X-linked myalgia, 245–246
  and myopathic stiffness, 244–247
  and tubular aggregates, 245, 245f

Cranial neuropathies/palsies, recurrent, 383b

Cranial volume and shape disorders, 403–422
  abnormal head shape in, 420–422, 420t
    craniosynostosis causing, 420–422, 421t
    extracranial forces causing, 420
    intracranial forces causing, 420
  macrocephaly as, 403–415, 405b
    communicating hydrocephalus as, 404–407
    metabolic megalencephaly and, 414–415

Cranial volume and shape disorders (Continued)
  noncommunicating Cranial volume and shape disorders hydrocephalus as, 407–412
  measuring head size in, 403, 404f
  microcephaly as, 415–420, 415b
    anencephaly in, 416
    chromosomal disorders and, 416
    defective prosencephalization as, 417–419
    encephalocele as, 416–417
    primary, 415–416
    secondary, 419–420
    vera (microcephaly primary hereditary), 415–416

Craniopharyngioma, 375–376

Craniosynostosis, 420–422, 421t

Creatine deficiency disorders, 151–152

Creatine kinase
  carnitine deficiency, 220
  dermatomyositis, 218
  lipid myopathies, 220
  spinal muscular atrophies, 211

Creatine, supplementation, 241

CRPS. See Complex regional pain syndrome

Cryptococcal meningitis, 137

Cryptorchidism, 189

CSF. See Cerebrospinal fluid

CT. See Computed tomography

CVAs. See Cerebrovascular accidents

Cyanotic syncope, 19
  epilepsy distinguished, 19

Cyproheptadine, 102

Cytochrome-c-oxidase deficiency, 196–197

Cytomegalic inclusion disease, 146–147

Cytomegalovirus infection, 146–147

Cytotoxic edema, 115

D

D-Amphetamines+ amphetamine, 434

Dandy-Walker malformation, 273
  noncommunicating hydrocephalus and, 408–409, 409f

Danon disease, 213

Daraprim, 148

Daydreaming, 30

Deafness
  acquired epileptiform aphasia, 37
  congenital, 393–395
  hearing impairment and, 391–397,
      395b
    anatomical considerations in, 391
    auditory dysfunction symptoms in,
        391–392
    congenital deafness in, 393–395
    specialized testing for, 392–393
    tests of hearing for, 391–392
  pontobulbar palsy with, 387–388
Deafness-dystonia-optic neuronopathy
    syndrome, 396
Debrancher enzyme deficiency, 219
Decerebrate posturing/rigidity, 3, 66
Decompressive craniectomy, 120
Decorticate rigidity, 66
Deep midline malformations, 129–130
Defective cellular migration, 418–419
Defective prosencephalization, 417–419
Dehydration, 81, 290
Delayed postanoxic encephalopathy, 67
Delirium
  diagnostic approach to, 64–65
  prescription drugs overdoses, 88
Delusions, 64
Demyelinating optic neuropathy,
    372–373
Dentatorubro pallidoluysian atrophy,
    176–177, 343
Dependency
  folinic acid, 14
  pyridoxine, 14
Depressed fracture, 92
Depression and suicidality
  clinical features, 424
  diagnosis, 424
  management, 424–425
Depression, headache, 105–106
Depressor anguli oris aplasia, 385
Dermal sinus, 304
Dermatomyositis, 217–218, 218f
Desvenlafaxine (pristiq), 434
Developmental amblyopia, 349
Developmental delay
  global, 143

Developmental delay (Continued)
  hemiplegia, 281
  in infants and young children,
      141–143
  language delay, 141–143
  motor development, 143
Deviation, eye, 66
Dexamethasone, for increased
    intracranial pressure, 121
DGS. See DiGeorge syndrome
Diabetes mellitus
  acute hemiplegia and, 287
  Wolfram syndrome and, 378
Diabetic ketoacidosis, 80–81
Dialysis encephalopathy, 85
Dialysis headache, 109
Diaminopyridine, congenital
    myasthenic syndromes,
    198–199
Diastematomyelia, 304
Diathesis, bleeding, 290–295
Diazepam, glycine encephalopathy, 11
Diencephalic gliomas, 376–377, 376f
Diencephalic syndrome, 376
Diet
  food additives, 107
  headache associated with, 98
  ketogenic, 54–55
Diffuse intrinsic pontine glioma
    (DIPG), 122
Diffusion-weighted images, 5, 10
DiGeorge syndrome (DGS), 8, 385
Diphenhydramine, 333–334
Diphtheria, facial weakness and, 389
Diplacusis, 393
Diplomyelia, 304, 305f
Diplopia, 116
Diskitis (disk space infection), 306
Dissociated nystagmus, 365
Diuretics, osmotic, 120
Divalproex, 22
Divergence nystagmus, 365
Dix-Hallpike test, 399
DMD. See Duchenne muscular
    dystrophy
D-methylmalonyl-CoA, 12–13
DOK7 gene, 212
Dopa-responsive dystonia, 336

Double hemiplegia, 315
Down syndrome, 302
Downbeat nystagmus, 364–365
Downward-beating nystagmus, 364
Doxycycline
  cat-scratch disease, 69
  Lyme disease, 70
  Rocky Mountain spotted fever, 71
Dravet syndrome, 22, 145
Drowsiness, benign physiologic
    myoclonus of, 343–344
Drug-induced chorea, 330–331
Drug-induced disorders
  accidental ingestion, 261
  acquired hearing impairment
      in, 396
  corticosteroid psychosis, 87
  headache, 107–108
  prescription drugs overdoses, 88–89
  pupils, fixed dilation, 66
  vertigo in, 399
  withdrawal, in newborns, 4–5
Drug-induced dystonia, 333–334
Drug-induced neuropathy, 224
Drug-induced nystagmus, 363–364
Drusen, 116–117, 117f
Duane syndrome, 350
Duchenne muscular dystrophy (DMD),
    213–216, 215f
Dup15q syndrome, 149
Dysesthesias, neuropathy and
    neuronopathy, 220–221
Dysferlinopathies, 225–226
Dyskinesias
  ADCY5 dyskinesia, 27
  facial weakness and, 381–391
    anatomical considerations in,
        381–382
    aplasia of facial muscles and,
        384–385
    approach to diagnosis for, 382–384
    from Bell palsy, 386–387
    from birth injury, 385–386
    causes of, 382b
    congenital syndromes causing,
        384–386
    depressor anguli oris aplasia in,
        385

Dyskinesias (Continued)
facial movement and, 381
from genetic disorders, 387–389
from hypertension, 389
from immune-mediated and
infectious disorders, 386–387
from infection, 389–390
from metabolic disorders, 390
motor unit disorders in, 383
neurological causes of, 383b
from polyneuritis cranialis, 387
pseudobulbar palsy in, 382–383
recurrent cranial neuropathies/
palsies in, 383b
sucking and swallowing in,
381–382
from syringobulbia, 390
from toxins, 390
from trauma, 391
from tumors, 391
familial paroxysmal nonkinesiogenic,
27
paroxysmal exertion-induced
dyskinesia, 27
paroxysmal kinesiogenic dyskinesia,
26–27
Dysphagia, congenital, 384
Dystonia, 333–340
acute reactions in, 333–334
blepharospasm in, 334
differential diagnosis of, in
childhood, 334b
dopa-responsive, 336
drug-induced, 333–334
focal, 334–335
generalized, 333
generalized genetic, 336–340
glutaric acidemia type I in, 336–337
hemifacial spasm in, 335–336
hepatolenticular degeneration
(Wilson disease) in, 337–338
hereditary genetic, 336–340
idiopathic torsion, 338
infantile bilateral striatal necrosis
in, 338
pantothenate kinase-associated
neurodegeneration in, 339,
339f

Dystonia (Continued)
rapid-onset dystonia-parkinsonism
in, 339
symptomatic generalized, 339–340
tardive, 334
torticollis in, 334–335, 334b
writer's cramp in, 335
Dystrophinopathies
Becker muscular dystrophy,
214–216
congenital, 202
Duchenne muscular dystrophy,
214–216, 215f
facioscapulohumeral dystrophy, 216,
216f
limb-girdle muscular dystrophies,
216
limb-girdle muscular dystrophy R1,
216–217
limb-girdle muscular dystrophy R2,
217
myotonic dystrophy 2, 217
proximal myotonic dystrophy,
217–218
sarcoglycanopathies, 217
Dystrophy, myotonic, 226

E
Early-onset childhood occipital
epilepsy, 38–39
Early-onset idiopathic torsion dystonia,
338
Early-onset severe retinal dystrophy,
377
Echocardiography, for mitral valve
prolapse, 289
Edema
cerebral, 80, 115
cytotoxic, 115
hypothyroidism, 161
optic disc, 116–117, 116b, 117f
Edrophonium chloride, 194
EEG. See Electroencephalography
EGR2 gene, 197
Electrical silence, cramps, 236
Electrical status epilepticus during slow
wave sleep (ESES), 40
Electrocardiogram (ECG), 277

Electrodiagnosis
hypotonia, 193
in neuropathy, 221t
Electroencephalogram, 425
Electroencephalography (EEG)
absence epilepsy, 31, 32f
anoxia and ischemia, 67
of autism/autistic spectrum
disorders, 142
benign familial neonatal seizures, 7
benign myoclonus of infancy, 25
brainstem aura, 263
cat-scratch disease, 68
concussion, 90
consciousness, altered states, 65, 67,
85
cyanotic syncope, 19
of encephalitis, 261
familial paroxysmal nonkinesiogenic
dyskinesia, 27
focal clonic seizures, 3
headache, 110–111
hemiconvulsions-hemiplegia
syndrome, 40–41
in hemiparetic seizure, 287
hemorrhagic shock and
encephalopathy syndrome, 70
hypernatremia, 81
hypoxic-ischemic encephalopathy, 9
infantile spasms, 23–24, 24t
juvenile myoclonic epilepsy, 34
Lafora disease, 36
Lennox-Gastaut syndrome, 34–35
Panayiotopoulos syndrome, 39
of progressive encephalopathies with
onset before age two, 152
pyridoxine dependency, 14
schizophrenia, 87
seizure patterns, 2
seizures, 2
split-screen video-EEG monitoring,
2–3
Electromyography (EMG)
of ataxia, 260
botulism, 198
of Brody myopathy, 245
centronuclear myopathy, 202
cramps, 236

Electromyography (EMG) (Continued)
  GM2 gangliosidosis, 212
  hypoxic-ischemic myelopathy, 192
  lipid myopathies, 220
  muscle stiffness, 237b
  of myotonia congenita, 239
  of myotonia fluctuans, 239
  neuropathy and neuronopathy,
      220–221
  in spinal muscular atrophies, 318
Electrophysiological studies, botulism,
    198
Eletriptan, headache, 100
ELISA. See Enzyme-linked
    immunosorbent assay
Emergent withdrawal syndrome, in
    chorea, 331
Emery-dreifuss muscular dystrophy,
    226–227
EMG. See Electromyography
Emotional stress, 100
Encephalitis
  versus aseptic meningitis, 70
  brainstem, 261–262
Encephalocele, 416–417
Encephalopathies
  acquired immunodeficiency
      syndrome, 152–153
  acute uremic encephalopathy, 84
  bilirubin encephalopathy, 7–8
  calcineurin inhibitor encephalopathy,
      87–88
  chronic nonprogressive
      encephalopathy, 189–190
  chronic uremic encephalopathy,
      84–85
  dialysis encephalopathy, 85
  glycine encephalopathy, 11
  Hashimoto encephalopathy,
      77–78
  hepatic encephalopathy, 82–83
  hypertensive encephalopathy,
      85, 85f
  hyponatremic encephalopathy, 82
  hypoxic-ischemic encephalopathy,
      9–10
  Lyme disease, 70
  metabolic (general), 66, 85–86

Encephalopathies (Continued)
  mitochondrial encephalopathy, lactic
      acidosis and stroke (MELAS),
      291
  myoclonic encephalopathy/
      neuroblastoma syndrome,
      266–267, 266f
  NMDA (anti-N-methyl-D-
      aspartate receptor antibody
      encephalopathy), 78–79
  organic, 64
  posterior reversible encephalopathy
      syndrome, 87
  postimmunization, 80
  progressive with onset after age two,
      171–179
    infectious disease, 175
    lysosomal enzyme disorders,
        171–179
  progressive with onset before age
      two, 152–158
    acquired immunodeficiency
        syndrome (AIDS)
        encephalopathy, 152–153
    amino acid metabolism disorders,
        153–156
    history and physical examination,
        152, 152f
    hypothyroidism, 161
    lysosomal enzyme disorders,
        156–158
    mitochondrial disorders, 161–163
    neurocutaneous disorders,
        163–166
    neuronal ceroid-lipofuscinosis,
        175–176
    subacute necrotizing
        encephalomyelopathy, 163
  recurrent, causes, 64b
  static, 145–152
    causes of apparent regression, 142b
  toxic, 87–89
Endocrine myopathies, 220
Endovascular embolization, 411
Enterovirus D68, 229
Enterovirus encephalitis, 73
Enterovirus infections, 229–230
Enteroviruses, 71

Enzyme replacement therapy, 205
Enzyme-linked immunosorbent assay
    (ELISA), 78
Ependymoma, 124
  ataxia, 270
  as spinal cord tumors, 313
Epidural empyema, 135
Epilepsia partialis continua, 40
Epilepsy, 412
  absence, 30–31, 34f
  autosomal dominant sleep-related
      hypermotor epilepsy, 37–38
  benign myoclonic, 25
  cerebral palsy and, 281–282
  childhood with occipital paroxysms,
      38–39
  cyanotic syncope distinguished, 19
  early-onset childhood occipital
      epilepsy, 38–39
  electrical status epilepticus during
      slow wave sleep, 40
  epileptic encephalopathy (early) with
      burst suppression, 25
  exacerbated by fever, 21–26
  with generalized tonic-clonic seizures
      on awakening, 42, 42b
  hemiplegia and, 287–288
  ictal vomiting associated with, 38
  idiopathic occipital epilepsy with
      photosensitivity, 39
  juvenile myoclonic, 33–34, 54f, 89–90
  late-onset/idiopathic childhood
      occipital epilepsy, 38–39
  myoclonic-astatic, 33
  with occipital paroxysms, 38–39
  post-traumatic, 92
  progressive myoclonus, 35–36, 35b
  reading, 41
  self-limited childhood epilepsy,
      39–40
  severe myoclonic, 25
  surgical approaches, 55–56
  temporal lobe, 41
Epileptic ataxia, 267
Epileptic encephalopathy (early) with
    burst suppression, 25
Episodic ataxia type 8 (EA8), 261
Episodic tension headache, 109

EPM2A gene, 35
Erythromelalgia, 251
Escitalopram (lexapro), 434
ESES. *See* Electrical status epilepticus during slow wave sleep
Esotropia, 348–349
Essential (familial) tremor, 344–345
Ethosuximide (antiepileptic)
    absence epilepsy, 31
    administration, 47
    adverse effects, 47
    indications for, 47
Ethylene glycol, 390
Exercise, as trigger factor for migraine, 98
Exercise intolerance, defined, 236–237, 241
Exertional headache, benign, 104
Exophoria, 349
Exotropia, 349
Expressive skills, in language development, 141–142
Extended migraine, 105
Extramedullary tumors, 255
Extraocular muscles, 349*t*
    congenital fibrosis of, 350–351
    pain from, 96
Extraventricular drain (EVD), 119
Eyelid myoclonia with/without absences, 31–33
Eye-of-the-tiger sign, in pantothenate kinase-associated neurodegeneration, 339, 339*f*
Eyes, examining, 65
Eyestrain, 109

F
Facial asymmetry, congenital, 384–386
Facial movement, 381
Facial muscles, aplasia of, 384–385
Facial nerve palsies, 385
Facial weakness and dysphagia, 381–391
    anatomical considerations in, 381–382
    aplasia of facial muscles and, 384–385
    approach to diagnosis for, 382–384

Facial weakness and dysphagia (*Continued*)
    from Bell palsy, 386–387
    from birth injury, 385–386
    causes of, 382*b*
    congenital syndromes causing, 384–386
        congenital bilateral Perisylvian syndrome, 384, 384*f*
        congenital dysphagia, 384
        congenital facial asymmetry, 384–386
    depressor anguli oris aplasia in, 385
    facial movement and, 381
    from genetic disorders, 387–389
        CLCN7-related osteopetrosis, 388
        facioscapulohumeral dystrophy in, 387–388
        Melkersson Rosenthal syndrome in, 388–389
        riboflavin transporter deficiency, 388
    from hypertension, 389
    from immune-mediated and infectious disorders, 386
    from infection, 389–390
        herpes zoster oticus (Ramsay Hunt syndrome), 389
        sarcoidosis, 389–390, 390*f*
    from metabolic disorders, 390
    motor unit disorders in, 383
    polyneuritis cranialis, 387
    pseudobulbar palsy in, 382–383
    recurrent cranial neuropathies/palsies in, 383*b*
    sucking and swallowing in, 381–382
    from syringobulbia, 390
    from toxins, 390
    from trauma, 391
    from tumors, 391
    unilateral, 281–282
Facioscapulohumeral dystrophy, 214–216
Fahr disease, in chorea, 332
Fainting, syncope, 29
Falx herniation, 118
Familial dysautonomia, 190
    newborns with, 383

Familial episodic pain syndromes, 252
Familial hemiplegic migraine (FHM), 97–98, 295–296
Familial hypokalemic periodic paralysis, 231–232
Familial infantile striatal degeneration, 338
Familial normokalemic periodic paralysis, 232
Familial paroxysmal choreoathetosis (FPC), 26–27
Familial paroxysmal nonkinesiogenic dyskinesia, 27
Familial recurrent brachial neuritis, 250
Familial tremor, 344
Familial X-linked myalgia, and cramps, 245–246
Fatigue
    and exercise, 236–237
    in neuromuscular disease, 208
Fazio-Londe disease, 388
Febrile seizures, 20–21
Felbamate (antiepileptic), 47
    selection, 45
Felnfluramine, 47–48
Fetal alcohol syndrome, 4–5
Fever illness refractory epileptic syndrome, 78–79
FHM. *See* Familial hemiplegic migraine
Fibroblast growth factor receptor (FGFR) gene, 408
Fibroblast growth factor receptor-associated craniosynostosis syndromes, 408
Fibromuscular dysplasia, 285
15q-related syndromes, 148–149
    Angelman syndrome, 149
    Dup15q syndrome, 149
    Prader-Willi syndrome, 148–149
FLAIR images, 67
Floppy infant, assessment of, 186–187
Fluoxetine (prozac), 213, 433
Fluvoxamine (luvox), 434
Focal clonic seizures, 3
Focal dystonias, 334–335
Focal familial recurrent neuropathy, 319
Focal inhibitory seizures, 287
Focal myoclonus, 342–343

Focal seizures
    in children, 36–41, 47
    with impaired awareness, 32–33
Folinic acid dependency, 14
Food additives, 107
Food and Drug Administration (FDA),
        101, 266
Foot deformities, spinal paraplegia, 300
Foramen magnum tumors, 255
Fosphenytoin sodium, 17, 49
FPC. *See* Familial paroxysmal
        choreoathetosis
Fractures
    compressed vertebral body, 310–312
    fracture dislocation and spinal cord
            transection, 311, 311*f*
    open head injuries, 92
Fragile X syndrome, 149–150
Friedreich ataxia, 276–277
Fukuyama congenital muscular
        dystrophy, 203
Fukuyama muscular dystrophy, 203
Fungal infections, 135–137, 135*b*
    candidal meningoencephalitis, 136
    coccidioidomycosis, 136–137, 138*b*
    cryptococcal meningitis, 137

G
Gabapentin
    for asthmatic amyotrophy, 319
    for complex regional pain syndrome,
        257
    for lumbar plexitis, 319
GAD-7 patient screening tool, 426*b*
Galactosemia (transferase deficiency),
        170
Gaucher disease type II
        (glucosylceramide lipidosis),
        156–157
Gaucher disease type III
        (glucosylceramide lipidosis),
        171–172
Gaze palsies, in ophthalmoplegia,
        359–361, 360*b*
GCS. *See* Glasgow Coma Scale
Gender differences
    headache, 97
    MECP2 duplication syndrome, 188

Generalized dystonia, 333
Generalized genetic dystonias,
        336–340
Generalized myasthenia, 355
Genetic disorders
    cerebral hypotonia, 190–192
    in chorea, 331–333
    congenital deafness from, 393–395
    familial dysautonomia, 190
    headache, 97–98
    hereditary autonomic and sensory
            neuropathy type III, 190
    later-onset, 395–396
    lipoprotein, 290–291
    metabolic defects, 192
    and migraine, 97–98
    oculocerebrorenal syndrome,
            190–191
    peroxisomal disorders, 191
    pyruvate carboxylase deficiency,
            191–192
    Zellweger spectrum disorder, 191
Genetic testing
    ataxia with oculomotor apraxia, 277
    congenital hypomyelinating
            neuropathy, 197
    emery-dreifuss muscular dystrophy,
            227
    familial dysautonomia, 190
    late-onset Pompe disease, 219
    in Lesch-Nyhan disease, 167–168
    oculocerebrorenal syndrome, 190
    peroxisomal disorders, 191
    in phenylketonuria, 156
    propionic acidemia, 13
    slow-channel congenital myasthenic
            syndrome, 213
Gentamicin, vertigo and, 399
Germ cell tumors, 125–126
Giant axonal neuropathy, 223
Gigantism, megalencephaly with, 413
Gigaxonin, 223
Glasgow Coma Scale (GCS), 91, 91*t*,
        119–120
Glial tumors, 122–124
Glianeuronal tumors, 122–124
Glioma, brainstem, in ophthalmoplegia,
        353–354, 354*f*

Global developmental delay, 143
    cerebral malformations, 145
    fragile X syndrome, 149–150
    intrauterine infections, 145–148
    perinatal disorders, 145
Globoid cell leukodystrophy (Krabbe
        disease), 223–224
Globulin, immune, 198
Glucose utilization disorders, 241–242
Glutaric acidemia type I, in dystonia,
        336–337
Glycoprotein degradation disorders,
        157–158, 158*b*
GM$_1$ gangliosidosis, 158, 158*b*
GM$_2$ gangliosidosis (juvenile Tay-Sachs
        disease), 171
    ataxia, 277
Gower sign, neuromuscular disease,
        209*f*
Gradenigo syndrome, in
        ophthalmoplegia, 354–355
Gram-negative sepsis, 69
Gray matter disorders
    infantile neuroaxonal dystrophy, 167
    infantile neuronal ceroid
            lipofuscinosis, 166–167
    Jansky-Bielschowsky disease,
            175–176
    juvenile Huntington disease, 176
    Lesch-Nyhan disease, 167–168
    magnetic resonance imaging of, 152,
            152*f*
    Menkes syndrome, 169
    mitochondrial encephalomyopathies,
            177
    myoclonic epilepsy and ragged-red
            fibers, 177
    neuronal ceroid lipofuscinosis,
            175–176
    Rett syndrome, 168
    syringomyelia and, 256
    xeroderma pigmentosum,
            177–178
GRIN1-related disorders, 151
GRIN2B-related neurodevelopmental
        disorder, 150–151
Group B *Streptococcus* (GBS), 130
Growing pains, 236

GTP cyclohydrolase 1-deficient dopa-responsive dystonia (DYT-GCH1), 336
Guanfacine, 435
Guillain-Barré syndrome, 386–387
Gum hypertrophy, 50

H
Hallervorden-Spatz syndrome, 339
Hallucinations, 28, 35–36, 64, 99
  auditory, 64
  visual, 64, 99
Haloperidol, 331
Hartnup disease, 262, 278
Hashimoto encephalopathy, 77–78
Hashimoto thyroiditis, 82
HBB gene, 292
Head circumference, 403
  measurement of, 115
Head elevation, increased intracranial pressure in, 119
Head injuries
  mild, ataxia, 267
  severe, 90–92
    closed, 91–92
    open, 92, 92f
Head size, measuring, 403, 404f
Head tilt, differential diagnosis of, 334b
Head trauma, 98, 119
Headache, 95–97
  analgesic rebound, 105
  approach to, 95–97
  benign exertional, 104
  caffeine, 105
  chronic, 96, 104, 111
  chronic low-grade non-progressive, 104–107
  chronic paroxysmal hemicrania, 104
  chronic progressive, 108
  cluster, 103–104
  connective tissue disorders, 108–109
  cranial structures (other), pain from, 109–110
  depression, 105–106
  drugs and foods associated with, 107–108

Headache (*Continued*)
  evaluation, 97
  eyestrain, 109
  generalized, acute, 96
  hemicrania continua, 104
  and hypertension, 109
  ice-pick, 99
  incidence in children, 97
  increased intracranial pressure in, 115
  indomethacin-responsive, 104
  localized, acute, 96
  low pressure/spinal fluid leak, 111
  pattern, 96
  post-traumatic, 106
  primary stabbing, 99
  psychogenic, 105–106
  recurrent, acute, 96
  seizure, 110–111
  sinusitis, 109–110
  sources of pain, 96, 96b
  stress, 105–106
  and systemic disease, 108–109
  temporomandibular joint syndrome, 110
  tension, 106–107
    episodic, 109
  vasculitis, 108
  whiplash/neck injuries, 110
Hearing impairment, 391–397
  from acoustic neuroma, 397, 397f
  acquired, 396–397
    drug-induced, 396
    from infectious disease, 396
    from metabolic disorders, 396
    from skeletal disorders, 396
    from trauma, 396
    from tumor, 396–397
  acquired epileptiform aphasia, 37
  and deafness, 391–397
    anatomical considerations in, 391
    auditory dysfunction symptoms in, 391–392
    congenital deafness in, 393–395
    specialized testing for, 392–393
    tests of hearing for, 392–393
  language delay, 142–143
  sensorineural, 391

Hearing tests
  brainstem auditory evoked response as, 393
  office testing in, 392
  pure-tone audiometry as, 392
  specialized testing for, 392–393
  speech tests, 393
Heart disease
  congenital, 288–289
  mitral valve disease, 289
  rheumatic, 289
Hematin infusions, acute intermittent porphyria, 255
Hemiconvulsions-hemiplegia syndrome, 40–41
Hemicrania continua, 104
  versus cluster headache, 103
Hemidystonia, 340
Hemifacial spasm, 335–336
Hemiparetic seizures, 287–288
Hemiplegia, 281–298
  acute, 283–296, 283b
    heart disease, 288–289
    migraine, 295–296
    trauma, 296
  alternating, 286–287
  chronic progressive, 281, 296–297
  diabetes mellitus, 287
  epilepsy, 287–288
  eye, 66
  heart disease, 288–289
  hypercoagulable states, 289–290
  hypocoagulable states, 290–295
  infections, 295
  migraine, 295–296
  in motor development, delayed, 143
  progressive, 296b
  Sturge-Weber syndrome, 296–297
  trauma, 296
  tumors, 296
Hemiplegic cerebral palsy, 281–283
Hemispherectomy, 55–56
Hemodialysis, 84
Hemoglobin electrophoresis, 293
Hemolytic-uremic syndrome, 84
Hemorrhage
  cerebellar, 268
  focal clonic seizures, 3

Hemorrhage (Continued)
  intracerebral, 91
  intracranial/intraventricular, 15–16
  neonatal, 283
  periventricular-intraventricular, in
     premature newborns, 126–
     128, 127b
  posterior fossa epidural, 91
  subarachnoid, 15–16
  subdural, 16, 91
Hemorrhagic shock and
     encephalopathy syndrome,
     69–70
Henoch-Schönlein purpura, 109
Hepatic encephalopathy, 82–83
Hepatolenticular degeneration, in
     dystonia, 337–338
Hereditary autonomic and sensory
     neuropathy type III, 190
Hereditary brachial plexopathy,
     319–320
Hereditary distal myopathies, 225
  autosomal recessive distal (dysferlin)
     myopathy, 225–227
  myotonic dystrophy, 226
Hereditary essential myoclonus, 342
Hereditary hyperekplexia (stiff infant
     syndrome), 20
Hereditary neuralgic amyotrophy,
     319–320
Hereditary neuropathies
  with liability to pressure palsy, 319,
     323–324
  metabolic, 254–255
Hereditary optic neuropathy, 377
  Bardet-Biedl syndrome and, 378
  Cockayne syndrome and, 378–379
  early-onset severe retinal dystrophy,
     377
  Laurence-Moon syndrome and, 378
  Leber congenital amaurosis as, 377
  retinoblastoma and, 378
  Wolfram syndrome and, 377–378
Hereditary sensory and autonomic
     neuropathies classification of,
     252–254
  type I (HSAN I), 252–253
  type II (HSAN II), 253

Hereditary sensory and autonomic
     neuropathies classification of
     (Continued)
  type III (HSAN III), 253
  type IV (HSAN IV), 253–254
  type V (HSAN V), 254
Hereditary spastic paraplegia (HSP),
     305–308
Herniation syndromes, 117–118, 118b
Heroin, 4–5
Herpes simplex encephalitis/herpes
     simplex virus (HSV), 14–15
  HSV-1 and HSV-2, 72
  in newborns, 14–15
Herpes simplex virus encephalitis, 72
Herpes zoster myelitis, 306–307
Herpes zoster oticus (Ramsay Hunt
     syndrome), 389
Heterophoria, 348
Heterotropia, 348
HEXA disorders, 158–171
Hiccupping, 11
HIE. See Hypoxic-ischemic
     encephalopathy
High-density lipoprotein (HDL)
     cholesterol, 291
High-performance liquid
     chromatography (HPLC), 293
Hippocampal cells, 67
Hippocampectomy, 55
History and physical examination, for
     vertigo, 398
History-taking
  delirium, 64–65
  headache, 96–97
  lethargy and coma, 65–66
  in progressive encephalopathies with
     onset before age two, 152,
     152f
HIV. See Human immunodeficiency
     virus
Holmes-Adie syndrome, 380
Holoprosencephaly, 417
Homeostasis, 119
Homeostasis, increased intracranial
     pressure in, 119
Homocystinuria, 153–154, 154f
Homovanillic acid (HVA), 266–267

Hopkins syndrome, 319
Horizontal gaze
  apraxia of, 359
  palsy, 361
Horizontal suspension, hypotonic
     infant, 185, 186f
Horner syndrome, 66, 379–380
HPLC. See High-performance liquid
     chromatography
HSP. See Hereditary spastic paraplegia
Human immunodeficiency virus (HIV)
  in acquired immunodeficiency
     syndrome encephalopathy,
     152
  intrauterine infections, 145
Human parechovirus encephalitis,
     72–73
Hunter syndrome (type II MPS),
     173–174
Huntington disease (HD), 166, 176
Hurler phenotype, 158b
Hurler syndrome (MPS I), 159–160
Hutchinson triad, in congenital syphilis,
     146
HVA. See Homovanillic acid
Hydranencephaly, 411
Hydrocephalus, 120–126
  causes of, 405b
  communicating, 404–407
     benign enlargement of
        subarachnoid space in, 404–
        406, 406f
     meningeal malignancy as, 406–407
  noncommunicating, 407–412
     congenital aqueductal stenosis in,
        407–408, 408f
     congenital brain tumors and, 410
     Dandy-Walker malformation and,
        408–409, 409f
     fibroblast growth factor receptor-
        associated craniosynostosis
        syndromes, 408
     hydranencephaly and, 411
     Klippel-Feil syndrome and,
        409–410
     porencephaly and, 411–412
     vein of Galen malformation and,
        410–411, 411f

Hydrocephalus (Continued)
  Walker-Warburg syndrome and, 411
  X-linked hydrocephalus (L1 syndrome) in, 408
  progressive, 171
  in toxoplasmosis, 147–148
Hyperacusis, 392
Hyperammonemia, 10b, 12–13
Hyperbilirubinemia, 7
Hypercarbia, in cerebral blood flow, 114
Hypercoagulable states, 289–290
Hypernatremia, 81
Hyperosmolar therapy, 120
Hyperosmolar therapy, for increased intracranial pressure, 120
Hyperparathyroidism, 82, 390
  maternal, 8
Hypersecretion, adrenal, 82
Hypersensitivity vasculitis, 109, 293
Hypertension
  facial weakness and dysphagia from, 389
  and headache, 109
Hypertensive encephalopathy, 85, 85f
Hyperthyroidism
  in chorea, 333
  in physiological tremor, 344
Hypertonia, 20
Hyperventilation, 119–120
  increased intracranial pressure in, 115
  panic disorder, 87
  paroxysmal disorders, 29
Hypnagogic hallucinations, 28
Hypnotics, 4–5
Hypoadrenalism, 239
Hypobetalipoproteinemia, ataxia, 275
Hypocalcemia, 239
  in newborns, 8
Hypocoagulable states, 290–295
  infections, 295
  lipoprotein disorders, 290–291
  mitochondrial encephalopathy, lactic acidosis and stroke, 291
  moyamoya disease, 291–292, 292f
  sickle cell disease, 292–293
  vasculopathies, 293–295

Hypocretin, 28
Hypoglycemia, 81
  blindness and, 372
  in newborns, 8–9, 8b
Hypomagnesemia, 86, 239
Hyponatremia, 81
Hyponatremic encephalopathy, 82
Hypoparathyroidism, 8
Hyporeflexia, muscular dystrophy, 209
Hypotension, 67
Hypothermia, 120
  therapy, 67–68
Hypothyroidism, 161, 390
Hypotonia, 185–186
  chorea and, 329
Hypotonic infant, 183–207
  appearance of hypotonia, 183–185
  approach to diagnosis of, 185–188
  benign congenital hypotonia, 188
  cerebral hypotonia, 188–192
  chromosomal disorders, 188–189
  differential diagnosis of, 184b
  genetic disorders, 190–192
  horizontal suspension, 185, 186f
  motor unit disorders. See Motor unit disorders
  spinal cord disorders, 192–193
  traction response, 184–185, 185f
  vertical suspension, 185, 186f
Hypoxia, prolonged, 66
Hypoxic-ischemic encephalopathy (HIE)
  approach to diagnosis of, 185–186
  consciousness, altered states, 67
  in newborns, 9–10
Hypoxic-ischemic myelopathy, spinal cord disorders, 192
Hypsarrhythmia, 23–24

I
Iatrogenic respiratory crisis, 194
Ibuprofen, headache, 100
I-cell disease, 159
Ice-pack test, in myasthenia gravis, 355–356
Ice-pick headache, 99
Ictal nystagmus, 364

Idiopathic basal ganglia calcification, in chorea, 332
Idiopathic cerebral venous thrombosis, 15
Idiopathic cranial polyneuropathy, 387
Idiopathic intracranial hypertension, 137–139
Idiopathic occipital epilepsy with photosensitivity, 39
Idiopathic torsion dystonia, 338
IEF. See Isoelectric focusing
Imaging
  of brain, 281
  echocardiography, 289
  spinal paraplegia, 299–315
Immunocompromised patients, cat-scratch disease, 68–69
Immunoglobulin, intravenous, 228
Immunosuppressive drugs, 87
Inborn errors of metabolism
  ataxia, 262–263
  consciousness, altered states, 83–84
  medium-chain acyl-coenzyme A dehydrogenase deficiency, 83–84
  in newborns, 6b, 83–84
Incontinentia pigmenti (Bloch–Sulzberger syndrome), 16
Increased intracranial pressure (ICP), 113–140
  age of child, 113
  bacterial meningitis. See Bacterial meningitis
  in brain tumors, 120–121
  cerebral blood flow in, 114
  cerebral edema, 115
  cerebrospinal fluid, 114
  in children, 115–117
  decompressive craniectomy in, 120
  diplopia and strabismus, 116
  features of, 114b
  fungal infections. See Fungal infections
  head elevation, 119
  headache, 115–116
  herniation syndromes, 117–118, 118b
  homeostasis, 119
  in hydrocephalus, 120–126

Increased intracranial pressure (ICP)
(Continued)
hyperventilation, 119–120
idiopathic intracranial hypertension,
137–139
in infancy, 115
intracranial hemorrhage. See
Intracranial hemorrhage
management of, 118–119
mass lesions, 115
medical treatment of, 118–120, 119b
monitoring, 119
normal, 114
optic disc edema, 116–117, 116b,
117f
osmotic diuretics for, 120
pathophysiology, 114–115
pentobarbital coma in, 120
presenting complaint, 113
symptoms and signs, 115–118
Indomethacin-responsive headache,
104
Infant, hypotonic, 183–207
Infantile bilateral striatal necrosis,
338–339
Infantile botulism, 198
Infantile esotropia, 349
Infantile neuroaxonal dystrophy, 167
Infantile spasms, 22–25
Infantile spinal muscular atrophy,
194–196, 195f
with respiratory distress type 1
(SMARD1), 196
Infants and young children
bacterial meningitis in, 131–133
benign myoclonic epilepsy, 25
biotinidase deficiency, 25–26
breath-holding spells, 18–19
developmental delay in, 141–143
epilepsy
epileptic encephalopathy (early)
with burst suppression, 25
severe myoclonic, 25
epileptic encephalopathy (early) with
burst suppression, 25
increased intracranial pressure in,
115
Lennox-Gastaut syndrome, 34–35

Infants and young children (Continued)
migraine, 26
paroxysmal disorders, 18–21, 18b
seizures in
apneic, 18
febrile, 20–21
myoclonic, 22–25
neurocutaneous disorders, 23b
nonfebrile, 22–26
Infarction
neonatal cord, 308–309
of optic nerve, 373
Infections, 326
facial weakness and dysphagia from,
389
intrauterine, congenital cataract
from, 368
ischemic arterial infarction and, 295
vertigo from, 399–401
Infectious disease, 175, 227–230
acute infectious myositis, 227–228
acute inflammatory demyelinating
polyradiculoneuropathy, 228
acute motor axonal neuropathy, 228
bacterial. See Bacterial meningitis
cervical infections, 285
chronic inflammatory demyelinating
polyradiculoneuropathy,
228–229
diskitis, 306
fungal. See Fungal infections
herpes zoster myelitis, 306–307
lupus myelopathy, 308
postinfectious/immune-mediated
disorders, 264–267
spinal paraplegia and, 306
tuberculous osteomyelitis, 307–308
Infectious disorders, 68–76
autoimmune encephalopathies, 76
bacterial infections, 68–76
Inflammation, inflammatory
myopathies, 217–219
Inflammatory myopathies, 217–219
Infratentorial epidural hematomas, 92
Injuries
birth, 385–386
brain, 190, 300
head, severe, 90–92

Injuries (Continued)
neck, 110
postnatal, 321–322
shaking, 90–91
spinal cord, 192–193
whiplash, 401
Inner ear
aplasia of, 394–395
definition of, 391
Inositol polyphosphate 5-phosphatase
(OCRL-1), 190
Insufficiency, convergence, 361
Insulin therapy, in Wolfram syndrome,
378
Intensive care unit weakness, 231
Interhemispheric commissurotomy, 56
International Classification of Headache
Disorders, 375
International League Against Epilepsy
(ILAE), 36
Internuclear ophthalmoplegia (INO),
360
Intoxications, in acute bilateral
ophthalmoplegia, 358
Intracranial arachnoid cysts, 126
Intracranial hemorrhage, 126–128
arterial aneurysms, 128–129
arteriovenous malformations,
129–130
cocaine abuse, 130
newborn, 15–16
intraventricular hemorrhage in,
126–128
at term, 128
perinatal, 126–128
Intracranial hypertension, causes of,
138b
Intracranial pressure, increased, 108
Intrauterine disorders, in secondary
microcephaly, 419
Intrauterine infections, 145–148
congenital lymphocytic
choriomeningitis, 147
congenital syphilis, 145–148
cytomegalovirus infection, 145
human immunodeficiency virus
(HIV), 145
rubella embryopathy, 147

Intrauterine infections *(Continued)*
    toxoplasmosis, 147–148
    Zika virus (ZIKV), 148
Intravenous botulism immune globulin
        (BabyBIG), 358
Intravenous immunoglobulin (IVIG),
        218, 228, 318–319, 328
Intraventricular hemorrhage, in
        newborn, 126–128
    at term, 128
Isaac syndrome (neuromyotonia), 238
Ischemia
    acute, 67
    hyperventilation and, 119–120
    retinal, 374–375
Ischemic exercise test, 241
Ischemic optic neuropathy, 373
Isoelectric focusing (IEF), 293
Isoniazid, neuropathy and, 224
Isovaleric acidemia, 12
Ixodes spp., 70

J
Jansky-Bielschowsky disease, 175–176
Jeavons syndrome, 31–33
Jerk nystagmus, 361–362
Jerks
    myoclonic, 3, 5
    reading epilepsy, 41
Jitteriness, newborns, 4
JME. *See* Juvenile myoclonic epilepsy
Joubert syndrome, 273, 273*f*
Juvenile Huntington disease, 176
Juvenile myoclonic epilepsy (JME),
        33–34, 34*f*, 89–90
Juvenile progressive bulbar palsy, 387
Juvenile-onset Parkinson disease, 345

K
Kawasaki disease, 268
Kayser-Fleischer ring, in
        hepatolenticular degeneration
        (Wilson disease), 337
KCNQ2 gene, 7
KCNQ3 gene, 7
Kearns-Sayre syndrome (KSS),
        in chronic bilateral
        ophthalmoplegia, 359

Kernicterus, 7
Ketoacidosis, diabetic ketoacidosis and,
        287
Ketogenic diet, 54–55
Klippel-Feil syndrome, 301
    noncommunicating hydrocephalus
        and, 409–410
Krabbe disease, 152*f*, 157, 308. *See also*
        Globoid cell leukodystrophy
    late-onset, 172
Krebs cycle, 240–241
KSS. *See* Kearns-Sayre syndrome

L
L1 syndrome, 408
Laboratory investigations
    delirium, 65
    lethargy and coma, 66
Labyrinthine disease, in vestibular
        nystagmus, 364
Lactate dehydrogenase deficiency
        (LDH), 241–242
Lactic acidosis, 291
Lafora disease, 35–36
Laing early-onset distal myopathy, 225
LAMA2 muscular dystrophy, 202–203
Lamotrigine (antiepileptic), 342
    absence epilepsy, 31
    acquired epileptiform opercular
        syndrome, 37
    administration, 48
    adverse effects, 48
    for erythromelalgia, 251
    generalized tonic-clonic seizures, 42
    indications for, 48
    juvenile myoclonic epilepsy, 34
    selection, 45
    temporal lobe epilepsy, 41
Lance-Adams syndrome, 342
Landau-Kleffner syndrome, 37, 142,
        429
Language delay, 141–143
Large-amplitude nystagmus, 365
Laser ablation, 55
Late-onset multiple carboxylase
        deficiency, 25–26
Late-onset Pompe disease, 219
    flaccid limb weakness, 219

Late-onset/idiopathic childhood
        occipital epilepsy, 38–39
Laurence-Moon syndrome, 378
LCMV. *See* Lymphocytic
        choriomeningitis virus
LDH. *See* Lactate dehydrogenase
        deficiency
Leber congenital amaurosis, 377
Legs, pain in, 236
Leigh syndrome, 163
Lennox-Gastaut syndrome, 25, 34–35,
        145
Lesch-Nyhan disease, 167–168, 252
Lesionectomy, 55
Lethargy, diagnostic approach to, 63*b*–
        64*b*, 65–66
Leucovorin (folinic acid), 148
Leukocoria, 378
Leukocytes, 75–76
Levetiracetam (antiepileptic), 102
    administration, 48
    adverse effects, 48
    benign myoclonic epilepsy, 25
    Dravet syndrome, 22
    drug withdrawal, 5
    generalized tonic-clonic seizures, 42
    indications for, 48
    infantile spasms, 24
    juvenile myoclonic epilepsy, 31
    newborns, treatment, 17
    selection, 45
    temporal lobe epilepsy, 41
    and zonisamide, 45
Light microscopy, Reye syndrome, 79
Limb pain, 254
Limb weakness
    flaccid, 208–235
    myotubular myopathy, 202
    neuromuscular disease, 208–210
    paraplegia, 299
Limb-girdle muscular dystrophies
        (LGMDs), 210, 213, 214*t*, 216
Limb-girdle muscular dystrophy R1,
        216–217
Limb-girdle muscular dystrophy R2,
        217
Limb-girdle myasthenia, 212
Lipid disorders, 223–224

Lipid myopathies, 220
Lipoma, 304
Lipoprotein disorders, ischemic
    arterial infarction and,
    290–291
Lisdexamfetamine (vyvanse), 434
Lissencephaly, 418, 419f
Listeria monocytogenes, 130
Live-attenuated virus vaccines, 80
Liver biopsy, Reye syndrome, 79
LMWH. *See* Low molecular weight
    heparin
Locked-in syndrome, 62
Low molecular weight heparin
    (LMWH), 286, 288
Low pressure/spinal fluid leak
    headache, 111
Low-amplitude physiological tremor,
    344
Lowe syndrome, 190. *See also*
    Oculocerebrorenal syndrome
Lower brainstem, and cranial nerve
    dysfunction, 381–402
Low-molecular-weight heparin
    (LMWH), 283
LSD. *See* Lysergic acid diethylamide
Lumbar plexitis, 319
Lumbar puncture, 65, 117–118
    for bacterial meningitis, 132
    for idiopathic intracranial
        hypertension, 137–139
Lupus erythematosus, in chorea, 333
Lupus myelopathy, 308
Lyme disease, 70
Lymphadenopathy, 65
    cat-scratch disease, 68–69
Lymphocytic choriomeningitis virus
    (LCMV), 147
Lymphocytosis, 69
Lysergic acid diethylamide (LSD), 89
Lysosomal enzyme disorders
    ATP7A-related copper transport
        disorders, 173
    congenital disorders of glycosylation,
        161
    Gaucher disease type II
        (glucosylceramide lipidosis),
        156–157

Lysosomal enzyme disorders
    (*Continued*)
    Gaucher disease type III
        (glucosylceramide lipidosis),
        171–172
    globoid cell leukodystrophy (Krabbe
        disease), 157, 172
    glycoprotein degradation disorders,
        157–158, 158b
    GM₁ gangliosidosis, 158, 158b
    GM₂ gangliosidosis (juvenile Tay-
        Sachs disease), 171
    Hunter syndrome (type II MPS),
        173–174
    I-cell disease, 159
    metachromatic leukodystrophy
        (late-onset lipidosis),
        172–173
    mucolipidosis type II, 159
    mucopolysaccharidoses, 159–160,
        173–174
    Niemann-Pick disease type A,
        160–161
    Niemann-Pick disease type B,
        160–161
    Niemann-Pick disease type C
        (sphingomyelin lipidosis),
        174–175
    occipital horn syndrome, 169
    in progressive encephalopathies
        with onset after age two,
        171–175
    in progressive encephalopathies with
        onset before age two, 156–158
    Sandhoff disease, 158
    Sly disease (type VII MPS), 174
    Tay-Sachs disease, 159

M
Machado-Joseph disease, 274–275
Macrocephaly, 403–415, 405b
    benign familial, 413
    communicating hydrocephalus as,
        404–407
    metabolic megalencephaly and,
        414–415
    noncommunicating hydrocephalus
        as, 407–412

Magnetic resonance angiography
    (MRA)
    in carotid and vertebral artery
        disorders, 286
    in hemiplegia, 281
Magnetic resonance imaging (MRI)
    of acoustic neuroma, 397, 397f
    of acute disseminated
        encephalomyelitis, 76–80,
        77f
    of anoxia and ischemia, 67
    of arachnoid cysts, 301
    of arteriovenous malformations, 301
    of astrocytoma, 312
    of ataxia, 260–261
    of atlantoaxial dislocation, 302
    of benign enlargement of
        subarachnoid space, 406, 406f
    of cat-scratch disease, 69
    of cerebral malformations, 145
    of cerebral palsy, 314
    of Chiari malformations, 302–303
    of childhood stroke, 284–285
    of chronic nonprogressive
        encephalopathy, 189–190
    of concussion, 90
    of congenital heart disease, 288
    of congenital hemisphere hypoplasia,
        272
    congenital syndrome, 384, 384f
    of consciousness, altered states, 67,
        90
    of diencephalic gliomas, 376f
    of diskitis (disk space infection), 306,
        307f
    of ependymoma, 270, 313
    of focal clonic seizures, 3
    of foramen magnum tumors, 255
    functional, 55
    in global developmental delay, 143
    of gram-negative sepsis, 69
    of headache, 95
    of hemiconvulsions-hemiplegia
        syndrome, 40–41
    in hemiplegia, 281
    of hereditary spastic paraplegia, 306
    of herpes simplex encephalitis/herpes
        simplex virus (HSV), 72

Magnetic resonance imaging (MRI) (Continued)
  of hypoxic-ischemic encephalopathy, 10
  in limb-girdle muscular dystrophy R2, 217
  of lumbar disc herniation, 256
  of lumbar plexitis, 319
  of multiple sclerosis, 265f
  of neurosarcoidosis, 390f
  of Pendred syndrome, 395
  of perinatal stroke, 282–283
  of postconcussion syndrome, 268
  of progressive encephalopathies with onset before age two, 152
  of shaking injuries, 90
  of spinal epidural hematoma, 312
  of spinal muscular atrophies, 318
  in spinal paraplegia, 300
  of sulfatide lipidosis, juvenile, 277
  supratentorial brain tumors, 120–121
  of syringomyelia, 256, 256f
  of Takayasu arteritis, 294–295
  of tethered spinal cord, 305
  of transverse myelitis, 310
  of tuberculous osteomyelitis, 307
  of X-linked cerebellar hypoplasia, 273
Magnetoencephalography (MEG), 55
Malignant hyperthermia (MH), 246
Mannitol, 120
Maple syrup urine disease (MSUD), 154–155
  ataxia, 262
  branched-chain amino acids disorders, 11–12
  intermittent, 262
  isovaleric acidemia mimicking, 12
Marcus-Gunn phenomenon, 351
Marie ataxia, 274–275
Marijuana, 4–5, 89, 107–108
Marinesco-Sjögren syndrome, 277
Marshall syndrome, 368
Mass immunization, 394
McArdle disease, 219, 241
McLeod syndrome, 332
MECP2 duplication syndrome, 150, 188

Medial longitudinal fasciculus (MLF), 360
Median neuropathy, 323
Medical treatment, ICP
  acutely increased ICP management, 119
  decompressive craniectomy, 120
  head elevation, 119
  homeostasis, 119
  hyperosmolar therapy, 120
  hyperventilation, 119–120
  hypothermia, 120
  ICP monitoring, 119
  pentobarbital coma, 120
  severe traumatic brain injury, 118–119
Medications
  immunosuppressive, 87
  status epilepticus, 51–54
Medium-chain acyl-coenzyme A dehydrogenase (MCAD) deficiency, 83–84
Medulloblastoma, 124
  ataxia, 271–272, 271f
MEG. See Magnetoencephalography
Megalencephalic leukoencephalopathy with subcortical cysts, 414–415
Megalencephaly (PIK3CA-related overgrowth spectrum), 412–414
  achondroplasia as, 412–413
  benign familial macrocephaly as, 413
  with gigantism, 413
  in glutaric acidemia type I, 337
  megalencephaly with gigantism as, 413
  metabolic, 414–415
  neurocutaneous disorders as, 413–414
Melkersson Rosenthal syndrome, 388–389
Meningeal malignancy, 406–407
Meningioma, 126
Meningismus, 65
  bacterial meningitis, 76
Meningitis
  aseptic, 75–76

Meningitis (Continued)
  bacterial, acquired hearing impairment from, 396
  basilar, 389
  common viruses causing, 75
Meningococcus, bacterial meningitis and, 133
Meningoencephalitis, 70
Menkes syndrome, 169
Menstrual cycle, migraine, 98
Mermaid syndrome, 302
Metabolic acidosis, 80–86
Metabolic disorders
  adrenomyeloneuropathy, 308
  arginase deficiency, 308
  spinal paraplegia and, 308
  and systemic disease, 80–86
Metabolic encephalopathies, 85–86
Metabolic megalencephaly, 414–415
Metabolic myopathies, 219–220
  acid maltase deficiency, 185–186
  carbohydrate myopathies, 219
  carnitine deficiency, 219–220
  enzyme deficiencies, 213
  late-onset Pompe disease, 219
Metabolic neuropathies, 254–255
Metabolism, long-chain fatty acid metabolism defects, 242–243
Metachromatic leukodystrophy, 172–173, 173f, 223
  juvenile, 277
Metastases, in brain, 125–126
Methadone, 4–5
Methylmalonic acidemia, 12–13
Methylphenidate, 4–5, 434
Methylprednisolone, 77
Metoclopramide, 331, 333–334
Mexiletine, for myotonia congenita, 239
MH. See Malignant hyperthermia
Michel defect, 394
Microcephaly, 415–420, 415b
  anencephaly in, 416
  chromosomal disorders and, 416
  defective prosencephalization as, 417–419
  encephalocele as, 416–417
  primary, 415–416
  secondary, 419–420

Microcephaly (Continued)
  vera (microcephaly primary
    hereditary), 415–416
Microsomal triglyceride transfer
    protein (MTTP), 275
Middle cerebral artery (MCA), 282
Middle ear, 391
Migraine
  acute attack, treating, 100–101
  ataxia, 263–264
  with aura, 99
  benign paroxysmal vertigo, 263–264
  with brainstem aura, 263
  in children, 26
  clinical syndromes, 98–99
  coma, 86
  complicated, 295–296
  diagnosis, 99–100
  equivalents, 98b
  exercise, 98
  extended, 105
  familial hemiplegic, 295–296
  genetic factors, 97–103
  head trauma, 98
  hemiplegia and, 295–296
  in infants and young children, 26
  management, 100–103
  menstrual cycle, 98
  ocular, 375
  ophthalmic, 375
  prophylaxis, 101–103
  retinal, 375
  stress, 98
  triggering factors, 98
  without aura, 99
Migraine coma, 98
Migraine prophylaxis, 101–103
  amitriptyline, 101
  botulinum toxin, 103
  calcitonin gene- related peptide
    receptor, 102
  calcitonin gene-related peptide
    molecule, 102
  calcitonin gene-related peptide
    receptor antagonists, 102
  cyproheptadine, 102
  levetiracetam, 102
  nerve blocks, 102–103

Migraine prophylaxis (Continued)
  propranolol, 102
  topiramate, 102
  valproate, 102
  zonisamide, 102
Miller Fisher syndrome, 264–265
Miller-Dieker syndrome, 418
Minocycline, vertigo and, 399
Mirror movements, 340
Mitchell and Pike OMS rating scale,
    341b
Mitochondrial disorders/myopathies
  clinical features, 244b
  decreased muscle energy, 243–244,
    243f, 244b
  mitochondrial encephalopathy, lactic
    acidosis and stroke, 291
  in progressive encephalopathies
    with onset before age two,
    161–163
Mitochondrial encephalomyopathies,
    177
Mitochondrial encephalopathy, lactic
    acidosis and stroke, 291
Mitral valve disease, 289
MLF. See Medial longitudinal
    fasciculus
Möbius syndrome, 350, 384–385
Modafinil, 28
Molecular genetic testing, 26
Mondini defect, 394
Monocular nystagmus, 363–365
Mononeuropathies, 322–324
Monoplegia, 317–324
  acute, differential diagnosis of, 318b
  approach to, 317
  arteriovenous malformations and,
    301
  lethargy and coma, 66
  monomelic amyotrophy (Hirayama
    disease), 317–318
  in painful limb, 250–252
  plexopathies. See Plexopathies
Monosynaptic reflex, 183
Morning glory disk, 370
Moro reflex, 4, 23, 187
Morquio syndrome, 301–302
Morvan syndrome, 238

Motor unit, 183
  continuous motor unit activity,
    237–238, 241
Motor unit disorders
  clues to, 187, 187b
  congenital myopathies, 199–202
  disorders of neuromuscular
    transmission, 198–199
  electrodiagnosis, 193
  evaluation of, 193b
  in facial weakness and dysphagia,
    383
  metabolic myopathies, 204–205
  milestones, failure to meet, 197
  muscle biopsy, 194
  muscular dystrophies, 202–204
  nerve biopsy, 194
  with perinatal respiratory distress,
    186b
  polyneuropathies, 197–198, 197b
  serum creatine kinase, 193
  spinal muscular atrophies, 194–197
  tendon reflexes, 187
  Tensilon test, 194
  transitory neonatal myasthenia, 199
Movement disorders, 325–347
  approach to the patient in, 325–326
  athetosis in, 328–333, 330b
  chorea in, 325, 328–333, 330b
  in drowsiness and sleep, 343
  dyskinesia in, 325
  dystonia in, 325, 333–340, 334b
  mirror movements in, 340
  paroxysmal, 325–326
  restless legs syndrome in, 343–344
  stereotypies in, 327–328
  tics and Tourette syndrome in,
    325–327
  tremor in, 325, 344–345
Moyamoya disease, 291–292, 292f
MRA. See Magnetic resonance
    angiography
MRI. See Magnetic resonance imaging
MS. See Multiple sclerosis
MSUD. See Maple syrup urine disease
MTTP. See Microsomal triglyceride
    transfer protein
Mucolipidosis type II, 159

Mucopolysaccharidoses, 159–160, 173–174
Multifocal clonic seizures, 3
Multifocal myoclonus, 342
Multi-minicore disease, 200–201
Multi-minicore myopathy, 246
Multiple sclerosis (MS), 309f
  ataxia, 265–266, 265f
  in transverse myelitis, 309
Muscle activity, abnormal, 237–240, 238b
  continuous motor unit activity, 237–238
  outline of diseases, 237b
  systemic disorders, 239–240
Muscle biopsy, 194
  hypotonia, 199
  progressive proximal weakness, 210
Muscle energy, decreased, 237b, 240–244, 240f
  carbohydrate utilization defects, 241–242
  clinical features, 241
  long-chain fatty acid metabolism defects, 242–243
  mitochondrial myopathies, 243–244, 243f, 244b
  myoadenylate deaminase deficiency, 244
Muscle fibers, structural protein, 213f
Muscle phosphoglycerate mutase deficiency (PGAM), 241–242
Muscle stiffness
  defined, 236
  electromyography, 237b
  myopathic, 244–247
Muscle weakness, 211
Muscle-eye-brain disease, 203–204
Muscular dystrophy
  Bethlem myopathy, 213–214
  collagen type VI-related dystrophy, 203
  congenital dystrophinopathy, 202
  congenital muscular dystrophy, 202
  congenital myotonic dystrophy, 185–186
  dystrophinopathies, 214–216

Muscular dystrophy (Continued)
  Emery-Dreifuss muscular dystrophy, 226–227
  Fukuyama congenital muscular dystrophy, 203
  Fukuyama muscular dystrophy, 203
  hyporeflexia, 209
  LAMA2 muscular dystrophy, 202–203
  spasticity, with hyperreflexia, 209
  tubulinopathies, 203
  Ullrich congenital muscular dystrophy, 203
Mutase deficiency, 13
Myasthenia gravis
  congenital, 351
  immune-mediated, 212
  mitochondrial disorders, 243–244
  in postviral cranial nerve VI palsy, 355–356
  symptoms, 237
Myasthenic crisis, 355
Myasthenic syndromes, 212–213
  limb-girdle myasthenia, 212
  slow-channel congenital myasthenic syndrome, 212–213
Mycoplasma pneumoniae, 285, 328
Myelin oligodendrocyte glycoprotein (MOG), 309–310
Myelomeningocele, congenital malformations and, 303–304
Myoadenylate deaminase deficiency, 244
Myoclonia, eyelid, 31–33
Myoclonic encephalopathy/ neuroblastoma syndrome, 266–267, 266f
Myoclonic epilepsy and ragged-red fibers, 177
Myoclonic seizures
  in children, 33–36
  clonazepam, 47
  in infants and young children, 22–25
  in newborns, 3
Myoclonic-astatic epilepsy, 33
Myoclonus, 340–343
  benign infantile, in newborns, 4
  chorea and, 331

Myoclonus (Continued)
  epileptic, 340
  hereditary essential, 342
  hypnagogic, 28
  in infants and young children, 22–25
  nonepileptic, 340
  opsoclonus-myoclonus-ataxia syndrome, 341–342
  palatal, 343
  persistent early-onset, 66
  physiological, 340
  postanoxic action myoclonus, 67
  posthypoxic, 342
  progressive myoclonus epilepsies, 35–36, 35b
  rhythmic, 340
  segmental (focal), 342–343
  spinal, 300
  symptomatic, 342–343
Myoedema, 240
Myoglobinuria, 241
Myokymia, 240
  and paroxysmal ataxia, 260
Myopathic stiffness, and cramps, 244–247
Myopathies, 183, 225–227
  autosomal recessive distal myopathy, 225–227
    dysferlinopathies, 225–226
    emery-dreifuss muscular dystrophy, 226–227
    myotonic dystrophy, 226
    nebulin myopathy, 226
  Brody myopathy, 245
  carbohydrate, 219
  endocrine, 220
  hereditary distal myopathies, 225
  inflammatory, 217–219
  Laing early-onset distal myopathy, 225
  lipid, 220
  metabolic, 219–220
  mitochondrial, 243–244, 243f, 244b
  myotubular (centronuclear) myopathy, 201–202
  nemaline (rod) myopathy, 199–200, 200f
Myophosphorylase deficiency, 241

Myotonia congenita, 238–239
Myotonia fluctuans, 239
Myotonic disorders, 238–239
Myotonic dystrophy, 226
Myotonic dystrophy 2, 217
Myotubular (centronuclear) myopathy, 201–202
Myozyme, 219

N

Naproxen, headache, 100
Narcolepsy, 27–28
Nausea, anticonvulsants, 45
NCV. *See* Nerve conduction velocity
Nebulin myopathy, 226
Neck injuries, 110
Neck muscles, weakness in, 209
Necrotizing fasciitis, 285
Needle electromyography (EMG), in spinal muscular atrophies, 318
Negative myoclonus, 340
Nemaline (rod) myopathy, 199–200, 200f
Neonatal abstinence syndrome, 4–5
Neonatal cord infarction, 308–309
Neonatal hemorrhage, 283
Neonatal traumatic brachial neuropathy, 320–321
Neostigmine, congenital myasthenic syndromes, 198–199
Nerve biopsy, hypotonia, 194
Nerve blocks, 102–103
Nerve conduction velocity (NCV), 76
Nerve root pain, 249
Nerve stimulation studies, repetitive, in myasthenia gravis, 355
Neuralgic amyotrophy, 318
Neuroacanthocytosis, 332–333
Neuroblastoma, 313
Neuroborreliosis, Lyme disease, 70
Neurocutaneous disorders, 413–414
epidermal nevus syndrome in, 414
hypomelanosis of Ito in, 413–414
in progressive encephalopathies with onset before age two, 163–166
seizures in infancy, 23b

Neuroferritinopathy, in pantothenate kinase-associated neurodegeneration, 339
Neurofibromatosis type 1 (NF1), 163–164, 164f
optic gliomas and, 376, 376f
Neurofibromatosis type I, 122
Neurogenic arthrogryposis, 196
Neuroleptic malignant syndrome, 246
Neuromuscular blockade, 230–231
Neuromuscular disease
clinical features of, 208–210
Gower sign, 209f
initial complaint, 208–209
physical findings, 209–210
signs of, 210b
symptoms of, 209b. *See also* Limb weakness
Neuromuscular transmission, disorders of, 198–199
Neuromyelitis optica (Devic disease), 372–373
Neuromyotonia, 238
Neuronal ceroid lipofuscinoses (NCLs), 166
Neuronal depression, migraine, 99
Neuronal excitability, decreased/increased, 62–63, 62t
Neuronal tumors, 122–124
Neuronitis, 400
Neuronopathy, 183, 222
diagnosis in, 220–221
juvenile amyotrophic lateral sclerosis, 222
Neuropathy, 183
acute ataxic neuropathy, 264
Charcot-Marie-Tooth inherited, 222–223
compressive optic, 375–377
congenital hypomyelinating neuropathy, 197–198
deafness-dystonia-optic neuronopathy syndrome as, 396
demyelinating optic, 372–373
diagnosis in, 220–221
drug-induced, 224
genetic, 223–224

Neuropathy (*Continued*)
hereditary, 249
with liability to pressure palsy, 319–320, 323–324
optic, 377
ischemic optic, 373
lipid disorders, 223–224
median, 323
metabolic, 254–255
metachromatic leukodystrophy, 223
neonatal traumatic brachial neuropathy, 320–321
optic, 372–373
peroneal, 323
polyneuropathies, 197–198
radial, 322–323
recurrent, causes of, 383b
sensory and autonomic, 252–254
with systemic disease, 224–225
toxic-nutritional optic, 373–374
ulnar, 323
uremia, 240
Neuroretinitis, 373, 373f
Neurosarcoidosis, 390f
Neurotoxicity, 88
Newborns
apnea, 4
benign nocturnal myoclonus, 4
bilirubin encephalopathy, 7–8
encephalopathies
bilirubin, 7–8
hypoglycemia, 8–9
hypoxic-ischemic, 9–10
with familial dysautonomia, 383
focal clonic seizures, 3
folinic acid dependency, 14
hemorrhage
intracranial/intraventricular, 3, 15–16
subarachnoid, 15–16
subdural, 16
herpes simplex encephalitis, 14–15
hypocalcemia, 8
hypoxic-ischemic encephalopathy, 9–10
idiopathic cerebral venous thrombosis, 15

Newborns *(Continued)*
  incontinentia pigmenti (Bloch–
    Sulzberger syndrome), 16
  intracranial/intraventricular
    hemorrhage in, 3, 15–16
  isovaleric acidemia, 12
  jitteriness, 4
  maple syrup urine disease, 11–12
  methylmalonic acidemia, 12–13
  multifocal clonic seizures, 3
  myoclonic seizures, 3
  neonatal abstinence syndrome, 4–5
  neonatal hemorrhage, 283
  neonatal traumatic brachial
    neuropathy in, 320–321
  organic acid disorders and
    aminoacidopathies, 10–16
  paroxysmal disorders, 2–5
  perinatal infections seizures, 14
  propionic acidemia, 13–14
  pyridoxine dependency, 14
  seizure-like events, 4–5
  seizures in
    benign familial, 7
    differential diagnosis, 5–8
    differential diagnosis by peak time
      of onset, 6b
    due to metabolic derangements,
      8–9
    duration of therapy for, 17–18
    inborn errors of metabolism, 6b
    patterns, 2–4, 2b
    treatment, 16–18
  spinal cord injury in, 192–193
  subarachnoid hemorrhage, primary,
    15–16
  subdural hemorrhage, 16
  tonic seizures, 3–4
  trauma, 15–16
  vitamin-dependent seizures, 14
Nicotinamide adenine dinucleotide
  (NAD), 240–241
Niemann-Pick disease type C
  (sphingomyelin lipidosis),
  174–175
Night cramps, 236
Night sleep, disturbed, 28
Night terrors, 28–29

Nitrofurantoin, neuropathy and, 224
NKX2.1-related choreiform disorders,
  331–332
Nodular heterotopia, bilateral
  periventricular, 418, 418f
Noncommunicating hydrocephalus,
  407–412
  congenital aqueductal stenosis in,
    407–408, 408f
  congenital brain tumors and, 410
  Dandy-Walker malformation and,
    408–409, 409f
  fibroblast growth factor receptor-
    associated craniosynostosis
    syndromes, 408
  hydranencephaly and, 411
  Klippel-Feil syndrome and, 409–410
  porencephaly and, 411–412
  vein of Galen malformation and,
    410–411, 411f
  Walker-Warburg syndrome and, 411
  X-linked hydrocephalus (L1
    syndrome) in, 408
Nonepileptic myoclonus, 340
Nonfixed torticollis, 334–335
Nonketotic hyperglycinemia, 11
Nonparalytic strabismus, 348–349
Nonrapid eye movement (non-REM)
  sleep, 28
Nonsteroidal antiinflammatory drugs,
  251
Nonstimulant medications
  atomoxetine (strattera), 435
  clonidine and guanfacine, 435
  viloxazine (qelbree), 435
Normal self-stimulatory behavior,
  19–20
Null point, in congenital nystagmus,
  362–363
Nystagmus, 361–363, 362t
  acquired, 363–365
  congenital, 361–363
  differential diagnosis of, 362b
  dissociated, 365
  divergence, 365
  downbeat, 364–365
  drug-induced, 363–364
  examination, 65

Nystagmus *(Continued)*
  ictal, 364
  jerk, 361–362
  monocular, 365
  pendular, 363–364
  physiological, 362
  see-saw, 365
  spasmus nutans in, 363
  upbeat, 365
  vestibular, 345

O
Obsessive-compulsive behavior in
  Sydenham (rheumatic)
  chorea, 329–330
Obsessive-compulsive disorder
  (OCD)
  clinical features, 426–427
  diagnosis, 427
  management, 427
  obsessions and compulsions, 427
  prevalence of, 426
  treatment, 431–433
Obsessive-compulsive traits, in autism/
  autistic spectrum disorders,
  142
Occipital fracture, 92
Occipital nerve blocks, 103
Octreotide, 103
Ocular alignment, in nonparalytic
  strabismus, 348
Ocular bobbing, 362
Ocular dysmetria, 362
Ocular flutter, 362
Ocular migraine, 375
Ocular motility disorders, 348–366
  assessment, in coma, 66
  nonparalytic strabismus in, 348–349
  nystagmus in, 362b, 362t
  ophthalmoplegia in, 349–361, 349t
Ocular motor apraxia, 359–360
Ocular myasthenia, 355
Oculocerebrorenal syndrome (Lowe
  syndrome), 190–191
Oculomotor apraxia type 1, with ataxia,
  276
Oculomotor apraxia type 2, with ataxia,
  276

Oculomotor nerve palsy/III cranial nerve, 349–350
Office testing, 392
OKT3 meningoencephalitis, 88
Olanzapine, 331
Olanzapine (zyprexa), 430
Olivopontocerebellar atrophy (OPCA), 274–275
Ondine curse, 65
One-and-a-half syndrome, 360
OPCA. *See* Olivopontocerebellar atrophy
Open head injuries, 92, 92*f*
Ophthalmic migraine, 375
Ophthalmoplegia, 349–361, 349*t*
  abducens nerve palsy/VI cranial nerve in, 350
  acquired, causes of, 352*b*
  acute bilateral, 357–358, 357*b*
  acute unilateral, 352–355, 353*b*
  aneurysm in, 353
  apraxia of horizontal gaze in, 359
  botulism in, 358
  brainstem glioma in, 353–354, 354*f*
  brainstem stroke in, 354
  Brown syndrome in, 350
  carotid-cavernous sinus fistula in, 354
  cavernous sinus thrombosis in, 354
  chronic bilateral, 358–359, 358*b*
  congenital, 349–352
  congenital fibrosis of the extraocular muscles in, 350–351
  congenital myasthenia gravis in, 351
  congenital ocular motor apraxia in, 359–360
  congenital ptosis in, 351–352, 352*b*
  congenital vertical ocular motor apraxia in, 361
  convergence paralysis in, 361
  gaze palsies in, 359–361, 360*b*
  Gradenigo syndrome in, 354–355
  horizontal gaze palsy in, 361
  internuclear, 360
  intoxications in, 358
  Kearns-Sayre syndrome in, 359
  oculomotor nerve palsy/III cranial nerve in, 349–350

Ophthalmoplegia *(Continued)*
  thyroid ophthalmopathy in, 358–359
  toxic-metabolic disorders in, 360
  trochlear nerve palsy/IV cranial nerve in, 350
  vertical gaze palsy in, 361
Opioid overdose, 88
Opisthotonos, 3, 66
Oppositional defiant disorder (ODD)
  clinical features, 430
  diagnosis, 430–431
  overview, 430
  treatment, 431
Opsoclonus, 362
Opsoclonus-myoclonus-ataxia syndrome (OMAS), 341–342
Optic disc edema, 116–117, 116*b*, 117*f*
Optic nerve hypoplasia, congenital, 369–370, 370*f*
Optic neuritis, 372–373
Optic neuropathies, 372–374
  compressive, 375–377
  demyelinating, 372–373
  hereditary, 377
  ischemic, 373
  toxic-nutritional, 373–374
Optic pathway gliomas, 376–377
Oral contraceptives, headache, 98
Orbital tumors, in postviral cranial nerve VI palsy, 357
Orexin (hypocretin), 28
Organ of Corti, 391
Organic acid disorders and aminoacidopathies, newborns, 10–16
  branched-chain amino acids disorders, 11–12
  folinic acid dependency, 14
  herpes simplex encephalitis, 14–15
  idiopathic cerebral venous thrombosis, 15
  incontinentia pigmenti, 16
  isovaleric acidemia, 12
  methylmalonic acidemia, 12–13
  nonketotic hyperglycinemia, 11
  perinatal infections seizures, 14

Organic acid disorders and aminoacidopathies, newborns *(Continued)*
  primary subarachnoid hemorrhage, 15–16
  propionic acidemia, 13–14
  pyridoxine dependency, 14
  trauma and intracranial hemorrhage, 15–16
  vitamin-dependent seizures, 14
Orthotopic liver transplantation, 191–192
Osmolality disorders, 80–82
Osmophobia, migraine, 99–100
Osteomyelitis-neuritis, 321
Otitis media, 396
Overshoot dysmetria, 360
Oxcarbazepine (antiepileptic)
  administration, 49
  adverse effects, 49
  carbamazepine compared, 38
  indications for, 49
  newborns, treatment, 17
  temporal lobe epilepsy, 41
Oxidation-phosphorylation coupling, 240–241

P
Pachygyria, 418, 419*f*
Pain
  arm, 320
  complex regional pain syndrome, 250–251
  congenital insensitivity to with anhidrosis, 253–254
  from cranial structures, 109–110
  in diskitis (disk space infection), 306
  growing pains, 236
  indifference to (central congenital insensitivity), 252–255
  limb, 250–252, 254
  SCN9A neuropathic pain syndromes, 251–252
  thalamic, 257
Palatal myoclonus, 343
Pallid syncope, 19
Panayiotopoulos syndrome, 39
Panic disorder, 87

Pantothenate kinase-associated neurodegeneration (PKAN), 176, 339, 339f
Papilledema, 116, 116b, 117f, 269–270
Paralysis
    convergence, 361
    sleep, 28
Paraplegia, 299–316. *See also* Quadriplegia
    approach to, 299
    cerebral, 313–315
    congenital malformations of, 300–305
    defined, 299
    hereditary spastic paraplegia, 305–308
    metabolic disorders, 308
    in motor development, delayed, 143
    neonatal cord infarction, 308–309
    spastic diplegia, 314–315
    spinal. *See* Spinal paraplegia
    transverse myelitis, 309–310
Parathyroid disorders, 82
Parents, telling bad news to, 143–152
Parinaud syndrome, 361
Parkinsonism
    in pathological tremors, 344
    in tremor, 344
Paroxetine (paxil), 434
Paroxysmal disorders, 1–60
    approach to, 1–2
    ataxia, and myokymia, 260
    of childhood
        eyelid myoclonia with/without absences, 31–33
        focal seizures, 36–41
        generalized seizures, 41–43
        hyperventilation syndrome, 29
        juvenile myoclonic epilepsy, 33–34, 54f
        myoclonic seizures, 33–36
        paroxysmal dyskinesias, 26–27
        progressive myoclonus epilepsies, 35–36, 35b
        sleep disorders, 27–29
        staring spells, 30–31
        stiff infant syndrome, 20
        syncope, 29–30

Paroxysmal disorders (Continued)
    in infants and young children
        apneic seizures, 18
        benign myoclonic epilepsy, 25
        benign spasms, 25
        biotinidase deficiency, 25–26
        breath-holding spells, 18–19
        epileptic encephalopathy (early) with burst suppression, 25
        febrile seizures, 20–21
        infantile spasms, 22–25
        Lennox-Gastaut syndrome, 34–35
        migraine, 26
        myoclonus, spasms and myoclonic seizures, 22–26
        normal self-stimulatory behavior, 19–20
        severe myoclonic epilepsy, 25
        syncope, 18–19
    ketogenic diet, 54–55
    in newborns
        apnea, 4
        benign familial neonatal seizures, 7
        benign nocturnal myoclonus, 4
        differential diagnosis of seizures, 5–8
        focal clonic seizures, 3
        folinic acid dependency, 14
        herpes simplex encephalitis, 14–15
        hypocalcemia, 8
        hypoglycemia, 8–9, 8b
        hypoxic-ischemic encephalopathy, 9–10
        idiopathic cerebral venous thrombosis, 15
        incontinentia pigmenti (Bloch–Sulzberger syndrome), 16
        isovaleric acidemia, 12
        jitteriness, 4
        methylmalonic acidemia, 12–13
        multifocal clonic seizures, 3
        myoclonic seizures, 3
        neonatal abstinence syndrome, 4–5
        organic acid disorders and aminoacidopathies, 10–16
        perinatal infections seizures, 14

Paroxysmal disorders (Continued)
        propionic acidemia, 13–14
        pyridoxine dependency, 14
        seizures due to metabolic derangements, 8–9
        subarachnoid hemorrhage, 15–16
        subdural hemorrhage, 16
        tonic seizures, 3
        trauma and intracranial hemorrhage, 15–16
        vitamin-dependent seizures, 14
    pathophysiology, 18–21, 18b
    status epilepticus, management, 51–54
    surgical approaches, 55–56
    vagal nerve stimulation, 55
Paroxysmal dyskinesias, in children, 26–27
Paroxysmal dystonic head tremor, 345
Paroxysmal exertion-induced dyskinesia, 27
Paroxysmal kinesiogenic dyskinesia, 26–27
Paroxysmal nonkinesiogenic dyskinesia (PNKD), familial, 27
Parsonage-Turner syndrome, 318–319
Patent foramen ovale (PFO), 288
Pediatric acute-onset neuropsychiatric syndrome (PANS), 328, 427
Pediatric autoimmune neuropsychiatric disorder related to streptococcal infection (PANDAS), 328
Pediatric infection triggered autoimmune neuropsychiatric disorders (PITANDS), 328
Pelizaeus-Merzbacher disease, 170–171
Pendred syndrome, 395
Pendular nystagmus, 363–364
Penetrating fracture, 92
Penicillin, Lyme disease, 70
Pentobarbital coma, 120
Perampanel (antiepileptic), 49
Perifascicular atrophy, dermatomyositis, 218, 218f
Perinatal brain injuries, in secondary microcephaly, 420
Perinatal disorders, 145

Periodic breathing, 4
Periodic lateralizing epileptiform
    discharges (PLEDs), 65
Periodic limb movements in sleep
    (PLMS), 20
Periodic paralyses, 231–233
    Andersen-Tawil syndrome, 232–233
    familial hyperkalemic periodic
        paralysis type 1, 232
    familial hypokalemic periodic
        paralysis, 231–232
    familial normokalemic periodic
        paralysis, 232
Periventricular-intraventricular
    hemorrhage, in premature
    newborns, 126–128, 127b
Peroneal neuropathy, 323
Peroxisomal biogenesis disorders, 191
Peroxisomal disorders, 191
Peroxisomes, 191
Persistent focal dystonias, 333
Persistent vegetative state (PVS), 68
PET. See Positron emission tomography
PFO. See Patent foramen ovale
Phasic tone, 183
Phencyclidine (angel dust), 89
Phenobarbital (antiepileptic)
    administration, 49
    adverse effects, 49
    indications for, 49
    neonatal abstinence syndrome, 4–5
    neonatal seizures, 17
    newborns, treatment, 17
    and primidone, 50
Phenothiazine, 331
Phenylethylmalonamide (PEMA), 50
Phenylketonuria, 155–156, 155f
Phenytoin (antiepileptic)
    administration, 49
    adverse effects, 49–50
    indications for, 49
    metabolism, 44
    neonatal seizures, 17
    newborns, treatment, 17
Phosphofructokinase deficiency (PFK),
    241–242
Photophobia, migraine, 99
PHQ-9 patient screening tool, 424b

Physical examination, of progressive
    encephalopathies with onset
    before age two, 152
Physiological myoclonus, 340
Physiological nystagmus, 362
Physiological tremor, 344
PIK3CA-related overgrowth spectrum
    (PROS), 412
Pineal region tumors, 125
Pituitary adenoma, 377
Pituitary apoplexy, blindness from, 374
Plagiocephaly, 420
Plasma exchange, 199
PLEDs. See Periodic lateralizing
    epileptiform discharges
Plexopathies
    acute idiopathic plexitis, 318–319
    acute symptomatic plexitis, 319–322
    asthmatic amyotrophy (Hopkins
        syndrome), 319
    brachial plexitis, 250, 318–319
    brachial plexus, 321–322
    hereditary brachial plexopathy,
        319–320
    lumbar plexitis, 319
    lumbar plexus, 322
    mononeuropathies, 322–324
    plexus tumors, 322, 322f
Plexus tumors, 322, 322f
PLMS. See Periodic limb movements
    in sleep
PNETs. See Primitive neuroectodermal
    tumors
Pneumococcus, bacterial meningitis
    and, 133
Poisoning, 89
Poland anomaly, 385
POLG-related disorders, 162–163
Polycystic ovary syndrome, 102
Polymyositis, 218–219
Pompe disease, 204–205. See also Acid
    maltase deficiency
Pontobulbar palsy with deafness,
    387–388
Porencephaly, 411–412
Positive myoclonus, 340
Positron emission tomography (PET),
    40–41

Postanoxic action myoclonus, 67
Postconcussion syndrome, 268
Posterior fossa
    decompression of, 303
    epidural hemorrhage, 91
    increased pressure in, 118
    primary tumors of, 120
Posterior reversible encephalopathy
    syndrome (PRES), 85
Posthypoxic myoclonus, 342
Postictal hemiparesis, 287–288
Postimmunization encephalopathy, 80
Postinfectious/immune-mediated
    disorders, 264–267
Postnatal injuries, 321–322
Postnatal systemic disease, in secondary
    microcephaly, 420
Post-traumatic epilepsy, 92
Post-traumatic headache, 106
Posttraumatic stress disorder (PTSD),
    431
Posttraumatic vision loss, 372–375
Postural orthostatic tachycardia
    syndrome (POTS), 29–30
Postural reflexes, 187
Postural tone, 183
Postviral cranial nerve VI palsy
    myasthenia gravis in, 355–356
    orbital inflammatory disease in,
        356–357
    orbital tumors in, 357
    recurrent painful ophthalmoplegic
        neuropathy, 356
    trauma in, 357
Prader-Willi syndrome, 148–149, 188–
    189, 189b
Prednisone
    for dermatomyositis, 218
    for Duchenne and Becker muscular
        dystrophy, 215
    for infantile spasms, 24–25
    for toxoplasmosis, 148
Pregabalin, 251, 318–319
Pregnancy, chorea in, 333
Premature newborns
    respiratory distress syndrome, 7
    tonic seizures, 3
    traction response in, 184–185

PRES. *See* Posterior reversible encephalopathy syndrome
Prescription drugs overdoses, 88–89
  general diagnostic principles, 88
  general management principles, 88–89
PRICKLE1-related disorders, 36
Primary carnitine deficiency, 83
Primary familial brain calcification, in chorea, 332
Primary microcephaly, 415–416
Primary subarachnoid hemorrhage, 15–16
Primidone (antiepileptic), 50
Primitive neuroectodermal tumors (PNETs), 124, 125*f*, 269–270
Prochlorperazine, 101
  headache, 101, 105
  in tardive dyskinesia, 331
Progressive cavitating leukoencephalopathy, 171
Progressive distal weakness, 220–227, 221*b*
  myopathies, 225–227
  neuronopathy, 222
  neuropathy, 222–225
Progressive hydrocephalus, 171
Progressive myoclonic epilepsy type 1, 36
Progressive proximal weakness, 210–220, 210*b*
  distinguishing features in, 211*t*
  endocrine myopathies, 220
  GM2 gangliosidosis, 212
  inflammatory myopathies, 217–219
  metabolic myopathies, 219–220
  muscular dystrophies, 213–217
  myasthenic syndromes, 212–213
Promethazine, 26, 101, 105
  headache, 101
Propionic acidemia, 13–14
Propranolol, migraine, 102
Prothrombotic states, 289–290
Proximal myotonic dystrophy, 217
Pseudobulbar palsy, 382–383
Pseudo-internuclear ophthalmoplegia, 360
Pseudoseizures, children, 42

Psychiatric disturbances, in hepatolenticular degeneration (Wilson disease), 337
Psychogenic gait disturbances (conversion reaction), 259–260
Psychogenic headache, 105–106
Psychogenic (functional) movement disorders
  biopsychosocial model, 433
  clinical features, 433
  diagnosis, 433
  management, 433
  pseudosleep, 433
Psychogenic nonepileptic spells (PNES), 42
Psychological disorders, 86–87
Psychomotor delay and regression, 141–182
  bad news, telling parents of, 143–152
    15q-related syndromes, 148–149
    autosomal dominant intellectual disability syndromes, 150–151
    autosomal recessive intellectual disabilities, 151–152
    cerebral malformations, 145
    child approach with developmental delay, 144–152
    COVID-19 (SARS-CoV-2), 148
    intrauterine infections, 145–148
    perinatal disorders, 145
    static encephalopathy, genetic causes of, 148
    X-linked developmental disorders, 149–150
  developmental delay, 141–143. *See also* Developmental delay
    delayed motor development, 143
    global, 143
    language delay, 141–143
  gray matter disorders. *See* Gray matter disorders
  progressive encephalopathies with onset after age two, 152–158
    infectious disease, 175
    lysosomal enzyme disorders, 171–175

Psychomotor delay and regression *(Continued)*
  progressive encephalopathies with onset before age two, 152–158
    acquired immunodeficiency syndrome (AIDS) encephalopathy, 152–153
    amino acid metabolism disorders, 153–156
    history and physical examination, 152, 152*f*
    hypothyroidism, 161
    lysosomal enzyme disorders, 156–158
    mitochondrial disorders, 161–163
    neurocutaneous disorders, 163–166
    neuronal ceroid-lipofuscinosis, early infantile, 166–168
    subacute necrotizing encephalomyelopathy, 163
    white matter disorders. *See* White matter disorders
Ptosis
  causes of, 352*b*
  congenital, 351–352
Pulseless disease (Takayasu arteritis), 294–295
Pupil
  disorders of, 379–380
    aniridia as, 379
    benign essential anisocoria as, 379
    examining, 65
    fixed, dilated pupil as, 379
    Horner syndrome as, 379–380
    tonic pupil syndrome (Adie syndrome) as, 380
  examining, 65
Pupillary disorders, Horner syndrome, 66
Pupillary reflex, absent in comatose patient, 66
Pure-tone audiometry, 392
Purkinje cells, 67
PVS. *See* Persistent vegetative state
Pyridostigmine, congenital myasthenic syndromes, 198–199

Pyridoxine
    dependency, 14
    for drug-induced neuropathy, 224
Pyrimethamine (Daraprim), 148
Pyruvate carboxylase deficiency,
        191–192
Pyruvate dehydrogenase deficiency
        (PDH), ataxia, 262–263
Pyschogenic nonepileptic spells (PNES)
    clinical features, 431–432
    diagnosis, 432
    overview, 431
    treatment, 432–433

Q
Quadriplegia, 299–316
    arginase deficiency, 308
    cerebral, 313–315
    cerebral palsy, 313–315, 314t
    defined, 299
    spastic, 315
Quetiapine, 331
Quinidine sulfate, 213

R
Rabies encephalitis, 73
Radial neuropathy, 322–323
Radiography, cervical spine, 110
Radioisotope bone scanning, in spinal
        paraplegia, 300
Ragged-red fibers
    in mitochondrial encephalopathy,
        lactic acidosis and stroke, 291
    mitochondrial myopathies, 244, 244f
Ramsay Hunt syndrome, 389. See also
        Herpes zoster oticus
Rapid eye movement (REM) sleep,
        27–28
Rapid-onset dystonia-parkinsonism,
        339
Rasmussen syndrome
        (hemiconvulsions-
        hemiplegia), 40–41
Reading epilepsy, 41
Receptive skills, in language
        development, 141–142
Recurrent painful ophthalmoplegic
        neuropathy, 356

Refixation reflex, 368
Reflex asystole, pallid syncope, 19
Reflex sympathetic dystrophy (complex
        regional pain syndrome), 250
Reflux, 18
Refractive errors, eyestrain, 109
Refsum disease, 278
Renal disorders
    consciousness, altered states, 84–85
    hypertension, 109
Repetitive nerve stimulation studies, in
        myasthenia gravis, 355
Respiratory chain (mitochondrial)
        myopathies, 243–244, 243f,
        244b
Respiratory distress, infantile spinal
        muscular atrophy with
        respiratory distress type 1
        (SMARD1), 196
Respiratory distress syndrome,
        premature newborns, 7
Responsiveness, lack of, 62
Restless legs syndrome, 343–344
    benign physiologic myoclonus,
        343–344
    rhythmic movement disorder, 344
Retinal disease, 374–375
Retinal ischemia, 374–375
Retinal migraine, 375
Retinal tear, 375
Retinitis pigmentosa, 275
Retinoblastoma, 378
Retinochoroidal colobomas, 370
Rett syndrome, 168
Reye syndrome, 79–80, 120
Rheumatic chorea, 329–330
Rheumatic heart disease, 289
Rhombencephalitis, 76
Rhythmic myoclonus, 340
Riboflavin transporter deficiency, 388
Rickettsial infections, 70–71
Rifampin, 69
Rigid spine syndrome, 246–247
Riley-Day syndrome, 190
Rinne test, 392
Rippling muscle disease
        (caveolinopathies), 247
Risdiplam, 195–196

Risperidone, 331
Risperidone (risperdal), 430
Rizatriptan, headache, 100
Rocky Mountain spotted fever, 70–71
Rubella embryopathy, 147
Rufinamide
    Dravet syndrome, 22
    selection, 45
RYR1 gene, mutations of, 200

S
Sandhoff disease, 158
Sanfilippo disease (MPS III), 160
Sarcoglycanopathies, 217
Sarcoidosis, 389–390, 390f
Scaphocephaly, 420
SCAs. See Spinocerebellar atrophies
Scheibe defect, 394
Schimmelpenning syndrome, 414
Schizophrenia, 64, 87
    and substance abuse, 89
School-age children, bacterial
        meningitis in, 133
Sciatica, 249
Scissoring, 187
SCN1A-related disorders, 21
SCN9A neuropathic pain syndromes,
        251–252
Scoliosis
    Duchenne and Becker muscular
        dystrophy, 215
    spinal paraplegia and, 300
Secondary microcephaly, 419–420
See-saw nystagmus, 365
Segmental (focal) myoclonus, 342–343
Seizure headache, 110–111
Seizure-like events, newborns
    apnea, 4
    benign infantile myoclonus, 4
    jitteriness, 4
Seizures
    apneic, 18
    benign familial neonatal, 7
    in children
        consciousness, altered states, 67
        febrile, 20–21
        focal clonic, 3
        focal inhibitor, 287

Seizures (Continued)
  generalized, 41–43, 63
  hemiparetic, 287–288
  in infants and young children
    apneic, 18
    febrile, 20–21
    myoclonic, 22–26
    neurocutaneous disorders, 23b
    nonfebrile, 22–26
    normal self stimulatory
      behavior, 19–20
  focal with impaired awareness, 32–33
  movements mimicking, 2b
  multifocal clonic, 3
  myoclonic, 3, 22–26, 33–36
  in newborns
    differential diagnosis, 5–8
    differential diagnosis by peak time
      of onset, 6b
    due to metabolic derangements,
      8–9
    duration of therapy for, 17–18
    inborn errors of metabolism, 6b,
      83–84
    patterns, 2–4, 2b
    seizure-like events, 4–5
    treatment, 16–18
  nonfebrile, 22–26
  parathyroid disorders, 82
  and spells, 1
  subtle, 2
  syncope mimicking, 1, 29–30
  tonic, 3–4
  uncontrolled, 2
Selective serotonin and norepinephrine
    reuptake inhibitors (SSNRIs),
    434
Selective serotonin reuptake inhibitors
    (SSRIs), 142, 433–434
  citalopram (celexa), 434
  escitalopram (lexapro), 434
  fluoxetine (prozac), 433
  fluvoxamine (luvox), 434
  headache, 106
  paroxetine (paxil), 434
  psychological disorders, 87
  sertraline (zoloft), 433
Self-limited childhood epilepsy, 39–40

Sensorineural hearing impairment,
    391–392
Sensory and autonomic disturbances,
    249–257
  central congenital insensitivity
    (indifference) to pain,
    252–255
  complex regional pain syndrome,
    250–251
  familial episodic pain syndromes,
    252
  painful limb, 250–252
  patterns of sensory loss, 250t
  SCN9A neuropathic pain syndromes,
    251–252
  sensation disturbances, 250b
  sensory symptoms, 249–250
  spinal disorders, 255–257
Sentaxin (SETX), 222
Sepiapterin deficiency (DYT-SPH), 336
Sepsis, gram-negative, 69
Septo-optic dysplasia, 369
Sertraline (zoloft), 433
Serum creatine kinase, motor unit
    disorders, 193
Setting-sun sign, 407
Severe generalized weakness, 199
Severe myoclonic epilepsy of infancy, 25
Severe traumatic brain injury, 118–119
SGCE myoclonus-dystonia, 342
Shaking injuries, 90–91
SIADH. See Syndrome of inappropriate
    antidiuretic hormone
    secretion
Sickle cell disease (SCD),
    hypocoagulable states,
    292–293
SIDS. See Sudden infant death
    syndrome
Single-photon emission computed
    tomography, 55
Sinusitis, 109–110
Skeletal disorders, acquired hearing
    impairment from, 396, 398b
Skull fracture, 92
SLC6A1-related neurodevelopmental
    disabilities, 151
SLC22A5 gene, 220

SLE. See Systemic lupus erythematosus
Sleep
  benign infantile myoclonus, 4
  benign physiologic myoclonus of,
    343–344
  disorders, 27–29
  rhythmic movement disorder, 344
Sleepwalking, 28–29
Slow channel syndrome, 198
Slow-channel congenital myasthenic
    syndrome, 212–213
Sly disease (type VII MPS), 174
Small-amplitude nystagmus, 365
Sodium benzoate, glycine
    encephalopathy, 11
Sodium loss, 82
Sonophobia, 99–100
Spasms
  defined, 236
  hemifacial, 335–336
Spasmus nutans, 334–335, 345, 363
Spastic diplegia, 314–315
Spastic paraplegia, 305
Spastic quadriplegia, 315
Spasticity, with hyperreflexia, 209
Speech tests, 393
Spells
  apneic, 4
  breath-holding, 18–19
  and seizures, 1, 19
  staring, 30–31
Spina bifida, spinal paraplegia and, 300
Spinal cord
  arachnoid cysts of, 301
  concussion, 311
  hypoxic-ischemic myelopathy, 192
  injuries, 192–193
    in breech presentation, 192
    in cephalic presentation, 192–193
  tethered, 304–305
  tumors, 312
Spinal disorders, 255–257
  lumbar disc herniation, 255–256
  syringomyelia, 256–257
Spinal epidural hematoma, 312
Spinal muscular atrophies, 211–212
  congenital cervical, 196
  infantile, 194–196, 195f

Spinal muscular atrophies *(Continued)*
 neurogenic arthrogryposis, 196
 with respiratory distress type 1
  (SMARD1), 196
 tendon reflexes in, 317
Spinal myoclonus, 300
Spinal paraplegia
 arachnoid cysts, 301
 arteriovenous malformations of, 301
 atlantoaxial dislocation, 301–302
 caudal regression syndrome, 302
 causes of, 299–315, 300*b*
 congenital malformations of,
  300–305
 hereditary spastic paraplegia,
  305–308
 infections, 306
 metabolic disorders, 308
 neonatal cord infarction, 308–309
 spina bifida, 300
 spinal cord tumors, 312
 symptoms and signs of, 300
 tethered spinal cord, 304–305
 transverse myelitis, 309–310
 trauma, 310–312
Spinocerebellar atrophies (SCAs),
  274–275
Spinocerebellar degenerations, 274–275
Sprengel deformity, 302
Staphylococcus aureus infections
 in diskitis (disk space infection), 306
 gram-negative sepsis, 69
Staring spells, 30–31
Static encephalopathy, 142*b*, 145–152
Status epilepticus
 adverse effects, 53
 defined, 41–42
 diazepam, 52
 hospital-based treatment, 53–54
 initial hospital management, 52
 management, 51–54
 midazolam, 53
 seizure clusters medication, 52
 seizure emergencies, in home, 52
Steppage gait, 209
Stereotypies, 327–328
Stevens-Johnson syndrome, 46, 49–50
Stiff infant syndrome, 20

Stimulant medications
 D-Amphetamines+ amphetamine,
  434
 lisdexamfetamine (vyvanse), 434
 methylphenidate, 434
Strabismus
 increased intracranial pressure in,
  116
 nonparalytic, 348–349
 Prader-Willi syndrome, 188–189
Streptococcus pneumoniae meningitis,
  acquired hearing impairment
  from, 396
Streptomycin, vertigo and, 399
Stress
 headache, 105–106
 as trigger factor for migraine, 98
Stretching of muscle, 236
Strokes
 acute hemiplegia and, 283
 brainstem, in ophthalmoplegia, 354
 causes of, 284*b*
 sickle cell disease, 292–293
Structural protein, of muscle fibers, 213*f*
Stumbling, 209
Sturge-Weber syndrome (SWS),
  296–297
Subacute necrotizing
  encephalomyelopathy, 163
Subacute sclerosing panencephalitis
  (SSPE), 175
Subarachnoid hemorrhage
 increased intracranial pressure, 116,
  128–129
 primary, 15–16
 seizures, differential diagnosis, 5–8
Subarachnoid space, benign
  enlargement of, 404–406, 406*f*
Subdural empyema, 135
Subdural hemorrhage, 91
 in newborns, 16
Substance abuse, 89
Sucking, anatomical considerations in,
  381–382
Sudden infant death syndrome (SIDS),
  84
Suicidal ideation, 424
Sulfadiazine, for toxoplasmosis, 148

Sulfatide lipidosis, 223
 juvenile, 277
Sumatriptan, 103
 headache, 100
Superior oblique palsy, 357
Supratentorial brain tumors, 120–121
Supratentorial epidural hematomas, 91
Supratentorial intracranial vessels, pain
  transmission from, 96
Supratentorial malformations, 130
Supratentorial tumors, 120
Surgical approaches, paroxysmal
  disorders, 55–56
Survival motor neuron 1 gene (SMN1),
  211
Swallowing, anatomical considerations
  in, 381–382
SWS. *See* Sturge-Weber syndrome
Sydenham chorea, 329–330
Symptomatic generalized dystonia,
  339–340
Symptomatic myoclonus, 340, 342–343
Syncope
 in children, 29–30
 cyanotic, in infants and young
  children, 19
 mimicking seizures, 1, 29
 pallid, in infants and young children,
  19
Syndrome of inappropriate antidiuretic
  hormone (SIADH), 81
SYNGAP1-related intellectual disability,
  150
Syphilis, congenital, 146
Syringobulbia, 390
Syringomyelia, 256–257
Systemic arterial pressure, 114
Systemic disorders, in chorea, 333
Systemic lupus erythematosus (SLE)
 consciousness, altered states, 78
 headache, 108
 hemiplegia and, 294

T
Tachycardia, apnea with, 4
Takayasu arteritis, 294–295
Tardive dyskinesia, 331
Tardive dystonia, 334

Tay-Sachs disease, 159

Telangiectasia, 275

Temporal lobe epilepsy, 41

Temporal lobectomy, 55

Temporomandibular joint syndrome (TMJ), 110

Tendon reflexes
   motor unit disorders, 187
   neuromuscular disease, 210
   neuropathy and neuronopathy, 220–221
   in spinal muscular atrophies, 317

Tensilon test, 66, 194

Tension headache, 106–107
   episodic, 109

Termination of pregnancy, *Toxoplasma gondii*, 148

Thalamic pain, 257

Theophylline, 331

Thomsen disease, 238

Thoracolumbar radiographs, in compressed vertebral body fractures, 310–312

Thymectomy, for myasthenia gravis, 356

Thyroid disorders, 82, 239–240

Thyroid ophthalmopathy, in chronic bilateral ophthalmoplegia, 358–359

Tiagabine (antiepileptic), 50

Tick paralysis, 230–231

Tics, 326–327

Tinnitus, 392

Todd paralysis, 287

Toe walking, in Duchenne muscular dystrophy, 209

Tolosa-Hunt syndrome, 387

Tone, 183

Tonic neck reflex, 187

Tonic pupil syndrome (Adie syndrome), 380

Tonic seizures, 3–4

Tonsillectomy, 328

Topiramate (antiepileptic), 50–51, 102
   generalized tonic-clonic seizures, 42
   infantile spasms, 24
   juvenile myoclonic epilepsy, 31
   migraine, 102

Topiramate (antiepileptic) *(Continued)*
   selection, 45

Torticollis, in dystonia, 334–335, 334*b*

Tourette syndrome, 326–327

Toxic encephalopathies, 87–89

Toxic shock syndrome, 71

Toxic-metabolic disorders, 360–361

Toxic-nutritional optic neuropathies, 373–374

Toxins
   facial weakness and dysphagia from, 390
   neuropathy, 224–225

Toxoplasma gondii, 147–148

Toxoplasmosis, 147–148

Traction response, hypotonia, 184–185

Transcranial Doppler (TCD) screening, for sickle cell disease, 293

Transitory lateral rectus palsy, 357

Transitory neonatal myasthenia, 199

Transplantation, renal, 85

Transverse myelitis, 309–310
   Devic disease (neuromyelitis optica), 372–373

Trauma
   altered states of consciousness, 65, 89–92
   to carotid artery, 285–286
   compressed vertebral body fractures, 310–312
   concussion, 90
   facial weakness and dysphagia from, 391
   fracture dislocation and spinal cord transection, 311, 311*f*
   head injuries, severe, 90–92
   hearing impairment from, 396
   hemiplegia, 296
   organic acid disorders, newborns, 15–16
   physical examination, 65
   in postconcussion syndrome, 268
   post-traumatic epilepsy, 92
   post-traumatic headache, 106
   in postviral cranial nerve VI palsy, 357
   retinal, 375
   shaking injuries, 90–91

Trauma *(Continued)*
   spinal cord concussion, 311
   spinal epidural hematoma, 312
   spinal paraplegia and, 310–312
   as trigger factor for migraine, 98
   to vertebral artery, 286
   vertigo from, 401

Traumatic brain injury (TBI), 118–119

Tremor, 344–345
   essential (familial), 344–345
   paroxysmal dystonic head, 329–330

Trichloroethylene, 390

Tricyclic antidepressants, 88–89

Trigeminal nerve, 96, 115–116

Trochlear nerve palsy/IV cranial nerve, 350

Tuberculous meningitis, 133–134

Tuberculous osteomyelitis, 307–308

Tuberous sclerosis, 122, 164–166, 165*f*, 166*b*

Tuberous sclerosis complex (TSC), 166*b*

Tubular aggregates, and cramps, 245, 245*f*

Tubulinopathies, 203

Tumors, 108
   of cauda equina, 313
   facial weakness and dysphagia from, 391
   hearing impairment from, 396–397
   hemiplegia, 287, 296
   negative, 341
   plexus, 322, 322*f*
   of spinal cord, 312

Tyrosine hydroxylase deficiency (DYT-TH), 336

U

Ullrich congenital muscular dystrophy, 203

Ulnar neuropathy, 323

Ultrasound, focal clonic seizures, 3

Unfractionated heparin (UFH), 286

Unilateral esotropia, 348–349

Unilateral ophthalmoplegia, acute, 352–355
   causes of, 353*b*

Unilateral (uncal) transtentorial herniation, 118

Upbeat nystagmus, 365
Uremia, 240
    neuropathy, 225
Usher syndrome, 394–395

V

Vaccine-associated poliomyelitis,
    229–230
Vaccine-preventable encephalitis, 75
Vaccines, postimmunization
    encephalopathy, 80
Vagal nerve stimulation (VNS), 55
    Lennox-Gastaut syndrome, 31
Valproate (antiepileptic), 102
    administration, 51
    adverse effects, 51
    benign myoclonus of infancy, 25
    generalized tonic-clonic seizures, 42
    indications for, 51
    infantile spasms, 24
    juvenile myoclonic epilepsy, 34
    migraine, 102
    selection, 45
    stiff infant syndrome, 20
Vanillylmandelic acid (VMA), 266–267
Vanishing white matter disease, 178
Varicella, 79, 295, 306
Vascular disorders
    ataxia and, 268
    vascular headache, post-traumatic,
        106
Vasculitis
    headache associated with, 108
    hypersensitivity, 293
    neuropathy, 225
Vasculopathies
    ischemic arterial infarction and,
        293–295
    isolated angiitis of CNS, 293–294
    neuropathy, 225
    systemic lupus erythematosus, 294
    Takayasu arteritis, 294–295
VCFS. *See* Velocardiofacial syndrome
VDRL, 146
Vein of Galen malformation,
    noncommunicating
    hydrocephalus and, 410–411,
    411*f*

Velocardiofacial syndrome (VCFS), 8
Venlafaxine (effexor), 434
Ventriculoperitoneal (VP) shunt, for
    hemiplegia, 283, 290
Vermal aplasia, 272–273
Vertebral artery, trauma to, 286
Vertebrobasilar occlusion, 268
Vertical gaze palsy, 361
Vertical pendular nystagmus, 363
Vertical suspension, hypotonic infant,
    185, 186*f*
Vertigo, 397–401
    anatomical considerations of,
        397–398
    approach to, 398–399
    benign paroxysmal vertigo, 263–264
    causes of, 398*b*, 399–401
        bacterial infections as, 399–400
        drugs as, 399
        epilepsy as, 399
        Ménière disease as, 400–401
        migraine as, 401
        motion sickness as, 401
        trauma as, 401
        viral infections as, 400
    history and physical examination
        for, 398
    peripheral *versus* central, 398*t*
    special tests for, 399
        caloric testing in, 399
        Dix-Hallpike test, 399
Very-long-chain acyl coenzyme A
    dehydrogenase deficiency,
    242–243
Vestibular neuritis, 400
Vestibular nystagmus, 364
VGKC. *See* Voltage-gated potassium
    channel
Vigabatrin (antiepileptic)
    administration, 51
    adverse effects, 51
    indications for, 51
    infantile spasms, 24
Viloxazine (qelbree), 435
Vincristine, neuropathy and, 224
Viral encephalitis, 71–72
Viral infections, 229–230
    aseptic meningitis, 75–76

Viral infections *(Continued)*
    ataxia, 264
    enterovirus infections, 229–230
    enteroviruses, 71
    herpes simplex encephalitis/herpes
        simplex virus, 72
    in newborns, 14–15
    meningoencephalitis, 70
    rubella embryopathy, 147
    West Nile virus, 230
Vision loss
    acute, causes of, 371*b*
    progressive, 375–377
        causes of, 371*b*
        from compressive optic
            neuropathy, 375–377
        from craniopharyngioma, 375–376
        from hereditary optic neuropathy,
            377
        from Leber congenital amaurosis,
            377
        from optic pathway and
            diencephalic gliomas, 376–
            377, 376*f*
        from pituitary adenoma, 377
        from retinoblastoma, 378
        from Wolfram syndrome, 377–378
Visual evoked response, 368
Visual hallucinations, 64, 99
Visual system, disorders of, 367–380
    blindness as. *See* Blindness
    disorders of pupil in, 379–380
    hereditary optic neuropathy in, 377
    optic neuropathies as, 372–374
        compressive, 375–377
        demyelinating, 372–373
        ischemic, 373
        toxic-nutritional, 373–374
    progressive loss of vision in, 375–377
    retinal degeneration, symptoms of,
        378–379
    retinal disease in, 374–375
    visual acuity and, assessment of,
        367–368
        clinical, 367–368
        visual evoked response for, 368
Vitamin K supplementation, for
    neonatal hemorrhage, 283

VMA. *See* Vanillylmandelic acid
VNS. *See* Vagal nerve stimulation
Voltage-gated potassium channel
  (VGKC), 238
Vomiting
  anticonvulsants, 45
  increased intracranial pressure
    in, 116
  migraine, 99
Von Hippel-Lindau disease, 270.
    See also Cerebellar
    hemangioblastoma
VPS13A disease, 332–333

W
Waardenburg syndrome, 394
Wada test, 55
Walker-Warburg syndrome, 203
  noncommunicating hydrocephalus
    and, 411
Weakness
  facial, 381–391
    anatomical considerations in,
      381–382
    aplasia of facial muscles and,
      384–385
    approach to diagnosis for,
      382–384
    from Bell palsy, 386–387
    from birth injury, 385–386
    causes of, 382*b*
    congenital syndromes causing,
      384–386
    depressor anguli oris aplasia in,
      385
    facial movement and, 381
    from genetic disorders, 387–389
    from hypertension, 389
    from immune-mediated and
      infectious disorders, 386–387
    from infection, 389–390
    from metabolic disorders, 390

Weakness *(Continued)*
    motor unit disorders in, 383
    from polyneuritis cranialis, 387
    pseudobulbar palsy in, 382–383
    recurrent cranial neuropathies/
      palsies in, 383*b*
    sucking and swallowing in,
      381–382
    from syringobulbia, 390
    from toxins, 390
    from trauma, 391
    from tumors, 391
  hypotonia
    central core disease, 200
    congenital fiber-type
      disproportion myopathy, 201
    limb, 208–235
    myotubular myopathy, 202
    paraplegia, 299
    unilateral, 281–282
Weber test, 392
West Nile virus, 230
West syndrome, 24
WFS1-spectrum disorder, 377–378
Whiplash/neck injuries, 110, 401
White forelock, 394
White matter disorders
  aspartoacylase deficiency (Canavan
    disease), 169–170
  cerebrotendinous xanthomatosis,
    178–179
  galactosemia (transferase deficiency),
    170
  Pelizaeus-Merzbacher disease,
    170–171
  progressive cavitating
    leukoencephalopathy, 171
  in progressive encephalopathies
    with onset before age two,
    169–171
  progressive hydrocephalus, 171
  X-linked adrenoleukodystrophy, 178

Wilson disease, 173
Wilson disease, in dystonia, 337–338
Wobble chairs, 428
Wolfram syndrome, 377–378
World Health Organization (WHO),
  95, 122
Writer's cramp, 335

X
Xeroderma pigmentosum, 177–178
X-linked adrenoleukodystrophy, 178
X-linked cerebellar hypoplasia, 273
X-linked developmental disorders,
  149–150
  alpha-thalassemia X-linked disability
    syndrome, 150
  fragile X syndrome, 149–150
  MECP2 duplication syndrome,
    150
X-linked hydrocephalus (L1
  syndrome), 408
X-linked inheritance, 278
X-linked McLeod syndrome, 332
X-linked muscular dystrophies, 213
X-linked myotubular myopathy, 202
Xp21 gene site, 214, 214*b*

Z
Zellweger spectrum disorders, 191, 393
Zellweger syndrome (ZS), 191
Zika virus (ZIKV), 148
  in secondary microcephaly, 419–420
Zolgensma, 196, 212
Zolmitriptan, headache, 100
Zonisamide (antiepileptic), 51, 102
  benign myoclonus of infancy, 25
  Dravet syndrome, 22
  infantile spasms, 24
  Lafora disease, 34
  selection, 45
  Unverricht-Lundborg syndrome, 36
ZS. *See* Zellweger syndrome